Kohlhammer

Florian Heinen (ed.)

NeuroKids

Child Neurology Workbook

Diagnosis and Therapy
Mind Maps

W. Kohlhammer

Notice concerning pharmacological statements:

Pharmacological data is constantly changing due to clinical experience, pharmacological research and changes to production processes. The publisher and authors have taken great care to ensure that all statements made in this book conform to the current state of knowledge. However, the publisher and authors cannot provide a guarantee in this respect. Therefore, each reader is required to check the statements which have been made, in particular in relation to medicine names, contained substances, specific areas of use and dosages on the basis of the medicine packaging label and the corresponding specialist information, and to only act on his or her own responsibility in the area of patient supply. The choice of medicines which are often used shall not give rise to a claim to completeness. The compounds which are listed under "sources" with names are only recorded in alphabetical order. These do not reflect frequency of prescription or preferences.

Legal notice

We have carefully checked all statements in the book. Despite the care, no liability or guarantee for the correctness, completeness and up-to-dateness of the data can be assumed. This also applies to all other websites which are referred to with hyperlinks. W. Kohlhammer GmbH is not responsible for the content of websites which are reached via such a link. We reserve the right to carry out updates, changes or additions to the provided information and data.

The structure and content of this publication are subject to copyright protection. No part of this publication may be reproduced, stored in retrieval systems, or transmitted, in any form or by any means, without the prior permission in writing W. Kohlhammer GmbH, or as expressly permitted by law or licence.

1st edition 2017

All rights reserved:
© 2017 by W. Kohlhammer GmbH, Stuttgart
Production: W. Kohlhammer GmbH, Stuttgart

Print:
ISBN 978-3-17-032161-8

E-Book-Format:
pdf: ISBN 978-3-17-032162-5

Preface of the editor and co-editors

"Make things as simple as possible, but not simpler." (Albert Einstein)

Paediatric Neurology is becoming a core discipline in clinical paediatrics. Combining child neuroscience, understanding of development, and real world hands-on-practice with continually advancing genetics, imaging techniques, metabolic control and therapy approaches creates a unique discipline where experienced clinical skills, compassion and theoretical background are coming together.

We developed the **"Paediatric Clinical Scout – PCS"** to allow an immediate point-of-care orientation, a kind of graphical clinical guidance, in short: a cognitive map. The Paediatric Clinical Scout guides you through diagnosis and treatment until you arrive at a definitive diagnosis or therapy – right in front of the patient, where your clinical work is being done: YOUR smart medicine with YOUR smart mobile phone for YOUR smart decisions.

The Paediatric Clinical Scout – PCS provides:

- bedside orientation
- a mind map
- guidance in conjunction with your own judgements and your in-house plans of action
- guidance to pharmacotherapy (with references from Germany, UK, USA)
- a selection of topics that extend your in-depth knowledge and know-how
- a patient-centered reference point
- an educational tool

The Paediatric Clinical Scout – PCS is not:

- a classical textbook
- a medical cookbook
- releasing you from thinking for yourself
- releasing you from making responsible and well-founded decisions
- releasing you from the daily dialogue with colleagues and mentors

We strongly support and fully acknowledge every child's individual self, and we make every effort to achieve the best possible for every child's health and well-being.

The world famous painter Gerhard Richter generously allowed us to use the portrait of his daughter Ella (Ella 2007), reflecting childhood, development, self-consciousness and vulnerability ... besides all the other characteristics of a child that are so much better expressed in a painting than described in hundred words.

We believe that the Paediatric Clinical Scout is a useful tool for paediatricians all over the world, possibly requiring some local adjustments, and we do hope for a lively feedback.

May 2017

Florian Heinen, Ludwig-Maximilians-University Munich, Germany
and the group of co-editors
Lucia Gerstl, Munich, Germany
Michaela Bonfert, Munich, Germany
Sandro Krieg, Munich, Germany
Alenka Pecar, Munich, Germany
Jens Böhmer, Gothenborg, Sweden

and

Steffen Berweck, Munich, Vogtareuth, Germany
Ingo Borggräfe, Munich, Germany
Kajal Chhaganlal, Beira, Mozambique
Hans-Jürgen Christen, Hannover, Germany
Urban M Fietzek, Munich, Germany
Andreas Hufschmidt, Wittlich, Germany
Matthias Kieslich, Frankfurt, Germany
Mirjam N. Landgraf, Munich, Germany
Volker Mall, Munich, Germany
Wolfgang Müller-Felber, Munich, Germany
Moritz Tacke, Munich, Germany
Uta Tacke, Freiburg, Germany

Preface of the EPNS

Introduction NeuroKids-App and -Workbook

From App-Idea to Ideal-App

Times are changing. And very fast in the field of transferring medical knowledge to doctors-in-training and medical students. Currently, at many universities, we still see the sterile traditional model where plenary lectures are given *ex-cathedra* to full auditoria of (falling asleep) medical students with little or no interaction. The medical knowledge can then afterwards be found back in standard textbooks, which, as we all know, are often outdated at the time of publishing.

But times are indeed changing. Already for some years now, the world wide web allows fast and online access to tons of data. The majority of knowledge, papers, research results, guidelines, … became accessible fast, easily and almost effortless, real but also sometimes 'alternative' facts. Teaching finally becomes more active and more interactive, on line, in small groups and with immediate feedback. In parallel, we also see an increased patient empowerment, so that the patient becomes a real partner in his relationship with professional health care providers. Patient organizations become more and more professional in their way to inform their members/patients, using exactly the same www materials.

This immense increase of virtual possibilities possibly comes at a price. Especially in the field of medicine, we still need some scientific guidance and control. We cannot leave everything run on its own and rely on social control. Medicine cannot be reduced to Wikipedia pages.

And this is exactly what the makers of this new NeuroKids initiative have understood very well. After many years of careful consideration and trying, this new app and workbook is now ready for worldwide use. In these changing times, it encompasses best of both worlds. Medical students, doctors-in-trainings and teachers will find an user-friendly and intuitive app. Confronted with a problem in clinic, the app on their mobile device can guide them through better diagnostic or treatment options. Completely different to a classic textbook, the search starts with a clinical problem or question. The scientific content is up to date, well controlled and will not remain passive and standard for years to come. The strength of this initiative will be the continuous updating of information, based on the everyday use of the app and on immediate feedback of the users. And this is unique.

The editor, Professor Florian Heinen, has to be congratulated with this wonderful new initiative. He pursued this app idea for years because he rightly felt this is the way forward in teaching our younger colleagues. I am very happy that NeuroKids was endorsed and supported by the board of the European Paediatric Neurology Society (EPNS). We sincerely believe this is a major step forward in training and educating young and old paediatric neurologists and are therefore extremely happy to collaborate in this project. This initiative will become a core instrument in the educational program of the EPNS. Indeed, times are changing …

Lieven Lagae
President European Paediatric Neurology Society

Credits

The app und belonging workbook is the result of tremendous, past and present, effort and input from an interdisciplinary group of people (in alphabetical order):

Renate Berger, Thomas Brandt, Hans Christoph Diener, Marianne Dieterich, Mechthild M., Felicitas, Gemma M. and Augustin M. Heinen, Elmar Heinen, Richard Michaelis (†), Ruprecht Poensgen, Ulrike Döring and the team of W. Kohlhammer Publishers, Dietrich Reinhardt, Otto and Liselotte Rothenfusser, Kathrin Schneider (Concept & Desing), Gerd Schulte-Körne, Jörg Urban.

Gabriele Stecher as secretary and personal assistant to the editor had a pivotal role that helped to consolidate the entire project.

Cooperations

European Paediatric Neurology Society (EPNS)
President: Prof. Lieven Lagae, Leuven, Belgium
Secretary Sue Hargreaves
Homepage: www.epns.jmre.es/

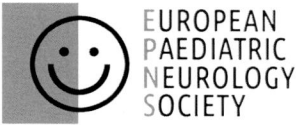

Ludwig-Maximilians-University Munich, Germany
Paediatric Neurology and Developmental Medicine
Children's Hospital
Head: Prof. Dr. med. Prof. h. c. Florian Heinen, MD, Munich, Germany
Homepage: www.ispz-muenchen.de

Ludwig-Maximilians-University Munich, Germany
Institute for Medical Education
Director: Prof. Dr. Martin Fischer, MD, Munich, Germany
Homepage: www.klinikum.uni-muenchen.de

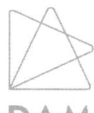

Ludwig-Maximilians-University Munich, Germany
Center for International Health
Speaker: Prof. Dr. Katja Radon, Munich, Germany
Homepage: www.international-health.uni-muenchen.de

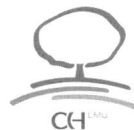

List of authors

Editor

Heinen, Florian, Prof. Dr. med. Prof. h.c.
Hauner Children's Hospital of the Ludwig-Maximilians-University of Munich,
Department of Paediatric Neurology and Developmental Medicine
Lindwurmstr. 4, 80337 München, Germany

Co-editors

Gerstl, Lucia, Dr. med.
Hauner Children's Hospital of the Ludwig-Maximilians-University of Munich,
Department of Paediatric Neurology and Developmental Medicine
Lindwurmstr. 4, 80337 München, Germany

Bonfert, Michaela, Dr. med.
Hauner Children's Hospital of the Ludwig-Maximilians-University of Munich,
Department of Paediatric Neurology and Developmental Medicine
Lindwurmstr. 4, 80337 München, Germany

Krieg, Sandro, PD Dr. med.
Technical University of Munich, Department of Neurosurgery
Ismaningerstr. 22, 81675 München, Germany

Pecar, Alenka, Dr.
University Hospital München, Campus Großhadern, Pharmacy,
Department of Drug Information
Marchioninistr. 15, 81377 München, Germany

Böhmer, Jens, Dr. med.
Queen Silvia Childlren's Hopsital, Sahlgrenska University Hospital
Smörslottsgatan 1, 41685 Göteborg, Sweden

Berweck, Steffen, Prof. Dr. med.
Schön Klinik Vogtareuth, Department of Neuropaediatrics, Rehabilitation
Krankenhausstr. 20, 83569 Vogtareuth, Germany

Borggräfe, Ingo, PD Dr. med.
Hauner Children's Hospital of the Ludwig-Maximilians-University of Munich,
Department of Paediatric Neurology and Developmental Medicine
Lindwurmstr. 4, 80337 München, Germany

Chhaganial, Kajal
Universidade Católica de Mozambique
Beira, Mozambique

Christen, Hans-Jürgen, Prof. Dr. med.
Hospital for Paediatrics and Adolescent Medicine
Janusz-Korczak-Allee 12, 30173 Hannover, Germany

Fietzek, Urban, Dr. med.
Schön Klinik München Schwabing, Department of Neurology and Clinical Neurophysiology
Parzivalplatz 4, 80804 München, Germany

Hufschmidt, Andreas, PD Dr. med.
St. Elisabeth Hospital, Department of Neurology
Koblenzer Straße 91, 54516 Wittlich, Germany

Kieslich, Matthias, PD Dr. med.
University Hospital Frankfurt, Centre of Paediatrics and Adolescent Medicine,
Department of Neuropaediatrics
Theodor-Stern-Kai 7, Haus 32, 60590 Frankfurt/M., Germany

Landgraf, Mirjam, Dr. med., Dipl.-Psych.
Hauner Children's Hospital of the Ludwig-Maximilians-University of Munich,
Department of Paediatric Neurology and Developmental Medicine
Lindwurmstr. 4, 80337 München, Germany

Mall, Volker, Prof. Dr. med.
kbo Children's Centre Munich, Technical University Munich
Heiglhofstr. 63, 81377 München, Germany

Müller-Felber, Wolfgang, Prof. Dr. med.
Hauner Children's Hospital of the Ludwig-Maximilians-University, Department of
Paediatric Neurology and Developmental Medicine
Lindwurmstr. 4, 80337 München, Germany

Tacke, Moritz, Dr. med.
Hauner Children's Hospital of the Ludwig-Maximilians-University of Munich,
Department of Paediatric Neurology and Developmental Medicine
Lindwurmstr. 4, 80337 München, Germany

Tacke, Uta, Dr. med. Dipl. Psych.
University Chidlren's Hospital Basel, Department of Neuro- und Developmental
Paediatrics
Spitalstr. 33, 4056 Basel, Switzerland

Authors

Bast, Thomas, PD Dr. med.
Epilepsy Centre Kork, Department of Children and Adolescents
Landstr. 1, 77694 Kehl-Kork, Germany
Chapter E.07, E.09, E.10, E.11, *E.01*

Bernius, Peter, Dr. med.
Schön Klinik München Harlaching, Department of Paediatric and Neuro Orthopaedics
Harlachinger Str. 51, 81547 München, Germany
Chapter Q.02

Berweck, Steffen, Prof. Dr. med.
Schön Klinik Vogtareuth, Department of Neuropaediatrics, Rehabilitation
Krankenhausstr. 20, 83569 Vogtareuth, Germany
Chapter G.01, I.01, *A.08, M.01*

Bidlingmaier, Christoph, PD Dr. med.
Hauner Children's Hospital of the Ludwig-Maximilians-University of Munich,
Department of Haemostaseology
Lindwurmstr. 4, 80337 München, Germany
Chapter A.09.3, *A.09.1, A.09.4, A.09.5*

Blaschek, Astrid, Dr. med.
Hauner Children's Hospital of the Ludwig-Maximilians-University of Munich,
Department of Paediatric Neurology and Developmental Medicine
Lindwurmstr. 4, 80337 München, Germany
Chapter H.01, J.01, *H.01, J.02*

Bode, Harald, Prof. Dr. med.
University Hospital Ulm, Hospital for Paediatrics and Adolescent Medicine, Department
of Neuropaediatrics and Centre of Social Paediatrics
Schillerstraße 15, 89077 Ulm, Germany
Chapter *D.01*

Böhmer, Jens, Dr. med.
The Queen Silvia Childlren's Hopsital, Sahlgrenska University Hospital
Smörslottsgatan 1, 41685 Göteborg, Sweden
Chapter C.03, C.05, D.05, L.08, N.02, P.04, R, U, *A.09.1, C.01, C.02, M.02, M.03*

Bonfert, Michaela, Dr. med.
Hauner Children's Hospital of the Ludwig-Maximilians-University of Munich,
Department of Paediatric Neurology and Developmental Medicine
Lindwurmstr. 4, 80337 München, Germany
Chapter *A.01, E.05*

Borggräfe, Ingo, PD Dr. med.
Hauner Children's Hospital of the Ludwig-Maximilians-University of Munich,
Department of Paediatric Neurology and Developmental Medicine
Lindwurmstr. 4, 80337 München, Germany
Chapter E.01, E.04, E.05, E.06, *A.01, A.02, B.01,E.02, E.03, G.02, U*

Brandl, Ulrich, Prof. Dr. med.
University Hospital Jena, Hospital for Paediatrics and Adolescent Medicine, Department
of Neuropaediatrics and Centre of Social Paediatrics
Kochstr. 2, 07740 Jena, Germany
Chapter *E04*

Brockmann, Knut, Prof. Dr. med.
University Hospital Göttingen, Hospital for Paediatrics and Adolescent Medicine,
Department of Neuropaediatrics and Centre of Social Paediatrics
Robert-Koch-Str. 40, 37075 Göttingen, Germany
Chapter *H.01*

Brückmann, Hartmut, Prof. Dr. med.
University Hospital München, Campus Großhadern, Institute for Radiology,
Department of Neuroradiology
Marchioninistr.15, 81377 München, Germany
Chapter *A.09.2, A.09.4, A.09.5*

Christen, Hans-Jürgen, Prof. Dr. med.
Hospital for Paediatrics and Adolescent Medicine
Janusz-Korczak-Allee 12, 30173 Hannover, Germany
Chapter J.03, N.02

Debus, Otfried, PD Dr. med.
St. Clemens Hospital
Düesbergweg 124, 48153 Münster, Germany
Chapter E.04

Dichgans, Martin, Prof. Dr. med.
Feodor-Lynen-Str. 17, 81377 München, Germany
Chapter A.09.1

Ebinger, Friedrich, PD Dr. med.
St. Vincence Hospital, Hospital for Paediatrics and Adolescent Medicine
Am Busdorf 2, 33098 Paderborn, Germany
Chapter K.01

Elger, Christian E., Prof. Dr. med.
University Hospital Bonn, Department of Epileptology
Sigmund-Freud-Str. 25, 53105 Bonn, Germany
Chapter E.11

Enders, Angelika, Dr. med.
Hauner Children's Hospital of the Ludwig-Maximilians-University of Munich,
Department of Paediatric Neurology and Developmental Medicine
Lindwurmstr. 4, 80337 München, Germany
Chapter L.06, L.08

Ensenauer, Regina, PD Dr. med.
University Hospital Düsseldorf, Hospital for Paediatrics and Adolescent Medicine,
Department of Paediatric Metabolic Disorders
Moorenstr. 5, 40225 Düsseldorf, Germany
Chapter A.07, N.01

Faber, Fabienne Lara, Dr. med.
Hauner Children's Hospital of the Ludwig-Maximilians-University of Munich,
Department of Paediatric Neurology and Developmental Medicine
Lindwurmstr. 4, 80337 München, Germany
Chapter N.01

Fietzek, Urban, Dr. med.
Schön Klinik München Schwabing, Department of Neurology and Clinical Neurophysiology
Parzivalplatz 4, 80804 München, Germany
Chapter A.03, M.01

Führer, Monika, Prof. Dr. med.
Hauner Children's Hospital of the Ludwig-Maximilians-University of Munich,
Department of Paediatric Palliative Care
Lindwurmstraße 4, 80337 München, Germany
Chapter C.04

Gasser, Thomas, Prof. Dr. med.
University Hospital Tübingen, Department of Neurology
Hoppe-Seyler-Straße 3, 72076 Tübingen, Germany
Chapter L.01

Gerstl, Lucia, Dr. med.
Hauner Children's Hospital of the Ludwig-Maximilians-University of Munich,
Department of Paediatric Neurology and Developmental Medicine
Lindwurmstr. 4, 80337 München, Germany
Chapter A.01, A.09.1, E.02, A.02, A.09.4, A.09.5, E.01, E.03, E04, E.05, E.06, L.04

Heinen, Florian, Prof. Dr. med. Prof. h.c.
Hauner Children's Hospital of the Ludwig-Maximilians-University of Munich,
Department of Paediatric Neurology and Developmental Medicine
Lindwurmstr. 4, 80337 München, Germany
Chapter C.01, C.02, A.03, A.04, A.12, C.03, C.05, D.01, E.01, E.06, G.01, G.02, F.01, R, U

Hermanns-Clausen, Maren, Dr. med.
Toxicity Information Centre Freiburg
Mathildenstr. 1, 79106 Freiburg, Germany
Chapter A.13

Hernáiz Driever, Pablo, PD Dr. med.
Charité Hospital for Paediatrics and Adolescent Medicine, Department of Oncology and Haematology
Augustenburger Platz 1, 13353 Berlin, Germany
Chapter K.01

Hilgendorff, Anne, PD Dr. med.
Hauner Children's Hospital of the Ludwig-Maximilians-University of Munich,
Department of Paediatric Neurology and Developmental Medicine
Lindwurmstr. 4, 80337 München, Germany
Chapter *B.02*

Hübner, Johannes, Prof. Dr. med.
Hauner Children's Hospital of the Ludwig-Maximilians-University of Munich,
Department of Infectious Diseases
Lindwurmstr. 4, 80337 München, Germany
Chapter J.04

Hufschmidt, Andreas, PD Dr. med.
St. Elisabeth Hospital, Department of Neurology
Koblenzer Straße 91, 54516 Wittlich, Germany
Chapter *C.05*

Huppke, Peter, Prof. Dr. med.
University Hospital Göttingen, Hospital for Paediatrics and Adolescent Medicine,
Department of Neuropaediatrics and Centre of Social Paediatrics
Robert-Koch-Str. 40, 37075 Göttingen, Germany
Chapter L.05

Ikonomidou, Hrissanthi, Prof. Dr. med.
University of Wisconsin School of Medicine and Public Health, Pediatric Neurology
Clinic
600 Highland Ave, Madison,, 53792 Wisconsin, USA
Chapter *B.01*

Jahn, Klaus, Prof. Dr. med.
Schön Klinik Bad Aibling, Department of Neurology
Kolbermoorer Str. 72, 83043 Bad Aibling, Germany
Chapter F.01

Jansson, Annette, PD Dr. med.
Hauner Children's Hospital of the Ludwig-Maximilians-University of Munich,
Department of Rheumatology
Lindwurmstr. 4, 80337 München, Germany
Chapter *J.02*

Kieslich, Matthias, PD Dr. med.
University Hospital Frankfurt, Centre of Paediatrics and Adolescent Medicine,
Department of Neuropaediatrics
Theodor-Stern-Kai 7, Haus 32, 60590 Frankfurt/M., Germany
Chapter A.08, A.10, L.01, L.04, *U*

Kirschner, Janbernd, Prof. Dr. med.
University Hospital Freiburg, Hospital for Paediatrics and Adolescent Medicine,
Department of Neuropaediatrics and Neuromuscular Disorders
Mathildenstr. 1, 79106 Freiburg, Germany
Chapter O.05, *Q.01*

Kluger, Gerhard, Prof. Dr. med.
Schön Klinik Vogtareuth, Department of Neuropaediatrics, Epileptology
Krankenhausstr. 20, 83569 Vogtareuth, Germany
Chapter *A.12*

König, Rainer, Prof. Dr. med.
University Hospital Frankfurt, Institute of Human Genetics
Theodor-Stern-Kai 7, 60590 Frankfurt/M., Germany
Chapter *L.06*

Korinthenberg, Rudolf, Prof. Dr. med.
University Hospital Freiburg, Hospital for Paediatrics and Adolescent Medicine,
Department of Neuropaediatrics and Neuromuscular Disorders
Mathildenstraße 1, 79106 Freiburg, Germany
Chapter A.06, O.02, *O.03*

Krieg, Sandro, PD Dr. med.
Technical University of Munich, Department of Neurosurgery
Ismaningerstr. 22, 81675 München, Germany
Chapter A.09.4, A.09.5, P.01, P.02, *A.05, A.09.2, P.04, L.04, U*

Kurnik, Karin, PD Dr. med.
Hauner Children's Hospital of the Ludwig-Maximilians-University of Munich,
Department of Haemostaseology
Lindwurmstr. 4, 80337 München, Germany
Chapter *A.09.1, A.09.3*

Landgraf, Mirjam, Dr. med., Dipl.-Psych.
Hauner Children's Hospital of the Ludwig-Maximilians-University of Munich,
Department of Paediatric Neurology and Developmental Medicine
Lindwurmstr. 4, 80337 München, Germany
Chapter A.10, C.01, C.02, C.03

Langhagen, Thyra, Dr. med.
University Hospital München, Campus Großhadern, Department of Otorhinolaryngology and Department of Paediatric Neurology and Developmental Medicine
Marchioninistr. 15, 81377 München, Germany
Chapter F.01

Liese, Johannes, Prof. Dr. med.
University Hospital Würzburg, Hospital for Paediatrics and Adolescent Medicine of the Bavarian Julians-Maximilians-University, Department of Infectious Disease and Immunology
Josef-Schneider-Str. 2, 97080 Würzburg, Germany
Chapter J.04

Linn, Jennifer, Prof. Dr. med.
University Hospital Dresden, Department of Neuroradiology
Fetscherstr. 74, 01307 Dresden, Germany
Chapter J.02

Maier, Esther, PD Dr. med.
Hauner Children's Hospital of the Ludwig-Maximilians-University of Munich,
Department of Inborn Errors of Metabolism and Department of Paediatric Neurology and Developmental Medicine
Lindwurmstr. 4, 80337 München, Germany
Chapter N.01, N.03

Mall, Volker, Prof. Dr. med.
kbo Children's Centre Munich
Heiglhofstr. 63, 81377 München, Germany
Chapter A.04, A.13, U

Michaelis, Richard, Prof. Dr. med. (†)
Beethovenweg 33, 72076 Tübingen, Germany
Chapter R

von Moers, Arpad, PD Dr. med.
DRK Kliniken Berlin Westend, Hospital for Paediatrics and Adolescent Medicine
Spandauer Damm 130, 14050 Berlin, Germany
Chapter P.03

Muhle, Hiltrud, PD Dr. med.
University Hospital Schleswig-Holstein, Department of Neuropaediatrics
Schwanenweg 20, 24105 Kiel, Germany
Chapter E.06

Müller-Felber, Wolfgang, Prof. Dr. med.
Hauner Children's Hospital of the Ludwig-Maximilians-University of Munich,
Department of Paediatric Neurology and Developmental Medicine
Lindwurmstr. 4, 80337 München, Germany
Chapter D.04, H.01, N.03, O.03, O.06, O.07, A.04, O.01, O.04, O.08, R

Müller-Schunk, Stefanie, Dr. med.
University Hospital München, Campus Großhadern, Institute of Radiology, Department of Neuroradiology
Marchioninistr. 15, 81377 München, Germany
Chapter A.09.5

Münch, Hans-Georg, Dr. med.
Hauner Children's Hospital of the Ludwig-Maximilians-University of Munich,
Department of Neonatology
Lindwurmstr. 4, 80337 München, Germany
Chapter B.02

Neubauer, Bernd A., Prof. Dr. med.
University Hospital Gießen and Marburg, Department of Neuropaediatrics, Social Paediatrics and Epileptology
Feulgenstr. 12, 35392 Gießen, Germany
Chapter E.05, E.02

Niemann, Gerhard, PD Dr. med.
Hospital for Paediatrics and Adolescent Medicine Schömberg
Römerweg 7, 75328 Schömberg, Germany
Chapter E.03

Noterdaeme, Michele, Prof. Dr. med.
Klinik Josefinum, Department of Child and Adolescent Psychiatry
Kapellenstr. 30, 86154 Augsburg, Germany
Chapter D.02, D.03, D.05

Olivieri, Martin, Dr. med.
Hauner Children's Hospital of the Ludwig-Maximilians-University of Munich,
Department of Haemostaseology
Lindwurmstr. 4, 80337 München, Germany
Chapter *A.09.1, A.09.3, A.09.4, A.09.5*

Omran, Heymut, Prof. Dr. med.
University Hospital Münster, Hospital for Paediatrics and Adolescent Medicine
Albert-Schweitzer-Campus 1, 48149 Münster, Germany
Chapter *P.02*

Pecar, Alenka, Dr.
University Hospital München, Campus Großhadern, Pharmacy, Department of Drug
Information
Marchioninistr. 15, 81377 München, Germany
Chapter *U*

Peraud, Aurelia, PD Dr. med.
University Hospital München, Campus Großhadern, Department of Neurosurgery
Marchioninistr.15, 81377 München, Germany
Chapter *A.05, A.09.2, P.01, P.02, L.04*

Pfister, Hans-Walter, Prof. Dr. med.
University Hospital München, Campus Großhadern, Department of Neurology
Marchioninistr. 15, 81377 München, Germany
Chapter *J.04*

Pohl-Koppe, Anette, PD Dr. med.
Paediatric Office
Seybothstraße 17, 81545 München, Germany
Chapter *J.03*

Poschmann, Michael, Dr. med.
Schön Klinik München Harlaching, Department of Paediatric and Neuro Orthopaedics
Harlachinger Str. 51, 81547 München, Germany
Chapter *Q.02*

Reiter, Karl, PD Dr. med.
Hauner Children's Hospital of the Ludwig-Maximilians-University of Munich,
Department of Paediatric Intensive Care
Lindwurmstr. 4, 80337 München, Germany
Chapter *A.12, J.04, M.03*

Rona, Sabine, Dr. med.
University Hospital Tübingen, Department of Neurosurgery
Hoppe-Seyler-Str. 3, 72076 Tübingen, Germany
Chapter *A.02*

Rosenbaum, Thorsten, Prof. Dr. med.
Hospital Duisburg, Department of Paediatrics and Adolescent Medicine
Zu den Rehwiesen 9, 47055 Duisburg, Germany
Chapter *L.03*

Rost, Imma, Dr. med.
Centre of Human Genetics and Laboratory Medicine
Lochhamer Straße 29, 82152 Martinsried, Germany
Chapter *L.06, L.08*

Rostásy, Kevin, PD Dr. med.
Hospital for Paediatrics and Adolescent Medicine Datteln, Centre of Neuropediatrics,
Developmental Medicine and Social Paediatrics
Dr.-Friedrich-Steiner-Str. 5, 45711 Datteln, Germany
Chapter *H.01, J.01*

Schara, Ulrike, Prof. Dr. med.
University Hospital Essen, Hospital for Paediatrics, Department of Neuropaediatrics and
Centre of Social Paediatrics
Hufelandstr. 55, 45147 Essen, Germany
Chapter *O.01, O.04, O.08*

Schlamp, Dieter, Dr. med.
kbo-Heckscher Klinikum München, Hospital for Child and Adolescent Psychiatry
Deisenhofenerstr. 28, 81539 München, Germany
Chapter *D.02, D.03*

Schmitz, Bettina, Prof. Dr. med.
Vivantes Humboldt-Hospital, Department of Neurology, Stroke Unit and
Centre of Epilepsy
Am Nordgraben 2, 13509 Berlin, Germany
Chapter *E.06*

Schröder, Sebastian, PD Dr. med.
Hauner Children's Hospital of the Ludwig-Maximilians-University of Munich,
Department of Paediatric Neurology and Developmental Medicine
Lindwurmstr. 4, 80337 München, Germany
Chapter *G.02, M.01, R, G.01, I.01*

Stehr, Maximilian, Prof. Dr. med.
Hospital Hallerwiese, Cnopf Children's Hospital, Department of Paediatric Surgery and Urology
St.-Johannis-Mühlgasse 19, 90419 Nürnberg, Germany
Chapter M.02

Straube, Andreas, Prof. Dr. med.
University Hospital München, Campus Großhadern, Department of Neurology
Marchioninistr. 15, 81377 München, Germany
Chapter *C.01, C.02, C.03*

Stücker, Ralf, Prof. Dr. med.
Children's Hospital Altona, Department of Paediatric Orthopedics
Bleickenallee 38, 22763 Hamburg, Germany
Chapter Q.01

Steinbeis von Stülpnagel, Celina, Dr. med.
Schön Klinik Vogtareuth, Department of Neuropaediatrics
Krankenhausstr. 20, 83569 Vogtareuth, Germany
Chapter Support Groups

Tacke, Uta, Dr. med. Dipl. Psych.
University Chidlren's Hospital Basel, Department of Neuro- und Developmental Paediatrics and Department of Paediatric Neurology and Developmental Medicine
Spitalstr. 33, 4056 Basel, Switzerland
Chapter D.01, *D.03, L.03, L.05,*

Tacke, Moritz, Dr. med.
Hauner Children's Hospital of the Ludwig-Maximilians-University of Munich, Department of Paediatric Neurology and Developmental Medicine
Lindwurmstr. 4, 80337 München, Germany
Chapter J.02

Vlaho, Stefan, Dr. med.
District Hospital Altötting-Burghausen, Department of Paediatrics and Adolescent Medicine
Vinzenz-von-Paul-Str. 14, 84503 Altötting, Germany
Chapter *A.07, D.04*

Weigand, Heike, Dr. med.
Hauner Children's Hospital of the Ludwig-Maximilians-University of Munich, Department of Paediatric Neurology and Developmental Medicine
Lindwurmstr. 4, 80337 München, Germany
Chapter *P.03*

Wiater, Alfred, Dr. med.
Hospital Porz am Rhein, Children's Hospital
Urbacher Weg 19, 51149 Köln, Germany
Chapter D.06

Wilken, Bernd, Prof. Dr. med.
Hospital Kassel, Department of Neuropaediatrics and Centre of Social Paediatrics
Mönchebergstr. 48e, 34125 Kassel, Germany
Chapter *J.04*

Willichowski, Ekkehard, Prof. Dr. med.
University Hospital Göttingen, Hospital for Paediatrics and Adolescent Medicine, Department of Neuropaediatrics and Centre of Social Paediatrics
Robert-Koch-Str. 40, 37075 Göttingen, Germany
Chapter *N.03*

Wohlrab, Gabriele, Dr. med.
Children's Hospital Zürich, Department of Neurphysiology and Neuropaediatrics
Steinwiesstrasse 75, 8032 Zürich, Switzerland
Chapter B.01

Wolff, Markus, Dr. med.
University Hospital Tübingen, Department of Paediatrics and Adolescent Medicine
Hoppe-Seyler-Str. 1, 72076 Tübingen, Germany
Chapter A.02, E.03

Content

Preface of the editor and co-editors	5
Preface of the EPNS	7
Credits	9
Cooperations	11
List of authors	13
Abbreviations	23

A Emergency and intensive care ... 25
- A.01 Febrile seizures ... 26
- A.02 Status epilepticus (SE) ... 30
- A.03 Acute dystonic reaction ... 32
- A.04 Acute Ataxia ... 34
- A.05 Acute increased intracranial pressure (ICP) ... 37
- A.06 Guillain-Barré Syndrome (GBS) ... 41
- A.07 Neurometabolic dysfunction ... 44
- A.08 Traumatic brain injury (TBI) ... 50
- A.09 Paediatric stroke ... 52
  - A.09.1 Thromboembolic events ... 56
  - A.09.2 Intracranial haemorrhage/bleeding ... 62
  - A.09.3 Cerebral venous sinus thrombosis ... 70
  - A.09.4 Dissection (cerebrovascular) ... 74
  - A.09.5 Arteriovenous malformations ... 77
- A.10 Battered child ... 85
- A.11 Coma ... 87
- A.12 Brain death ... 98
- A.13 Intoxications ... 99

B Neonatology ... 105
- B.01 Neonatal seizures ... 106
- B.02 Neonatal hypoxic-ischaemic encephalopathy (HIE) ... 108

C Pain ... 113
- C.01 Headache ... 114
- C.02 Primary Headache ... 116
- C.03 Secondary Headache ... 121
- C.04 Pain management in palliative care ... 122
- C.05 Idiopathic intracranial hypertension (IIH) ... 128

D Development ... 133
- D.01 Developmental disorders ... 135
- D.02 Hyperkinetic disorder ... 138
- D.03 Education entrance qualification (school maturity) ... 141
- D.04 Tic disorder and Tourette syndrome ... 142
- D.05 Autism spectrum disorder (ASD) ... 144
- D.06 Fetal alcohol spectrum disorders (FASD) ... 145

E Epilepsy ... 149
- E.01 Epilepsy ... 150
- E.02 First seizure ... 153
- E.03 Paroxysomal events (non-epileptic) ... 154
- E.04 West-Syndrome ... 160
- E.05 Benign epilepsy with centrotemporal spikes (BECTS, Rolandic epilepsy) . 161
- E.06 Absence epilepsy ... 163
- E.07 Juvenile myoclonic epilepsy ... 164
- E.08 Localizing signs in epilepsy ... 166
- E.09 Therapeutic strategies in different electroclinical epilepsy syndromes ... 170
- E.10 Epilepsy surgery ... 176

F Vertigo ... 183
- F.01 Vertigo and dizziness ... 185

G Movement disorders ... 191
- G.01 Cerebral palsy ... 192
- G.02 Dystonia ... 200

H Cranial nerves ... 207
- H.01 Facial palsy ... 208
- H.02 Optic neuritis ... 212

I Rehabilitation ... 217
- I.01 Rehabilitation (inpatient) ... 219

J Inflammation and infection ... 223
- J.01 Multiple sclerosis/ADEM ... 225
- J.02 Cerebral vasculitis ... 230
- J.03 Lyme disease ... 236
- J.04 Meningitis and encephalitis ... 238

K Oncology 243
K.01   Neoplasm of the CNS 244

L Genetics 253
L.01   Genetics 254
L.02   Neurocutaneous syndromes 256
L.03   Craniosynostosis 262
L.04   Rett syndrome 264
L.05   Microdeletion syndromes 266
L.06   Trisomy 21 270

M Autonomic nerve system 275
M.01   Hypersalivation and dysphagia 276
M.02   Bladder dysfunction 279
M.03   Sleep disorders 280

N Neurometabolic and neurodegenerative disorders 285
N.01   Neurometabolic disorders 286
N.02   Neurodegenerative disorders 294
N.03   Mitochondrial disorders 296

O Neuromuscular disorders 305
O.01   Neuromuscular disorders 306
O.02   Muscle dystrophies 309
   O.02.1 Duchenne-Becker muscular dystrophy (DMD, BMD) 310
   O.02.2 Limb-girdle muscular dystrophy (LGMD) 312
   O.02.3 Emery-Dreifuss Syndrome 314
   O.02.4 Myotonic dystrophy, Dystrophia myotonica (DM) 316
   O.02.5 Facio-scapulo-humeral muscular dystrophy (FSHD) 318
   O.02.6 Distal muscular dystrophy 320
   O.02.7 Congenital muscular dystrophy (CMD) 322
O.03   Myopathies 324
O.04   Myositis 330
O.05   Spinal muscular atrophy (SMA) 333
O.06   Neuromuscular transmission 336
O.07   Peripheral nerve lesions 338
O.08   Neuropathies 340

P Hydrocephalus, Myelomeningocele (MMC), Chiari Malformations 345
P.01   Hydrocephalus in infants 346
P.02   Management of the shunted hydrocephalus 348
P.03   Myelomeningocele (MMC) 350
P.04   Chiari malformations (CM) 352

Q Neuro-Orthopaedics 357
Q.01   Hip joint 358
Q.02   Scoliosis 360

R Neurological examinations 365
R.01   Neurological examinations (from 2 years of age) 366
R.02   6 minutes neurological examination 368
R.03   Developmental assessment – overview & orientation 370
R.04.1 Basic developmental assessment – up to 20 days 372
R.04.2 Basic developmental assessment – 4th to end of 8th week 374
R.04.3 Basic developmental assessment – 3rd to end of 4th months 376
R.04.4 Basic developmental assessment – 6th to end of 8th months 378
R.04.5 Basic developmental assessment – 11th to end of 13th months 380
R.04.6 Basic developmental assessment – 17th to end of 19th months 382
R.04.7 Basic developmental assessment – 21st to end of 26th months 384

Medication 389

Abbreviations

ACIP	Advisory Committee on Immunisation Practices
AV	withdrawn from market
BNFC (UK)	British National Formulary for Children (BNF for Children 2011–2012; www.bnf.org)
bid	bis in die / twice a day
BSA	body surface area
d	day
D5W	Dextrose/Glucose 5 %
DD	daily dose
ECMO	extracorporeal membrane oxygenation
h	hours
IU	International unit
LMWH	low molecular weight Heparins
MAOI	Monoamine oxidase inhibitor
max.	maximum
min	minutes
Mio	Million
NS	Normal saline (NaCl 0.9 %)
NSAID	Non-steroidal anti-inflammatory drugs
Off-label	Off-label use
SD	single dose
sec	seconds
SPC (Germany)	Summary of Product Characteristics
SWE	Sterile water for injection
T (USA)	Taketomo (Paediatric Dosage Handbook. Carol K. Taketomo, Pharm D, 18th Ed., Lexicomp, publication 2011; www.lexi.com)
U	Unit

A Emergency and intensive care

A.01 Febrile seizures | PCS-Diagnosis 1/2

Emergency and intensive care

History
- Age (1–72 months of age; peak: 18 months)
- Seizure type
- History of fever and infectious diseases
- Drug history
- Developmental history
- Past medical history (seizures?)
- Perinatal history
- Immunization status
- Family history (e. g. febrile seizures)

Physical examination
- Acute
  - Infectious focus? Focal neurological symptoms/ Cranial nerve palsies
  - Meningeal signs (Neck stiffness, Kernig or Brudzinski signs, …)
  - Irritability, behaviour
- Post-acute:
  - Developmental delay?

Course
- Complete (neurological) recovery within approx. 1–2 hours after a simple febrile seizure

Clues to diagnosis
Simple febrile seizure?
- Seizure type: generalized, tonic clonic > atonic
- 70 % of simple febrile seizures stop spontaneously within less than 5 minutes
- Duration < 15 minutes

Complex febrile seizure?
- Focal onset seizure (which secondarily generalizes)
- Duration > 15 minutes
- Seizure clusters:
  - Reccurent seizures within 24 hours
- No complete neurological recovery in the postictal period

Metabolic disorders?
- Dehydration with eletrolyte imbalance
- Lasting decreased consciousness

Meningitis/Encephalitis?
- Decreased consciousness, headache, photophobia
- Neck stiffness, meningeal signs (pitfalls: may be absent or more subtle in children < 12–24 months of age)
- Irritability
- Vomiting
- Petechiae/purpuric rash
- Bulging fontanelle

Other reasons?
- Traumatic brain injury (TBI)
- Battered child

- \> 18 months of age
- Obvious infectious focus

- \< 18 months of age
- No obvious infectious focus
- Child is pretreated with antibiotics
- Recurrent medical consultation during the same period of fever

Investigations/ Laboratory
- Blood
  - Full blood count and differential
  - Blood culture, PCR: HSV
  - CRP
- CSF[1]
  - White cell count, protein, glucose
  - Culture, PCR: HSV
- Urine analysis
  - Cytology
  - Culture

See chapter A.07 Neurometabolic dysfunction
- GLUT1-Deficiency Syndrome

See chapter J.04 Meningitis and encephalitis

See chapter A.08 Traumatic brain injury and A.10 Battered child

---

- Obvious infectious focus
- CSF normal
- Child in no obvious distress
- Complete (neurological) recovery

- **NO** obvious infectious focus
- Child critically ill
- CSF pleocytosis
- Lasting neurological symptoms or decreased conciousness

- Developmental delay

- Simple febrile seizure

- Further investigations

A.01 Febrile seizures

A.01 Febrile seizures | PCS-Diagnosis 2/2

Emergency and intensive care

Developing epilepsy?
- ▶ Recurrent febrile seizures
- ▶ Afebrile seizures
- ▶ Developmental delay

See chapter E Epilepsy
- ▶ Dravet-Syndrome Spectrum (SCN1A mutation testing; if negative: SCN9A and PCDH19)

1 Recommended for children < 18 months of age; strongly recommended for children < 12 months of age (please follow the national guidelines)

A.01 Febrile seizures | PCS-Therapy 1/1

Emergency and intensive care

▶ Continuing febrile seizure (> 3 minutes)	▶ Diazepam rectally (< 15 kg 5 mg, > 15 kg 10 mg) ▶ Diazepam (as IV injection over 3–5 minutes) 0,25 mg/kg/single dose	Continuing seizure: ▶ Midazolam IV 0,1–0,2 mg/kg/single dose Or ▶ Lorazepam IV 0,05–0,1 mg/kg/single dose Or ▶ Diazepam 0,25 mg/kg/single dose In case of continuing seizure: ▶ Phenobarbital IV 10 mg/kg/single dose	Continuing seizure: Switch to the treatment algorithm of convulsive status epilepticus (see chapter A.02 Status epilepticus (SE))

▶ Spontaneously stopped febrile seizure	▶ Physical examination (complete neurological recovery within approx. 1–2 hours?)
	▶ Monitoring
		Continuing fever: antipyretic treatment
		▶ Physical methods
		▶ Antipyretic drug treatment
		  – Paracetamol rectally: 75 mg < 6 months, 125 mg 6–24 months, 250 mg 2–8 years, 500 mg > 8 years every 6–8 hours
		    oraly: 10–15 mg/kg/single dose every 6 h;
		    IV: 10–15 mg/kg/single dose oraly every 6 h (max. 60 mg/kg/d)
		  – Ibuprofen 2,5–10 mg/kg/single dose (max. 600 mg/single dose) every 6–8 h oraly
		  – Metamizole 10 mg/kg/single dose every 4–6 h p.o./IV	

Questions, you should discuss with the parents:
▶ Diagnosis?
▶ How often can a febrile seizure occur?
▶ Does a simple febrile seizure have adverse effects on neurocognition or development?
▶ Is a febrile seizure the beginning of a (lifelong) epilepsy?
▶ Are there effective preventive procedures? (E. g. is antipyretic treatment working as a relapse prophylaxis?)

Consultation after a febrile seizure
▶ At which date?
▶ Which consultant?
▶ Which examinations?

Drug treatment in case of a relapse
▶ Diazepam rectally (< 15 kg 5 mg, > 15 kg 10 mg)
  – How to use?
  – How to preserve?

A.01 Febrile seizures

A.02 Status epilepticus (SE) 1/2

Emergency and intensive care

- ▶ The correct diagnosis leads to the correct treatment algorithm
  - – Generalized convulsive status epilepticus
  - – Focal status epilepticus
  - – Absence status epilepticus, myoclonic status epilepticus

Treatment algorithm for generalized convulsive status epilepticus

Duration (in min)	Management	Investigation	Treatment
3–5	▶ Recovery position ▶ Open and maintain airway ▶ Time keeping ▶ Preparing phone contact ▶ Prepare IV line	▶ Measure temperature	Diazepam rectally: 0,5–0,7 mg/kg; < 15 kg: 5 mg; > 15 kg: 10 mg Or Midazolam nasal: 0,2 mg/kg (of the IV solution) Or Midazolam buccal: 6 months to 1 year: 2,5mg 1 year to < 5 years: 5 mg 5 years to < 10 years: 7,5 mg 10 years to < 18 years: 10 mg Or *Vascular access:* Lorazepam IV: 0,05–0,1 mg/kg (over 30–60s)

5–20	▶ Check your diagnosis (DD acute dystonia, status dystonicus, other "non-epileptic" status …)
	▶ Physical examination (signs for increased intracranial pressure, meningeal signs, conscious level, pupils …)
	▶ Take a brief history
	  – Traumatic brain injury
	  – Infectious disease
	  – Drugs
	  – Intoxication
	  – AED and withdrawal of AED
	  – (Drug) Allergies
	▶ Supportive medical management:
	  – Monitor airway, breathing and circulation
	  – Give oxygen
	  – Maintain normoglycemia and electrolyte balance
	  – Look for vascular access
	▶ Contact the intensive care unit
		▶ Blood:
		  – Glucose
		  – pH and base excess
		  – Full blood count and differential
		  – Electrolytes
		  – Urea, creatinine
		  – CRP
		  – Level of AED
		  – Toxicological tests
		  – Blood culture (if fever)
		▶ Coagulation factors (if fever)
			Lorazepam IV: 0,05–0,1 mg/kg (injection over 30–60s)
			If not available:
			Clonazepam IV: 0,01–0,05 mg/kg (injection over 1–5 minutes) (max. 0,5 mg/min)
			Or
			Diazepam IV: 0,2–0,5 mg/kg (injection over 1–3 min) (max. 5 mg/min)
			Children < 2 years consider: Additionally Pyridoxin IV: 100 mg

A.02 Status epilepticus (SE)

A.02 Status epilepticus (SE) 2/2

Emergency and intensive care

20–60	▶ Further treatment and monitoring in an intensive care setting ▶ Intubate if necessary ▶ Supportive medical management (see above)	▶ Fever: lumbar puncture ▶ No obvious reason: CT	Valproic acid IV: 20–40 mg/kg (injection over 3–5 min) (max. 6 mg/kg/min) Or Phenobarbital IV: 15–20 mg/kg (injection over 8–10 min) (2 mg/kg/min, max. 100 mg/min) Or Phenytoin IV: 15–20 mg/kg (injection over 15–20 min) (1 mg/kg/min, max. 50 mg/min) Or Levetiracetam 15–20 mg/kg (injection over 15 min)
> 60	▶ Supportive medical management at intensive care unit ▶ EEG-Monitoring		**Midazolam Infusion:** bolus 0,2–0,5 **mg/kg, then** infusion rate 5–**30 mcg/kg**/min (0,3–1,8 mg/kg/h) (titration **to patterns on EEG**) Or Thiopental Infusion: bolus 5 mg/kg, then infusion rate 3–5 mg/kg/h (titration to patterns on EEG) **Propofol Infusion:** bolus 1–2 mg/kg, then **infusion** rate 1–4 mg/kg/h (titration **to patterns on** EEG)

Addendum – Focal status epilepticus
The treatment algorithm for a focal status epilepticus is equivalent to those of a generalized status epilepticus, but you're not so pressed for time.

Addendum – Diagnostic approach	Addendum – treatment
▶ A complete and exact diagnostic approach is even necessary for patients with a confirmed diagnosis of epilepsy, especially if the ictal phenomenology is new. ▶ In children presenting with confusion and loss of awareness, only an EEG can help to confirm the epileptic aetiology or to detect an absence status epilepticus.	▶ The effect of drug treatment may be different in different children. So look for individual treatment algorithms in children with recurrent status epilepticus. ▶ Argument for Phenytoin over Phenobarbital – there's a lower risk for respiratory depression. ▶ Levetiracetam IV may be an effective treatment option. Reports show a good response in treating a focal status epilepticus

Addendum: Treatment algorithm for Absence Status epilepticus and generalized myoclonic status epilepticus

Physical exam	Investigation	Treatment
▶ Clinical presentation: extended status of confusion, maybe only mildly decreased consciousness, rarely agitation. Maybe associated with automatisms (Absence SE) or subtle generalized myoclonia (myoclonic SE) ▶ EEG: generalized 3Hz spike-and-wave complexes, rhythmic delta-activity, spike-slow-wave-complexes, polyspike-slow-wave-complexes	▶ Only the correct diagnosis of Absence SE and generalized myoclonic status epilepticus allows an efficient drug treatment! ▶ Confirm the clinical diagnosis on the EEG (generalized spike-wave-complexes or polyspike-wave-complexes)! ▶ Notice: The inadequate drug treatment of generalized epilepsies (e.g. with Carbamazepin, Vigabatrin or Phenytoin) can cause an Absence SE and generalized myoclonic status epilepticus!	▶ Withdrawal of inadequate AED ▶ Benzodiazepine (oral or IV) e.g. Lorazepam ▶ Valproic acid IV ▶ Maybe Levetiracetam IV (there are no studies)

A.03 Acute dystonic reaction | PCS-Diagnosis 1/1

Emergency and intensive care

Medical history
- Concomitant medication
  - Neuroleptics or other antidopaminergic medication
  - Serotonin reuptake inhibitor
  - Biperiden
- Cocaine abuse
- HIV
- Previous dystonic reactions
- Pathognomonic, typical somatic experience
  - Dysphagia
  - Sense of tightness in the throat
  - Swollen tongue
  - Oculogyric crisis

Physical examination
- Cranial nerves and oculomotor examination
- Intraoral inspection
- Identification of typical movement patterns

Symptoms
- Laryngeal spasm
- Dysarthria
- Dyspnea

▶ Acute dystonic reaction with a vital indication for treatment

Symptoms
- Oro-bucco-lingual dyskinesia
- Cervical dystonia
- Pharyngeal dystonia
- Limb dystonia
- Truncal dystonia
- Oculogyric crisis

▶ Acute dystonic reaction with an urgent indication for treatment

▶ Frequent Biperiden intake

Consider DD bodily distress disorder
- ▶ Otherwise start symptomatic treatment

▶ Spontaneous remission, when patient is unobserved

Consider DD bodily distress disorder
Dystonic symptoms per se exacerbate in emotionally charged situations, and often remit upon relaxation. This characteristic of dystonic syndromes should not be used as diagnostic proof of a "Psychogenic" disorder.

A.03 Acute dystonic reaction

A.03 Acute dystonic reaction | PCS-Therapy

Emergency and intensive care

Urgent treatment indication (frequent)	▶ Anticholinergic (e.g. Biperiden slow IV 0.05–0.1 mg/kg [max. 5 mg/6 hrs]) Or ▶ Antihistaminergic (e.g. Promethazine IV 0.5–1 mg/kg/single dose [max. four times daily])	▶ If symptoms persist after 30 min – Repeat treatment ▶ If symptoms persist after 60 min – Change medication ▶ Dose escalation only in intensive care setting ▶ If patients do not respond to treatment – Correct diagnosis? – Consider differential diagnosis
Vital treatment indication (extremely rare!)	▶ Supply oxygen ▶ Benzodiazepines (e.g. Diazepam 5–10 mg or Lorazepam 0.1 mg/kg [in fractions of 2 mg, max. 4 mg/single dose]) And ▶ Anticholinergic (e.g. Biperiden slow IV 0.05–0.1 mg/kg [max. 5 mg/6 h]) ▶ Monitoring of vital signs for 24 h	▶ If symptoms persist – Repeat treatment after 15–30 min ▶ Dose escalation in intensive care setting ▶ If patients do not respond to treatment – Correct diagnosis? – Consider differential diagnosis

A.04 Acute Ataxia | PCS-Diagnosis 1/2

Emergency and intensive care

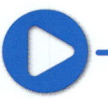

Medical history
▶ Progression
  – Acute (hours – days)
  – Subacute (weeks – few months)
  – Chronic (months – years)
  – Paroxysmal/recurrent
▶ Medication
▶ Family history
▶ Accompanying symptoms

Clinical findings
Cerebellar versus sensory
▶ Cerebellar
  – Hypotonia
  – Asynergy, dysmetria
  – Nystagmus
  – Dysarthria
  – Tremor (intention)
▶ Sensory
  – Position and vibration sensations ↓
  – Areflexia
  – Romberg's test worsening when eyes closed (darkness)
Cerebellar localization
▶ Cerebellar hemisphere syndrome (CHS)
  – Unilateral/bilateral
  – Nystagmus
  – Dysarthria
  – Coordination disorder:
    ▶ Upper extremities + lower extremities + trunk + gait
▶ Rostral cerebellar vermis syndrome (rCVS)
  – Hypotonia
  – Coordination disorder:
    ▶ Lower extremities + trunk + gait

Differential diagnosis
Vascular diseases [see chapter A.09.5 Arteriovenous malformations]
▶ Infarction (CHS – see below. acute, possibly recurrent)
▶ Haemorrhage
▶ Transient ischaemic attack
▶ Basilar-type migraine/migraine with brain stem aura (MBA)
▶ Vascular malformation
▶ Systemic vasculitis (e. g. Lupus erythematodes)

Cerebellar tumors (see chapter K.01 Neoplasm of the CNS)
▶ Medulloblastoma (cCVS, see below. subacute, symptoms of intracranial pressure, cranial nerve failure)
▶ Astrocytoma (cCVS, see below. mostly WHO I, subacute-chronic, visual field failure)
▶ Ependymoma (cranial nerve failure, subacute)
▶ Other (hemangioblastoma, metastases, …)

Infectious/parainfectious diseases
▶ Acute cerebellar ataxia in childhood (cCVS or PS, see below. acute, days–weeks) after infection (often: varicella, others), duration weeks to a few months, rarely protracted. Note: Opsoclonus Myoclonus Syndrome
▶ Viral encephalitis (brain stem encephalitis with cerebellar involvement)
▶ Bacterial infection, abscess, tuberculosis/tuberculoma
▶ Chronic panencephalitis

Autoimmune disorders
▶ Multiple sclerosis (see chapter J.01 Multiple sclerosis/ADEM)
▶ Acute disseminated encephalomyelitis
▶ Miller-Fisher syndrome (special type of acute Guillan-Barré syndrome with characters of polyneuritis, ophthalmoplegia, see chapter A.06 Guillain-Barré syndrome (GBS)

Paraneoplastic diseases
▶ Opsoclonus myoclonus (ataxia) syndrome (see chapter G Movement disorders)
▶ Chronic, adulthood: paraneoplastic cerebellar degeneration

Medication/toxic substances (subacute, chronic)
▶ Anticonvulsants (phenytoin, carbamazepine, barbiturates)
▶ hemotherapeutic substances (5-flouracil, cytosine arabinoside)
▶ Heavy metals (lead, thallium, mercury)

Others
▶ Trauma
▶ Benign paroxysmal torticollis of infancy (paroxysmal, recurrent, typical beginning in the 1st year of life, absence of symptoms 3rd–5th year of life, under certain circumstances torticollis not in the foreground but trunk- and gait ataxia, migraine in family history, discussed as migraine precursor)

Working hypothesis managed diagnostics
▶ MRI
▶ Laboratory parameters
▶ Lumbar puncture
▶ Sonography including colour duplex sonography of extra-/intracranial vessels
▶ Clinical neurophysiology

A.04 Acute Ataxia

A.04 Acute Ataxia | PCS-Diagnosis 2/2

Emergency and intensive care

- ▶ Caudal cerebellar vermis syndrome (cCVS)
  - Nystagmus (variable) +/- Hypotonia
    - ▶ Coordination disorder: +/- lower extremities + trunk + gait
- ▶ Pancerebellar syndrome (PS)
  - Hypotonia, nystagmus, dysarthria
  - Coordination disorder

A.05 Acute increased intracranial pressure (ICP) | PCS-Diagnosis

Emergency and intensive care

- ▶ Medical history
  - Trauma
  - Resuscitation
  - Fever
  - Meningism
  - Clotting disorder
  - Metabolic disturbances
- ▶ Clinical findings (MRI for …)
  - Headaches
  - Psychomotor disturbance
  - Unspecific signs
  - Abdominal discomfort
  - Hypertonia
  - Bradycardia
  - Torticollis
  - Vomiting (posterior fossa!)
  - Visual disturbance
  - Prominent optic disc (fundoscopy[1])
  - Disturbance of pupillary reaction
  - Decreased consciousness level
  - Cheyne-Stokes breathing
  - Abnormal extensor posturing

- ▶ CT in acute phase to rule out
  - Haemorrhage
  - Infarction
  - Hydrocephalus
  - Swelling
  - Tumor
- ▶ MRI for further evaluation

- ▶ GCS 13–15
- ▶ GCS 9–12
  Or
- ▶ Vasospasm
  Or
- ▶ Pseudotumor cerebri
- ▶ GCS ≤ 8

- ▶ No ICP-monitoring required
- ▶ Non-invasive ICP-monitoring[2]
  - Transcranial doppler sonography (TCD) with pulsatility index[3]
- ▶ Invasive ICP-monitoring
  - Ventricular catheter[4] for continuous ICP-monitoring and CSF drainage to treat increased ICP
  - Parenchymal ICP probe[5]: additional measurement of pO_2 and pH
- ▶ if drainage of CSF not possible
  - Epi- or subdural ICP probes ("old fashioned")

- ▶ Acutely increased ICP of different aetiologies

---

1 Prominent optic discs can develop with a delay of several days
2 Continuous monitoring or measurement of ICP peaks is not possible
3 Pulsatility index = quotient systolic blood flow (linked to systolic blood pressure)/intracranial diastolic blood flow (linked to ICP); normal 0,7–1. Source of error: stenosis, altered flow with changing blood viscosity and circulation
4 Ventricular catheter; source of error: no reliable measurements in case of over-drainage and slit ventricles; complications: infection, daily CSF lab test required, bleeding in catheter trajectory
5 Parenchymal probe: low risk for infection or bleeding, small parenchymal defect; but limited reliability of measurements

A.05 Acute increased intracranial pressure (ICP) | PCS-Therapy 1/2

Emergency and intensive care

Basic Therapy
- Head above bed in 30°
- Neutral position of head
- Sedation (Pentobarbital as continuous infusion, Thiopental (2–4 mg/kg) as bolus)
- Relaxation
- Mechanical ventilation, PCO_2 at max. 35 mmHg (4.6 kPa)
- Normo- to mild hypovolemia
- Fluid balance
- Electrolyte balance
- Normo- or hypothermia

Monitoring
- Systemic blood pressure, pulse
- Arterial PO_2, PCO_2, pH
- Body weight, urine output
- CBC, electrolytes, urine analysis, glucose
- Exclude fever and sepsis
- CT

▶ Trauma	▶ Diffuse swelling	▶ Evaluation and resuscitation
		▶ Normalize blood pressure
		▶ Intubation and ventilation
			▶ Escalated therapy
			  – External ventricular CSF drain (EVD)
			  – Mannitol (0,25 g/kg/single dose 4–8 h),
			  NOTE: rebound effect
			  – Alternatively hyperosmolar NaCl-solution
			  – Moderate hyperventilation, PCO_2 32–35 mmHg (4.2–4.6 kPa)
			▶ Monitoring
			  – EVD
			  – Central venous pressure
			  – Serum osmolality, electrolytes
			
			▶ Intensified regimen for refractory ICP↑
			  – Barbiturate with burst-suppression in EEG
			  – Moderate hyperventilation, PCO_2 < 32 mmHg (4.2 kPa)
			▶ Monitoring
			  – Continuous EEG
			  – Serum level of barbiturates
			  – Jugular venous saturation
			  – Cerebral perfusion pressure (CPP)

	▶ Bleeding (epi-, subdural, intraparenchymal) ▶ Contusion	▶ Decompression of acute sub- or epidural haematoma ▶ In case of massive cerebral swelling: decompressive craniectomy with dural patch ▶ Surgical resection of growing contusions	
▶ Space occupying lesion	▶ Tumor oedema	▶ Dexamethasone 0,3 mg/kg/d ▶ Mannitol (as bolus in severe swelling, dosing see above)	
	▶ Impaired CSF circulation	▶ GCS ≤ 8 And ▶ Hydrocephalus	▶ Extraventricular drainage
		▶ Occlusive hydrocephalus Or ▶ Malresorptive hydrocephalus	▶ Ventriculoperitoneal shunt
		▶ Space occupying cyst	▶ Internal shunt
		▶ Aqueductal stenosis	▶ Endoscopic third ventriculostomy
	▶ Tumor	▶ Tumor resection	
▶ Hypoxia	▶ Infarction	▶ Decompressive craniectomy	
	▶ oedema	▶ See therapy for "Trauma" → "diffuse swelling"	
▶ Metabolic disturbances	▶ Symptomatic therapy		
▶ Vascular cause	▶ Infarction	▶ Space occupying infarction	

A.05 Acute increased intracranial pressure (ICP) | PCS-Therapy 2/2

Emergency and intensive care

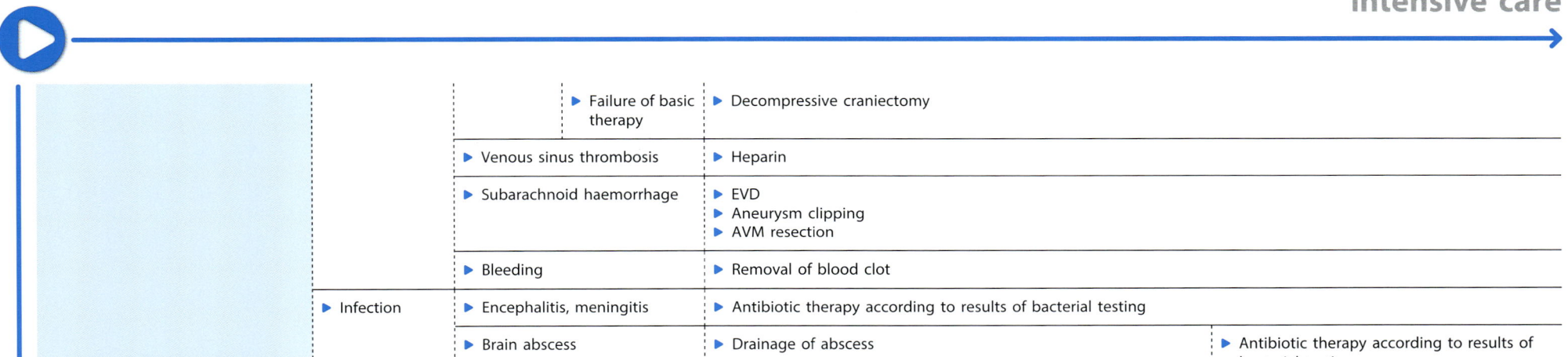

		▶ Failure of basic therapy	▶ Decompressive craniectomy	
		▶ Venous sinus thrombosis	▶ Heparin	
		▶ Subarachnoid haemorrhage	▶ EVD ▶ Aneurysm clipping ▶ AVM resection	
		▶ Bleeding	▶ Removal of blood clot	
	▶ Infection	▶ Encephalitis, meningitis	▶ Antibiotic therapy according to results of bacterial testing	
		▶ Brain abscess	▶ Drainage of abscess	▶ Antibiotic therapy according to results of bacterial testing

A.06 Guillain-Barré Syndrome (GBS) | PCS-Diagnosis 1/1

Emergency and intensive care

Clinical clues to the diagnosis of GBS	Basal diagnostics		Further diagnostic work-up		
▶ Acute, flaccid, usually symmetric ascending paresis ▶ Loss of deep tendon reflexes ▶ Mild ataxia ▶ Neuropathic pain, but no sharply delineated segmental sensory loss ▶ Involvement of cranial nerves ▶ Autonomic involvement (cardiocirculatory and bladder dysfunction) ▶ Progression for 1–4 weeks[1]	▶ LP – Clues for GBS: increased CSF protein[2]; normal or only slightly increased CSF cell count < 50/mm³ – Clues against GBS: more than 50 mononuclear cells/mm³; increased neutrophils in CSF; CSF protein > 2,5 g/l	▶ Anamnestic, clinical and laboratory clues to GBS	▶ Electroneurography and electromyography ▶ Determination of antibodies in serum[3]: IgG against GM1, -GM1b, -GD1a, -GalNac-GD1a; Campylobacter jejuni serology	▶ At least 1 electrodiagnostic feature of demyelinating neuropathy – Motor NCV < 80 % of lower limit of normal – Distal latency > 110 % of upper limit of normal – Amplitude-ratio of proximal/distal stimulation < 0.5 – F-wave-latency > 120 % of upper limit of normal	▶ GBS (AIDP)
				▶ Electrodiagnostic clues to axonal neuropathy – CMAP-amplitude at distal stimulation < 80 % of lower limit of normal – Electromyographic signs of acute denervation – No findings indicative of demyelination	▶ GBS (AMAN)
Clinical arguments against a diagnosis of GBS ▶ Distinct, persistent asymmetry of paresis ▶ Sphincter dysfunction as an initial sign ▶ Persistent bladder-/rectal dysfunction ▶ Sharply defined segmental sensory loss				▶ Electrodiagnostic evidence of demyelination with secondary axonal involvement – Signs of demyelination ▶ And – Signs of axonal dysfunction	▶ GBS (AIDP with secondary axonal damage)
				▶ Electrodiagnostic findings normal (at least 2 weeks after onset of symptoms)	▶ GBS improbable ▶ Consider differential diagnoses
		▶ Anamnestic, clinical and laboratory clues to a hereditary, metabolic or toxic neuropathy			Further diagnostic work-up

1 If progression > 4 weeks, consider subacute inflammatory demyelinating polyneuropathy (SIDP) if progression > 8 weeks diagnosis chronic inflammatory demyelinating polyneuropathy (CIDP).
2 Can be normal during the first 10 days after onset of symptoms!
3 The determination of antigangliosid antibodies is not part of the basic diagnostic work-up; in Germany only 5 % of children with GBS (AMAN) can be expected to show positive findings.

A.06 Guillain-Barré syndrome (GBS) | PCS-Therapy, part 1 1/1

Emergency and intensive care

▶ Continuing deterioration with imminent loss of ability to walk

Or

▶ After loss of ability to walk

Intravenous immunoglobulins (IVIG)[1]
▶ 0,4 g/kg body weight on five successive days

Or

Plasma exchange (PE)[1]
▶ 200–250 ml/kg body weight in 3–5 sessions during 7–14 days

▶ Response to IVIG/PE

▶ No response to IVIG/PE

▶ Repetition of IVIG or plasma exchange can be considered after 3–4 weeks (evidence class IV)

Rehabilitation
▶ As in-patient in a paediatric rehabilitation hospital
  – Generally indicated for all severely affected patients
  – Especially indicated until return of ability to walk and at school-age
▶ As out-patient, involving physiotherapists and occupational therapists experienced in treatment of children
  – After discharge from hospital in less severely affected patients, at pre-school age and in families able to cope with the therapeutic efforts
  – After discharge from rehabilitation hospital until functional recovery

---

▶ Progression

Or

▶ Secondary deterioration 4–6 weeks after onset of GBS (suggesting the possible presence of subacute or chronic inflammatory demyelinating polyneuropathy, SIDP or CIDP)

▶ Continuous treatment with Prednisone 1 mg/kg body weight/d

Or

▶ Pulsed treatment with Methylprednisolone 20 mg/kg body weight/d for 3–5 days

Or

▶ Single trial with IVIG 1 g/kg body weight for 2 days; if relapsing to be repeated every 4 weeks, slowly tapering the dosage to the least effective level

▶ Rehabilitation: see above

---

1 IVIG and PE can be regarded equivalent concerning efficacy, but IVIG is superior concerning tolerability (evidence class I)

A.06 Guillain-Barré syndrome (GBS) | PCS-Therapy, part 2

Emergency and intensive care

Management of GBS		
Cardiovascular monitoring and treatment	▶ ECG monitoring ▶ Periodic measurements of blood pressure	▶ In all patients with severe GBS due to the risk of hypertensive crises and cardiac dysrhythmias ▶ In patients with vegetative instability, use special caution when applying invasive diagnostic or therapeutic measures (such as pharyngeal suctioning) because these can provoke critical arrhythmia
Respiratory monitoring and treatment	▶ Periodic measurements of peak flow and forced vital capacity (fVC) ▶ Periodic measurements of blood gases	▶ In all patients with severe GBS, especially when the upper extremities and cranial nerves are involved ▶ In some patients, abnormal blood gases do not occur before acute respiratory decompensation ▶ Therefore, do not wait until patients show abnormal blood gas values! Intubation and artificial ventilation are indicated when fVC < 25 % of normal
Pain management and psychological guidance	▶ Use age-appropriate pain scales, observe and consider pain behaviour	▶ Pain treatment should be liberal, including use of opioids ▶ See chapter C Pain ▶ Paralyzed and ventilated patients are in an exceptional psychological situation. Therefore, liberal sedation is indicated. ▶ Do not use benzodiazepines in not-intubated patients; they induce muscular relaxation and can give rise to respiratory failure! ▶ If artificial ventilation is necessary for more than 7 days, consider early tracheotomy to terminate deep sedation and enable communication
Positioning, physiotherapy	▶ Prophylaxis of decubitus ulcers and contractures	▶ During the acute paralytic phase, apply passive movement exercises (CAUTION: cases with severe neuropathic pain) ▶ After onset of improvement, gradually increase active exercises
Anticoagulation treatment	▶ Usually low molecular weight heparins (LMH), discuss with experts for coagulation disorders, see chapter S Medication	▶ Consider in immobile patients

A.07 Neurometabolic dysfunction | PCS-Classification 1/2

Emergency and intensive care

Classification according to dysfunction

Type I:	Endogenous intoxication provoked by catabolism	Urea cycle defects Organic acidurias Aminoacidopathies Disorders in the transport and oxidation of fatty acids
Type II:	Disorders in the availability of glucose, without endogenous intoxication	Glycogen storage diseases
Type III:	Dysfunction in energy acquisition of glucose	Mitochondriopathies

Classification according to specific organs

Liver	Galactosemia, hypertyrosinemia type I
Cardiovascular	Disorders in the transport and oxidation of fatty acids, respiratory chain defects
CNS	Urea cycle defects, organic acidurias, cofactor deficiencies

Classification according to time of manifestation of neurometabolic dysfunction

Type	Characteristics	Examples	Peak manifestation
Type Intoxication	Initially often clinically silent interval (hours–2 d) Increasing intoxication with "septic" clinical picture, apathy/coma Patients may also show signs and symptoms associated with: ▶ Neurotoxicity ▶ Cardiotoxicity ▶ Hepatotoxicity	Protein degradation disturbance ▶ Aminoacidopathies ▶ Organic acidurias ▶ Urea cycle defects Disorders in the transport and oxidation of fatty acids; Disorders of carbohydrate metabolism: galactosemia	At birth and in the first week of life with typical symptom-free interval
Hypoglycemia with prolonged fasting periods	Hypoglycemia after exceeding the disease-specific fasting tolerance Convulsions	Reduced fasting tolerance: increased glucose consumption, e.g., congenital hyperinsulinism Reduced or longer fasting tolerance: disturbed glucose availability, e.g., glycogen storage disease type I	Neonatal period and late infancy
Disturbed neurotransmission	Neonatal epileptic encephalopathy Epilepsy resistant to treatment	Non-ketotic hyperglycinemia Vitamin-B_6-dependent epilepsy	Often prenatal, neonatal period

A.07 Neurometabolic dysfunction

44

A.07 Neurometabolic dysfunction | PCS-Classification 2/2

Emergency and intensive care

Disturbed energy metabolism	Energy-dependent organs are predominantly affected ▶ Muscle: hypotension ▶ Heart: cardiomyopathy ▶ Brain: encephalopathy ▶ Liver: hepatopathy ▶ Kidneys: tubulopathy Lactic acidosis	Mitochondriopathies	Depends on severity, predominantly neonatal period but also possible in "late adulthood"
Metabolic disorders of complex molecules	No acute decompensation but progressive deterioration	Lysosomal storage diseases	Age of several months to years

A.07 Neurometabolic dysfunction | PCS-Acute intervention 1/1

Emergency and intensive care

As the outcome depends essentially on the rapid control of the metabolic crisis, a simultaneous start of emergency treatment and diagnostic work-up is required in most cases.
Initial therapy is therefore non-specific and becomes more specific in the course of the diagnostic work-up (acute intervention – confirmation of suspected diagnosis – specific therapy):

Evidence of metabolic causes ▶ Clinical picture of sepsis with exclusion of an infection ▶ Hyperexcitability/convulsions ▶ Altered level of consciousness, clinical picture of encephalopathy ▶ Comatose state	**Simultaneous approach (points 1–3); imperative to contact local metabolic centre/transfer**	**1. Tests**	Blood tests: ▶ Basic metabolic tests: blood gas analysis, glucose, lactate, ammonia (on ice) ▶ General basic diagnostic work-up: complete blood count, CRP, clotting screen, CK, transaminases, creatinine, uric acid, urea, electrolytes ▶ Reserve: EDTA-blood, serum, dried blood spot on filter card Urine: ▶ Basic diagnostic work-up: urine dipstick (ketones/glucose/infection) ▶ Store: approximately 4–10 ml (in refrigerator) If lumbar puncture to exclude meningitis: ▶ Cytology/status ▶ Store: 1–3 ml (-80°C) (see Chapter N.01 Neurometabolic disorders)
If required, additional evidence on: **History** ▶ Reduced/increased movements of baby in pregnancy ▶ Consanguinity of parents ▶ Intrauterine/postnatal death of siblings ▶ Temporary disturbances of consciousness of unknown cause ▶ Dietary history (aversion/avoidance)		**2. Initiate forced anabolism**	▶ Corresponding to glucose production rate ▶ Glucose infusion: Usually 10 mg/kg/min (e.g.: 10 % glucose solution: 12 ml/kg in 2 h) or more, with adequate electrolyte supplements. ▶ If necessary, additional administration of insulin (e.g.: 0.1–1 IU/kg × h with blood sugar > 200 mg/dl {11 mmol/l})

Physical examination
▶ Muscular hypotension
▶ Irritability
▶ Micro-/macrocephaly
▶ Failure to thrive
▶ Delayed development
▶ Intrauterine growth retardation
▶ Dysmorphic stigmata
		3. Stop exogenous supply	▶ No dietary proteins
			▶ No dietary fats
			▶ If suspected galactosemia/hereditary fructose intolerance: no galactose/fructose
			▶ In the case of an emergency:
			  – Administer intravenous fluids, glucose and electrolytes, stop food supply
			  – This limited regime should not be continued for longer than 12 h

Clinical confirmation of the working diagnosis	**Diagnostic work-up** ▶ Overall profile (basic diagnostic work-up + store specimens that can now be used for specific tests, e.g., organic acids in urine, amino acids in plasma etc.) ▶ Possibly challenge test in a symptom-free interval (e.g. glucose) ▶ Enzyme analyses ▶ Genetic analyses	**Specific therapy** ▶ Dietetic therapy ▶ Specific supplements (e.g. carnitine) ▶ Adjuvant therapy (e.g. radical scavengers for mitochondriopathy) ▶ Enzyme replacement therapy	**Follow-up at metabolic outpatient clinic** ▶ Education/counselling ▶ Clinical/laboratory follow-ups ▶ Social paediatrics/rehabilitation

A.07 Neurometabolic dysfunction

A.07 Neurometabolic dysfunction | PCS-Therapy following: confirmation of suspected diagnosis 1/1

Working diagnosis	Course of action
Type I: Metabolic disease Intoxication Type	Achieve anabolism! ▶ > 100 kcal/kg/d applied as glucose 15–20 mg/kg × min, ▶ Additionally insulin, start with 0.1 IU/kg × h ▶ If necessary, fat 1–2 g/kg × d (*warning:* avoid if disorder in the transport and breakdown of fatty acids is suspected)
	Detoxification: ▶ Specific treatment (e.g. sodium benzoate for hyperammonaemia) ▶ Increase diuresis ▶ Remove toxic substances (e.g. glycine, carnitine) ▶ If necessary, dialysis
Type II: Metabolic disease With disturbed glucose availability	Ensure glucose supply ▶ Adjusted to glucose production rate (glucose 7–8 mg/kg × min) ▶ Hyperinsulinism: > 10 mg/kg × min
	Specific treatment: ▶ E.g. carnitine in organic acidurias ▶ Diazoxide in hyperinsulinism
Type III: Metabolic disease With dysfunction in energy acquisition from glucose	Limit glucose administration ▶ Glucose 3–4 mg/kg × min, ▶ Additional energy supply from fat 2–4 g/kg × d
	Specific instructions ▶ Sodium bicarbonate/sodium citrate ▶ Coenzyme supplementation ▶ Alpha lipoic acid ▶ Renal/cardiac protection

A.07 Neurometabolic dysfunction | PCS-Specific therapy: Type I 1/1

Emergency and intensive care

Type I: Endogenous intoxication provoked by catabolism

Recommended basic therapy:
▶ Glucose 15–20 mg/kg × min, additionally insulin (individual adjustment, start with 0.1 IU/kg × h)
▶ Fat 1–2 g/kg × d (warning: contraindicated in fatty acid oxidation disorders)

Disorder	Leading signs	Advanced diagnostic tests	Specific therapy	Contraindicated
Urea cycle defects e.g. ▶ Carbamoylphosphate synthase I deficiency (CPSI) ▶ N-acetylglutamate synthase deficiency (NAGS) ▶ Ornithine carbamoylphosphate transferase deficiency (OCT) ▶ Argininosuccinate synthase deficiency (ASS), citrullinemia ▶ Argininosuccinate lyase deficiency (ASL), argininosuccinic aciduria ▶ Arginase deficiency (ARG), hyperargininemia	Ammonia ↑	▶ Specific amino acid profile (plasma) ▶ Orotic acid (urine)	NH_3 detoxication: ▶ Forced diuresis: – Furosemide 1–2 mg/kg and dose ▶ NH_3 detoxication: – Sodium benzoate: 250(–500) mg/kg × d – Additionally sodium phenylbutyrate: 250(–500) mg/kg × d ▶ If necessary, dialysis Replacement of urea cycle intermediates: ▶ L-arginine IV (except for ARG): 2 mmol/kg × d Support of the mitochondrial metabolism with L-Carnitine (100 mg/kg × d) If necessary, administration of anti-emetics, e.g. Ondansetron 0.15 mg/kg and dose IV	Administration of protein or amino acids IV Start after an initial pause (not > 12 h) e.g. with 1 g/kg × d
Organic acidurias e.g. ▶ Methylmalonic aciduria (MMA) ▶ Isovaleric acidemia (IVA) ▶ Propionic acidemia (PA)	Metabolic acidosis with enlarged anion gap, lactate ↔/↑; ammonia↑; ketonuria; possible neutropenia, thrombocytopenia; pancytopenia	Organic acids in urine, acyl-carnitine profile in blood or plasma	Forced diuresis: ▶ Furosemide 1–2 mg/kg and dose ▶ L-Carnitine (100 mg/kg × 3 IV or p.o.) ▶ Correction of acidosis ▶ When diagnosis is confirmed add specific conjugating substances or coenzymes, e.g. – IVA: L-Glycine 150–250 mg/kg × d; – MMA: Vit B_{12} 1 mg/d	Administration of protein or aminoacids IV Start after an initial pause (not > 12 h) e.g. with 1 g/kg × d
Aminoacidopathies e.g. Maple syrup urine disease (MSUD)	In contrast to standard organic acidurias there is no accumulation of activated CoA compounds – acidosis and hyperammonemia are therefore less pronounced	▶ Amino acids in plasma or dried blood drop on filter card ▶ Organic acids in urine	Forced diuresis: ▶ Furosemide 1–2 mg/kg (with further dose adjustment) ▶ Correction of acidosis	Administration of protein or amino acids IV Initially stop (not > 12 h), then begin, e.g. with 1 g/kg × d
Fatty acid oxidation disorders (long chain) e.g. ▶ Very-long-chain acyl-CoA dehydrogenase deficiency (VLCAD) ▶ Long-chain-3-hydroxy acyl-CoA dehydrogenase deficiency (LCHAD) ▶ Mitochondrial trifunctional protein-(TFP-)deficiency	Blood sugar, lactate, free fatty acids, ketones, ammonia	▶ Acylcarnitine profile in plasma or dried blood drop on filter card ▶ Organic acids (dicarboxylic acids)	Medium-chain triacylglyceroles (MCT fats)	Carnitine (increases the formation of potentially toxic acylcarnitines); fat (can be administered at a low dose)

A.07 Neurometabolic dysfunction

A.07 Neurometabolic dysfunction | PCS-Specific therapy: Type II/III

Emergency and intensive care

Type II: Disorders in the availability of glucose, without endogenous intoxication

Recommended basic therapy:
- Glucose 10 g mg/kg × min

Disorder	Leading signs	Advanced diagnostic tests	Specific therapy	Contraindicated
Hyperinsulinism	Hypoglycemia	▶ Glucose requirement > 10 mg/kg × min ▶ Analysis of insulin/C-peptide ▶ Glucose/insulin index (hypoglycemia with insulin > 3 mU/l)	▶ Increase glucose to 15–20 mg/kg × min ▶ Glucagon: 5–10 mcg/kg × h IV ▶ Diazoxide: 15 mg/kg, 3 times per day	
Fatty acid oxidation disorder of medium-chain fatty acids (MCAD deficiency)	Blood sugar, lactate, free fatty acids, ketones	▶ Acylcarnitine profile in plasma or dried blood drop on filter card ▶ Organic acids in urine ▶ Molecular genetics	Administration of L-Carnitine (controversial): (e.g. 20 mg/kg, 3 times IV or p.o. per day)	Limited fat supply (controversial)
Glycogen storage disease	Hypoglycemia, uric acid ↑, lactate ↑, triglycerides ↑	▶ Enzyme analysis ▶ Molecular genetics		

Type III: Dysfunction in energy acquisition from glucose

Recommended basic therapy:
- Limit glucose supply
  - Reduce glucose to 3–4 mg/kg × min,
  - Fat 2–4 g/kg × d

Disorder	Leading signs	Advanced diagnostic tests	Specific therapy	Contraindicated
Mitochondriopathies	▶ Elevated lactate ▶ Metabolic acidosis	▶ Alanine/lysine ratio > 3 ▶ CSF lactate ▶ Lactate in urine (single sample or 24-h-sampling) ▶ Acylcarnitine/carnitine status in plasma or dried blood drop on filter card ▶ If necessary, challenge test ▶ ECG, echocardiography, MRI + spectroscopy ▶ Muscle biopsy (analysis of respiratory chain complexes, analysis of mitochondrial DNA depletion) ▶ Genetics (mitochondrial-/nuclear-encoded diseases)	Symptomatic: ▶ Correction of acidosis, anticonvulsant medication Supplements with reported clinical efficacy: ▶ Quinone (Coenzyme Q, Idebenone): Coenzyme Q_{10} deficiency ▶ Idebenone +/- Vit E: Friedreich ataxia, +/- cardiomyopathy ▶ Ketogenic diet, thiamine: PDHC E1-deficiency ▶ Riboflavin: Complex I deficiency mitochondrial myopathy ▶ L-Carnitine: Mitochondriopathies, independent of any biochemical deficiency with secondary carnitine deficiency ▶ Creatinine, aerobic exercise: mitochondrial myopathy, independent of any biochemical deficiency	High glucose supply

A.08 Traumatic brain injury (TBI) | PCS-Diagnosis 1/1

Emergency and intensive care

History
- Location and time of accident
- Course and mechanism of accident
- Primary care at accident
- Clinical symptoms (initial and during the further course)
- Initial lowest Glasgow Coma Scale
- Duration of vigilance disturbance
- Nausea, vomiting (when and how often)
- Cephalgia, dizziness/vertigo (character and time of occurrence)
- Pre-existing diseases
- Medication

Clinical findings
- Vigilance and behaviour
- Respiration
- Sport Concussion Assessment Tool 5 (SCAT5)
- Child-SCAT5
- Glasgow Coma Scale
- Haematomas, fractures
- Muscle reflexes, pyramidal signs
- Cranial nerve function tests (incl. oculomotoric, pupil light reaction)
- Coordination tests
- Sensibility test
- Signs for cervical spine injury
- Antero-/retrograde amnesia (time of occurrence and duration)

Optional laboratory
- Blood count
- Coagulation tests
- Blood gas analysis
- Electrolytes, glucose
- Liver and renal function tests
- AB0 typing for optional transfusion

▶ Initial GCS 13–15 points

▶ Check risk factors:
- Prolonged vigilance disturbance (> 5 min)
- Prolonged amnesia (retrograde amnesia > 5 min)
- Serious/increasing cephalgia or vertigo
- Recurrent vomiting
- Bulging fontanelle
- Post traumatic seizure
- Focal neurological deficit
- Visual disturbance (for example diplopia)
- Coagulation disorder
- Suspicious impression fracture (palpation)
- Suspicious skull base fracture (monocular haematoma, haematotympanon)
- Suspicious dural injury (CSF leak)
- Accident mechanism (for example high velocity accident, battered child, height of fall > 3 m)

▶ Mild traumatic brain injury *without* risk factors

▶ Possible: Admission for Neuromonitoring:
- Heart rate
- Respiratory rate
- Blood pressure
▶ Cerebral ultrasound
▶ EEG (optional)

▶ Clinical worsening

▶ Mild traumatic brain injury *with* risk factors (grade I)

▶ Initial GCS 9–12 points

▶ Moderate traumatic brain injury (grade II)

▶ Initial GCS < 9 points

▶ Severe traumatic brain injury (grade III)

▶ Computed tomography (CT)

Depending on existing risk factors and co-existing injuries add:
▶ CT/conventional x-ray of the cervical spine
▶ Detailed orbital CT
▶ Duplex sonography
▶ MRI with DWI, T2* and angiography sequences to detect diffuse axonal injuries or additional vascular injuries
▶ Ear-nose-throat, ophthalmological, plastic surgical, neurosurgical consultation

In case of polytrauma add:
▶ Trauma CT (Pan-Scan) und abdominal sonography

See chapters
▶ A.05 Acute increased intracranial pressure (ICP)
▶ A.09.2 Intracranial haemorrhage/ bleeding

A.08 Traumatic brain injury (TBI)

A.08 Traumatic brain injury (TBI) | PCS-Therapy 1/1

Emergency and intensive care

- GCS < 9 or significant midline shift or brain oedema
- Intracranial pressure (ICP) monitoring
- Anticonvulsive prophylaxis (for example Phenytoin, Levetiracetam)
- Intubation
- Intensive care neuromonitoring:
  - Vital functions
  - ICP
  - Laboratory
  - Clinical neurological examination
  - EEG
  - AEP, SEP
  - Duplex sonography
  - CT, MRI
- Increased intracranial pressure (ICP)
- For details see chapter A.05 Acute increased intracranial pressure (ICP)
- All
- No posttraumatic deficits at the end of the intensive care period
- Follow-up:
  - Clinical neurological examination
  - EEG (Caution: development of posttraumatic epilepsy)
  - In case of a suspicious growing skull fracture native skull x-ray
  - Optional CT/MRI
  - Neuropsychological examination
  - Endocrinological examination

- Impression fracture (at least skull width)
- Epidural haematoma (EDH), subdural haematoma (SDH)
- Neurosurgical intervention
- See chapter A.09.2 Intracranial haemorrhage/bleeding
- Standard neuromonitoring:
  - Heart rate, respiration rate, blood pressure
  - Parenteral nutrition
- Cerebral sonography
- Optional electroencephalography (EEG)
- Clinical deterioration
- Complications:
  - Sinus vein thrombosis
  - Traumatic vascular injury
  - Stroke
  - Seizure
  - Hydrocephalus
  - Cerebral infection
  - Diabetes insipidus centralis
  - SIADH
  - Salt Wasting Syndrome
  - Posttraumatic epilepsy
  - Posttraumatic hypopituitarism
- Posttraumatic deficits at the end of the intensive care period:
  - Neurological
  - Neuropsychological
  - Physically
  - Constitutionally
- Transfer to rehabilitation unit (see chapter I.01 Rehabilitation)

- Combined skeletal, soft tissue, facial and ocular injuries
- Other surgical interventions
  - Traumatology
  - Plastic surgery
  - Ophthalmology
  - Ear-nose-throat (ENT)

A.09 Paediatric stroke | PCS-Diagnosis, part 1 1/1

Emergency and intensive care

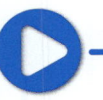

History
- Time of onset of symptoms
- Main symptoms
  - Headache
  - Hemiparesis
  - Facial palsy
  - Decreased consciousness level
  - Visual impairment
  - Dysarthria/Aphasia
  - Ataxia
  - Epileptic seizures
- Further course (i.e. progressive alteration of consciousness)
- Pre-existing conditions (cardiac, vascular, renal, hemato-oncological, metabolic, infectious, vasculitis, fibromuscular dysplasia, coagulation disorder)
- Trauma
- Drugs
- Family history (Stroke? Coagulation disorder?)

Internal examination/neurological examination
- Brainstem symptoms
- Pathological reflexes
- Meningism
- Heart murmur

Paediatric NIH stroke scale
- 1 Level of consciousness (LOC)
- 2 Horizontal extraocular movements
- 3 Visual fields
- 4 Facial palsy
- 5 Arm motor drift (left and right)
- 6 Leg motor drift (left and right)
- 7 Limb ataxia
- 8 Sensation
- 9 Language/aphasia
- 10 Dysarthria
- 11 Extinction/inattention

Basic diagnostic work-up
- Routine laboratory tests
  - Blood cell count and differential, glucose, electrolytes, retention parameters, TSH, CRP, CK, CK-MB, LDH, Troponin T, blood gas
- Coagulation
  - Prothrombin time (PT), international normalized ratio (INR), activated partial thromboplastin time (aPTT), fibrinogen, antithrombin, D-Dimers
- Blood pressure, ECG
- Temperature
- Oxygen saturation

Technical investigations
- Consider Doppler/duplex ultrasound extra- and intracranial
- MRI, MRI-angiography
  - MRI is the most sensitive, preferred investigation
- CT
- Chest X-ray

A.09 Paediatric stroke

52

A.09 Paediatric stroke | PCS-Diagnosis, part 2

▶ Indicators for cerebral ischaemia – Loss of corticomedullary differentiation – Space occupying processes – Hypoperfusion	
▶ Additional indicators for thrombo-embolism – Angiographic detection of stenosis – Hyperdense media sign	See chapter A.09.1 Thromboembolic events
▶ Additional indicators for intracranial bleeding – CT: hyperdensity	See chapter A.09.2 Intracranial haemorrhage/bleeding
▶ Additional indicators for cerebral venous sinus thrombosis – Congestion bleeding – General or local oedema – Fresh thrombus might show increased density – After administration of contrast "empty-delta-sign" – Occluded veins visible as hyperdense strips	See chapter A.09.3 Cerebral sinus venous thrombosis
▶ Additional indicators for dissection (Duplex-Ultrasound) – Direct imaging of extracranial vessel wall haematoma and of extra- and intracranial stenosis – Low density helical vessel wall structure – Tapered stenosis or occlusion – Intraluminal membranes – Local ectasia – Increased sheer velocity	See chapter A.09.4 Cerebrovascular dissection
▶ Additional indicators for vasculitis (high-resolution, contrast-enhanced MRI) – Vessel wall thickening and wall enhancement – Arterial wall irregularities	See chapter J.02 Cerebral vasculitis
▶ Additional indicators for cerebrovascular malformation in MRI/CT – Pathological vascular structures – Possible calcification – Possible perifocal oedema – Fresh or old intracerebral blood remnants	See chapter A.09.5 Arteriovenous malformations
Differential diagnosis: migraine, transitory ischaemic attack (TIA)	

A.09 Paediatric stroke | PCS-Acute therapy 1/1

Emergency and intensive care

Basic diagnostic work-up/Monitoring
- Glucose (Serum)
- Blood pressure
- Heart rate
- Temperature
- Respiratory rate, oxygen-saturation
- Electrolytes
- Fluid balance
- Neurological examination (Paediatric NIH Stroke Scale)

- See chapter A09.1 Thromboembolic events
- **Specific/recanalization therapy:**
  - Rare, highly specialized centers with a (paediatric) stroke unit

Post-acute
- Hydration: ensure adequate fluid supply (*NOTE:* assess fluid balance, especially in cardiac insufficiency)
- Gastric ulcer protection (e.g. Esomeprazole 1 mg/kg/d)
- Mobilization
  - As early as possible
  - Exclusion: fresh subarachnoid haemorrhage (SAB) with untreated aneurysm
- Specific anti-infectious therapy

Poor ventilation	Breathing therapy
Initial attempt to swallow unsuccessful	Gastric tube

Epileptic seizures	Antiepileptic therapy
	  – Acute: benzodiazepines, e.g. Lorazepam 0,1 mg/kg IV
	  – Post-acute: e.g. Levetiracetam IV, aim for 30 mg/kg
	  → see chapter E.09 Therapeutic strategies in different electroclinical epilepsy syndromes
	Duration of treatment: depends on each individual case; stop medication as early as clinically justifiable, e.g. after 6–8 weeks

High risk for deep vein thrombosis (DVT) or pulmonary embolism (PE)	Low molecular weight heparin Compression stockings as early as possible, tailored

- **Rehabilitation** See chapter I Rehabilitation
- Start with physiotherapy, occupational therapy, speech therapy
- Involve caregiver/family members

Secondary prophylaxis:
See specific chapter

A.09 Paediatric stroke

A.09.1 Thromboembolic events | PCS-Diagnosis, part 1 1/1

Emergency and intensive care

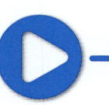

- ▶ Time of onset of symptoms
- ▶ Main symptoms
  - – Hemiparesis
  - – Facial palsy
  - – Dysarthria/Aphasie
  - – Impaired consciousness
  - – Epileptic seizures
  - – Headache
  - – Ataxia
  - – Visual impairment
- ▶ Further course (i.e. progressive alteration of consciousness)
- ▶ Pre-existing conditions (cardiac, vascular, renal, haemato-oncology, metabolic, infectious, vasculitis, fibromuscular dysplasia, coagulation disorder)
- ▶ Trauma
- ▶ Drugs (hormonell contraceptive?)
- ▶ Family history (Stroke? Coagulation disorder?)

Internal examination/neurological examination
- ▶ Brainstem symptoms
- ▶ Pathological reflexes
- ▶ Meningism
- ▶ Heart murmur

Paediatric NIH stroke scale
- ▶ 1 Level of consciousness (LOC)
- ▶ 2 Horizontal extraocular movements
- ▶ 3 Visual fields
- ▶ 4 Facial palsy
- ▶ 5 Arm motor drift (left and right)
- ▶ 6 Leg motor drift (left and right)
- ▶ 7 Limb ataxia
- ▶ 8 Sensation
- ▶ 9 Language/aphasia
- ▶ 10 Dysarthria
- ▶ 11 Extinction/inattention

Basic diagnostic work-up
- ▶ Routine laboratory tests
  - – Blood cell count and differential, glucose, electrolytes, retention parameters, TSH, CRP, CK, CK-MB, LDH, Troponin T, blood gas
- ▶ Coagulation
  - – Prothrombin time PT/ international normalized ratio INR, activated partial thromboplastin time aPTT, fibrinogen, antithrombin, D-Dimers
- ▶ Blood pressure, ECG
- ▶ Temperature
- ▶ Oxygen saturation

Technical investigations
- ▶ Consider doppler/duplex ultrasound of the extra- and intracranial vessels
- ▶ MRI, MRI-angiography (including neck vessels)
  - – MRI is the most sensitive, preferred investigation
- ▶ CT
- ▶ Chest X-ray

A.09.1 Thromboembolic events

A.09.1 Thromboembolic events | PCS-Diagnosis, part 2 1/1

Emergency and intensive care

- ▶ MRI/MRI-angiography[1] (incl. neck vessels)
  - Diffusion weighted sequences: detection of ischaemia, characterisation of stroke (territory infarction, lacunar infarction, hemodynamic watershed stroke; multiple strokes), perfusion weighted imaging (PWI; hypoperfusion?)
  - MRI angiography (detection of intracranial stenosis)
  - Gradient echo MRI [T2*]: detection bleeding arteriopathies of extra-/intracranial vessels
- ▶ CT/CT-angiography (incl. neck vessels)
  - Loss of cortico-medullary differentiation
  - Space occupying processes
  - Hypo-perfusion
  - Angio-CT detection of stenosis
  - Hyperdense media sign
- ▶ 24h-ECG: arrhythmia?
- ▶ Transthoracic and transesophageal echocardiogram: cardiac sources of embolism
- ▶ Laboratory investigation:
  - Status of lipids incl. lipoprotein(a)
  - Factor VIII
  - Protein C, protein S
  - Lupus anticoagulant
  - Factor V Leiden-mutation
  - Prothrombin mutation
  - Fasting homocysteine
  - MTHFR mutation
  - Anticardiolipin-/beta 2-glycoprotein antibodies
  - Anti-nuclear antibodies ANA
  - Anti-neutrophile cytoplasmic antibodies ANCA

---

[1] Diffusion and perfusion weighted MRI may give further information to decide on the risks and benefits of revascularisation therapy

A.09.1 Thromboembolic events | PCS-Therapy, part 1 1/1

Emergency and intensive care

Monitoring
- Serum glucose
  - Glucose > 200 mg/dl (11.1 mmol/l): consider continous insulin infusion
- Blood pressure
- Heart rate
- Body temperature
- Respiratory rate
- Oxygen-saturation
- Electrolytes
- Fluid balance
- Neurological status
- Paediatric NIH Stroke Scale

Thrombolysis
- Contact specialized paediatric stroke unit in time (narrow therapy window)
- No evidence-based guidelines

No additional platelet inhibitors or anticoagulants

No thrombolysis	Bleeding in CT or MRI	No additional platelet inhibitors or anticoagulants

	No bleeding in CT or MRI[1]	**Neonates**
		- Depending on severity, either no therapy or Heparin (unfractionated Heparin (UFH), low molecular weight Heparin (LMWH) or Acetylsalicylic acid (ASA)
		
		Children
		- LMWH SC
		  - First year of life: $2 \times 1,5$ mg/kg/d
		  - After first year of life: $2 \times 1,0$ mg/kg/d
		Or
		- UFH IV
		  - No initial bolus
		Or
		- ASA (3–5 mg/kg)

- Proven dissection of cerebral arteries
Or
- Brain stem symptoms with proven basilar artery stenosis[1]
Or
- Progressive brain stem symptoms
Or
- Fluctuating thrombus
	- Unfractionated Heparin UFH IV
	- 200–600(–800) U/kg/d
	- aPTT ~ 50–60 sec
	Or
	- Low molecular weight heparin LMWH
	  - First year of life: $2 \times 1,5$ mg/kg/d
	  - After first year of life: $2 \times 1,0$ mg/kg/d

1 Therapy: Consider: IV lysis RTPA 0,9mg/kg (10 % within 10 min, 90 % within 1-3 hours)

A.09.1 Thromboembolic events

A.09.1 Thromboembolic events | PCS-Therapy, part 2

Emergency and intensive care

▶ Severe symptoms	▶ Oxygen
▶ Impaired breathing	▶ Oxygen ▶ Intubation and ventilation
▶ Profoundly increased blood pressure (> 95th Percentile)	▶ Decrease blood pressure slowly to normal ranges ▶ IV: Urapidil IV, Dihydralazin IV, also Labetalol where appropriate ▶ Titrate according to the required blood pressure reduction
▶ Lysis planned Or ▶ Cardiac infarction Or ▶ Cardiac insufficiency Or ▶ Acute renal failure Or ▶ Aortic aneurysm	▶ Careful monitoring of blood pressure levels ▶ Decrease blood pressure slowly to normal ranges ▶ IV: Urapidil IV, Dihydralazin IV, also Labetalol where appropriate

▶ Arterial hypotension	▶ After exclusion of cardiac congestion by echocardiography
	  – Consider to increase blood pressure with catecholamines
	  – Volume deficiency: assess fluid balance and administer the appropriate quantity of isotonic fluids
	  – Consider central venous access device (CVAD) and invasive blood pressure measurements

▶ Elevated intracranial pressure	▶ See chapter A.05 Acute increased intracranial pressure (ICP) ▶ In case of space consuming stroke: Consider early decompression surgery

A.09.1 Thromboembolic events | PCS-Secondary prophylaxis 1/1

Emergency and intensive care

▶ Unknown aetiology	▶ Screening for thrombophilia	Consider underlying diseases, such as ▶ Vasculitis: see chapter J.02 Cerebral vasculitis ▶ M. Fabry: test for alpha-galactosidase activity in serum/plasma; genetic analysis ▶ Sickle cell disease: hemoglobin electrophoresis ▶ Marfan's syndrome: physical examination (Beighton criteria) ▶ Ehlers-Danlos syndrome Type IV: fibroblast-culture; genetic testing ▶ Mitochondriopathy: muscle biopsy, genetic analysis, lactate (serum and cerebral fluid) ▶ Homocystinuria and aminoacidopathies: amino acids (urine) ▶ Drugs: drug screening (urine) ▶ Moyamoya disease: MRI angiography, digital subtraction angiography ▶ Neurocutaneous syndromes: see chapter L.02 Neurocutaneous syndromes		▶ Treat underlying disease ▶ Anticoagulation according to underlying disorder

		▶ Etiology not yet clarified (→ consider secondary prophylaxis until aetiology is known)
		Or
		▶ Persistent unknown aetiology (cryptogenic stroke)
			▶ Consider LMWH SC (neonates and children)
			▶ Consider ASA p.o.[1] (3–5 mg/kg/d).
			  – Monitor with PFA-100 or multiplate
			  – Inhibition of platelet aggregation with a combination of two drugs (ASA and dipyramidole) is rarely used in children. The most likely use would be in children with moyamoya disease
			  – Length of ASA therapy in accordance with clinical course and underlying disease (weeks – months – years)
				▶ ASA intolerance (rare)[2]
				  – Clopidogrel (1 mg/kg/d)

▶ Known aetiology	▶ Chronic (persistent) atrial fibrillation			▶ Oral anticoagulation with cumarines
				  – If there are no contraindications (risk of falling, compliance etc.), aim for an INR of 2.0–3.0
				  – May be started already after 3–5 days in patients with minor infarction

	▶ Mechanical valvular transplant			▶ Oral anticoagulation with cumarines[3]: INR 2.5–3.5
	▶ Biological valvular transplant			▶ Oral anticoagulation with cumarines[3]: INR 2.0–3.0 – Generally for 3 months (interdisciplinary coordination with cardiologists)
	▶ Persistent foramen ovale (PFO)			▶ Secondary prophylaxis with 3–5 mg ASA/kg (no data for children available) ▶ Specialists (cardiology, neurology and hemostaseology) consider to close the PFO to avoid recurrent events and long-term anticoagulation with its potential side effects.

1 Data for dosage and agreeability of ASA in neonates are lacking.
2 There is generally no problem concerning intolerance of antihypertensives and statins in children.
3 Oral anticoagulation with cumarines in children is generally only used if there is an indication for long-term anticoagulation (years or lifelong). Otherwise the use of low molecular weight heparin (LMWH) is preferred because of better controllability, better compliance, and fewer complications.

A.09.1 Thromboembolic events

A.09.2 Intracranial haemorrhage/bleeding | PCS-Diagnosis 1/2

Emergency and intensive care

Medical history
- Dependence on location of apoplectiform paresis

Symptoms
- Sensory deficits
- Speech problems
- Headache
- Epileptic seizures

Imaging
- CT

Signs for AVM
- History
  - Cardiac and haemodynamic detoriation in newborns
  - Blood flow murmur over fontanelle
  - In older children mostly asymptomatic until the occurrence of AVM bleeding
- Symptoms
  - Haemodynamic deterioration in 50 % of patients
  - Signs of increased intracranial pressure (ICP)

- CT in emergency situation with angiography
- Gold standard: conventional cerebral angiography (for diagnosis and treatment planning)

- Arteriovenous malformation

Signs for cavernous malformations
- History
  - Positive family history
  - Genetic condition
  - Cranial nerve deficits
- Symptoms
  - Focal neurological deficits (paresis, speech problems)
  - Epileptic seizures (Bleeding is rarely fatal)

- CT (detection of acute bleeding)
- MRI with gradient echo sequences (detection of older bleeding as well as more recent bleeding components)

Cavernomas are typically occult on angiography

- Cavernous malformation/ cavernoma

Signs for cerebral aneurysm
- History/risk factors
  - Positive family history
  - Trauma
  - Aortic coarctation
  - Polycystic kidneys
  - Tuberous sclerosis
  - Ehlers-Danlos disease
  - Syphilis
  - Moyamoya disease
  - HIV
  - Thalassemia minor, sickle cell disease
  - Glucose-6-phosphatase deficiency
- Symptoms
  - Subarachnoid haemorrhage (SAH) (in 74 % of patients)
    - Sudden onset of severe headaches
    - Nausea
    - Vomiting
    - Disturbed consciousness
  - Rarely focal neurological deficits as a consequence of aneurysmatic space-occupying lesions (18 %) or thromboembolic infarction

Signs for subarachnoid haemorrhage (SAH)
- Sudden headache
- Nausea
- Vomiting
- Impaired consciousness
- Epileptic seizures

- CT
  - Basal SAH
  - Concomitant hydrocephalus
- MRI with MRA
- Cerebral angiography (gold standard) → exact evaluation of aneurysmal configuration and concomitant vascular malformations; treatment planning

- Aneurysm with SAH

Signs for aneurysm without SAH
- Solely focal neurological deficits

- CT (to exclude SAH, might be negative after 2 days)
- MRI with angiography (visualization of aneurysm)
- Cerebral angiography (gold standard) → exact evaluation of aneurysmal configuration and concomitant vascular malformations; treatment planning

- Aneurysm without SAH

A.09.2 Intracranial haemorrhage/bleeding | PCS-Diagnosis 2/2

Emergency and intensive care

Signs for moyamoya disease/syndrome	▶ MRI with MRA	▶ MRI findings for Moyamoya disease	▶ Conventional angiography for final diagnosis (stenosis and occlusion of carotid artery, anterior cerebral artery (ACA), collaterals/characteristic moyamoya vessels (puff of smoke)	▶ Moyamoya

▶ History
  – Symptomatic in first decade of life
  – Asian origin
  – Associated disorders
    ▶ Neurofibromatosis
    ▶ Down's syndrome
    ▶ Sickle cell disease
  – Congenital heart defect
  – Previous radiation therapy of the head
▶ Symptoms
  – 80 % (40 % TIA, 40 % stroke) symptomatic with ischaemic signs (paresis, sensory deficits, speech problems, visual field defects)
		– Multiple small ischaemic lesions (water shed infarcts, basal ganglia, periventricular lacunes)
		– Atrophy of involved cerebral hemisphere
		– Gyral contrast enhancement
		– Flow voids in vessels of circus of Willis
			▶ SPECT and PET as perfusion studies	

A.09.2 Intracranial haemorrhage/bleeding | PCS-Therapy 1/1

Emergency and intensive care

Arteriovenous malformations (AVM)	▶ Lesions deep-seated or in eloquent areas of the brain	▶ Embolization
	▶ Standard procedure	▶ Optional: presurgical embolization ▶ Surgical resection of AVM including blood clot ▶ Optional: radiosurgery (so far no long-term experience in children)
Cavernous malformations/cavernomas	▶ Symptomatic And ▶ Progressive enlargement ▶ Brain stem	▶ Surgical resection with intra-operative electrophysiological monitoring in eloquent location or brain stem
	▶ Non-symptomatic/incidental finding And/or ▶ Stable in size (and below 1 cm in size)	▶ Close follow-up with MRI ▶ Compared to supratentorial cavernomas, brain stem cavernomas are associated with a far higher risk of recurring bleeds with severe neurological consequences
	Alternative	▶ Stereotactic radiosurgery with Cyberknife/Gamma-Knife therapy
Paediatric aneurysm	▶ Favourable location/anterior circulation And ▶ Ideal configuration (neck/dome relationship!)	▶ Microsurgical aneurysm clipping
	▶ Unfavourable location/posterior circulation	▶ Interventional treatment – Coiling – Stenting
	▶ Giant aneurysm	Clipping or interventional occlusion of carrier vessel
	▶ Mycotic aneurysm	Antimycotic/antibiotic treatment
	▶ Persistent hydrocephalus	Ventriculo-peritoneal (VP) shunting
Moyamoya disease/syndrome	▶ Therapy of choice	▶ Drugs – Anticoagulatory drugs – Calcium channel blocker ▶ Surgical therapy – STA-MCA-bypass (dependent on vessel size, reserved for older children) – Encephalomyosynangiosis – Encephaloduroarteriosynangiosis – Pial synangiosis – Multiple burr-hole surgery ▶ Treatment of clinically leading side first

A.09.2 Intracranial haemorrhage/bleeding

A.09.2 Intracranial haemorrhage/bleeding | PCS-Diagnosis (Trauma) 1/3

Emergency and intensive care

Medical history ▶ Preterm baby before 34 gestational week ▶ Traumatic birth ▶ Prolonged delivery ▶ Trauma ▶ Shaken baby? **Symptoms** ▶ Lethargy ▶ Irritability ▶ Epileptic seizures ▶ Focal deficits ▶ Respiratory or cardiovascular problems **Imaging** ▶ Ultrasound ▶ CT ▶ MRI	▶ Newborn – Preterm (non-traumatic)	**Signs of ventricular bleeding** ▶ History – Preterm baby before 34 gestational week – Prolonged delivery ▶ Symptoms – Increasing head circumference – Lethargy – Epileptic seizures	▶ Ultrasound through anterior fontanelle, findings – I: subependymal bleeding – II: < 50 % occlusion of lateral ventricle – III: > 50 % occlusion of lateral ventricle with ventricular enlargement – III with intraparenchymal bleeding – Bleeding in the posterior fossa can be missed on transfrontellar ultrasonography	▶ Ventricular bleeding
		Signs of posterior fossa bleeding ▶ History – Birth trauma after prolonged labor – Assisted labor (forceps or vacuum extraction) – Subgaleal haematoma – Palpable skull fracture ▶ Symptoms – Mostly within first 24 hours of life – Lethargy, irritability, coma – Bulging fontanelle – Epileptic seizures – Opisthotonus – Cranial nerve deficits – Bradykardia – Coma	▶ MRI/CT findings – Skull fracture – Acute blood is hyperdense on CT and, depending on age of haemorrhage, hyper- or hypointense on T1- and T2-spinecho sequences on MRI	▶ Posterior fossa bleeding
		Signs of supratentorial bleeding ▶ History – Subdural haematoma as birth trauma – Mostly temporal – Occasionally cortical contusions ▶ Symptoms – Focal neurological deficits – Epileptic seizures – Lethargy, irritability – Bulging fontanelle	▶ CT findings: acute, supratentorial bleeding (hyperdense) ▶ MRI-finding: depending on age of haemorrhage, hyper- or hypointense on T1- and T2-Spinecho sequences on MRI	▶ Supratentorial bleeding
	▶ Infants	**Signs of acute subdural haematoma** ▶ History – Trauma – Child abuse/shaken baby (retinal haemorrhage, long-bone fractures) – Coagulation disorder ▶ Symptoms – Disturbed level of consciousness – Respiratory problems	▶ Fundoscopy: prominent optic disc, retinal haemorrhage ▶ Skeletal survey: fractures of skeleton ▶ CT findings – Hyperdense areas – In infants often interhemispheric haematoma – In older children frontoparietal haematoma with convex-concave configuration – Midline shift – Compression of lateral ventricle	▶ Acute subdural haematoma

A.09.2 Intracranial haemorrhage/bleeding | PCS-Diagnosis (Trauma) 2/3

Emergency and intensive care

– Epileptic seizures – Anemia	▶ MRI-findings: depending on age of haemorrhage, hyper- or hypo-intense on T1- and T2-spinecho sequences on MRI in acute phase	

Signs of chronic subdural haematoma
▶ History
  – Moderate trauma with delay
  – Repetitive child abuse
  – CSF shunt (overdrainage?)
  – Developmental disturbances
  – Coagulation disorder
▶ Symptoms
  – Macrocephalus
  – Irritability
  – Vomiting
  – Epileptic seizures
  – Retinal haemorrhages
	▶ CT-findings
	  – Hypodense, in case of rebleeding also hyperdense areas
	  – Multiple haematoma membranes frequently present
	  – Prominent haematoma membrane
	  – Calcifications
	  – Contrast enhancement of haematoma capsule and septae
	▶ MRI-findings (also help to differentiate from external hydrocephalus)
	  – Inhomogeneous signal
	  – Contrast enhancement of haematoma capsule and septae
		▶ Chronic subdural haematoma

School-aged children

Children older than 10 y

Signs of epidural haematoma
▶ History
  – Traumatic skull fracture
  – Bleeding from middle meningeal artery
  – Venous sinus injury
  – Additional haematoma of scalp
▶ Symptoms
  – No or mild clinical signs, headache
  – Decreased consciousness level, irritability
  – Vomiting
	▶ CT-findings
	  – Hyperdense in acute phase
	  – Mostly temporal or parieto-occipital
	  – Limited to cranial sutures, biconvex
	  – Crossing the midline is possible
	  – Midline shift
	  – Ventricular compression
	▶ MRI-findings
	  – Depending on age of haemorrhage, hyper- or hypointense on T1- and T2-spinecho sequences on MRI in acute phase
		▶ Epidural haematoma

Signs of parenchymal bleeding
▶ History
  – High velocity trauma
▶ Symptoms
  – Mostly with severe head injuries
  – Epileptic seizures
  – Focal neurological deficits
  – Loss of consciousness
	▶ CT findings
	  – Hyperdense during first days
	  – Hypodense perifocal oedema
	  – Contrast enhancement in subacute phase
	  – Mostly temporal and frontal
		▶ Parenchymal bleeding

Signs of acute subdural haematoma
▶ History
  – Trauma
  – Child abuse (retinal haemorrhages, long-bone fractures)
  – Coagulation disorder
▶ Symptoms
  – Altered consciousness
	▶ Fundoscopy: prominent optic disc, retinal haemorrhage
	▶ Skeletal survey: fractures of skeleton
	▶ CT-findings
	  – Hyperdense
	  – In infants under 2 y often interhemispheric haematoma
	  – In older children frontoparietal haematoma with convex-concave configuration
		▶ Acute subdural haematoma

A.09.2 Intracranial haemorrhage/bleeding

A.09.2 Intracranial haemorrhage/bleeding | PCS-Diagnosis (Trauma) 3/3

Emergency and intensive care

- Respiratory problems
- Epileptic seizures
- Anemia

- Midline shift
- Ventricular compression
▶ MRI-findings hypointense on T1- and T2-spinecho sequences on MRI in acute phase

A.09.2 Intracranial haemorrhage/bleeding | PCS-Therapy (Trauma) 1/1

Emergency and intensive care

Intraventricular haemorrhage in pre-term and term infants	▶ Without ventricular enlargement	▶ Clinical surveillance (check head circumference)
	▶ With ventricular enlargement (grade III- and IV-bleeding)	▶ Repetitive lumbar or ventricular puncture ▶ Ventricular drainage via Ommaya-reservoir
Bleeding in the posterior fossa	▶ Clinically stable child	▶ Clinical surveillance (check head circumference)
	▶ Clinically instable child	▶ Decision on surgical decompression depends on size of bleeding and on clinical condition of the individual child
	▶ Hydrocephalus occlusus	▶ External ventricular drainage
Supratentorial bleeding in the new-born	▶ Small haematoma	▶ "Watchful waiting" ▶ If applicable, burr hole drainage of liquefied haematoma
	▶ Large haematoma with neurological deficits	▶ Surgical decompression
Acute subdural haematoma		▶ Emergency decompression and removal of haematoma
Chronic subdural haematoma		▶ Surgical intervention indicated when the condition is clinically or radiologically progressive ▶ External ventricular drain ▶ Ligation of ventricular drain if appropriate
Epidural haematoma	▶ Not symptomatic	▶ Clinical surveillance
	▶ Space occupying ▶ Symptomatic	▶ Craniotomy and haematoma evacuation ▶ If necessary, elevation of depressed skull fracture
Parenchymal bleeding, contusions		▶ Therapy if increased intracranial pressure is of paramount importance ▶ External ventricular drain ▶ Hematoma evacuation in case of growing and space-occupying clot ▶ Decompressive craniectomy with dural enlargement and temporal decompression if increasing intracranial pressure remains refractory to above measures

A.09.2 Intracranial haemorrhage/bleeding

A.09.3 Cerebral venous sinus thrombosis │ PCS-General approach to diagnosis, part 1 1/1

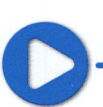

Emergency and intensive care

- ▶ Time of onset of symptoms
- ▶ Main symptoms
- ▶ Headache
- ▶ Hemiparesis
- ▶ Facial palsy
- ▶ Impaired consciousness
- ▶ Visual impairment
- ▶ Dysarthria
- ▶ Ataxia
- ▶ Epileptic seizures
- ▶ Further course (i.e. progressive alteration of consciousness)
- ▶ Pre-existing conditions (cardiac, vascular, renal, haemato-oncology, metabolic, infectious, vasculitis, fibromuscular dysplasia, coagulation disorder)
- ▶ Trauma
- ▶ Drugs
- ▶ Family history (Stroke? Coagulation disorder?)

Examination
Paediatric NIH stroke scale[1]
- ▶ 1 Level of consciousness (LOC)
- ▶ 2 Horizontal extraocular movements
- ▶ 3 Visual fields
- ▶ 4 Facial palsy
- ▶ 5 Arm motor drift (left and right)
- ▶ 6 Leg motor drift (left and right)
- ▶ 7 Limb ataxia
- ▶ 8 Sensation
- ▶ 9 Language/aphasia
- ▶ 10 Dysarthria
- ▶ 11 Extinction/inattention
- ▶ Heart murmur
- ▶ Brain stem symptoms

Basic diagnostic work-up
- ▶ Routine laboratory tests
  - Blood cell count and differential, glucose, electrolytes, retention parameters, TSH, CRP, CK, CK-MB, LDH, Troponin T, blood gas
- ▶ Coagulation
  - Prothrombin time (PT), international normalized ratio (INR), activated partial thromboplastin time (aPTT), fibrinogen, antithrombin, D-Dimers
- ▶ Blood pressure, ECG
- ▶ Temperature
- ▶ Oxygen saturation

Technical investigations
- ▶ Consider Doppler/duplex ultrasound of extra- and intracranial vessels as initial screening
- ▶ MRI, MRI-angiography/veniography
  - MRI is the most sensitive, preferred investigation
- ▶ CT
- ▶ Chest X-ray

1 For neurological assessment in adults, the NIH Stroke Scale has proven useful {Lyden, 1994 935/id}. An adapted version can be used for children over two years of age.

A.09.3 Cerebral venous sinus thrombosis

A.09.3 Cerebral venous sinus thrombosis | PCS-General approach to diagnosis, part 2

- ▶ Indicators for cerebral ischaemia
  - Loss of corticomedullary differentiation
  - Space consuming processes with ventricular affection
  - Hypoperfusion

- ▶ Clinical signs for cerebral venous sinus thrombosis
  - Infection
  - Dehydration
  - papilloedema
  - Headache
  - Seizures
- ▶ Additional indicators for cerebral venous sinus thrombosis in MRI/MRA:
  - Occlusion of veins
  - "Empty-delta-sign"
  - Enlarged veins showing an intensified signal
  - Acute thrombus: hypointense in T2
  - Subacute thrombus: hyperintense in T1 and T2
- ▶ Angiography:
  - May be required in rare cases to confirm diagnosis
- ▶ Additional indicators for cerebral venous sinus thrombosis in CT:
  - Congestion bleeding
  - General or local edema
  - Fresh thrombus might show increased density
  - After administration of contrast "empty-delta-sign"
  - Occluded veins visible as hyperdense strips

Cerebral venous sinus thrombosis

A.09.3 Cerebral venous sinus thrombosis | PCS-Therapy 1/1

Emergency and intensive care

Basic therapy
- Treat underlying disorder
- Supportive care
- Screen for thrombophilia → treatment of inhibitor deficiency if possible

- Cerebral venous sinus thrombosis with bleeding
  - Consider anticoagulation

  Acute therapy
  - None
  - Consider 100–200 U/kg/d of UFH[1]

  Secondary prohylaxis
  - If no bleeding or stable situation: LMWH[1]
  - Duration according to risk factors and patency

- Cerebral venous sinus thrombosis without bleeding
  - Anticoagulation

  Acute therapy
  - 200–400–600 U/kg/d UFH IV (aim at aPTT 50–60 s)
    - If stable, switch to LMWH in therapeutic doses
    - Aim at Anti-factor-Xa level of 0.6–0.8

  - Newborns/infants: e.g. 2 × 1,5 mg/kg Enoxaparine/d SC[1,2]

  - Children > 1 year: e.g. 2 × 1 mg/kg Enoxaparine/d SC[1,2]

  Secondary prophylaxis
  - Change to 1x/d
    - Aim at Anti-factor-Xa-level: 0.2–0.6
    - Duration according to risk factors and patency

  - Newborns/infants: e.g. 1 × 1 mg/kg Enoxaparine/d SC[1,2]

  - > 1 year: e.g. 1 × 0.75 mg/kg Enoxaparine/d SC[1,2]

1 UFH = unfractionated heparin ("IV-heparin"); LMWH = low molecular weight heparin
2 NOTE: No approval for LMWH in children, no evidence based studies

A.09.3 Cerebral venous sinus thrombosis

A.09.4 Dissection (cerebrovascular) | PCS-Diagnosis 1/2

Emergency and intensive care

Medical history
- Exact onset of symptoms
- Further course (e.g. progressive impaired consciousness)
- Headache
- Previous medical conditions (heart, vascular, renal, oncological, metabolic, infections, fibromuscular dysplasia)
- Trauma
- Medication
- Epileptic seizures

Symptoms[1]
- Consciousness
- Brain stem symptoms
- Pathol. reflexes
- Hemiparesis
- Aphasia, dysarthria
- Visual field defect
- Gaze palsy
- Meningism
- Cardiac murmur (endocarditis?)

Basic diagnostic work-up
- Routine blood tests
  - Full blood count, glucose, electrolytes, renal parameters, TSH, CRP, CK, CK-MB, LDH, troponin
- Clotting
  - International normalized ratio (INR), aPTT, Fibrinogen, antithrombin, D-dimer

Evidence for cerebrovascular dissection

History
- Acute onset of single-sided pain in the head or neck
- Previous trauma (50 %)
- Previous (40 % of patients) or current (20 %) transitory ischaemic attack (TIA)
- Fibromuscular dysplasia (FMD)

Physical examination
- Local signs of cerebral ischaemia
  - Carotid artery dissection (75 %)
  - Vertebral artery dissection (97 %)
- Horner's syndrome (30 %)
- Ipsilateral cranial nerve deficit
  - Facial palsy
  - Collet-Sicard syndrome
  - Dysgeusia
- Amaurosis fugax
- Acute onset of pulse synchronous tinnitus (10–15 %)
- Signs for classic connective tissue disease

Evidence for other causes
- Nausea
- Vomiting
- Decreased consciousnesss level
- Epileptic seizures
- Known aneurysm
- Marked signs of cerebral ischaemia
- History of cardiac disease
- Dehydration
- Papillary oedema

Signs for dissection of the carotid artery
- Acute onset of single-sided pain in the neck, face and orbita
- Ipsilateral Horner's syndrome (peripheral cause)
- Amaurosis fugax

Signs of vertebral artery (VA) dissection
- Acute onset of single-sided pain especially in arm, neck and occiput (C2, 3)
- History of chiropractic manipulation
- Wallenberg's syndrome
- Radicular lesion (C4), C5, C6, (C7), may be only motorial
- Subarachnoidal haemorrhage (SAH) symptoms

See chapter A.09 Paediatric stroke

- Duplex sonography[2]
  - Direct proof of extracranial haematoma of the arterial wall and extra- and intracranial stenosis > 50 %
  - Helical structure in the vessel wall with reduced echo[3]
  - Sharply tapered stenosis or obliteration
  - Intraluminal membrane
  - Local ectasia
  - "Swash phenomenon"[4]
  - Current blood flow acceleration
  - Obliteration plus "swash"
  - Any abrupt vertebral artery dilation could be a sign of dissection

Proof of arterial wall haematoma and/or stenosis		
No clear proof of arterial wall haematoma and/or stenosis	▶ Time-of-flight-MRA (TOF-MRA)	▶ Suspected dissection
		▶ No new information

- T1 fat suppressed MRI[5]
  - After 2–3 days, the arterial wall haematoma appears as hyperintense sickle in the arterial wall
  - Renal artery duplex sonography (exclusion of stenosis due to fibromuscular dysplasia (FMD))

- Intraarterial angiography
  - Direct proof of intimal rupture (rare)
  - High-grade stenosis
  - Obliteration with wedge-shaped course and consecutive collapsed vessel ("string sign")

- Cerebrovascular dissection

A.09.4 Dissection (cerebrovascular)

A.09.4 Dissection (cerebrovascular) | PCS-Diagnosis 2/2

Emergency and intensive care

- Blood pressure, ECG
- Temperature
- Oxygen saturation (pulse oximetry)

---

1. For neurological examination in adults, the NIH Stroke Scale has proven to be useful {Lyden, 1994 935/id}. An adapted version can be used for children older than 2 years
2. Highly appropriate for dissections of the extracranial carotid and complete vertebral artery. For dissections of the petrous part of the A. carotis interna, MRA is more appropriate.
3. "Helical": alternating between proximal and distant probe position in a proximal-distal course.
4. By alternating current bidirectional signal with little orthograd or without any current.
5. Less reliable for vertebroarterial dissections. While contrast agents would improve visualization of the vessel wall (e.g. for follow-up examinations), any vessel wall haematoma may appear isointense and therefore would be even more difficult to detect.

A.09.4 Dissection (cerebrovascular) | PCS-Therapy 1/1

Emergency and intensive care

▶ Confirmed dissection of an extra- or intracranial vessel without subarrachnoid haemorrhage (SAH)	▶ Cerebrovascular dissection without signs of cerebral ischaemia	**Acute** ▶ Platelet aggregation inhibitor		**During follow-up** ▶ Platelet aggregation inhibitor for 1 year ▶ Longer with fibromuscular dysplasia (FMD) or connective tissue disease						
	▶ Carotid artery dissection with signs of cerebral ischaemia	**Acute** ▶ LMH IV ▶ PTT 2–3 times increased	**Subacute** ▶ Heparin IV or SC ▶ PTT 2–3 times increased **Heparin induced Thrombocytopenia** ▶ HIT Typ II[1]: Danaparoid-Na or Lepirudine	Stroke consolidation without complications	▶ Oral anticoagulation[2] – Phenprocoumon or Warfarin – INR 2–3 – Until regression of the obstruction – Not shorter than 3 months ▶ Sonographic control[3] after 3 months	▶ Persisting obliteration/stenosis	▶ Without cliric al symptoms	▶ Oral anticoagulation for another 3 months ▶ Sonographic control after 3 months	▶ Persisting vascular pathology	▶ Switch to platelet aggregation inhibitor
	▶ Distal thromboembolism in cerebral arteries	**Acute** ▶ Local intra-arterial lysis if possible								
	▶ Recurrent symptoms in patients under conservative therapy Or ▶ Severe hemodynamic impairment	**Acute** ▶ Surgery or stenting if possible[4]					▶ With clinical symptoms	▶ Vascular/cerebral diagnosis	▶ Individual therapy	
▶ Symptomatic dissecting aneurysm with SAH (most commonly V4 segment)		**Acute** ▶ Endovascular coil embolisation – Premise: adequate collateralization (baloon occlusion) – Affected vessel will be occluded – See chapter A.09.2 Intracranial haemorrhage/bleeding								

1 Due to lacking evidence this approach is extrapolated from adult guidelines.
2 Secondary prophylaxis of intracranial dissections without subarrachnoid haemorrhage (SAH) follows the same anticoagulation regimen and has to be adapted to the local vascular pathology in order to reduce the risk of bleeding.
3 Highly appropriate for dissections of the extracranial carotid and complete vertebral artery. For dissections of the petrous part of the A. carotis interna, magnetic resonance angiography (MRA) is more appropriate.
4 There are no controlled studies for surgery or stenting in paediatric patients. Concerning endovascular techniques there are only case reports available (Malek 2000, Lylyk 2001).

There are no controlled studies for the treatment of thrombosis in children. All therapeutic options are extrapolated from adult guidelines. The therapy in paediatric patients is individual and has to be modified according to the specific clinical situation and complicating factors (e.g. haemorrhage). Most drugs are not approved for children and their application has to be seen as an individual approach that requires the informed consent of both parents.

A.09.4 Dissection (cerebrovascular)

A.09.5 Arteriovenous malformations | PCS-Diagnosis cerebral, part 1

Emergency and intensive care

History
- Time of onset of symptoms
  - Main symptoms
  - Headache
  - Hemiparesis
  - Facial palsy
  - Decreased consciousness level
  - Visual impairment
  - Dysarthria
  - Ataxia
  - Epileptic seizures
  - Further course (i.e. progressive alteration of consciousness)
- Pre-existing conditions (cardiac, vascular, renal, haemato-oncological, metabolic, infectious, vasculitis, fibromuscular dysplasia, coagulation disorder)
- Trauma
- Drugs

Examination
Paediatric NIH stroke scale[1]
- 1 Level of consciousness (LOC)
- 2 Horizontal extraocular movements
- 3 Visual fields
- 4 Facial palsy
- 5 Arm motor drift (left and right)
- 6 Leg motor drift (left and right)
- 7 Limb ataxia
- 8 Sensation
- 9 Language/aphasia
- 10 Dysarthria
- 11 Extinction/inattention
- Heart murmur
- Brain stem
- Meningism

Basic diagnostic work-up
- Routine laboratory tests
  - Blood cell count and differential, lactate, ammonia glucose, electrolytes, retention parameters, TSH, CRP, CK, CK-MB, LDH, Troponin T, blood gas
- Coagulation
  - Prothrombin time (PT), international normalized ratio (INR), activated partial thromboplastin time (aPTT), fibrinogen, antithrombin, D-Dimers
- Blood pressure, ECG
- Temperature
- Oxygen saturation

Technical investigations
- Consider Doppler/duplex ultrasound of extra- and intracranial vessels as initial screening
- MRI, MRI-angiography
  - MRI is the most sensitive, preferred investigation
- CT
- Chest X-ray

---

1 For neurological assessment in adults, the NIH Stroke Scale has proved useful {Lyden, 1994 935/id}. An adapted version can be used for children over two years of age.

A.09.5 Arteriovenous malformations │ PCS-Diagnosis cerebral, part 2 1/2

Emergency and intensive care

▶ No evidence for cerebral ischaemia in CT/MRI[1]	▶ Evidence for cerebrovascular malformation in CT/MRI – Pathological vascular structures – Possible calcification – Possible perifocal oedema – Recent or old intracerebral blood remnants ▶ Epileptic seizures (focal/generalized) ▶ Focal neurological deficit ▶ Cardiovascular sequelae due to shunting	▶ MRI (if not already performed instead of CT) And ▶ Digital subtraction arteriography (DSA)[2]	▶ AV shunt	▶ Evidence for AVM – Arteriovenous shunts with nidus – Contrast uptake	▶ AVM
				▶ Evidence for vein of Galen malformation (VGAM) – Aneurysmatically dilated vein of Galen with fistulas – Contrast uptake	▶ VGAM
				▶ Evidence for dural arteriovenous fistula (dAVF) – Transdural arteriovenous shunt with fistulas – No nidus – Contrast uptake	▶ dAVF
			▶ No AV shunt	▶ Evidence for cavernoma – "Popcorn-like" – Heterogeneous core surrounded by hypointense hemosiderin – Surrounding oedema with fresh blood – Partial uptake of contrast medium	▶ Cavernom
				▶ Evidence for developmental venous anomaly (DVA) – Venous star with draining vein ("caput medusae") – Contrast uptake	▶ DVA
				▶ Evidence for capillary teleangiectasia: – Abnormally dilated capillaries surrounded by parenchyma – Hyperintense in T2 – Frequently within the brain stem – Uptake of contrast medium	▶ Capillary teleangiectasia
				Further differential diagnosis ▶ Hypervascularized tumor (maybe with AV shunt; differential diagnosis: impaired blood-brain barrier)	
	▶ Evidence for differential diagnoses – Cerebroarterial dissection (see chapter A.09.4 Dissection (cerebrovascular)) – Intracranial haemorrhage (see chapter A.09.2 Intracranial haemorrhage/bleeding) – Migraine (see chapter C.02 Primary headache) – Transient ischaemic attack (see chapter A.09.1 Thromboembolic events) – Vasculitis (see chapter J.02 Cerebral vasculitis)			Go to the appropriate chapter	

A.09.5 Arteriovenous malformations

A.09.5 Arteriovenous malformations | PCS-Diagnosis cerebral, part 2

- ▶ Evidence for cerebral ischaemia on CT
  - No cortico-subcortical differentiation
  - Space-occupying effects due to oedema (ventricular compression, shift, midline shift, herniation)
  - Lesion fits anatomically to a vascular territory
  - Reduced perfusion on perfusion-CT/MRI
  - (Impaired diffusion on MRI)

Possible reasons
- ▶ Thromboembolism (see chapter A.09.1 Thromboembolic events)
- ▶ Cerebroarterial dissection (see chapter A.09.4 Dissection (cerebrovascular))
- ▶ Cerebral venous sinus thrombosis (see chapter A.09.3 Cerebral venous sinus thrombosis)

Go to the appropriate chapter

---

1 NOTE: CT performed during the first 3 h may give false negative results for ischaemia. Neither CT, nor diffusion MRI without any pathologic findings can exclude stroke with sufficient certainty. If necessary repeat imaging later in the course of the disorder.
2 First, MR angiography; DSA only in centers that can also provide specialized therapy.

A.09.5 Arteriovenous malformations | PCS-Therapy cerebral 1/1

Emergency and intensive care

AVM	▶ Individual interdisciplinary therapeutic approach in a specialized center with consideration of each patient's specific pathology and risk profile. No general guidelines available.	
Dural arteriovenous fistula (dAVF)	▶ Therapeutic options (also in combination) 　– Observation 　– Surgery 　– Endovascular therapy 　– Radiosurgery	
Cavernoma	▶ Surgery if indicated 　– Consult a neurosurgeon	
Vein of Galen aneurysmal malformation (VGAM)	▶ Prenatal diagnosis	▶ Sustain pregnancy as long as possible ▶ Delivery in a center with paediatric intensive care unit (cardiology and neurology) ▶ Postnatal endovascular therapy according to the clinical status and as late as possible
	▶ Postnatal diagnosis	▶ Endovascular therapy with relation to the clinical score, commencing as late as possible and clinically reasonable
Developmental venous anomaly (DVA)	No therapy	
Capillary teleangiectasia		

A.09.5 Arteriovenous malformations

A.09.5 Arteriovenous malformations | PCS-Diagnosis spinal 1/2

Emergency and intensive care

Medical history
- Exact onset of symptoms
- Further course (e.g. progressively impaired consciousness)
- Headache
- Previous medical conditions (cardial, vascular, renal, oncological, metabolic, infection, fibromuscular dysplasia)
- Trauma
- Medication
- Epileptic seizures

Symptoms
- Consciousness
- Brain stem symptoms
- Pathol. reflexes
- Hemiparesis
- Aphasia, Dysarthria
- Visual field defect
- Gaze palsy
- Seizures
- Meningism
- Cardiac murmur (Endocarditis?)

Basic diagnostic workup
- Routine lab **(B)**
  - Blood count, glucose, lactate, ammonia, electrolytes, renal parameters, TSH, CRP, CK, CK-MB, LDH, Troponin
- Coagulation
  - PT (Quick), aPTT, fibrinogen, antithrombin, D-dimer
- Blood pressure, ECG
- Temperature
- Oxygen saturation (pulse oximetry)
- Consider lumbar puncture after cranial imaging to exclude space occupying lesion

---

- Simultaneous cerebral symptoms
  - Headache
  - Epileptic seizures
  - Decreased consciousness level
  - Brain stem symptoms
  - Hemiparesis
  - Aphasia, Dysarthria
  - Visual field defect
  - Gaze palsy
  - Meningism

Go to PCS Stroke (see chapter A.09 Paediatric stroke)

- No cerebral symptoms
- Spinal MRI
  - T1 +/- contrast medium, T2
  - If possible, chronic MRA
- Spinal digital substraction arteriography DSA[1]

Vascular malformation with AV shunt	Evidence for spinal AVM – Pathologic flow voids/vascular structures with nidus within or surrounding the spinal cord – Occasionally space-occupying vascular lesion – New/old remnant of haemorrhage (hemosiderin) – Spinal cord oedema	Spinal AVM
	Evidence for dAVF (dural arteriovenous fistula) – Spinal cord oedema (congestion oedema), frequently with conal involvement – Pathologic flow voids within the subarachnoid space	dAVF
Vascular malformation without AV shunt	Evidence for cavernoma – "Popcorn-like" – Heterogeneous core surrounded by hypointense hemosiderin – Surrounding oedema with fresh blood – Partial uptake of contrast agent	Cavernoma
No vascular malformation	Evidence for myelitis – MRI: spinal cord oedema +/- uptake of contrast medium – No pathologic flow voids – Evidence for infection in CSF and blood	Myelitis (CSF, Serology?)
	Evidence for malignant growth – Space-occupying lesion +/- uptake of contrast medium – No pathologic flow voids	Malignancy
	Evidence for spinal ischaemia – Spinal cord oedema +/- uptake of contrast medium in a vascular territory – No pathologic vasculature	Spinal Ischaemia

A.09.5 Arteriovenous malformations

A.09.5 Arteriovenous malformations | PCS-Diagnosis spinal 2/2

Emergency and intensive care

▶ Evidence for spinal haemorrhage:
  – Clear evidence of haematoma

▶ Spinal haemorrhage

1 Only if AV malformation is strongly suspected and therapeutic relevance is given, in a specialized center

A.09.5 Arteriovenous malformations | PCS-Therapy spinal 1/1

Emergency and intensive care

Arteriovenous malformation (AVM)

Dural arteriovenous fistula (dAVF)

▶ Individual interdisciplinary therapeutic approach in a specialized center with consideration of each patient's specific pathology and risk profile. No general guidelines available.
▶ Options for therapy (also in combination)
 – Observation
 – Surgerys
 – Endovascular therapy

A.09.5 Arteriovenous malformations

A.10 Battered child | PCS-How to proceed in case of suspected child abuse

Emergency and intensive care

Medical history
- Birth and developmental history
- Social and family history (*Caution:* any siblings?)
- Detailed course of "accident" (When? Where? Who? What? Witness?)

Physical examination
- General condition, state of care and nutrition
- Size, bodyweight, head circumference
- Neurological and developmental examination
- Ophthalmoscopy
- Thorough whole body inspection (especially mouth, genital and anal region)
- Smear for DNA diagnosis
- Optional vaginal smear/anal smear for microbiological investigations and DNA diagnosis
- Detailed documentation of all lesions (morphology, size, colour, localization, consistence); prepare sketches or preferably take photos
- Behavioral observation and documentation
- If there are any reasonable findings suspecting child abuse, admission to hospital ward and initiation of official custody withdrawal

Diagnostic work-up
- Laboratory (e.g. coagulation tests, creatine kinase, myoglobin, blood cell count, liver function tests)
- X-ray of suspect body areas (especially thorax und head)
- Scintigraphy
- CT or MRI
- EEG (optional evoked potentials)
- Psychological evaluation
- Ophthalmologic consultation
- Optional storage of vomit, urine, blood for toxicological investigations
- Optional gynaecological consultation
- Optional medicolegal consultation

Criteria suggesting child abuse
- Implausible history and injury pattern
- Inconsistent description of events that supposedly caused the symptoms/lesions
- Delayed medical consultation despite severe injuries
- Retinal haemorrhages
- Spiral fracture of long tubular bones, humerus fractures and dorsal serial rip fractures in infants
- Bilateral symmetric fractures
- Injuries/lesions of different ages
- Implausible pattern of burns and scalding

Diagnostic criteria
- Significant injury patterns (for example "shaken infant")
- Confession
- Exclusion of other possible diagnoses (differential diagnosis)

In case of suspected non-accidental injury/battered child
- Inform the family doctor
- Inform the community youth welfare office, also called Child Protective Services or Children and Family Court Advisory and Support Service in some countries
- Interdisciplinary case conference to evaluate the significance of the injuries/findings
- Optional confrontation of the parents concerning the suspected non-accidental injuries
- Decisions about further course of action
  - Report the offence to police
  - Specific plan of action and possible orders issued by the youth welfare office
  - Official custody withdrawal (incl. possible siblings)
  - Discharge from hospital ward (When? Where to?)

A.11 Coma | PCS-Diagnosis overview 1/1

Emergency and intensive care

	▶ PLUS	▶ Specific PCS
▶ Clinical setting: comatose patient	Altered vital signs	"Coma plus altered vital signs"
	Focal neurological signs	"Coma plus focal neurological signs"
	Specific history/clinical signs	"Coma plus specific history/clinical signs"
	No coma-related medical history ("empty history")	"Coma plus empty history"
	Secondary detorioration	"Coma – secondary detorioration"

A.11 Coma | PCS-Diagnosis Coma plus altered vital signs 1/2

Emergency and intensive care

► Coma PLUS ► Altered vital signs	► Respiration	► Cheyne-Stokes respiration	► Laboratory investigation[1] ► CT		Possible DD ► Bilateral hemispheric lesions ► Late sign of herniation ► Cardiac insufficiency (reported in adults)		
		► Apneustic, atactic or cluster breathing	► Laboratory investigation[1] ► MRI		► Brain stem lesion		
		► Slow, irregular or periodic breathing	► Laboratory investigation[1] ► Toxicology screen ► CT		Possible DD ► Intoxication ► Raised intracranial pressure		
		► Kussmaul's respiration	► Laboratory investigation[1]		Possible DD ► Diabetic ketoacidosis ► Severe dehydration		
		► Hyperventilation	► Laboratory investigation[1] ► NH_3 ► Salicylate plasma level (depending on history)		Possible DD ► Liver failure ► Metabolic acidosis ► Salicylate intoxication ► Functional		
	► Hemodynamics	► Compromised peripheral perfusion/ arterial hypotension/shock	► Laboratory investigation[1] ► Work-up shock (blood count, blood culture etc.) ► Chest x-ray ► Echocardiography		Possible DD ► Sepsis ► Cardiogenic shock ► Haemorrhage ► Dehydration		
		► Bradycardia	► Body temperature ► Laboratory investigation[1] ► Toxicologic screen ► Thyroid function ► Cortisol ► ECG	Possible DD: ► Hypothermia ► Intoxication ► Hypothyroidism ► Addison's disease			
				► No conclusive result or associated with arterial hypertension (cushing phenomenon)	► CT ► Work-up raised intracranial pressure	Possible DD ► Raised intracranial pressure

A.11 Coma

A.11 Coma | PCS-Diagnosis Coma plus altered vital signs 2/2

Emergency and intensive care

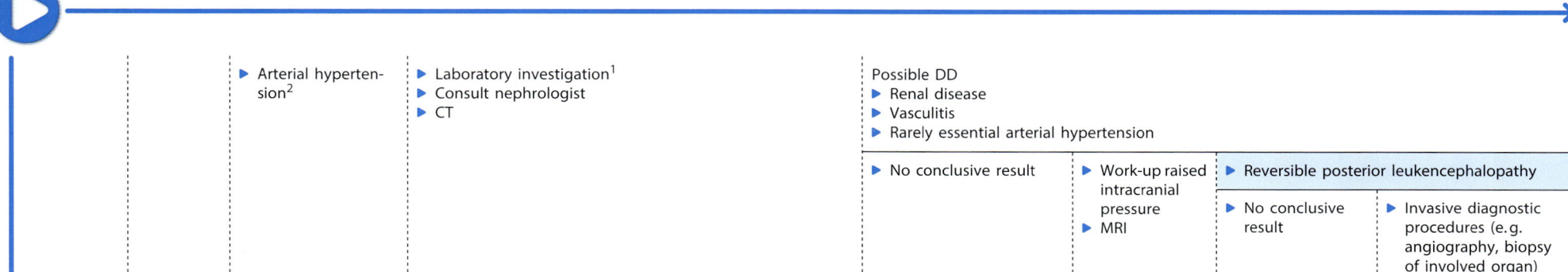

- ▶ Arterial hypertension[2]
- ▶ Laboratory investigation[1]
- ▶ Consult nephrologist
- ▶ CT

Possible DD
- ▶ Renal disease
- ▶ Vasculitis
- ▶ Rarely essential arterial hypertension

- ▶ No conclusive result
- ▶ Work-up raised intracranial pressure
- ▶ MRI
- ▶ Reversible posterior leukencephalopathy
- ▶ No conclusive result
- ▶ Invasive diagnostic procedures (e.g. angiography, biopsy of involved organ)

1 Laboratory investigations: Mandatory serum Glucose, arterial blood gas analysis incl lactate, electrolytes incl Mg, full blood count; urea, creatinine; liver enzymes, bilirubin, CRP. Consider: cortisol; urine porphyrins; TSH/T3/T4. Without conclusive coma aetiology: NH3; toxicologic screen. Suspected inborn errors of metabolism: plasma amino acids; Carnitine/acylcarnitine profile.
2 Arterial hypertension rarely caused by isolated CNS pathology (except pre-herniation)

A.11 Coma | PCS-Diagnosis Coma plus focal neurological signs 1/1

Emergency and intensive care

▶ Coma PLUS
▶ Focal neurological signs
	▶ Unilateral dilated, unreactive pupil	▶ Laboratory investigations[1]
		▶ CT
			Possible DD
			▶ Uncal herniation caused by space-occupying supra-tentorial lesion
			   – Tumor
			   – Haemorrhage
			   – Inflammatory/toxic oedema

	▶ Focal motor signs without brain stem signs	▶ Laboratory investigations[1]
		▶ CT/MRI with contrast[2]
			Possible DD
			▶ Postictal (Todd's paresis)
			▶ Supratentorial
			   – Tumor
			   – Haemorrhage
			   – Infarction
			   – Abscess
			   – Venous sinus thrombosis
			   – Vasculitis

	▶ Brain stem signs	▶ Laboratory investigations[1] ▶ CT/MRI[2]	Possible DD ▶ Cerebral herniation ▶ Infratentorial haemorrhage ▶ Brain stem encephalitis ▶ Bickerstaff brain stem encephalitis

1 Laboratory investigations: Mandatory serum Glucose, arterial blood gas analysis incl lactate, electrolytes incl Mg, full blood count; creatinine; liver enzymes, bilirubin, CRP. Consider: cortisol; urine porphyrins; TSH/T3/T4. Without conclusive coma aetiology: NH3; toxicology screen. Suspected inborn errors of metabolism: plasma amino acids; carnitine/acylcarnitine profile. Prolactin (postictally increased).
2 Preferably MRI, if immediately available

A.11 Coma

A.11 Coma | PCS-Diagnosis Coma plus specific history/clinical signs 1/3

Emergency and intensive care

▶ Coma PLUS ▶ Specific history/clinical signs	▶ History of trauma	▶ Laboratory investigation[1] ▶ CT/MRI[2]			Possible DD ▶ Subdural, epidural, subarachnoidal or parenchymal haemorrhage, cerebral contusion, diffuse axonal injury
		▶ Laboratory investigation[1] ▶ CT/MRI[2]			Possible DD ▶ Haemorrhage, oedema, hydrocephalus ▶ "Delayed" encephalopathy
	▶ Shock	▶ Laboratory investigation[1], incl. CK, troponin ▶ Diagnostic work-up for possible infections	▶ Signs of sepsis	▶ CT, followed by lumbar puncture if not contraindicated	Possible DD ▶ Meningitis/encephalitis ▶ Sepsis w/o meningitis
			▶ No signs of infection		Hypoxic-ischaemic injury
	▶ History of diabetes	▶ Laboratory investigation[1]			Possible DD ▶ Hypoglycemia ▶ Ketoacidosis
	▶ Hospitalized patient with intravenous maintenance infusion	▶ Iatrogenic hyponatriemia caused by hypotonic solution; hypoglycemia			
	▶ Icterus	▶ Laboratory investigation[1] ▶ NH_3			▶ Fulminant hepatic failure
	▶ Young child given aspirin				
	▶ History of unspecific viral infection	▶ Laboratory investigation[1] ▶ Lumbar puncture ▶ NH_3 ▶ MRI			Possible DD ▶ Acute disseminated encephalomyelitis ▶ Brain stem encephalitis ▶ Reye-like metabolic disease; mitochondriopathy ▶ Fulminant hepatic failure
	▶ Cough	▶ Laboratory investigation[1] ▶ Chest radiography			Possible DD ▶ Encephalitis or parainfectious encephalitis (e.g. Mycoplasma, Tb)
	▶ Headache	▶ Laboratory investigation[1] ▶ CT/MRI[2]			Possible DD[3] ▶ Subarrachnoid haemorrhage SAH ▶ Migraine, familial hemiplegic migraine ▶ Hydrocephalus ▶ Tumor

A.11 Coma

A.11 Coma | PCS-Diagnosis Coma plus specific history/clinical signs 2/3

Emergency and intensive care

A.11 Coma

	▶ Medication	▶ Verify medication and check on correct and regular administration		▶ Intoxication
		▶ Ciclosporin A		▶ Reversible posterior leucoencephalopathy
		▶ Medication history doubtful	▶ Plasma levels of sedatives, antiepileptics	Possible DD ▶ Inadvertent dosage error ▶ Intentional overdosing
	▶ Ventriculo-peritoneal shunt	▶ Check valve function, radiological shunt series ▶ CT, abdominal sonography		▶ Shunt dysfunction
	▶ Post-cardiosurgery using extracorporeal bypass ▶ Positive pressure ventilation	▶ Laboratory investigation[1] ▶ CT		▶ Cerebral arterial gas embolisation
	▶ Intracardiac shunt	▶ Laboratory investigation[1] ▶ CT		Possible DD ▶ Abscess ▶ Infarction
▶ Coma PLUS ▶ Specific history/clinical signs	▶ Malignancy	▶ Laboratory investigation[1] incl. schistocytes (helmet cells) ▶ MRI ▶ Bone marrow biopsy		Possible DD ▶ Hemophagocytic lymphohistiocytosis ▶ Thrombotic trombocytopenic purpura ▶ CNS metastases ▶ Sinus venous thrombosis ▶ Infection
	▶ Rescued from smoke-filled, enclosed space	▶ Laboratory investigation[1] ▶ Pulse oximetry ▶ Carboxy-Hb ▶ Cyanide	▶ Emergency treatment	Carbon monoxide or cyanide intoxication
	▶ Pathological findings at fundoscopy	▶ Bleeding	▶ Laboratory investigation[1] ▶ CT/MRI[2]	Possible DD ▶ Battered child ▶ After cardiac massage
		▶ Papilloedema	▶ Laboratory investigation[1] ▶ CT/MRI[2]	Increased intracranial pressure[4]
	▶ Cutaneous manifestations	▶ Signs of trauma	▶ Laboratory investigation[1] ▶ CT	Possible DD ▶ Traumatic brain injury (see chapter A.08 Traumatic brain injury) ▶ Battered child
		▶ Petechiae	▶ Laboratory investigation[1] ▶ CT (with sepsis after stabilization if focal signs)	Possible DD ▶ Sepsis

A.11 Coma | PCS-Diagnosis Coma plus specific history/clinical signs 3/3

Emergency and intensive care

		▶ MRI/Angio when infarction/vasculitis suspected	▶ Cerebral haemorrhage or infarction in ITP[5] ▶ Vasculitis
	▶ Cafe-au-lait spots, facial naevus flammeus	▶ Laboratory investigation[1] ▶ CT ▶ EEG	Possible DD: ▶ Intracranial tumor ▶ Seizure in neurocutaneous syndrome
▶ Foetor ex ore	▶ Alcohol plasma level ▶ Laboratory investigation[1]		Possible DD ▶ Alcohol intoxication ▶ Diabetic ketoacidosis ▶ Other inborn errors of metabolism (e.g. aminoacidopathy)
▶ Fever	▶ Laboratory investigation[1], thyroid hormones ▶ Diagnostic work-up for possible infections ▶ NH_3 ▶ MRI ▶ EEG ▶ Lumbar puncture (after CT)		Possible DD ▶ CNS-infection ▶ Parainfectious encephalitis ▶ Autoimmune disease ▶ Heat stroke ▶ Hyperthyroidism
▶ Abdomen	▶ Rebound tenderness ▶ Tumor ▶ Bloody stools	▶ Laboratory investigation[1] ▶ Ultrasound ▶ Abdominal radiography, abdominal CT ▶ Colon-contrast enema	Possible DD ▶ Invagination ▶ Volvulus ▶ Vasculitis ▶ Hemolytic uremic syndrome HUS/thrombotic thrombocytopenic purpura (TTP)
	▶ Enteritis	▶ Laboratory investigation[1] ▶ Enteroviral PCR ▶ Stool: EHEC, Shigella ▶ Schistocytes (helmet cells) ▶ ADAMTS13 mutation	Possible DD ▶ Hypo/hypernatremia ▶ Encephalitis ▶ Hemolytic uremic syndrome HUS/TTP

1 Laboratory investigations: mandatory serum Glucose, arterial blood gas analysis incl lactate, electrolytes incl Mg, full blood count; urea, creatinine; liver enzymes, bilirubin, CRP. Consider: cortisol; urine porphyrins; TSH/T3/T4. Without conclusion coma aetiology: NH3; toxicology screen. Suspected inborn error of metabolism: plasma amino acids; carnitine/acylcarnitine profile. Prolactin (postictal increase)
2 MRI if immediately available.
3 +/- Ataxia, genetics
4 Papillae show changes indicative of increased intracranial pressure after 2–3 days. CT < 24 h after intracranial pressure increase
5 Decreased ADAMTS13 plasma level

A.11 Coma | PCS-Diagnosis Coma without relevant medical history 1/1

Emergency and intensive care

▶ Coma PLUS ▶ No relevant medical history ("empty history")	▶ Sudden presentation	▶ Laboratory investigation[1] ▶ CT			Possible DD ▶ Battered child ▶ SAH
		▶ EEG			▶ Postictal ▶ Non-convulsive status epilepticus
		▶ Laboratory investigation[1] ▶ ECG			▶ Cardiac rhythm disturbance (e.g. long-QT syndrome)
	▶ Rapid deterioration of consciousness from a state of complete health	▶ Place patient's arm above his face ▶ Pull eyelids open	▶ Arm falls onto face ▶ Eyelids close in slow movement	▶ Toxicologic screen	▶ Intoxication (diverse agents)
			▶ Arm does not fall onto face ▶ Eyelids do not close in slow movement		▶ Psychogenic/functional
	▶ Increasing deterioration of consciousness in the course of hours to days	▶ Laboratory investigation[1] ▶ Urine: organic acids, ketones ▶ CT/MRI ▶ Consider thyroid hormone levels			Possible DD ▶ Diverse inborn errors of metabolism (deterioration often precipitated by mild unspecific infections) ▶ Hashimoto encephalopathy

1 Laboratory investigations: Mandatory serum Glucose, arterial blood gas analysis incl lactate, electrolytes incl Mg, full blood count; creatinine; liver enzymes, bilirubin, CRP. Consider: cortisol; urine

A.11 Coma | PCS-Diagnosis Coma secondary deterioration 1/1

Emergency and intensive care

▶ Coma PLUS ▶ Secondary deterioration in	▶ Trauma, haemorrhage, infarction	▶ Laboratory investigation[1] ▶ CT	Possible DD ▶ Secondary haemorrhage ▶ Cerebral oedema ▶ Raised intracranial pressure ▶ Hydrocephalus (see chapter P.01 Hydrocephalus in infants)
	▶ Meningitis ▶ Encephalitis	▶ Laboratory investigation[1] ▶ CT	Possible DD ▶ Hydrocephalus ▶ Abscess ▶ Cerebral oedema, raised intracranial pressure (see chapter A.05 Acute increased intracranial pressure (ICP))
	▶ Hyponatremia[2]	▶ Laboratory investigation[1] ▶ CT	Possible DD ▶ Cerebral oedema ▶ Central pontine myelinolysis
	▶ Diabetes[2,3]		▶ Cerebral oedema

[1] Laboratory investigations: Mandatory serum Glucose, arterial blood gas analysis incl lactate, electrolytes incl Mg, full blood count; urea, creatinine; liver enzymes, bilirubin, CRP. Consider: cortisol; urine porphyrins; TSH/T3/T4. Without conclusive coma aetiology: NH3; toxicology screen. Suspected inborn errors of metabolism: plasma amino acids; Carnitine/acylcarnitine profile.
[2] CAUTION: avoid rapid changes in plasma sodium concentration
[3] The blood glucose level was lowered too rapidly

A.11 Coma | PCS-Treatment 1/2

Emergency and intensive care

▶ Compromised vital functions	▶ GCS < 9 Or ▶ Compromised protective reflexes Or ▶ Pathological breathing[1]		▶ Intubation
	▶ Shock	▶ Resuscitation (volume, vasopressors, inotropes)	▶ Proceed according to aetiology[2]
▶ Hypoglycemia Or ▶ No available blood glucose measurements			▶ Glucose 20 % 2 ml/kg, rapid infusion
▶ Coma w/o apparent cause (adolescents)	▶ Opiate-intoxication possible (often small pupils, not obligatory)		See chapter A.13 Intoxications
▶ Unilateral dilated pupil unreactive to light[3]		▶ Acute treatment of increased intracranial pressure	See chapter A.05 Acute increased intracranial pressure (ICP)
▶ Rapidly progressive impairment of breathing, pupillary reaction, consciousness and motor signs[4]			
▶ Localized clinical and/or CT-signs	▶ Haemorrhage ▶ Tumor ▶ Cerebral contusion	▶ Neurosurgical consultation	See corresponding chapters
	▶ Infection ▶ Venous sinus thrombosis ▶ Multifocal Infarctions	▶ Aciclovir until HSV ruled out	
	▶ Vasculitis ▶ Thrombotic thrombocytopenic purpura	▶ Immunosuppression ▶ Plasmapheresis	
▶ Non-focal signs	▶ Hypoxic-ischaemic[5]	▶ General prophylaxis and treatment of increased intracranial pressure[6]	See chapter A.05 Acute increased intracranial pressure (ICP)
	▶ Infection	▶ Aciclovir until HSV ruled out ▶ Antibiotics	See chapter J. Inflammation and infection
	▶ Acute disseminated encephalomyelitis	▶ High-dose steroids	See chapter J.01 Multiple sclerosis/ADEM

A.11 Coma | PCS-Treatment 2/2

Emergency and intensive care

	▶ Carbon monoxid intoxication	▶ Hyperbaric O_2	See chapter A.13 Intoxications
	▶ Other intoxications (cyanide, alcohol)	▶ Specific antidotes; glucose to counter ethyl alcohol intoxication	
	▶ Hypertensive crisis	▶ Antihypertensive treatment	
	▶ Shunt dysfunction	▶ General prophylaxis and treatment of raised intracranial pressure[7]	See chapter A.05 Acute increased intracranial pressure (ICP) and P.02 Management of the shunted hydrocephalus
	▶ Inborn error of metabolism	▶ In the absence of a specific diagnosis, administer high-dose intravenous glucose, no amino acids, no fat	See chapter A.07 Neurometabolic dysfunction
▶ Status epilepticus	See chapter A.02 Status epilepticus (SE)		
▶ No diagnosis despite extensive investigation		▶ Consider steroids (e.g. Prednisone 2 mg/kg/d)	

1 Hyperkapnia, pathologic or borderline oxygen saturation (pulse oximetry)
2 Consider hypothermia after cardiac arrest
3 Uncal herniation
4 Suspect transtentorial herniation
5 Hypothermia after cardiac arrest
6 ICP-measurement not indicated
7 Cave: cautious reduction of blood pressure (goal: decrease of MAP by 20–25 % in 15 min to 2 hrs)

A.12 Brain death | PCS-Diagnosis Brain death 1/1

Emergency and intensive care

Fundamental criteria for the diagnosis "brain death"	Validation of irreversibility by *observation time*	Primary brain damage, supratentorial	Children from 2 years on	Experienced paediatric neurologist See national guidelines	Diagnosis brain death: after 12 h
1. Acute severe brain damage And **2. Clinical findings** (all 3) ▶ Coma ▶ Wide and fixed pupils (r/l) ▶ Absence of oculo-cephalic/vestibulo-ocular reflexes ▶ Absence of corneal reflexes (r/l) ▶ Absence of pain reactions (trigeminal and non-trigeminal) ▶ Absence of pharyngeal and trachial reflexes ▶ Apnea (Apnoe-test) And **3. Confirmed irreversibility**			Children younger than 2 years		Diagnosis brain death: after 24 h
			Newborns		Diagnosis brain death: after 72 h
		Secondary brain damage			Diagnosis brain death: after 72 h
	Validation of irreversibility by *additional findings* ▶ Isoelectric (flatline) EEG (obligatory in cases of infratentorial brain damage and in children under 2 years of age) Alternatively ▶ Extinct evoked potentials (only accepted in cases of supratentorial and secondary brain damage) Or ▶ Confirmed complete absence of cerebral blood flow, e.g. by sonography/Doppler follow-up or radionuclide cerebral blood flow scan.				Diagnosis brain death

A.12 Brain death

A.13 Intoxications | PCS-Leading symptoms 1/1

Emergency and intensive care

Medical history
- Empty medication package
- Suicide note
- Industrial accident
- Substance abuse
- Psychiatric medical history
- Neurological symptoms (cephalgia, syncopes, vertigo or similar) in the patient's past or in family members

Clinical findings
- Abnormal pupils/puppillary reflexes
- Neurological findings
- Punctures
- Specific halitosis (fetor oris)

Laboratory parameters
- Blood glucose
- Blood gas analysis (acidosis?)
- Creatinine
- Electrolytes
- Urinalysis
- Drug screening and toxicological analysis

Evidence for specific noxious agent	▶ See specific chapter ▶ *CAUTION:* also consider possible combinated (multiple) intoxications!
Low blood glucose	▶ Sulfonylurea, (long-lasting) insulin, metformin
Acidosis, anion gap (Na-Cl-HCO$_3$ > 16 mEq/L)	▶ Ethylene glycol (ethanediol) ▶ Methanol, substances metabolized to methanol ▶ Ethylene glycol monoalkyl ethers ▶ Salicylate or similar, NSAIDs incl.; mefenamic acid
Acidosis, lactate ↑	▶ Metformin ▶ Alpha lipoic acid ▶ Propylene glycol (notably after IV application) ▶ Zidovudine and other nucleoside reverse transcriptase inhibitors (NRTI)
Ketoacidosis	▶ Ethanol, *CAUTION:* consider undiagnosed diabetes
COHb? MetHb? MetHb ↑: blood colored like chocolate *NOTE:* often only slight acidosis	▶ *NOTE:* often only mild acidosis ▶ Carbon monoxide ▶ Met-Hb-forming substances – Aniline and other aromatic amines, nitrite, nitrobenzene, 4-DMAP overdosage, nitroglycerine, overdosage of some local anesthetics
Acidosis (in some patients only mild)	▶ Hydrogen cyanide (HCN) ▶ Hydrogen sulfide (e. g. cesspit)
Ammonia ↑	▶ Valproic acid overdosage ▶ DD metabolic disorder ▶ Toxic liver failure [e. g. paracetamol (acetaminophen)]
Miosis, drooling, perspiration	▶ Nicotine poisoning, muscarinic syndrome, cholinergic syndrome
Miosis, coma	▶ Opiate syndrome
Miosis with deep coma	▶ Hypnotics syndrome, opiate syndrome
Mydriasis, dry skin	▶ Anticholinergic syndrome
Mydriasis, hyperthermia, CK ↑, metabolic acidosis	▶ Malignant neuroleptic syndrome ▶ Serotonin syndrome

A.13 Intoxications | PCS-General measures 1/2

Emergency and intensive care

Step 1	Acute patient-centered care	Emergency medical aid according to ABC rule, if necessary	
Step 2 (attend to step 3 in parallel if appropriate)	Primary elimination of poison	Gastric lavage Should only be considered in potentially life-threatening intoxications	Gastric lavage (if necessary 0,5 mg Atropine for prevention of reflex laryngospasm); recovery (lateral) position for patients with full or reduced consciousness and with appropriate protective reflexes; for patients with failing protective reflexes use intubation Lavage with 5–10(–20) l lukewarm H_2O (in portions of 10 ml × kg) via a flexible, orally inserted tube brushed with adhesive Lidocaine gel 2 % (infant ø 11 mm) Terminal, 0,5–1 g/kg Activated charcoal (carbo med.) dissolved in water and applied via a gastric tube. Clamp off and remove tube. Contraindication: unprotected respiratory ducts, risk factors for intestinal bleeding or perforation, liquid hydrocarbons, surfactants, caustic substances
		Activated charcoal Within the first hour after ingestion of potentially toxic dosages. Only if toxic substance binds well to Activated charcoal.	Activated charcoal in powder or tablet form suspended in 50–200(–300) ml water, juice or soft drink, carefully stirred until obtaining a reasonably homogeneous suspension Let the child drink the suspension independently; if necessary, application via gastric tube (see above) Not effective in intoxications with metallic salts such as Lithium, Potassium, iron supplements, and with alcohols Contraindication: unprotected respiratory ducts, gastrointestinal tract lesions
		Whole bowel irrigation Iron tablets, drug clusters, potentially toxic ingestions of sustained – release or enteric – coated drugs, drugs not absorbed by Activated charcoal and for removal of illiat drugs in "body packers".	Procedure: Isotonic polyethylene glycol solution (e. g. 40 ml/kg/h to max. 1 l/h) Use max. 500 ml/h in children aged 6 months to 6 years, max. 1 000 ml/h in children aged 6–12 years Use 1 500–2 000 ml/h in adolescents. Best via nasogastric tube until clear liquid appears rectally or until radiologically seen drug clusters or iron tablets are eliminated. Contraindication: intestine obstruction or perforation, ileus, cardiovascular instability, unprotected respiratory ducts
		Aperients like Glauber's salt Not as initial treatment or in combination with Activated charcoal. Can be necessary in the course of further treatment. (Exception: Glauber's salt without Activated charcoal in intoxications with barium nitrate)	Contraindication: absence of peristaltic sounds, intestine obstruction or perforation, ionic shift, intravascular volume depletion, caustic substances
Step 3	Special pharmacotherapy	Antidote If necessary before Step 2!	Lorazepam or Diazepam in seizures e. g. cholinergic syndrome – Atropine therapy see chapter for individual noxa

A.13 Intoxications

A.13 Intoxications | PCS-General measures 2/2

Emergency and intensive care

Step 4	Secondary measures of poison elimination	Recurrent charcoal application Indication: Theophyllin, Phenobarbital, Quinine, Quinidine, Chloroquine, Carbamazepine	6 g (until 12 years) or 10 g (12–18 years) of Activated charcoal 1(–4) hourly; additional application of aperient if required; avoid ready-made mixtures with laxatives
		Indication for alkalization of urine: salicylate intoxication	Initially sodium bicarbonate 8,4 % (= 1 molar) 0,5–1 ml/kg BW; aim for urine pH 7,5–8,5; if necessary repeat sodium bicarbonate application, monitor serum levels of Na and K and serum pH
		Hemodialysis/-filtration Severe intoxication with e.g. salicylates, methanol, glycols, ethanol, isopropanol, metformin, Theophyllin and others	In (impending) life-threatening intoxications. Consultation with poison emergency center recommended.
		Intermittent hemoperfusion Intoxication with e. g. Phenobarbital, Carbamazepine	Secondline alternative to haemodialysis if the latter is unavailable

Notes

Notes

B Neonatology

B.01 Neonatal seizures | PCS-Diagnosis 1/1

Neonatology

Medical history
- Pregnancy
- Risk factors
- Medication/cigarettes/illegal drugs/alcohol
- Childbirth/placenta
- APGAR score/umbilical cord pH
- Birth weight, head circumference
- Family history

Clinical findings
- Vital signs
- Neurological findings
- Dysmorphic features
- Preterm/full term
- DD epileptic/non-epileptic events
  - Wakefulness/sleep
  - Eyes open/closed
  - Movements can be provoked/interrupted
- EEG (60-min recording including polygraphy)
- Laboratory check-up
  - Exclude acute metabolic dysfunction
  - Glucose, Calcium, Sodium, Magnesium, Ammonia, Lactate
  - Blood gas analysis, red and white blood cell count, thrombocytes
- CNS sonography

Laboratory check-up
- Infectious diseases
  - Blood, CSF, incl. HHV6, TORCH
- Metabolic diseases
  - Amino acids/organic acids in blood, urine
  - Exclude glucose transporter 1-deficiency (glut-1)
- Additionally (depending on clinical symptoms)
  - Neurotransmitter/amino acids (CSF), pipecolic acid (plasma, CSF) or alpha-AASA (plasma)
  - Genetic work-up

Hypoglycemia	► Fructose biphosphatase deficiency (FBD) ► Glucose-6-phosphatase deficiency (von Gierke's disease) ► Maple syrup urine disease (MSUD) ► Hyperinsulinism (Beckwith-Wiedemann syndrome) ► And others
Hypocalcemia	► Hypoparathyroidism ► Maternal hyperparathyroidism
Hyperammonemia	► Argininosuccinic aciduria ► Carbamoyl phosphate synthetase deficiency ► Citrullinemia ► Methylmalonic acidemia ► MCAD (Medium-chain acyl-CoA dehydrogenase deficiency) ► Propionic acidemia ► Ornithine transcarbamylase deficiency
Lactic acidosis	► Fructose biphosphatase deficiency (FBD) ► Glucose-6-phosphatase deficiency (von Gierke's disease) ► MCAD (Medium-chain acyl-CoA dehydrogenase deficiency) ► Mitochondriopathies
Metabolic acidosis	► Fructose biphosphatase deficiency (FBD) ► Glucose-6-phosphatase deficiency (von Gierke's disease) ► Maple syrup urine disease (MSUD) ► Methylmalonic acidemia ► MCAD (Medium-chain acyl-CoA dehydrogenase deficiency) ► Propionic acidemia

EEG
- Long-term video-EEG monitoring
- Amplitude-integrated EEG (a-EEG)

MRI
- MRI spectroscopy

Ophthalmologic examination
- Fundus examination (mydriasis)

► Depending on findings: diagnosis and treatment

B.01 Neonatal seizures

B.01 Neonatal seizures | PCS-Therapy

Neonatology

Basic measures	Step 1: causal treatment		Seizure control unsuccessful	Step 2: treatment with anticonvulsants	No successful seizure control	Step 3: treatment of status epilepticus (SE)
Stabilization of respiration, circulation, pulse, blood pressure	Hypoglycemia	▶ Initially 2 ml/kg Dextrose 10 % IV ▶ Maintenance up to 8 ml/kg/day		**Phenobarbital** ▶ Loading dose 10 (maximum 40) mg/kg/d ▶ Response: maintenance dose 3–5 mg/kg/d ▶ **Permanent response: step 4** If no response, give additionally **Lorazepam** ▶ 0,05–0,10 mg/kg IV Or **Midazolam** ▶ 0,1–0,2 mg/kg IV Or **Levetiracetam** ▶ (10–)20(–60) mg/kg/day IV Or **Phenytoin** ▶ Loading dose 15–20 mg/kg (1 mg/kg/min IV) ▶ *CAUTION:* blood level control, non-linear kinetics ▶ Response: stop PHT, no oral application		**Midazolam** (consider as step 2) ▶ Loading dose: 0,15 mg/kg IV, followed by continuous IV appl. of 1 μg/kg/min, stepped up by 0,5–1 μg/kg every 2 min until onset of clinical response (max. dose 18 μg/kg/min) ▶ Persisting status epilepticus: second loading dose of 0,10–0,15 mg/kg about 15–10 min after 1. loading dose Or **Lidocaine** ▶ Loading dose: 2 mg/kg IV within 10 min ▶ Followed by continuous application in reduced dosage: – 6 mg/kg/h for 6 h – 4 mg/kg/h for 12 h – 2 mg/kg/h for 12 h with repeated monitoring of blood levels Or **Thiopental** ▶ 10 mg/kg IV
	Hypocalcemia	▶ 2 ml/kg Calcium gluconate 10 % IV (10 min) ▶ Maintenance up to 8 ml/kg/day				
	Hypomagnesemia	▶ 0,25 ml/kg magnesium sulfate 50 % IM ▶ Maintenance: 0,25 ml/kg IM every 12 h or Magnesium 0,15 mmol/kg slowly IV ▶ Infusions are stopped when normal Magnesium levels have been reached				
	Clinical signs for Pyridoxine dependent seizures **Pyridoxine** ▶ 3 × 100 mg IV per day (ideal with continous aEEG/EEG) *CAUTION:* monitor vital parameters (apnea possible) ▶ or maintenance 15–30 mg/kg/day oral appl. for 7 days **Pyridoxal phosphate** ▶ 30 mg/kg/day in 3 doses oral appl. for 5 days **Folinic acid** ▶ 3–5 mg/kg/day in 3 doses oral appl./IV for 5 days					

Oral medication	Stop antiepileptic drug (AED) treatment as soon as possible Drug withdrawal		
Phenobarbital ▶ Maintenance: 3–5 mg/kg/day ▶ Recurrent seizures ▶ Frequent seizures/status epilepticus level 2–3 ▶ Single clinical/subclinical seizures **Topiramate, Carbamazepine, Lamotrigine** ▶ Few cases, single case reports	**Dependent on** ▶ Aetiology ▶ Neurological examination ▶ EEG	**Stop treatment (Step 4)** ▶ 2 weeks after last seizure evaluate if treatment can be stopped ▶ In seizure-free children with abnormal EEG and abnormal neurological examination, continued treatment until the age of 3 months may be justifiable	

B.02 Neonatal hypoxic-ischaemic encephalopathy (HIE) | PCS-Diagnosis 1/1

Neonatology

Intrapartum history
- Heart rate decelerations
- Umbilical cord complications
- Placental complications
- Apgar 10 min < 5
- Cord blood gas or any within 1 h – pH < 7,0
- Obstructed labor
- Prolonged resuscitation (10 min)

Neurological presentation[1]
- Level of consciousness
  - Lethargy/stupor/coma
- Activity
  - Decreased
  - None
- Posture
  - Distal flexion
  - Complete extension
  - Decerebrate
- Tone
  - Hypotonia/hypertonus
- Primitive reflexes
  - Weak or absent suck
  - Incomplete or absent or exaggerated Moro
- Autonomic system
  - Pupils: constricted/dilated-non-reactive
  - Bradycardia
  - Respiration: periodic/apnea/hyperventilation
- Seizures

- a-EEG

- Lower activity > 5 µV
And
- Higher activity > 10 µV

- Lower activity < 5 µV AND Higher activity < 10 µV (moderate asphyxia)
Or
- Higher activity < 5 µV (severe asphyxia)
Or
- Burst suppression (severe asphyxia)

- No asphyxia

- At least one of the fetal distress signs listed in column 1 of the table (Intrapartum history)
And
- Neurological signs of encephalopathy (column 1)
  - At least one sign in three of six categories[1]
    - Consciousness
    - Activity
    - Posture
    - Tone
    - Primitive reflexes
    - Autonomic system
Or
- Abnormal aEEG
Or
- Seizures

- Hypoxic-ischaemic encephalopathy

- Above criteria are not met

- Check possible differential diagnosis

- Neonatal encephalopathy of other origin

See corresponding chapter

1 for detailed information see: Sarnat HB, Sarnat MS. (1976). Neonatal encephalopathy following fetal distress. A clinical and electroencephalographic study. Arch Neurol,33(10):696–705.

B.02 Neonatal hypoxic-ischaemic encephalopathy (HIE)

B.02 Neonatal hypoxic-ischaemic encephalopathy (HIE) | PCS-Therapy

Basic medical support
- Maintenance of oxygenation
  - Controlled ventilation
- Prevention of both hyper- and hypocapnia
  - Controlled ventilation
  - Neuromuscular blockade if necessary
- Prevention of hypotension
  - Intravenous fluid if hypovolemia is suspected
  - Catecholamines
- Prevention of hypertension
  - Sedation/analgesia
- Prevention of hyperviscosity
  - Partial exchange transfusion if hematocrit > 70 %
- Maintenance of glucose supply
  - Intravenous glucose
- Management of intracranial pressure
  - Avoid fluid excess
  - Aim for upper limit of normal blood pressure
  - Midline head posture
  - Maintain upper body in raised position (≈ 45°)
- Management of seizures (see chapter B.01 Neonatal seizures)

▶ Moderate asphyxia (Lower activity < 5 µV And higher activity < 10µV)

▶ Severe asphyxia (Higher activity < 5 µV Or burst suppression)

▶ Hypothermia 33 – 34°C for 72 hours (evidence grade 1B)

▶ Consider contraindications such as
  - Severe bleeding
  - Thrombosis
  - Ongoing bradycardia
  - Hypotonia resistant to therapy
  - Severe tissue necrosis

Notes

Notes

C Pain

C.01 Headache | PCS-Orientation 1/2

Pain

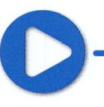

History
Headache-specific history
▶ Acute headache
  – Time of onset
  – Duration
  – Localization
  – Quality
  – Intensity (disabling vs. tolerable, VAS[1])
  – Prodromes
  – Aura
  – Vegetative symptoms
  – Associated symptoms (e.g. hemiparesis)
  – Impairment of daily routine
  – Triggers (physical/psychological …)
  – Factors possibly associated with onset
  – Ameliorating factors
  – Aggravating factors
  – Efficacy of medications taken
▶ Additional features in recurrent headaches
  – Number of headache types
  – Frequency chronic-static, chronic-progressive, episodic (headache diary 2-3 w)
  – Sequence of typical episode
  – Impairment of quality of life

General paediatric history including
▶ Former head trauma (sports concussion)
▶ Comorbidity/symptoms other than headache
▶ Medication, CAM[2]
▶ Daily fluid intake
▶ Nicotine, alcohol (and other drugs)

Psychosocial history including
▶ Structure of day, day-night rhythm
▶ School performance/bullying
▶ Hobbies and sports
▶ Media consumption
▶ Signs of anxiety or depression

Physical examination
▶ General paediatric status including
  – Weight
  – Height
  – Head circumference
  – Blood pressure
  – Nuchal rigidity
  – Dysmorphism
  – Neurocutaneous features
  – Oromandibular system (masseter)
  – Musculoskeletal system (C_1–C_3; trapezius)
  – Stage of puberty
  – Features of systemic process
▶ Neuropaediatric status including
  – Mental state
  – Cranial nerves
  – Visual assessment
    ▶ Pupil response
    ▶ Acuity of vision
    ▶ Temporal visual fields
    ▶ Eye movements
    ▶ Appearance of optic disc
  – Muscle tendon reflexes
  – Motor system
  – Sensory system
  – Coordination (Minor Neurological Dysfunction – MND)
▶ Evaluation of pericranial musculature

Signs of myofascial trigger points (MTrP)
  – Taut band
  – Twitch response
  – Jump sign
  – Referred pain
  – Indicator muscle C_1–C_3: trapezius muscle

5 Dimensions of headache
▶ Localization/topography
▶ Phenomenology
▶ Etiology
▶ Severity
▶ Others (development, participation, hints pointing to other diseases, social dimension)

Red flags:
▶ Continious progressive headache
▶ Sudden severe headache
▶ Recent onset of severe headache (< 4–8 weeks)
▶ Occipital headache
▶ Cluster headache
▶ Early morning headache
▶ Pain that wakes the child (to be distinguished from pain present on awakening)
▶ Worsening of headache in recumbency and/or during straining, coughing and/or other forms of Valsalva maneuver
▶ Changing character of headache in patients diagnosed with primary headache
▶ (Morning/fasting) nausea or vomiting (not associated with typical migraine)
▶ Neurologic dysfunction (other than typical aura associated with migraine)
▶ Confusion
▶ Seizure(s)
▶ Changes of behaviour and/or personality
▶ Cognitive decline
▶ Polyuria, polydipsia
▶ Behavioural decline, avoiding behaviour, missing school

Working diagnosis: Primary headache (ICHD-3 Beta[3])
1. Migraine
1.1 Migraine without aura
1.2 Migraine with aura
1.3 Childhood periodic syndromes (commonly precursors of migraine)
1.4 Retinal migraine
1.5 Complications of migraine
1.6 Probable migraine
2. Tension Type Headache (TTH)
2.1 Infrequent episodic TTH
2.2 Frequent episodic TTH
2.3 Chronic TTH
2.4 Probable TTH
3. Mixed forms

Working diagnosis: chronic daily headache
Headache >15 days/month independent of the main diagnosis but especially if migraine type, warrants referral to tertiary headache center due to high risk of both exacerbation and chronification; DD: chronic migraine

Working diagnosis: secondary headache
See chapter C.03 Secondary headache

Working diagnosis: Bodily distress syndrome (BDS)
Overlap to psychiatric disorders (depression, anxiety)

C.01 Headache

C.01 Headache | PCS-Orientation 2/2

Family history including
- Headaches
- Neurological and psychiatric conditions

1 VAS = visual analogue scale
2 CAM = complementary and alternative medicine
3 ICHD: International Headache Classification, 3rd Beta

C.02 Primary Headache | PCS-Diagnosis Tension-Type Headache vs. Migraine 1/1

Pain

History and physical examination
See chapter C.01 Headache
	▶ No signs and symptoms of symptomatic headaches	**Criteria of the ICHD-3 Beta**[1]
		▶ Headache lasting 30 minutes to 7 days
		▶ Headache has at least 2 of the following 4 features
		  – Bilateral location
		  – Pressing/tightening (non-pulsating) quality
		  – Mild or moderate intensity (VAS < 6)
		  – Not aggravated by routine physical activity
		▶ No nausea or vomiting (anorexia may occur)
		▶ No more than one of photophobia or phonophobia
			▶ Most common primary headache. Pathophysiology, concept as well as wording "not fully understood"	▶ Tension-type headache (TTH)

		Criteria of the ICHD-3 Beta[1]
		▶ Headache attack lasting 2 to 72 hours
		▶ Headache has at least 2 of the following 4 features
		  – Bilateral or unilateral (frontal/temporal) location
		  – Pulsating quality
		  – Moderate to severe intensity (VAS > 6)
		  – Aggraviation by or causing avoidance of routine physical activity (e.g. climbing stairs)
		▶ At least one of the following accompanies headache:
		  – Nausea and/or vomiting
		  – Photophobia and phonophobia (may be inferred from patient's behaviour)
			▶ Premonitory symptoms
			  – Change in mood
			  – Bulimia
			  – Yawning
			  – Pallor
			  – Hypo-/hyperactivity
			  – Disturbance of speech and reading skills
			  – Others
			▶ Abdominal symptoms common in (pre-)school aged children
			▶ Interruption of daily activities
			▶ Child seeks rest
			▶ Imperative urge to sleep
			▶ Restitution after sleep
				▶ Migraine without aura

		▶ Aura consists of at least one of the following features
		  – Visual
		  – Sensory
		  – Speech and/or language
		  – Motor
		  – Brainstorm
		  – Retinal
		▶ At least 2 of the following 4 features characterise the aura
		  – At least one aura symptom spreads gradually over ≥ 5 minutes and/or two or more symptoms occur in success on
		  – Each individual aura symptom lasts 5–60 minutes
		  – At least one aura symptom is unilateral
		  – The aura is accompanied, or followed within 60 minutes, by headache
		Headache that meets the criteria "migraine without aura" (see above) begins during the aura or follows aura within 60 minutes
				▶ Migraine with aura

1 ICHD-3 Beta: the international classification of Headache Disorders

C.02 Primary Headache

116

C.02 Primary Headache | PCS-Therapy Tension-Type Headache

Symptomatic treatment of acute episodes **Non-pharmacologic measures** ▶ Distraction ▶ Relaxation procedures ▶ Damp cloth on forehead ▶ Peppermint oil on forehead or temples **Symptomatic drugs** ▶ Ibuprofen (10–15 mg/kg/SD) ▶ Acetaminophen (10–20 mg/kg/SD; max. 60 mg/kg/d) ▶ Acetylsalicylic acid (< 12 yr: 10 mg/kg/SD, 25 mg/kg/d; > 12 yr: 500–1000 mg/SD)	Counseling of patients and caregivers	**Basic** ▶ Education on the basis of the biopsychosocial pain model ▶ Headache diary ▶ Trigger minimization ▶ Sleep pattern normalisation ▶ Fluid intake ▶ Consumption of alcoholic drinks, caffeine and nicotine ▶ Media consumption ▶ Day structure to cope with or avoid stress ▶ Physical activity on a regular basis ▶ Psychological evaluation
	▶ > 2 days a week suffering disabling or prolonged headaches: discuss prophylaxis (prefer non-pharmacological measures over prophylactic drugs)	**Non-pharmacologic** ▶ Biobehavioural programs ▶ Physical therapy – "trigger point concept" for pericranial and neck muscles ▶ Biofeedback ▶ Acupressure/-puncture ▶ TENS (transcutaneous electrical nerve stimulation) **Prophylactic drugs** ▶ Magnesium 400 (200–600) mg/d (absent/weak evidence) ▶ Amitriptyline 0,5–1(-2) mg/kg/d (absent/weak evidence) – Trial over 1–4 weeks, (especially if pericranial muscles are "tense") ▶ Topiramate 0.5–1(–2) mg/kg/d (absent/weak evidence)

C.02 Primary headache | PCS-Therapy Migraine 1/2

Pain

Goals
- Fast relief of pain
- Fast return to normal function (< 1–2 hours)
- No recurrence
- Low frequency of attacks
- Low impact on participation and quality of life
- Prevention of chronification and abuse of analgesics

Options
- Multimodal regimen
  - Education
  - Life-style management
  - Acute pharmacotherapy
  - Prophylactic pharmacotherapy
  - Bio-behavioural treatment
  - Functional therapies (physiotherapy-trigger-point therapy, manual therapy and others)
  - Complementary and alternative medicine (CAM)

Step 1
Basic measures
- Retreat/sleep
- Protection against stimuli
- Damp cloth on forehead
- Peppermint oil on forehead and temples
- If nausea dominates the attack: Domperidone 1 gtt/kg, max. 30 gtt per dose Dimenhydrinate supp. 40 mg 8–15 kg 1 ×/day 15–25 kg 2×/day > 25 kg 3×/day

Step 2
Analgesics and anti-inflammatory drugs
- Ibuprofen 10–15 (15 mg/kg) p.o./supp.
- Acetaminophen 15 mg/kg p.o./supp.
- Naproxen 5–7.5 mg/kg; max. 500 mg p.o.
- Metamizole 10–20 mg/kg p.o.
- Acetylsalicylic acid (ASA) 10–15 mg/kg p.o.
- Diclofenac 50 mg p.o.
- Take drug without delay after onset (within 30 min)
- Dose adequately high for age/weight
- Repeat after 3–4 hours if necessary

Step 3
Migraine-specific drugs
- Rizatriptan 5–10 mg buccal, oral
- Sumatriptan 10–20 mg nasal
- Zolmitriptan 2.5–5 mg nasal
- Almotriptan 6.25–12.5 mg oral
- Stratified strategy: Determine severity at headache onset, take NSAID or triptan if severity surpasses the individually determined triptan threshold
- Repeat not more than once, not before 2 hours after first dose, and only if first dose did have an effect
- Exclude contraindications for triptans prior to prescription: vascular conditions (e.g. stroke, TIA, hypertension, angina pectoris, myocardial infarction, peripheral artery occlusive disease, Raynaud's syndrome), presence of vascular risk factors, intake of MAO inhibitors (within past 2 weeks) or ergotamines, impaired renal or liver function, pregnancy and lactation
- Consider combination: Rizatriptan AND Naproxen

Step 4
Emergency treatment
Specialized center!
- Intravenous analgesics (ASA, Acetaminophen, Metamizole)
- Subcutaneous Sumatriptan 0.05–0.2 mg/kg; max. 6 mg

Evidence-based non-pharmacologic prophylactic measures:
- Education
- Headache diary
- Sleep-pattern normalization
- Avoidance of caffeine, alcohol and nicotine
- Regular exercise
- Autogenic training
- Progressive relaxation of muscles (Jacobsen)
- Biofeedback

Pharmacoprophylaxis
- Mg^{2+} 400 (200–600) mg/d
- Topiramate 0.5–1(–2) mg/kg (max. 100 mg)
- Amitriptyline 0.5–1(-2) mg/kg, max. 100 mg
- Propranolol 0.5–2 mg/kg/d
- Flunarizine (< 40 kg 5 mg/d, > 40 kg 10 mg/d)
- Acetylsalicylic acid (ASA) 2–3 mg/kg/d

Phytotherapeutics
- Butterbur extract 2 × 25 mg/d

Note
- "Check and balance" in dialogue with the patient: prophylactic drugs are frequently prescribed and taken evidence is weak or absent or inapropriate to age or no superiority to placebo is shown
- Re-evaluate diagnosis, psychology and non-pharmacotherapy (including trigger-point physiotherapy)
- Choose drug in view of the patient's clinical features, comorbidities and drug profiles
- Start at a low dose
- Titrate slowly over 4(-12) weeks
- If a trend of improvement is seen, adjust dose for optimal control
- If sustained, satisfying response is achieved, continue therapy for 4–6 months

C.02 Primary headache | PCS-Therapy Migraine 2/2

▶ Wean slowly (not during "stressful" times; e.g. preferably during vacations)

Severely disabling, treatment-resistant chronic migraine:
Botulinum toxin (specialized center, off label)

C.03 Secondary Headache | PCS-Overview 1/1

Pain

History (details see chapter C.01 Headache)
- Medical history
- Family history
- Headache history
- Impact of the headache on the child's and family's life
- Missed school days/leisure activities because of headache
- Self-explanation of the headache
- Analgesic use
- Complementary and alternative medicine

Physical examination
- Complete examination

Red flags
- See chapter C.01 Headache"

- Respiratory tract infection: viral pharyngitis, otitis, streptococcal infection and (less common) sinusitis are the most common causes of headache in the paediatric population.
- Intracranial neoplasm: headache but unlikely in the absence of red flags (see chapter K.01 Neoplasm of the CNS)
- Meningitis/encephalitis: see chapter J.04 Meningitis and encephalitis
- Subarachnoid/intracranial haemorrhage: see chapter A.09.2 Intracranial haemorrhage/bleeding
- Post-lumbar puncture headache
- Hypertension: uncommon but treatable cause of headache, mostly secondary
- Symptomatic chiari malformation: see chapter P.04 Chiari malformations (CM)
- Lyme disease: see chapter J.03 Lyme disease
- Pseudotumor cerebri: see chapter C.05 Idiopathic intracranial hypertension (IIH)
- Hydrocephalus/shunt dysfunction: see chapter P.01 Hydrocephalus in infants
- Hypercapnia/hypoxia/hypoventilation: hypercapnia (e.g., due to cystic fibrosis), hypoxia (e.g., due to obstructive sleep apnea syndrome) and hypoventilation (e.g. due to neuromuscular disease) can lead to headache
- Stroke: see chapter A.09 Paediatric stroke
- Cerebrovascular dissection: see chapter A.09.4 Cerebrovascular dissection
- Posttraumatic (head/neck) incl. trauma-triggered migraine
- Poisoning: alcohol, caffeine, lead, carbon monoxide, iron deficiency
- Epilepsy headache: can be ictal as well as post-ictal, common comorbidity with migraine
- Medication induced headache including rebound-headache from analgesics

Consider
- Primary headache
- Bodily distress syndrome

Pitfalls
- Secondary headache needs to be treated lege artis, just recognizing the underlying cause is no treatment per se
- Especially chronic daily headache patients (> 15 days/month with headache) need referral to a headache center

C.04 Pain management in palliative care | PCS-Diagnosis 1/2

Pain

Patient with emerging pain or with changes in existing pain requiring therapy

Medical history	Basic diagnostic work-up	Extended diagnostic work-up
Underlying disease (UD) and complications and accompanying diseases; Therapy of UD including any side effects (e.g. neuropathy after vincristine)	Check medical reports, surgery reports, reports of therapists (physiotherapy, psychotherapy etc.).	Re-evaluation of previous imaging procedures Focus on pain-associated findings, e.g. causal/palliative medical interventions
Pain Localization: Encourage the child and/or the parents to describe the pain and show where it hurts (use transitional objects or drafts). Localize the pain on a body map or the patient's own body.	Comprehensive physical examination, observe and document visible and palpable phenomena (trophic disorders, relieving posture/respiration to avoid pain, abnormal positions, spontaneous movements, behaviour/facial expression in daily routine, visible and palpable lesions/tumors, skin/soft tissues lesions from bedding etc.). Document localisation of pain in standardized fashion, e.g. body map	Stepwise diagnostic imaging with strictest consideration of burden *vs.* possible benefits for the patient (decisive is the actual burden of repositioning or transportation of the patient while radiation exposure is of only secondary importance): ▶ Sonography ▶ X-rays (skeleton, e.g. pathological fractures) ▶ CT or MRI, particularly if, e.g., palliative radiotherapy for pain relieve is possible
Intensity of pain: Assessment and documentation of actual pain intensity Self-rating is the gold standard. Ask the patient/parents to describe current pain intensity as compared with previously experienced pain.	Pain assessment: Self-rating Instruments: Faces Pain Scale from 3 years, Visual Analog Scale (VAS) from school age, Numeric Analog Scale (NAS) approximately from 12 years of age External assessment: Paediatric Pain Profile, Premature Infant Pain Profile (PIPP), Neonatal Infant Pain Scale (NIPS)	
Time course of pain: During the course of the day Pain during the night Pain experienced directly after waking up in the morning (opiate dosage intervals too long? end of dose failure?) Suddenly or gradually increasing pain Duration of pain (incident pain, episodic pain, persistent pain with exacerbations)	Pain diary with colour codes for the intensity of pain to document the course of pain over 24h	
Quality of pain: Ask the patient/parents to describe the quality of pain in comparison with previously experienced pain. Suggest distinct quality features based on specific examples (e.g., sharp, burning, dull, gnawing, or dysaesthetic pain).	Pain diary: Use specific symbols for different qualities of pain (e.g. burning or sharp pain) with the possibility of localizing the experienced pain on a body map	Imaging procedures, e.g. if neuropathic pain or pain through pathologic fractures may be alleviated by radiotherapy or surgery
Co-reactions, e.g. physical and psychological symptoms: Anxiety Restlessness Sweating Sensations of heat/cold Reactions of defense and avoidance (young and disabled children)	Pain diary: Record coexisting symptoms (e.g. anxiety, dyspnea, nausea) in the pain diary	

C.04 Pain management in palliative care | PCS-Diagnosis 2/2

Trigger and/or booster of pain: Ask specifically whether pain coincided with ▶ Particular body positions ▶ Nursing care (procedures like changing clothes, baths, transfers) ▶ Food intake ▶ Passing stool or urine – Intake of medication ▶ Therapy (e.g. physiotherapy) ▶ Presence of any persons or anyone in particular?	In consideration of the data recorded in the pain diary, schedule daily routine with periods for care provision (e.g. changing clothes), food intake, school, therapy, hobbies etc. Identify strategies for avoiding pain and for a better pain tolerance (e.g. by anticipating procedure-related pain and administering a breakthrough dose before commencing the procedure)	
Drugs, duration and dosage of previous pain medication	Analysis of medical reports, or previous pain diaries or personal records (e.g. of the parents) for limitations of sufficient pain therapy: Compliance? Fears and reservation against pain medication, especially opioids (e.g. adverse effects, risk of addiction)	Consider laboratory tests for liver and renal function, electrolytes and blood counts to avoid adverse effects of pain drugs in case of organ impairment.
Effects and adverse effects of previous pain medication	Analysis of ▶ Previous medical and nursing reports on adverse effects (e.g. pruritus, hallucinations, or other adverse effects, difficult to treat) that may influence the selection of appropriate opioids ▶ Previous/current medication? Possible interactions? ▶ Reports of the parents or the child on poor experiences/aversions or adverse effects with certain medications; experiences with self-medication/ alternative therapies	
Type and outcome of non-pharmacological interventions	Analysis of ▶ Reports (nursing, physiotherapy etc.) on helpful position, temperature, relaxation techniques and other interventions; ▶ Reports of the parents or children on preferences/wishes, previously successful/unsuccessful strategies and interventions	
Impact of pain on the child's environment (family, friends, peers and teachers, activities)	Analysis of previous reports (nursing, psychosocial advisors, rehabilitation for families, children's hospices) on specific strains and resources of the family: Who is in close contact with the child (parents, siblings, grandparents, friends)? Who belongs to the care team (nursing, therapists, teachers, spiritual advisers, physicians etc.)? How do the parents/the helpers evaluate the situation? What is felt to be their main burden? What are their fears related to the child's pain (helplessness, disease progress, imminent death)?	

C.04 Pain management in palliative care | PCS-Therapy 1/2

Integration of pain therapy into a palliative medical treatment plan facilitates the perception and improvement of these conditions.

Multimodal adjustment

Principles of therapy:
1. Two-step strategy (WHO)
2. Doses are administered at regular intervals
3. Appropriate route of administration
4. Treatment is adapted to the individual child
- Use only a few, well known drugs; be aware of drug interactions and side effects as well as miscibility (in SC or IV application)
- Oral route of administration for all patients who do swallow, for the other patients use subcutaneous application
- Treatment on regular intervals, do not treat only on demand
- To allow for an undisturbed sleep, switch to long-acting formulations as soon as possible after dose-titration with immediate release formulations (e.g. Morphine solution) is completed
- In addition to baseline therapy, prescribe an fast-acting opioid (e.g. Morphine solution, transmucosal Fentanyl) as rescue/break-through medication
- Anticipatory application of fast-acting opioid prior to painful procedures (e.g. changing clothes, change of posture)
- Regular reassessment and documentation of pain and pain therapy to check on compliance and therapeutic success
- Close contact between pain therapist and patient/parents/caregivers to allow early adjustment of pain therapy in response to changing conditions (stronger pain, adverse effects, increasingly impaired organ function)

Nociceptive Pain:
Stimulation of peripheral nociceptors
Conduction along sensitive nerve fibers

Quality:
- Visceral: fuzzy, dull, pressing, diffuse, hard to localize
- Somatic: sharply restricted, can be well localized, nagging

WHO guidelines on the pharmacological treatment of persisting pain in children with medical illnesses no longer list Codeine and Tramadol and switched to a two-step approach (WHO, 2012) (dosage see supplementary tables):
- Step I: Mild pain: Non-opioid analgesics, e.g. Ibuprofen, Paracetamol
- Step II: Opioid-analgesics[1]

Important: In cases of severe pain start with step II.

Weaning from opioids after short-term treatment in 5–10 days, after long-term treatment within weeks.

The choice of the analgesic within one step primarily follows the profile of adverse effects in relation to individual patient's situation. Morphine should be considered as first-line strong opioid as there is a great level of experience in paediatrics. It is available in a wide variety of formulations and application forms.

Opioid treatment according to nociceptive pain + Dexamethasone
Very good efficacy of Methadone (NMDA receptor)
NOTE: Long and highly variable half-life, monitoring by a pain specialist recommended!

Anticonvulsants (Gabapentin, Carbamazepine), antidepressants (Amitriptyline),
Ketamine, Lidocaine
Therapy by pain specialists!

Neuropathic pain:
By infiltration/compression of other lesions (toxic/medication) of peripheral nerves, less frequent central lesions; up to 30 % of the patients in outpatient clinics for pain in oncology

Osseous pain (e.g. in skeletal metastases, infiltration by leukemia):
Non-steroidal anti-inflammatory drugs, steroids, bisphosphonates;
always in combination with opioids
Palliative radiotherapy (few sessions with higher doses in case of limited life expectancy, even in children),
Radionuclide therapy (e.g. mIBG-therapy in osseous metastases in neuroblastoma)

Headache caused by increased intracranial pressure or hypocapnia
See chapter A.05 Acute increased intracranial pressure (ICP)
If pharmacologic treatment unsuccessful: Neurosurgical intervention e.g. liquor shunt OP

- Selection of alternative opioids according to their adverse effects and individual patient characteristics; Particularly suitable for
  - Renal failure: Tilidine, Methadone, Fentanylpiritramid
  - Restricted hepatic function: Hydromorphone

Unsuccessful pain therapy due to:
- Inadequate pain assessment
- Inexperienced physicians in dealing with analgesics (particularly opioids!)
- Low compliance
- Avoid non-compliance[2] by open communication about anxieties and fears, comprehensive information to all persons concerned about the effects and adverse effects, as well as the importance of a good pain therapy for the child's quality of life.

Failure of pain therapy: Interventional treatment:
In less than 10 % of the children, pain is not sufficiently controlled with non-invasive treatment in the terminal phase. For these children, an individual concept including interventional treatment (peripheral nerve blocking, epidural/intrathecal application of Morphine and local anesthetics, intraventricular Morphine) may be considered.

C.04 Pain management in palliative care | PCS-Therapy 2/2

Muscle cramps, forced postures, spasticity	Trial with Baclofen p.o., intrathecal administration by specialists. Benzodiazepines and cannabinoids may be used in addition	Botulinum toxins injections by specialists
Colicky pain caused by bile, gastrointestinal, or urinary tract obstruction	Midazolam p.o. or IV/SC Butylscopolamine	Relief (puncture, catheter, fistula treatment etc.), since colicky pain often cannot be treated sufficiently with drugs

1 Do not forget prophylactic treatment with laxatives during opioid therapy
2 Patient: inappropriate route of administration, i.e. no IM injections; attention to preference/reluctance for solution or tablets, avoid short dosing intervals (after dose-titration) to allow undisturbed sleep; adverse effects (fatigue, drowsiness) are sometimes perceived as worse as pain; fear of addiction. Parents: Fear of "doing wrong" with "dangerous" drugs, fear of causing addiction in the child, fear of acceleration of death. Caregivers: Lack of experience, fear of being responsible for a dying child, particularly, when the medical prescriptions are not concise

C.04 Pain management in palliative care | PCS-Therapy in acute pain crisis 1/1

Pain

During an acute pain crisis, the treatment of the palliative patient has priority. **Medical history and diagnostic work-up serve to exclude any complications requiring immediate treatment and to assess previous pain therapy**	**Opioid titration in an acute pain crisis**[1] **Important:** Maintain opioid antagonist (Naloxone) in case of respiratory depression antihistamines, antiemetics	**Opioid naive child** ▶ Pain assessment ▶ Starting dose (Morphine 0,05 mg/kg) IV, slow infusion for at least 5 minutes ▶ Careful observation of the patient, monitor pulse oximetry ▶ Pain re-assessment after 5 min (time for receptor binding) ▶ Repeat starting dose after 10 min, if not yet free of pain, repeat to complete pain relieve at rest! ▶ Determine the daily dose
	Consider alternative opioids (Hydromorphone, Fentanyl) in case of renal or liver impairment	**Child under opioid therapy** ▶ Pain assessment ▶ First dose: IV equivalence dose of 1/6 of the established daily dose ▶ Careful observation of the patient, monitor pulse oximetry ▶ Pain re-assessment after 5 min. (time for receptor binding) ▶ Repeat initial opioid dose after 10 min, if not yet free of pain, repeat to complete pain relieve at rest! ▶ Determine the daily dose

1 Caution:– Do not use weak opioids (ceiling effect)– Buprenorphine is not easily antagonized by naloxone; risk of respiratory depression, ceiling effect!– Note regarding Pethidine: Avoid accumulation of the metabolite norpethidine (risk of seizures!) – Levomethadone is unsuitable for titration due to its long half-life.

C.04 Pain management in palliative care

C.05 Idiopathic intracranial hypertension (IIH) │ PCS-Diagnosis 1/1

Pain

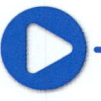

See chapter C.01 Headache and C.02 Primary headache

History
- Body weight (obesity BMI > 25, rapid weight gain)
- Medication
  - Somatotropic hormone
  - Hypervitaminosis A
  - Steroids, Interferon alpha
  - Cytosin-arabinoid, Ciclosporin
  - Acitretin
  - Tetracycline
  - Thyroxine, rhGH
  - Thiopenton
  - Sorbitol-overdosing
  - Oral contraception
- History of bleeding
- Endocrine disorders
  - Morbus Addison, Morbus Cushing
  - Hypothyreosis
  - Hypoparathyreoidism
  - Adenoma of hypophysis, acromegaly
- Hematologic disorders: anemia (iron deficieny anemia, pernicious anemia, polycythemia vera)
- Metabolic disorders
  - Enzymatic deficiency (galactosemia, antichymotrypsin-deficiency)
  - Cystic fibrosis
  - Hyper-/Hypovitaminosis (Vitamin A, D)

Symtpoms
- Headaches (75–100 %)[1]
- Decline of vision (30–50 %)
- Persistent vomiting (20–30 %)
- Double vision (20–30 %)
- Other visual symptoms[2]
- Associated features: tinnitus, meningism, torticollis-like head posture
- Inactivity, irritability, somnolence

Diagnostics
- Fundoscopy: papilloedema (50–100 %), enlarged blind spot
- Perimetry: narrowing of visual field
- MRT (incl. thin layers of N. opticus)
  - Space occupying lesion
  - Ventricle configuration normal or even tight
  - Flattering of the posterior aspect of the globe (80 %)
  - "Empty sella" sign (70 %)
  - Contrast enhancement of the pars prelaminaris n. optici (50 %)
  - Dilatation of the sheets of N.opticus (45 %)
  - Vertical wriggling of N. opticus (40 %)
  - Intraocular protrusion of N. opticus (30 %)
- Lumbar puncture[3]
  - Measurement of CSF opening pressure
  - Standard chemical analyses
  - B. burgdorferi serology

- MRT without specific finding
And
- CSF opening pressure at lumbar puncture > 25 cm (up to 60 cm) H_2O (lying aside)
And
- CSF normal

- Findings not consistent with diagnosis of IIH

- IIH

- Possible differential diagnosis
  - Hydrocephalus
  - Neuroborreliosis
  - Tumor
  - Other structural or vascular lesion in cMRT

---

1 Mainly pulsatile, frontal or occipital-nuchal, often onset on one side, sometimes retrobulbar pain or pain associated to eye movements; often amelioration after lumbar puncture
2 Occasionally episodically blurred vision, mono- or binocular, duration about 1 minute ("transient obscuration"), or short photopsia
3 A herniation after lumbar puncture has not been described (hypothesis: increased brain stiffness due to chronically raised ICP)

C.05 Idiopathic intracranial hypertension (IIH)

C.05 Idiopathic intracranial hypertension (IIH) | PCS-Therapy

Step 1
Treatment of associated underlying cause:
- Overweight
- Medication
- Internal disorders

Progression or insufficient regression with respect to
- Optical nerve/ocular fundus
- Vision/visual field
- Headaches
- Cognitive/neuro-psychological deficits

Step 2
LP:
- Aim to an opening pressure of < 15 cm H_2O
- Drain 20–60 ml

Reduction of CSF production: Acetazolamide
- Children: Start 25 mg/kg/d, elevation in steps of 25 mg/kg/d (max. 100 mg/kg/d or 2 g/d)
- Adolescents: 250 mg/SD × 4 or 500 mg/SD × 2 (max. 4 g/d)

Step 3
LP:
- Aim to an opening pressure of < 15 cm H_2O
- Drain 20–60 ml

Reduction of CSF production: Acetazolamide
- Children: Start 25 mg/kg/d, elevation in steps of 25 mg/kg/d (max. 100 mg/kg/d or 2 g/d)
- Adolescents: 250 mg/SD × 4 or 500 mg/SD × 2 (max. 4 g/d)
- Reduction of extracellular volume: diuretics:

Furosemide 1 mg/kg/d in the morning

Step 4
LP:
- Aim to an opening pressure of < 15 cm H_2O
- Drain 20–60 ml

Steroids
- Dexamethasone 1–2 mg/kg/d for 3–5 days, max. 16–32 mg/d

Or
- Methylprednisolone 20–30 mg/kg/d for 3–5 days, max. 500–1 000 mg/d

Step 5
Mechanical reduction of ICP
- Recurrent therapeutic lumbar puncture (20–60 ml/LP)

Step 6[1]
Mechanical reduction of ICP
- Recurrent therapeutic lumbar puncture (20–60 ml/LP)
- Surgical procedures with decompression of N. opticus and/or mechanical reduction of ICP
- Fenestration of the sheets of N. opticus if persistent loss of vision is impending
- Ventriculoperitoneal shunt

[1] Rarely indicated

Notes

Notes

D Development

D.01 Developmental disorders | PCS-Orientation, part 1

Medical history
- Developmental delay[1]
- Developmental disorders[2]
- Presentation:
  - Why?
  - Why now?
  - Why here?
  - Onset of symptoms?

Patient's history
- Pregnancy
- Delivery
- Newborn period/newborn screening
- Nutrition
- Milestones of development
  - Motor
  - Speech
  - Social
- Family history

Examination
- Paediatric examination
- Neurological examination
- Detailed developmental assessment
- Dysmorphic features
- Minor neurological dysfunction (MND)

Testing
- Ophthalmological examination
- Otological examination
- EEG/Wake- & Sleep recording
- Psychological/psychiatric assessment of
  - Cognition
  - Mind
  - Behavior
  - Emotions

Laboratory assessment
- Basic data including
  - Thyroid function
  - Metabolism: selective/screening
  - Genetics: selective/screening
- CSF (problem oriented)

Imaging
- Sonography
- CT
- MRI

Working hypothesis
- Primary global developmental delay
- Justifications
  - Cerebral morphology
  - Genetics
  - Metabolism
  - Infection
  - Dysfunction (e.g. electrical status epilepticus during sleep ESES)
- Unexplained

To do
- Working hypothesis?
- Counseling/management/education
  - Prognosis
  - Treatment goals
  - Supportive treatment
  - Developmental follow-up
  - Comorbidities?[3]
  - Diagnostic revision/escalation
  - Healthcare/welfare system: medical care (paediatrician/neuropaediatrician & social paediatric center, child & adolescent psychiatrist), handicapped ID, tax
  - Educational system: support, kindergarten, school, institution

---

1 Developmental delay: decreasing gap to normal development; probable developmental catch-up.
2 Developmental disorder: increasing gap to normal development; no developmental catch-up.
3 Wilson GN, Cooley WC (Hrsg.) (2006). Preventive Health Care for Children with Genetic Conditions. 2. Ed. Cambridge, New York, Melbourne, Madrid, Cape Town, Singapore, Sao Paulo: Cambridge University Press 2006:151–193.

D.01 Developmental disorders | PCS-Orientation, part 2 1/2

Development

Introduction/Definitions

Global developmental delay (GDD): ≥ 2 domains out of
- Gross and fine motor
- Speech/language
- Cognition
- Social/personal
- Activities of daily living are significantly affected.

Specific Developmental Delay:
1 domain is affected
Significant delay: ≥ 2 SD below age appropriate norms
- "GDD" applies for children below 4–5 years, and often predicts "Intellectual disability" (ID) for older children when IQ tests are feasible.

GDD/ID Prevalence: 1–3 %
Diagnostic yield 10–81 %
Risk factors for GDD
- Gender: male
- Familiy history of intellectual disability (ID)

Medical History:

At presentation:
- Onset of symptoms
- Course of symptoms
- Comorbidities
- Medical treatment

Prenatal
- Drugs, alcohol, teratogens
- Maternal illness

Peri-postnatal
- Gestational age
- Infections/TORCH
- Neonatal seizures
- Hypotonia
- Feeding problems
- Metabolic screening
- Previous illness
- Previous treatments

Deveopmental "milestones"
Family history (3 generations)
- Consanguinity
- Stillbirths
- Socioeconomic factors (related to mild delay)
- ID (recurrence 8–12 %)

Examinations

Physical exam
- Growth
- Skin, neurocutaneous signs
- Hepatosplenomegaly
- Vision
- Hearing

Neurological exam
- see chapter R Neurological examination

Dysmorphologic exam
- Take photos/videos

Exam for Minor Neurological Dysfunctions (MND)
Developmental evaluation
- Questionnaires
- Standardized tests

Testing

- Ophthalmological exam
- Hearing exam
- EEG wake/sleep recordings
- (speech or developmental regression, seizures)
- Genetic evaluation
- Consider neurophysiology
- Consider cardiology

Psychological/psychiatric tests of
- Cognition/adaptive skills
- Mind
- Behavior
- Emotions
- Autism Spectrum Disorders

Consider further multidisciplinary assessment
- Speech & language therapy
- Autism Spectrum Disorder service
- Physiotherapy
- Occupational therapy

Laboratory Assessment

- Full blood counts
- Glucose
- Thyroid hormones
- Vit B12
- Urea, electrolytes
- Ferritin
- Creatinkinase
- Lactate
- (Lead)

Metabolic tests (yield 0.2–5 %)
- In urine:
  - Organic/amino acids in urine
  - Oligosaccharides
  - GAA/creatine metabolites
  - Mucopolysaccharides
  - Uric acid
  - Purines/pyrimidines
  - Guanidinoacatate
- In blood
  - Ammonia (1st line when vomiting, coma)
  - Homocysteine
  - Acylcarnitines
  - Amino acids
  - Cholesterol
  - 7, 8 Dehydrocholesterol
  - Sialotransferrins (CDG syndromes)
  - VLCFA

Specific metabolic tests depending on clinical symptoms
CSF evaluation (problem oriented)
Genetics:
- Chromosome Microarray (1st line)
- DNA for Fragile in all
- In males X-linked ID panel
- In females MECP2
- FISH/cytogenetics
- Multigene panel investigations
- Exome
- Genome

To Do

Conclusion/Diagnosis/Working Hypothesis:
- Focal/anatomical area involved?
- Treatability
- Severity of the problem
- Aetiology
- Prognosis

Unknown diagnosis:
- Clinical re-evaluation, re-tests further diagnostic approach
- Counselling, management, education
  - Goal definition
  - Education/academic education
  - Familial resources
  - Social support
  - Medical resources
  - Social services, tax
  - Institutions, pre-school, school

D.01 Developmental disorders | PCS-Orientation, part 2 2/2

Imaging
- Cerebral MRI (1st line)
- Consider MRI spectroscopy
- CT for bones and calcifications
- Sonography in infancy

D.02 Hyperkinetic disorder | PCS-Diagnosis 1/2

Development

Medical history
- Child
- Parents
- School
- Kindergarten
- Peers
- Neurological examination
- Minor neurological dysfunction (MND)
  - Simple MND
  - Complex MND

Diagnostic Procedures
- Psychological testing
- EEG, incl. sleep-EEG

A. Inattentive
(at least six of the following symptoms for at least 6 months, to a degree that is maladaptive and inconsistent with the expected level of the child's development)
- Fails to give close attention to details, or makes careless errors in schoolwork or other activities
- Often fails to sustain attention in tasks or play activities
- Often appears not to listen to what is being said
- Often fails to follow through on instructions or finishing schoolwork, chores or duties
- Deficits in organizing tasks and activities
- Often avoids or strongly dislikes tasks that require sustained mental effort
- Often loses things
- Is often easily distracted by external stimuli
- Is often forgetful in the course of daily activities

B. Hyperactive
(at least three of the following symptoms for at least 6 months, to a degree that is maladaptive and inconsistent with the expected level of the child's development)
- Often fidgets with hands or feet or squirms on seat
- Leaves seat in classroom or in other situations in which remaining seated is expected
- Often runs around or climbs excessively in inappropriate situations
- Unduly noisy in playing, exhibits a persistent pattern of excessive motor activity

C. Impulsive
(at least one of the following symptoms for at least 6 months, to a degree that is maladaptive and inconsistent with the expected level of the child's development)
- Often blurts out answers before questions have been completed
- Often fails to wait in lines
- Often interrupts or intrudes on others
- Often talks excessively without appropriate response to social constraints

---

All criteria A, (B), C, D fulfilled without any of the comorbidities below

- Further diagnostic assessment to exclude somatic and neurological disorders (e.g. epilepsy, multiple sclerosis, systemic lupus erythematosous, adrenoleukodystrophy etc)
- Prepare for pharmacotherapy:
  - Laboratory investigations including full blood count, liver and kidney function, thyroid status, CRF and erythrocyte sediment
  - ECG
  - Blood pressure
  - Growth charts

All criteria A, B, C, D fulfilled
Diagnosis: Attention deficit hyperactivity disorder ADHD (F90.0)

Criteria A, C, D fulfilled, no hyperactivity
Diagnosis: Attention deficit disorder without hyperactivity ADD (F98.8)

Presence of A, (B), C, D symptoms but also
- Minor neurological dysfunction (MND)
- Development coordination disorder (DCD)
- Neurological deficits
- Dysmorphic signs
- Fetal alcohol syndrome (FAS), fetal alcohol spectrum disorder (FASD)
- Genetic syndrome
- (Extreme) prematurity
- Regression
- Episodic lethargy, cyclic vomiting
- Epilepsy
- (Severe) mental retardation

- Children with known comorbidites may exhibit symptoms of ADHD severely impairing function and participation
- Consider focused treatment of ADHD when indiciated

All criteria A, B, C, D fulfilled, associated
- Learning deficits

- Assessment and standardized tests of intelligence

Diagnosis based on level of intelligence

- Assessment and standardized tests of reading, spelling, arithmetic and language

- Assessment positive: comorbidity F90.0 with language deficits (F80) and/or deficits in school performance (F81)

D.02 Hyperkinetic disorder

138

D.02 Hyperkinetic disorder | PCS-Diagnosis 2/2

Development

D. Additional criteria			
D. Additional criteria ▶ Onset of the disorder is no later than the age of 7 years ▶ Pervasiveness (criteria should be met for more than a single situation e.g. the combination of inattention and hyperactivity should be present at home and at school) ▶ There must be clear evidence of clinically significant impairment in social, academic or occupational functioning	All criteria A, B, C, D fulfilled, associated ▶ Deficits in social interaction, qualitative speech and communication deficiencies, restricted, repetitive and stereotyped behavioural patterns (see chapter D.05 Autism spectrum disorder (ASD)) ▶ Anxiety ▶ Depression, fatigue ▶ "Unusual" behaviour ▶ Tics	▶ Assessment of autism (see chapter D.05 Autism spectrum disorder (ASD)) ▶ Assessment psychosis	▶ Assessment positive: pervasive developmental disorder (F84) or schizophrenia (F20)
		▶ Assessment depression, anxiety, Tic disorder (see chapter D.04 Tic disorder and Tourette syndrome)	▶ Assessment positive: F90.0, co-morbidity with depression (F32), anxiety (F40, F41) or Tic disorder (F95)
	All criteria A, B, C, D fulfilled, associated ▶ Aggressive or oppositional aggressive behaviour ▶ Temper tantrums ▶ Drug abuse	▶ Assessment conduct disorder, assessment substance abuse	▶ Positive assessment: Hyperkinetic conduct disorder (F90.1)
	Not all criteria (A, B, C, D) fulfilled	All criteria were met at some point in the patient's history	Hyperkinetic disorder in remission

D.02 Hyperkinetic disorder | PCS-Therapy 1/1

Development

Multimodal therapy of hyperkinetic disorder ▶ **Basics** ▶ **Psycho-education and counseling** ▶ **Parents** ▶ **Child** ▶ **Environment** **NOTE: It is a team approach to treat ADHD. Child neurologist, Child psychiatrist, psychologist and functional therapists.**	Hyperkinetic symptoms, mainly in school setting	Psycho-education and counseling in school setting ▶ Reinforcement programs ▶ Positive reinforcement ▶ Time-out techniques	Pharmacotherapy, if counseling not sufficient	(Long-acting) Methylphenidate formulations/norepinephrine reuptake inhibitor (Atomoxetine)
	Hyperkinetic symptoms, mainly in family setting	Parent training, interventions in family setting ▶ Positive reinforcement ▶ Setting limits ▶ Adequate negative consequences	Pharmacotherapy, if parent training not sufficient	(Long-acting) Methylphenidate formulations/norepinephrine reuptake inhibitor (Atomoxetine)
	Hyperkinetic symptoms, severe even under optimal conditions	Behavioral therapy → Self-instructional training → Self-management Requires reflection capability, introspection necessary. Can be used in school-aged children, not in pre-school-aged children.	Pharmacotherapy, if behavioural therapy not sufficient	(Long-acting) Methylphenidate formulations/norepinephrine reuptake inhibitor (Atomoxetine) Pre-school-aged children only in severe cases (off-label); in this age group, parent instruction and counseling is preferred
	Hyperkinetic symptoms, with comorbidities	Learning problems ▶ Behavioral therapy ▶ Treatment of learning problems (reading, spelling, arithmetic, language)	Pharmacotherapy, if behavioural therapy not sufficient	(Long-acting) Methylphenidate formulations/norepinephrine reuptake inhibitor (Atomoxetine)
		Tic disorder, anxiety disorder, substance abuse	Pharmacotherapy, if behavioural therapy not sufficient	First line: norepinephrine reuptake inhibitor (Atomoxetine)
		Conduct problems ▶ Behavioral therapy Social competence training	Pharmacotherapy, if behavioural therapy not sufficient	(Long-acting) Methylphenidate formulations/norepinephrine reuptake inhibitor (Atomoxetine)
	Marked pervasive hyperkinetic symptoms with acute crisis-ridden situations (e.g. school exclusion)	Pharmacotherapy	First line: stimulants (Methylphenidate, amphetamine) Rapid onset of effect (Dose: max. 60 mg/d or 2 mg/kg × d), gradual dose titration every week	
			Second line: norepinephrine reuptake inhibitor (Atomoxetine) Onset of effect within 2–4 weeks; start dose: 500 mcg/kg/d 1 SD, increase dose gradually every week over 4–6 weeks (Dose: 0,8–1,2 mg/kg/d), increase dose gradually every 2–4 weeks	

D.02 Hyperkinetic disorder

D.03 Education entrance qualification (school maturity) | PCS-Diagnosis

Development

Medical history
- Parents
- Child

Family history
- School achievement
- Academic/professional career

Environmental data

Examination of the child

Psychological tests

A. Somatic development
- Weight und height
- Hearing and vision
- Gross and fine motor skills
- Headaches
- Sleeping, eating, toilet training
- Chronic conditions (e.g. allergies)

B. Cognitive development
- Interest in (pre-)school skills
- Interest in symbols e.g. letters, digits, figures
- Language development (vocabulary, grammar, comprehension)
- Speaking in full sentences, is able to report about daily events
- Phonological awareness (rhymes, segmentation)
- Ability to compare sets, to count
- Attention, perseverance
- Endures frustration
- Short-term memory (repeats simple sentences, words or digits)

C. Social development
- Integration in peer group with adequate social play, empathy, acceptance within a group
- Cooperation in group setting
- Adequate initiation of and response to social overtures
- Ability to regulate social contacts, to carry small conflicts
- Understands instructions (rules of a game)
- Independence, autonomy (dresses himself)

D. Emotional development
- Stable relations with caregivers
- Accepts separation from caregivers
- Expresses emotions, wishes
- Adequate self-esteem, self awareness
- Explores new situations without fear
- Copes with small failures
- Can distinguish between reality and imagination
- Enjoys compliments

E. Additional information
- Therapeutic interventions
- Life events in the child's environment (migration, separation or divorce of the parents, social status of the parents, mental illness of the parents)

F. Early maturity in all domains and supportive environment

Problem	Assessment	Outcome
Somatic/physical deficits	Neurological and somatic examination, EEG, hearing test, vision tests	No abnormalities — School maturity
		Abnormal findings — Further diagnostic assessment of the underlying condition, its course, and re-evaluation
Cognitive deficits	Cognitive assessment	▶ No significant cognitive delay = IQ > 85 = school maturity
		IQ 70–85 learning disability
		IQ < 70 mental retardation
	Assessment of specific skills (reading, writing, arithmetic, language)	▶ No specific delay in scholastic skills = school maturity
		If screening indicates deficits — Assessment of neuro-developmental disorders
Social deficits	Screening for behavioural problems, internalized vs. externalized behaviour, emotional problems, pervasive developmental disorders. Assessment of environmental risk factors	▶ No abnormalities = school maturity
		If screening positive, check for specific externalising conditions such ADHD, conduct disorder
Emotional deficits		▶ No abnormalities = school maturity
		If screening positive, check for specific internalising conditions such as anxiety and depressive disorder, attachment disorders
Psychosocial problems	Check for risk factors such as child abuse, mistreatment or neglect	▶ No abnormalities = school maturity
		Deficits present — Further assessment and intervention
		▶ Early maturity for school enrolment should be considered

D.04 Tic disorder and Tourette syndrome | PCS-Diagnosis 1/1

Development

Medical history
- Sensation preceding/following motor phenomenon
- Transition to compulsive behaviour?
- Suppressibility
- Absence of tics during sleep
- Motor and/or vocal tics?
- Simple or complex tics?
- Drug history

Tics
- Phenomenology
- Frequency
- Intensity
- Complexity
- Impairment due to tics

Rating
- Yale Global Tic Severity Scale (YGTSS)

Psychopathological findings
- Hyperkinetic disorder
- Obsessive-compulsive disorder
- Depression
- Fear
- Autoaggressive behaviour
- Neuropsychological testing
- Psychiatric consultation

Laboratory workup
- Basic laboratory investigations: white blood cells, acanthocytosis, CRP, sedimentation rate, thyroid function, CK, Cu, coeruloplasmin, antineuronal antibodies, antiphospholipid antibodies, antistreptolysin antibodies, anti-DNase-B antibodies
- MRI
- EEG
- CSF work-up
- Ophthalmologic examination; slit lamp

Evidence of primary tic disorder	▶ Onset < 18 years ▶ Duration < 12 months	▶ Transient tic disorder of childhood	
	▶ Onset < 18 years ▶ Duration > 12 months ▶ Simple motor or vocal tics	▶ Chronic motor or vocal tic disorder	During the course of the disorder, the patient shows both motor and vocal tics (optional coprolalia/copropraxia; echolalia/echopraxia) ▶ Tourette syndrom
Evidence of secondary tic disorder ▶ Drug treatment (e.g. Carbamazepine, Lamotrigine, Methylphenidate) ▶ Drug abuse		Drug-induced disorder	
Evidence of co-morbidity	Obsessive compulsive disorder Sociophobia Hyperkinetic disorder (see chapter D.02 Hyperkinetic disorder) Stutter Asperger's syndrome Depression Fear	Diagnosis and treatment	
Evidence of symptomatic tic disorder	Brain tumor Encephalitis (see chapter J.04 Meningitis and encephalitis) Dystonias Ballism Myoclonus Chorea Evidence of streptococcal infection	Diagnosis and treatment of the underlying disease	
	Conversion disorder/functional/psychogenic	Diagnosis and treatment	

D.04 Tic disorder and Tourette syndrome

D.04 Tic disorder and Tourette Syndrome | PCS-Therapy

Basic treatment
- In-depth advice and counseling to patients and their families
- Strategies for coping with symptoms, concomitant disorders, stress situations, feelings of guilt
- Parenting instruction and support

▶ Transient tic disorder of childhood	No further treatment is necessary
▶ High level of distress ▶ Strong psychosocial stress ▶ Chronic tic disorder ▶ Tourette syndrome	▶ Symptom-oriented behavioural therapy: "Habit reversal training" ▶ Gradually increase dosage of all medications (increase in weekly intervals) ▶ Tiapride 2–5(–10) mg/kg bid Or ▶ Risperidone 0.5–2(–4) mg bid Or ▶ Sulpiride 0.5–1(–2.5) mg/kg bid Or ▶ Pimozide 0.5–2(–4) mg bid Or ▶ Haloperidol 0.25–2(–4) mg bid

If there are any comorbidities (especially obsessive-compulsive disorder, OSD) provide appropriate complementary therapy

D.05 Autism spectrum disorder (ASD) | PCS-Diagnosis 1/1

Development

Clues to diagnosis

1. Deficits in social interaction
- "Theory of mind": Prefers adults to peers, "no friends", tends to avoid eye contact, no reciprocal emotion, difficulties to share joy and interests, little social smile, "undemanding child", too much/too little distance, impaired empathy

2. Qualitative impairments in language and communication
- No or delayed speech development, echolalia, monotone language, pronominal inversion ("you" instead of "I")
- Severe nonverbal communication deficiencies, difficulties to start or maintain dialogue
- Inability for playful social imitation

3. Restricted, repetitive and stereotyped behavioural patterns
- Restricted interests and activities, "too many" rituals
- Toe-walking, hand-flapping
- Inability to accept even small changes of daily routines
- Perpetual arranging of objects

Medical history
- Pregnancy/perinatal
- Preexisting conditions (such as Trisomy 21, TSC, FRAXA)
- Psychomotor development, seizures, behavioural abnormalities
- Family history including psychosocial history and history for ASD, mental retardation, epilepsy, genetic/unclear syndromes

Physical examination
- Complete examination incl. Wood light

Investigations
- Laboratory
  - Must-do: full blood count, electrolytes, liver enzymes, creatinine, creatine kinase, thyroid function
  - Can-do: amino acids, urine organic acids, ammonium ions, lactate/pyruvate, TORCH titers, lumbar puncture, genetics
- Technical
  - Must-do: AEP
  - Can-do: Ophthalmological examination (incl. VEP), EEG, MRI

- Presence of symptoms of all main categories (social interaction, language/communication and behaviour)
- Normal findings on medical examination
- No hints pointing to symptomatic autism

Working diagnosis: idiopathic autism spectrum disorder (autistic disorder, Asperger's disorder, childhood disintegrative disorder, pervasive developmental disorder not otherwise specified)
- Differential diagnosis: ADHD, schizophrenia, psychic trauma, child abuse, neglect, obsessive-compulsive disorder all can go with autistic symptoms that improve on treatment of the underlying disorder
- Referral to child psychiatry for further evaluation

Presence of autistic symptoms but also
- Neurological deficits
- Dysmorphic signs
- Regression
- Episodic lethargy, cyclic vomiting
- Epilepsy
- Severe mental retardation
- Hereditary disorders in the family history
- Skin abnormalities pointing to neurocutaneos syndromes
- Preexisting condition

Working diagnosis: symptomatic autism
- Diseases that can go with autistic symptoms include many neurodegenerative, neuromuscular, neurometabolic and mitochondrial disorders, genetic conditions, severe epilepsies and acquired conditions such as post-hemorrhagic hydrocephalus, stroke and traumatic brain injury
- See chapters on respective leading symptoms for further investigation/treatment
- Symptomatic autism that does not improve on treatment of the underlying condition warrants referral to child psychiatry!

D.05 Autism spectrum disorder (ASD)

D.06 Fetal alcohol spectrum disorders (FASD)

Abnormalities of:	Fetal alcohol syndrome – FAS German S3-Guideline, Landgraf & Heinen, 2013.	Partial Fetal alcohol syndrome – pFAS Canadian Guideline, Chudley at al. 2005	Alcohol related neurodevelopmental disorder – ARND Canadian Guideline, Chudley at al. 2005
Growth Birth- or body weight Or Birth- or body length Or Body mass index ≤ 10. percentile	Present	Not present or present	Not present or present
Face: (1) Short palpebral fissure length ≤ 3. percentile, (2) Smooth philtrum (rank 4 or 5 Lip-Philtrum Guide) (3) Thin upper lip (rank 4 or 5 Lip-Philtrum Guide)	All 3 abnormalities	2 of 3 abnormalities	Less than 2 of 3 abnormalities
CNS functional and structural	Global intellectual deficit or significant combined developmental retardation Or At least 3 areas: ▶ Speech ▶ Fine motor skills ▶ Spatial-visual perception or spatial-constructive skills ▶ Learning or memory skills ▶ Executive functions ▶ Maths ▶ Attention ▶ Social skills/behaviour Or Head circumference at least ≤ 10. percentile	At least 3 areas: ▶ Hard or soft neurological signs (incl. sensory-motor signs) ▶ Brain structure (head circumference, MRI etc.) ▶ Cognition (IQ) ▶ Communication: receptive und expressive ▶ School performance ▶ Memory ▶ Executive functions and abstract thinking ▶ Attention deficit/hyperactivity ▶ Adaptive behaviour, social skills, social communication	At least 3 areas: ▶ Hard or soft neurological signs (incl. Sensory-motor signs) ▶ Brain structure (head circumference, MRI etc.) ▶ Cognition (IQ) ▶ Communication: receptive und expressive ▶ School performance ▶ Memory ▶ Executive functions and abstract thinking ▶ Attention deficit/hyperactivity ▶ Adaptive behaviour, social skills, social communication
Maternal alcohol consumption during pregnancy	Not confirmed or confirmed	Confirmed	Confirmed

Notes

Notes

E Epilepsy

E.01 Epilepsy | PCS-Orientation 1/2

Epilepsy

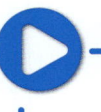

Medical history	EEG/Video-EEG	MRI	Patient-centered classification of epilepsy[2]		Tentative diagnosis	Therapy
▶ Presentation – Semiology – Duration – Lateralization phenomena? ▶ Video? **Medical Examination** ▶ Neurological examination ▶ Developmental state	▶ Awake-EEG ▶ Sleep-EEG[1] ▶ Sleep-deprived EEG ▶ Long-term EEG-video monitoring	▶ High resolution MRI (3.0 Tesla)	Dimension 1 – Localisation/epileptogenic zone/epilepsy syndrome Dimension 2 – Semiology Dimension 3 – Etiology Dimension 4 – Frequency of seizures Dimension 5 – Other medical or psychosocial features	1. *Where* is the lesion? 2. *How* does the seizure start and proceed? 3. *What* is the cause? 4. *How severe* is the epilepsy? 5. Are there *other medical* or *social* features? Does the epilepsy interfere with development?	▶ Summary of dimension 1–5 ▶ Epilepsy syndrome?	▶ Counseling ▶ Pharmacotherapy – Which AED? – Duration of therapy? – Emergency medication? ▶ Specific rules ▶ Seizure diary ▶ Factors about adherence

Dimension 1 – Epileptogeníc zone

▶ Not classifiable	Focal	Multilobar	Hemispheric multifocal	▶ Generalized
	▶ Frontal ▶ Perirolandic ▶ Temporal ▶ Neocortical temporal ▶ Mesial temporal ▶ Parietal ▶ Occipital ▶ Other (i.e. insular, hypothalamic etc.)	▶ Frontotemporal ▶ Temporoparietal ▶ Frontoparietal ▶ Temporo-parieto-occipital ▶ Other	▶ Bifrontal ▶ Bitemporal ▶ Other	

Dimension 2 – Semiology, seizure lateralisation signs

Signs	Hemispheric localization of lesions	Specificity	Prevalence
Versive seizure	Contralateral	> 90 %	TLE[3] 35 % ETLE 40 %
Unilateral ictal dystonia	Contralateral	90–100 %	TLE 35 % ETLE 20 %
"Sign of four"	Contralateral to the extended arm	90 %	65 % of patients with secondary generalized GTCS
Ictal speech	Non-dominant	> 80 %	10–20 %
Unilateral eye blinking	Ipsilateral	80 %	Rare, 1,5 %
Ictal vomiting	Non-dominant	> 90 %	Rare

E.01 Epilepsy | PCS-Orientation 2/2

Postictal aphasia	Dominant	> 80 %	Ca. 20 %
Postictal nose-rubbing	Ipsilateral	80–90 %	TLE 40–50 % FLE 10 %

Dimension 3 – Etiology

Hippocampal involvement	Cortical dysplasia	Vascular malformations	Inflammatory CNS infection	Hypoxic-ischaemic brain damage	Traumatic brain injury	Genetic disorder	▶ Cryptogenic ▶ Idiopathic
▶ Mesial temporal sclerosis ▶ Glioma ▶ Dysembryoplastic neuroepithelial tumor DNET ▶ Ganglioglioma ▶ Other	▶ Focal cortical dysplasia ▶ Hemimegalencephaly ▶ Schizencephaly ▶ Lissencephaly ▶ Holoprosencephaly ▶ Cortical heterotopia ▶ Hypothalamic hamartoma ▶ Hypomelanosis of Ito ▶ Other	▶ Cavernous angioma ▶ Arteriovenous malformations ▶ Sturge-Weber-syndrome ▶ Other	▶ Meningitis ▶ Abscess ▶ Autoimmune encephalitis (Anti-NMDAR, VGKC, GAD, LGI) ▶ Rasmussen's encephalitis ▶ Vasculitis ▶ Other	▶ Ischaemic stroke ▶ Global hypoxia ▶ Periventricular leukomalacia ▶ Hemorrhagic stroke ▶ Venous sinus thrombosis ▶ Other	▶ Subdural effusions ▶ Epidural effusions ▶ Contusion	▶ Tuberous sclerosis complex ▶ Progressive myoclonic epilepsies ▶ Channel disorders ▶ Neurometabolic disorders ▶ Mitochondriopathies (see chapter N.03 Mitochondrial disorders) ▶ Chromosomal aberrations ▶ Other	

Dimension 4 – Frequency of seizures

Daily seizures	Ongoing seizures	Rarely	Undefined
1 or more seizures/day	Less than one seizure/day, at least one seizure during the past six months	Less than one seizure during the last six months	▶ Unknown ▶ New onset epilepsy within the last 12 months

1 EEG tracing e.g. at noon; Melatonin: 3–5 mg (1 to 5 years of age), 6–10 mg (6–15 years of age)
2 Epilepsy classification: Loddenkemper T, Kellinghaus C, Wyllie E, Najm IM, Gupta A, Rosenow F, Lüders HO A proposal for a five-dimensional patient-oriented epilepsy classification. Epileptic Disord. 2005 Dec;7(4):308–16
3 TLE = Temporal lobe epilepsy; ETLE = extra temporal lobe epilepsies; FLE = frontal lobe epilepsies; GTCS = generalized tonic clonic seizure

E.02 First seizure | PCS-Diagnostic work-up 1/1

Epilepsy

▶ Paroxysmal event History Family history Physical examination (e.g. skin ab- normalities?, dysmorphic features?) Neurological examination Parents or caregivers might be asked to perform videorecording of the episodes (see chapter E.01 Epilepsy)	Epileptic seizure	Provoked	▶ Febrile convulsions	See chapter A.01 Febrile seizure
			▶ Other causes (consider lumbar puncture or CT in the emergency depart-ment if clinical signs sug-gest acute illness)	Hypoglycemia Electrolyte imbalance CNS infection CNS haemorrhage Stroke
		▶ Unprovoked	▶ Epilepsy	▶ EEG[1] ▶ MRI[2]
	No epileptic seizure	▶ Syncope, spells etc.	See chapter E.03 Paroxysomal events (non-epileptic)	

1 EEG: sensitivity after the first seizure about 40–50 %; sensitivity is highest during the first 48 hours after seizure; hyperventilation and photic stimulation increases the sensitivity especially in generalized epilepsies; consider sleep EEG if routine EEG during wakefulness is not conclusive
2 Brain imaging: see chapter E.01 Epilepsy

E.03 Paroxysomal events (non-epileptic) | PCS-Orientation 1/6

Epilepsy

1. Motor plus-paroxysmal events

Age	Disorder	Symptoms	Duration, frequency, course	Further investigations	Therapy
Infancy	Hyperekplexia	▶ Startle reaction ▶ Triggered by acoustic or other stimuli ▶ Neonatal: stiffness ("stiff-baby syndrome"), feeding difficulties ▶ Epileptic seizures	Variable course, may also be symptomatic in adulthood	▶ Enhanced motor reflexes (i.e. Glabella-reflex) ▶ Genetics GLRA1 gene (glycinereceptor) ▶ EEG	▶ Clonazepam (0,1–0,2 mg/kg/d) ▶ Valproic acid
	Benign infant myoclonia	▶ As in infantile spasms (Blitz-Nick-Salaam seizures), often during feeding	▶ Frequency: several times daily ▶ Course: remission 1st, 2nd of life year	▶ EEG	Consider differential diagnosis epileptic spasms
	Shuddering attacks	▶ Shuddering/shivering as if freezing	▶ Duration: seconds ▶ Usually provoked by emotions	▶ EEG to exclude epilepsy ▶ Provocation for video documentation	
	Spasmus nutans	▶ Clinical triad of – Head tilt/nodding 2–3 hz – Nystagmus – Possibly torticollis	▶ Spontaneous remission within 2nd–4th year of life in non-symptomatic cases ▶ Symptomatic head nodding ("Bobble-head-doll syndrome"): third ventricle enlargement	▶ MRI to exclude third ventricle enlargement	Symptomatic head nodding ("Bobble-head-doll syndrome"): surgery usually relieves symptoms
	Benign paroxysmal torticollis	▶ Torticollis ▶ Possibly associated with nausea, vomiting and ataxia	▶ Duration: minutes-hours-days ▶ Frequency: weekly, monthly ▶ Remission 3rd–5th year of life ▶ May also develop paroxysmal vertigo or migraine (precursor)	▶ MRI to exclude posterior fossa tumor ▶ CACNA1A mutations have been described in affected families	Antiemetics might be useful in cases of significant nausea/vomiting
	Sandifer-syndrome	▶ Paroxysmal abnormal posturing, torticollis	Variable	▶ Gastro-esophageal reflux disease	▶ Omeprazole ▶ Fundoplication may be indicated in severe cases
	Self-stimulation, self-gratifying behaviour	▶ Rhythmic movements, might be associated with flush	Variable	Video recording of the episode usually confirms the diagnosis	

E.03 Paroxysomal events (non-epileptic)

E.03 Paroxysomal events (non-epileptic) | PCS-Orientation

School aged children and adolescents	Drug related dystonia (see chapter A.03 Acute dystonic reaction)	Torticollis, opisthotonus, oculogyric crisis, abnormal posturing, trismus	Minutes to hours	Drug history (dopamine antagonists, anti-emetics, neuroleptic drugs)	Anticholinergic agents (i.e. Biperiden 1–3 mg IV or IM)
	Hyperventilation tetany	Contraction of face, hands and feet, paresthesia	Minutes	▶ Serum electrolytes: low free calcium ▶ Psychological evaluation	▶ CO_2 retention techniques (e.g. breathing into a plastic bag) ▶ Psychological management if indicated
	Tic disorder (see chapter D.04 Tic disorder and Tourette syndrome)	Short, involuntary complex movements, jerks, vocalizations which can be suppressed only partially	Variable		Consider: Tiapride and other pharmacotherapy
	Myoclonic dystonia	Myoclonic jerks predominantly of arms and shoulders, associated with dystonia (i.e. writing cramps, cervical dystonia)	▶ Myoclonic jerks appear as early as during the 1st year of life (median 5 years), dystonia later (usually at the age of 8 years) ▶ Progression until adolescence, then usually stable course	▶ Molecular genetics of DYT11: Mutations in the epsilon-sarcoglycan gene (SGCE)	E.g. anticholinergics, consider deep brain stimulation of the globus pallidus internus
	Paroxysmal kinesigenic dystonia	Dystonic or choreatic movements, exaggerated by movements	▶ Seconds to minutes ▶ Usually many episodes/day		Carbamazepine (or Phenytoin) usually effective
	Paroxysmal non-kinesigenic dystonia	▶ Dystonic or choreatic movements, NOT exaggerated by movements ▶ Might be provoked by drowsiness	▶ Minutes to hours ▶ Weekly		Clonazepam, Valproic acid, Acetazolamide may be effective
	Functional/psychogenic/somatoform seizures	▶ Occur only with observers ▶ Last longer than epileptic seizures ▶ Eyes usually closed ▶ Can coincide with epileptic seizures	Variable	Video-EEG of the episode	

E.03 Paroxysomal events (non-epileptic) | PCS-Orientation 3/6

Epilepsy

2. "Motor minus"-paroxysmal events

Age	Disorder	Symptoms	Duration, frequency, course	Further investigations	Therapy
Infancy	Alternating hemiplegia	Paroxysmal paresis of one side, may occur with ophthalmoplegia and nystagmus, relief during sleep Epileptic seizures may also occur Developmental delay	▶ Minutes to days ▶ Developmental delay	CACNA1A mutations only in familial cases	▶ Acute: Chloral hydrate ▶ Prophylactic: Flunarizine, Memantine, Topiramate ▶ Usually difficult to treat
Early childhood	Cataplexy in narcolepsy	Sudden loss of postural tone, commonly triggered by emotions such as laughter	▶ Seconds ▶ Daily	▶ CSF hypocretin decreased ▶ MSLT (multiple sleep latency test) ▶ Cataplectic episodes also occur in Niemann-Pick Typ C, Coffin-Lowry syndrom, Prader-Willi syndrom and basilar ischaemia (Doppler, MRI with gadolinium contrast)	Consider antidepressive agents (SSRI)
	Episodic ataxia type 1	▶ Episodic attacks may be triggered by movement ▶ Myokymia of the hands	▶ Seconds to minutes ▶ Daily	▶ EMG ▶ Genetics: mutation in the KCNA1 gene	Acetazolamide may be helpful
	Episodic ataxia type 2	▶ Episodic attacks may be exertion induced, sudden falls, nausea, vertigo	▶ Minutes to days ▶ Weekly and monthly	▶ Genetics: mutation in the CACNA1A gene	Acetazolamide usually effective

School-aged children and adolescents	Episodic potassium-sensitive paralysis	▶ Hypokalemic form
		  – Triggered by: carbohydrate rich food, sleep, starvation, exercise
		  – Proximal paresis with lacking deep tendon reflexes; oliguria may be present during attack
		  – Andersen's syndrome: small stature, dysmorphism, prolonged QT time
		▶ Hyperkalemic form
		  – Triggered by potassium rich food, exercise
		  – Paresis predominantly of lower limbs, myotonia of face and hands
			▶ Hypokalemic form
			▶ Hours to days, monthly
			▶ Hyperkalemic form
			▶ Minutes to hours, daily to monthly
				▶ During attack
				▶ Potassium serum levels, ECG
				▶ Genetics
				▶ Hypokalemic: mutation in CACN1AS or SCN4A genes
				▶ Hyperkalemic. mutation in the SCN4A gene
					▶ Hypokalemic form
					▶ Prevention
					▶ Diet
					▶ During attack: potassium chloride (0,2–0,4 mmol/kg p.o.)
					▶ Acetazolamide
					▶ Hyperkalemic form
					▶ Hydrochlorothiazide (25–50 mg)

	Hemiplegic migraine (see chapter C.02 Primary headache)	Typical migraine headache with hemiplegia, aphasia when dominant hemisphere is affected; paresthesia may also be present	Minutes – hours (– days – weeks – months!)	▶ MRI of the brain with diffusion at onset Genetics: SCN1A or CACNA1A gene-mutation	Pharmacoprophylaxis: Topiramate, Flunarizine, Verapamil, Acetazolamide

E.03 Paroxysomal events (non-epileptic)

E.03 Paroxysomal events (non-epileptic) | PCS-Orientation

3. Impaired consciousness with or without motor phenomena

Age	Disorder	Symptoms	Duration, frequency, course	Further investigations	Therapy
Infancy	Reflex anoxic syncope	Pain – reflectory bradycardia/cardiac arrest – pallor –- tonic posturing – generalized clonic movements	Seconds, variable frequency	▶ Note: Ocular compression test should only be performed with standby resuscitation ▶ ECG and long term ECG to exclude cardiac arrhythmias, i.e. long QT syndrome	Pace maker implantation may be warranted in severe cases
	Breath holding spells	Trigger (i.e. broken toy) – screaming – apnea – cyanosis – tonic posturing – generalized clonic movements	Seconds to minutes	▶ Exclude anemia ▶ ECG to exclude cardiac arrhythmias, i.e. long QT syndrome	Explanation to the parents (oral iron substitution in case of underlying iron deficiency anemia)
	Fabricated/induced illness (Münchhausen syndrome by proxy)	Broad spectrum of symptoms		Cooperation psychiatry and child- and youth-psychiatry	
School-aged children and adolescents	Syncope	Typical history of orthostatic dysfunction, i.e. triggered by emotional stress: pallor, loss of postural tone, clonic movements ("convulsive syncope", miction may also occur)	Seconds to minutes	▶ ECG (long QT-syndrome), consider echocardiography to exclude aortic stenosis	▶ Adequate fluid substitution ▶ Exercise
	Daydreaming	Can always be interrupted	Seconds to minutes		
	Functional/psychogenic/somatoform seizures: see above				
	Intoxication and metabolic crisis (see chapter A.07 Neurometabolic dysfunction)	Usually history of transient or progressive impairment of consciousness after starvation, infection	Hours to days	▶ Neurometabolic and toxicologic evaluation	
	Complicated migraine with aura (see chapter C.02 Primary headache)	▶ Basilar migraine/migraine with brain stem aura: impaired consciousness with cranial nerve dysfunction and ataxia ▶ Acute confusional migraine (may occur after mild traumatic brain injury)	4–24 hours	EEG shows generalized slowing Exclude basilar thrombosis if it is the first attack (MRI/MR Angio, CT-Angio)	See chapter C.02 Primary headache

E.03 Paroxysomal events (non-epileptic) | PCS-Orientation 5/6

Epilepsy

4. Other symptoms (vegetative, sensory, cranial nerves)

Age	Disorder	Symptoms	Duration, frequency, course	Further investigations	Therapy
Infancy	Benign paroxysmal upward gaze	Tonic upward gaze, maybe associated with down-beat-nystagmus and ataxia, motor delay	▶ Minutes–hours–days ▶ Daily–weekly ▶ Remission by the age of > 6	Consider MRI to exclude affection of the upper brain stem	
	Benign paroxysmal vertigo (see chapter F.01 Vertigo and dizziness)	Vertigo, nausea, nystagmus, falls	▶ Seconds – minutes ▶ Daily – monthly ▶ Remission by the age > 3		Dimenhydrinate
	Cyclic vomiting	Recurrent vomiting during episode, mainly during the night, headache (migraine precursor)	▶ Hours ▶ Weekly-monthly ▶ Patients may develop migraine later in life		Antiemetics Consider Topiramate
School-aged children and adolescents	Migraine with aura (see chapter C.02 Primary headache)	Types of auras: sensible, sensory, visual, motor, dizziness/vertigo Typical migraine headache, dizziniess/vertigo, nausea	Minutes to hours Weekly, monthly		See chapter C.02 Primary headache

5. Sleep-related disorders

Age	Disorder	Symptoms	Duration, frequency, course	Further investigations	Therapy
Neonatal and infancy	Benign neonatal sleep myoclonus	Repetitive and rhythmic myoclonic jerks during phases of deep sleep, multifocal, always disappears on awakening	Minutes, remission within 3 months of age	Usually not necessary	
	Central hypoventilation	Recurrent apnea, flat breathing, excessive daytime sleepiness	Commonly progressive	▶ Polysomnography ▶ Idiopathic forms: consider congenital central hypoventilation syndrome (also known as Ondine's curse or Ondine's syndrome) ▶ Symptomatic forms (e.g. brain stem compression, Chiari malformations): MRI, neurometabolic screening	▶ Mechanical ventilation support

E.03 Paroxysomal events (non-epileptic) | PCS-Orientation

	ALTE (Apparent life-threatening event)	Apnea, cyanosis, pallor, loss of tone		Exclude infection Neurometabolic screening MRI ECG, echocardiography	According to aetiology
Infancy	Jactatio capitis/corporis	Stereotype rhythmic movements (head banging, body rocking during drowsiness)	Remission by the age of 5	Psychological evaluation	Counseling, psychology
	Night terrors	▶ Screaming, upset, tachycardia, amnesia ▶ Most commonly occurring during the first half of the night	▶ 1–3/night, 5–10 minutes ▶ Remission usually by the age of 6–8	▶ Video ▶ Long-term video-EEG monitoring might be considered in selected cases to exclude frontal lobe epilepsy (patients usually older, seizures are shorter than night terrors) ▶ Psychological evaluation	Counseling, psychology
School-aged children and adolescents	Restless Legs	Nocturnal rhythmic leg movements, excessive daytime sleepiness	Chronic	▶ Polysomnography ▶ Symptomatic forms: ferritin, folic acid, B_{12}, Creatinine nerve conduction studies, EMG, spinal MRI	▶ L-Dopa plus decarboxylase-inhibitor ▶ Dopamin-agonists (Ropinirol, Pramipexol and others) ▶ Note: cooperation with adult neurologist ▶ Iron substitution if deficient

E.04 West-Syndrome | PCS-Diagnostic work-up 1/1

Epilepsy

History
- Age between 3 and 12 months (2–18 months)
- Loss of eye contact
- Epileptic spasms
- History of i.e. neonatal insult in symptomatic forms

Seizures: epileptic spasms, Infantile spasms
- Sudden flexion, extension of predominantly truncal muscles
- Occurring in cluster
- Predominantly on awaking or drowsiness

Clinical findings
- Seizure semiology: see above
- Rapid tonic upward deviation of the bulbi may also occur as a seizure semiolgy
- Developmental delay
- Developmental regression

EEG
- Hypsarrhythmia: generalized slowing > 300 µV with multiregional spikes and polyspikes
- Periodic patterns may occur during sleep
- EEG seizure pattern: generalized sharp wave followed by generalized amplitude attenuation
- Sleep EEG and long term video EEG mandatory in cases with non-conclusive EEG during wakefulness
- Absence of hypsarrhythmia: consider "epileptic spasms outside West-syndrome"

- MRI
- Genetic testing
- Neurometabolic work-up (see chapter N01 Neurometabolic disorders)

Normal investigations	diopathic West-syndrome
Pathologic investigations	Symptomatic West-syndrome:

Symptomatic West-syndrome:
- Prenatal insult
  - Hypoxia
  - Infection
- Neurometabolic disorder
- Genetic disorder
- Brain malformation

E.04 West-Syndrome

E.05 Benign epilepsy with centrotemporal spikes (BECTS, Rolandic epilepsy)
PCS-Diagnostic work-up 1/1

Medical history
- Age 6–10 (3–13 years)
- History of febrile convulsions
- Normal cognitive performance at school
- Family history of epilepsy in childhood

Physical examination
- Neurological examination and developmental status

Seizure semiology
- Seizures occur mainly during sleep
- **Unilateral seizures**
  - Somatosensory auras
  - Hemifacial tonic or myoclonic seizures
- Other ictal features
  - Oropharyngeal motor seizures
  - Hypersalivation
  - Speech arrest
  - Preserved consciousness
  - Unilateral motor seizures of arm and leg
- **Secondary generalized seizures**

Typical seizure semiology
- No impairment of cognition/speech

Atypical seizure semiology
- High seizure frequency
- Postictal paresis
- Status epilepticus
- Seizures solely occurring in wakefulness

- Impairment of cognition/speech

EEG (awake and sleep, all patients)

Typical EEG for Benign epilepsy with centrotemporal spikes (BECTS)
- Normal background activity
- Benign epileptic discharges of childhood
  - Location: usually centrotemporal leads
  - Uni- and bilateral
  - Isolated or in groups
  - Marked increase in frequency during drowsiness and sleep (stage I and II)

Atypical EEG for BECTS
- Intermittent focal slowing
- High frequency of interictal epileptic discharges (IED) during wakefulness
- Background slowing
- Generalized IED
- Polyspikes
- Lack of increase in frequency during drowsiness and sleep (stage I and II)
- Atypical location of IED

ESES/CSWS
- Electrical status epilepticus in sleep (ESES)/continuous spikes and waves during slow sleep (CSWS) (> 85 % of Non-REM-sleep)
- May occur focal or bilateral or generalized

- **Neuropsychological investigation**

Likely diagnosis of BECTS — MRI optional

Differential diagnosis — MRI
- BECTS-status epilepticus
- Acquired epileptic opercular syndrome
- Atypical benign partial epilepsy
- Continuous spike-waves during sleep (CSWS)/epileptic status epilepticus during sleep (ESES)
- Landau-Kleffner syndrome
- Benign epilepsy of childhood with occipital spikes
- Focal epilepsy due to structural lesion
- Cryptogenic focal epilepsy

*****Benign epileptic discharges of childhood BEPC**
- Occur in 2–4 % of healthy children
- Only 10 % of patients with BEPC suffer from seizures
- For patients without neurological and cognitive impairment or seizures, further diagnostic work is optional

E.06 Absence epilepsy | PCS-Diagnostic work-up 1/1

Epilepsy

Medical history
- Absence
- Loss of contact
- Sudden interruption of speech/activities
- Amnesia for the time of the seizure
- Impairment of school performance (e.g. missing words when writing a dictation)

Seizure semiology
- Loss of contact
- Sudden onset and end
- Eyes wide open
  - Blank stare
  - Upward bulbus deviation
- Duration (3–)5–10(–20) s
- Hyperventilation during clinical investigation triggers typical seizure semiology

Diagnostics
- Video-EEG with hyperventilation

▶ 3Hz spike and wave pattern	▶ Absence epilepsy ▶ Early infantile absence epilepsy (exclude GLUT1 deficiency) ▶ Childhood abcence epilepsy (CAE) ▶ Juvenile absence epilepsy (JAE)		
▶ Lack of 3 Hz spike and wave pattern	▶ Sleep-EEG	Generalized spike and wave pattern	Consider other generalized epilepsy syndromes (see chapter E.01 Epilepsy)
		Focal interictal epileptic discharge in the absence of generalized spike and wave pattern	Consider dialeptic seizures (absences) in focal epilepsy
		Lack of interictal epileptic discharges	Long-term EEG video monitoring

E.07 Juvenile myoclonic epilepsy | PCS-Diagnosis 1/1

Epilepsy

Medical history and clinical findings	EEG: awake plus hyperventilation and photic stimulation	Sleep-EEG including falling asleep and awakening (Note: sleep deprivation may provoke GTCS)	Long-term video-EEG	Imaging	Diagnosis	Differential diagnosis
▶ (Bilateral) myoclonia especially in the first hour after waking up ▶ Self report: patients tend to trivialize myoclonic jerks ▶ Parents tend to report myoclonic jerks as clumsiness ▶ Patients may show generalized tonic-clonic seizures (GTCS), especially after waking up, potentially provoked by sleep deprivation or drinking alcohol ▶ Patients may show absence symptoms ▶ Patients may have a positive family history ▶ Normal development ▶ Normal neurological findings	Generalized polyspikes with or without myoclonia Possible and/or additional features: – Polyspike waves – Irregular fast spike-wave-complexes – Photoparoxysmal response with or without photoconvulsive reaction				JME	PME[1] JAE[2]
	Focal epileptic discharges	Additional polyspikes		MRI	JME possible	PME
		Focal epileptic discharges		MRI	Focal epilepsy possible	PME
	Normal	Generalized polyspikes with or without myoclonia Possible and/or additional features: – Polyspike waves – Irregular fast spike-wave-complexes – Photoparoxysmal response with or without photoconvulsive reaction			JME	PME JAE
		Focal epileptic discharges		MRI	Focal epilepsy possible	PME
		Normal	Possible and/or additional features: – Polyspike-waves – Irregular fast spike-wave-complexes – Photoparoxysmal response with or without photoconvulsive reaction		JME	PME JAE
			Focal epileptic discharges	MRI	Focal epilepsy possible	PME
			Normal	MRI	JME unlikely, Other epilepsy types possible	

1 PME: Progressive myoclonus epilepsy
2 JAE: Juvenile absence epilepsy

E.07 Juvenile myoclonic epilepsy | PCS-Therapy

Choice of drugs	Treatment strategies	Gender	1. Choice (with initial target dose)	2. Choice	Further options
Check for possible contraindications to specific drugs (for example Valproic acid: hepatopathy or coagulopathy). Consider individual factors like body weight (increase of body weight by Valproic acid, decrease of body weight by Topiramate). Psychotropic effects of several drugs should be avoided (Levetiracetam in ADHD) or used (antidepressive effects of Lamotrigine) as appropriate. The extent of stress caused by severe and frequent seizures may influence the choice of drugs (e.g. only slow titration of Lamotrigine possible).	The aim is seizure freedom with normalization of EEG and without intolerable side effects. If required, drug doses may be increased up to the first appearance of undesirable side effects. Consider drug interactions when changing from one to another drug or when treating with a combination of drugs.	Female	Lamotrigine 2–4 mg/kg/d	Combination with Levetiracetam	Valproic acid, Topiramate, Ethosuximide, Phenobarbital, Sulthiame
			Levetiracetam 30–40 mg/kg/d	Combination with Lamotrigine	Valproic acid, Topiramate, Ethosuximide, Phenobarbital, Sulthiame
		Male	Valproic acid 10–20 mg/kg/d	Combination with Lamotrigine	Levetiracetam, Topiramate, Ethosuximide, Phenobarbital, Sulthiame
			If there are any contraindications to Valproic acid, consider Lamotrigine 2–4 mg/kg/d or Levetiracetam 30–40 mg/kg/d	Combination of Levetiracetam + Lamotrigine	Valproic acid, Topiramate, Ethosuximide, Phenobarbital, Sulthiame

E.08 Localizing signs in epilepsy | PCS-Orientation 1/3

Time of onset in relation to the seizure	Category of symptoms	Type of sense or symptom	Lateralization	Relation to language-dominant hemisphere	Symptomatogenic zone	Typical epileptogenic zone	Diagnostic value
Preceding visible seizure onset, patient is able to report on onset	Aura	Abdominal aura	–	–	Insular	Mesio(temporal), insular, frontal, variable	Moderate
		Somatosensory aura with somatotopic march of paresthesia	Contralateral	–	Parietal	Parietal	High
		Somatosensory aura without any march	(Contralateral)	–	Parietal, supplementary motor area, insular	Variable	Moderate
		Pain	(Contralateral)	–	Insular, parietal	Insular, parietal	Moderate
		Gustatory aura	–	–	Temporal, parietal, insular	Variable	Low
		Olfactory aura	–	–	Frontobasal, limbic	Frontobasal, limbic	Moderate
		Acoustic aura	Possibly contralateral (when elementary), complex hallucinations without lateralization	–	G. temporalis superior	Temporal neocortical	High
		Elementary visual aura (flashes)	Contralateral	–	Visual cortex	Occipital	High
		Amaurosis	–	–	Parieto-occipital	Occipital, parietal, variable	Moderate
		Complex visual hallucination (colors, changes in size/shapes)	Possibly contralateral	–	Temporo-occipital, parieto-occipital	Occipital, temporal, parietal, variable	Moderate
		Psychic aura (fear, deja vu phenomenon)	–	–	Amygdalon	Temporal, variable	Moderate
		Vertigo	–	–	Parietal, insular, temporal, frontal	Parietal, insular, temporal, frontal, variable	Low
		Body scheme	Possibly contralateral	–	Parietal	Parietal, variable	Moderate

E.08 Localizing signs in epilepsy

E.08 Localizing signs in epilepsy | PCS-Orientation 2/3

Preceding visible seizure onset, patient is not able to report on onset (age, handicap)	Behavior	Change in behaviour: suggests focal onset	-	-	-	-	Low
		Looking for shelter: suggests focal onset	-	-	-	-	Low
		Crying: suggests focal onset	-	-	-	-	Low
		Rubbing stomach: suggests abdominal aura	-	-	-	Temporal, insular, frontal, variable	Low
		Rubbing eyes, seeking gaze, blinks: suggests visual aura	-	-	-	Occipital, temporal, parietal, variable	Low
		Grasping and kneading a limb: suggests somatosensory aura	Contralateral	-	-	Parietal, variable	Low
Visible ictal symptoms	Motor	Unilateral cloni	Contralateral	-	Precentral gyrus	Precentral gyrus, variable	High
		Version (forced eye/head version)	Contralateral	-	Supplementary motor area	Variable	Moderate
		Tonic extension of an extremity, unilateral dystonia	Contralateral	-	Supplementary motor area	Variable	Moderate
		Figure sign of 4 (extension of one arm, flexion of the other just before secondary generalization)	Contralateral to extended arm	-	Supplementary motor area	Variable	High
		Asymmetric spasms	Contralateral	-	-	-	Low
		Unilateral automatisms	Ipsilateral	-	-	Temporal, variable	Moderate
		Nystagmus (fast component)	Contralateral	-	-	Occipital, variable	Moderate
		Unilateral lid myoclonia	Ipsilateral	-	-	Frontal and occipital, variable	Moderate
		Ictal smile in infants	-	-	-	Parieto-occipital, temporal	Low
		Dysphagia	-	-	Opercular	Opercular, insular, variable	Low

E.08 Localizing signs in epilepsy | PCS-Orientation 3/3

	Language	Speech arrest and preserved responsiveness	-	Dominant	-	Temporal, variable	Moderate
		Paraphasia and preserved responsiveness	-	Dominant	-	Temporal, variable	Moderate
		Automatisms and preserved language function and responsiveness	-	Non-dominant	-	Temporal, frontal, variable	Moderate
		Dysprosodia	-	Non-dominant	-	Temporal, variable	Low
	Vegetative, other	Vomiting	-	Non-dominant	Insular	Temporal, parieto-occipital, insular, variable	Moderate
		Drinking	-	Non-dominant	-	Temporal, variable	Low
		Bradycardia	-	Dominant	Insular	Temporal, variable	Low
		Spitting	-	Dominant	-	Temporal, variable	Low
		Urination in focal seizure		Non-dominant	-	Temporal, variable	Low
Postictal symptoms	Motor	Unilateral paresis	Contralateral	-	-	Precentral gyrus, variable	High
		Unilateral nose rubbing	Ipsilateral	-	-	Temporal, variable	Low
	Language	Aphasia	-	Dominant	-	Temporal, variable	Moderate
	Vegetative, other	Unilateral headache	Ipsilateral	-	-	Temporal, parieto-occipital, variable	Low
		Recall of complete seizure situation	-	Non-dominant	-	Frontal, temporal, variable	Low
		Lateral tongue bite	Contralateral	-	-	-	Moderate

E.09 Therapeutic strategies in different electroclinical epilepsy syndromes | PCS-Therapy 1/6

Epilepsy

Typical age of manifestation	Electroclinical syndrome	Specific considerations before starting treatment	First choice (including first target dose)	Second choice	Further options	Established combinations	Deterioration possible/typically by …	Don't forget …	In case of two failed adequate treatment periods, consider …
Neonate	Neonatal seizures	-	Phenobarbital (starting dose 10 mg/kg, maintenance 5 mg/kg/d)	Levetiracetam, Topiramate	Phenytoin, benzodiazepines, Lidocaine	-	-	Pyridoxine 3 × 100 mg IV Pyridoxal phosphate 3 × 100 mg/kg p.o. Folinic acid 3–5 mg/kg in 3 SD IV	-
	Ohtahara syndrome, Early myoclonic encephalopathy	Avoid Valproic acid if metabolic aetiology can not be ruled out	Phenobarbital (starting dose 10 mg/kg, maintenance 5 mg/kg/d)	Levetiracetam, Topiramate, Valproic acid	Sulthiame, Vigabatrin, Lamotrigine, Bromides, Phenytoin Zonisamide	Phenobarbital + Phenytoin, Valproic acid + Lamotrigine, Topiramate + Levetiracetam	Carbamazepine/Oxcarbazepine, Lamotrigine, Sodium channel blockers may be very effective in some genetic etiologies (KCNQ1, SCN2A …), occasionally Vigabatrin (Myoclonia)		Pharmacoresistance usual, high mortality
1–18 months	Benign myoclonic epilepsy	Because of the generally good prognosis, drug-based treatment may not be necessary	Valproic acid (20–30 mg/kg/d)	Lamotrigine	Ethosuximide, Sulthiame, Topiramate	Avoid!	Carbamazepine/Oxcarbazepine	-	Reconsider the diagnosis: Myoclonic-astatic epilepsy? Focal epilepsy? Progressive myoclonus epilepsy?
	Benign familial/non-familial epilepsy of infancy	Because of the generally good prognosis, drug-based treatment may not be necessary	Carbamazepine/Oxcarbazepine (10 mg/kg/d)	Sulthiame, Levetiracetam	-	Avoid!	-	-	Reconsider the diagnosis: Focal epilepsy of other aetiology?
	Infantile spasms	Fast and aggressive therapy. Vigabatrin is the drug of choice in tuberous sclerosis complex.	Vigabatrin (> 100 mg/kg/d)	Corticosteroids (different regiments) ACTH	Sulthiame, Valproic acid, Topiramate, Levetiracetam, Zonisamide, Rufinamide, Lamotrigine, Ketogenic diet	-	Carbamazepine/Oxcarbazepine	Early onset: Consider Pyridoxine, Pyridoxalphosphate, Folinic acid as above	Pharmacoresistance common

E.09 Therapeutic strategies in different electroclinical epilepsy syndromes | PCS-Therapy 2/6

		Corticosteroids (different regiments) ACTH	Vigabatrin	Sulthiame, Valproic acid, Topiramate, Levetiracetam, Zonisamide, Rufinamide, Lamotrigine, Ketogenic diet	-	Carbamazepine/ Oxcarbazepine	Early onset: Consider Pyridoxin/PALP/Folinic acid as above	Pharmacoresistance common
Dravet syndrome	Consider early combination therapy. Seizure freedom is not the primary aim of therapy. Aggressive treatment of status epilepticus!	Valproic acid 20–30 mg/kg/d	Bromides, Topiramate	Clobazam, Stiripentol, Ketogenic diet	Valproic acid + Stiripentol + Clobazam Bromides + Valproic acid Bromides + Valproic acid + Clobazam Bromides + Valproic acid + Topiramate	Carbamazepine/ Oxcarbazepine, Lamotrigine, Phenytoin	-	Pharmacoresistance common
		Bromides (40–50 mg/kg/d)	Valproic acid, Topiramate	Clobazam, Stiripentol, Ketogenic diet	Valproic acid + Stiripentol + Clobazam Bromides + Valproic acid Bromides + Valproic acid + Clobazam Bromides + Valproic acid + Topiramate	Carbamazepine/ Oxcarbazepine, Lamotrigine, Phenytoin	-	Pharmacoresistance common
		Valproic acid (20–30 mg/kg/d) plus Clobazam (0,2–03 mg/kg/d) plus Stiripentol (30–50 mg/kg/D)	Bromides, Topiramate	Clobazam, Stiripentol, Ketogenic diet	Valproic acid + Stiripentol + Clobazam Bromides + Valproic acid Bromides+ Valproic acid + Clobazam Bromides + Valproic acid + Topiramate	Carbamazepine/ Oxcarbazepine, Lamotrigine, Phenytoin	-	Pharmacoresistance common

E.09 Therapeutic strategies in different electroclinical epilepsy syndromes | PCS-Therapy 3/6

18 months to 5 years								
Myoclonic astatic epilepsy (Doose syndrome)	If onset with generalized tonic-clonic seizures or in the case of failure after first step: Fast and aggressive therapy.	Valproic acid 20–30 mg/kg/d	Lamotrigine, Ethosuximide, Ketogenic diet	Topiramate, Levetiracetam, Zonisamide, Bromides, Rufinamide, Clobazam, Stiripentol	Valproic acid + Lamotrigine Valproic acid + Ethosuximide Valproic acid + Ethosuximide + Lamotrigine	Carbamazepine/ Oxcarbazepine, Phenytoin. In some cases Lamotrigine (Myoclonia)	Avoid side effects with fatigue because of the risk to aggravate seizures. 50 % fast response vs. 50 % pharmacoresistance	Pharmacoresistance common. Exclude GLUT-1 deficiency. Differential diagnosis Lennox-Gastaut syndrome, progressive myoclonus epilepsy
Lennox-Gastaut syndrome	Seizure freedom is not the primary aim of therapy. Aggressive treatment of convulsive and non-convulsive status epilepticus!	Valproic acid 20–30 mg/kg/d	Lamotrigine, Topiramate, Clobazam, Rufinamide	Felbamate, Zonisamide, Vagus nerve simulation, Levetiracetam, Bromides, Stiripentol, Ethosuximide, Methsuximide, Ketogenic diet	Valproic acid + Lamotrigine Valproic acid + Topiramate Valproic acid + Rufinamide	Atypical absences, myoclonia: Carbamazepine/Oxcarbazepine, Phenytoin, in some cases Vigabatrin, Lamotrigine; Rarely tonic seizure aggravation by Benzodiazepines	Avoid side effects with fatigue because of the risk to aggravate seizures. -	Pharmacoresistance usual. Differential diagnosis: neurodegenerative diseases. In case of focal features (MRI lesion and/or constant EEG focus) and/or one prominent focal seizure semiology: Presurgical evaluation.
Early onset absence epilepsy	Exclude GLUT1 deficiency (= Ketogene diet treatment of choice)	Valproic acid 20–30 mg/kg/d	Ethosuximide or Valproic acid depending on first step	Lamotrigine, Sulthiame, Levetiracetam, Topiramate, Ketogenic diet	Valproic acid + Ethosuximide Valproic acid + Lamotrigine	Carbamazepine/ Oxcarbazepine, Phenytoin, Vigabatrin	-	Differential diagnosis: frontal lobe epilepsy, neurometabolic disease
Panayiotopoulos syndrome	Because of the good prognosis, drug-based treatment may not be necessary	Carbamazepine/ Oxcarbazepine/ Ethosuximide 20 mg/kg/d	Sulthiame, Levetiracetam	Valproic acid, Topiramate, Lamotrigine	Avoid!	-	-	Reconsider diagnosis: focal epilepsy of other aetiology?
CSWS, Landau-Kleffner syndrome, Atypical partial epilepsy	Fast and aggressive therapy.	Sulthiame 4–6 mg/kg/d	Clobazam, Levetiracetam, Corticosteroids (various regiments)	Topiramate, Valproic acid, Ethosuximide, Zonisamide, Ketogenic diet	Valproic acid + Ethosuximide+ Clobazam	Carbamazepine/ Oxcarbazepine, Lamotrigine may aggravate CSWS and negative myoclonus	-	Diagnosis of structural aetiology, differential diagnosis: neurometabolic disease. Consider presurgical evaluation. Consider genetic testing for GRIN2A.

E.09 Therapeutic strategies in different electroclinical epilepsy syndromes | PCS-Therapy 4/6

Age	Syndrome	Notes	1st line		2nd line	Avoid	Alternative		Goal	Differential diagnosis
5 to 10 years	Childhood absence epilepsy	-	Ethosuximide 20 mg/kg/d	Valproic acid	Lamotrigine, Sulthiame, Topiramate, Levetiracetam	Ethosuximide + Valproic acid Valproic acid + Lamotrigine	Carbamazepine/ Oxcarbazepine, Phenytoin, Vigabatrin	-		Differential diagnosis: frontal lobe epilepsy, exclude GLUT1-deficiency
	Rolandic epilepsy (benign focal epilepsy with centrotemporal spikes, BECTS)	Because of the good prognosis, drug-based treatment may not be necessary	Sulthiame 4–6 mg/kg/d	Levetiracetam, Oxcarbazepine	Valproic acid, Lamotrigine, Topiramate	Avoid!	Carbamazepine/ Oxcarbazepine, Lamotrigine may provoke CSWS and negative myoclonus in atypical cases	-		Reconsider diagnosis: focal epilepsy of structural aetiology?
> 10 years	Juvenile myoclonic epilepsy (Janz syndrome), juvenile absence epilepsy	Check for possible contraindications to specific substances (e.g. Valproic acid: hepatopathy or coagulopathy). Consider individual factors like gender (possible teratogenic effects of Valproic acid), body weight (increase of body weight by Valproic acid, decrease of body weight by Topiramate). Psychotropic effects of several drugs should be avoided (Levetiracetam in ADHD) or used (anti-depressive effects of Lamotrigine) as appropriate. The extent of stress caused by severe and frequent seizures may influence the choice of drugs (e.g., only slow titration of Lamotrigine possible).	Lamotrigine 2–4 mg/kg/d	Combination with Levetiracetam	Valproic acid (if possible), Topiramate, Ethosuximide, Phenobarbital, Sulthiame	Levetiracetam+ Lamotrigine If possible: Valproic acid + Lamotrigine Valproic acid + Levetiracetam	Regarding myoclonia: Carbamazepine/Oxcarbazepine, Phenytoin and sometimes Lamotrigine	Treatment aims to achieve seizure freedom with normalization of EEG and without intolerable side effects.		Reconsider diagnosis: structural aetiology, frontal lobe epilepsy? Differential diagnosis: progressive myoclonus epilepsy
			Levetiracetam 30–40 mg/kg/d	Combination with Lamotrigine	Valproic acid (if possible), Topiramate, Ethosuximide, Phenobarbital, Sulthiame	Levetiracetam + Lamotrigine If possible: Valproic acid + Lamotrigine Valproic acid + Levetiracetam	Regarding myoclonia: Carbamazepine/Oxcarbazepine, Phenytoin and sometimes Lamotrigine	Treatment aims to achieve seizure freedom with normalization of EEG and without intolerable side effects.		Structural aetiology, frontal lobe epilepsy? Differential diagnosis: progressive myoclonus epilepsy
			Valproic acid 20 mg/kg/d	Combination with Levetiracetam or Lamotrigine	Topiramate, Ethosuximide, Phenobarbital, Sulthiame	Valproic acid + Lamotrigine Valproic acid + Levetiracetam Levetiracetam + Lamotrigine	Regarding myoclonia: Carbamazepine/Oxcarbazepine, Phenytoin and sometimes Lamotrigine	Treatment aims to achieve seizure freedom with normalization of EEG and without intolerable side effects.		Structural aetiology, frontal lobe epilepsy? Differential diagnosis: progressive myoclonus epilepsy
								-	-	

E.09 Therapeutic strategies in different electroclinical epilepsy syndromes | PCS-Therapy 5/6

Epilepsy

	Epilepsy with generalized tonic-clonic seizures on awakening	Check for possible contraindications to specific substances (e.g. Valproic acid: hepatopathy or coagulopathy). Consider individual factors like gender (possible teratogenic effects of Valproic acid), body weight (increase of body weight by Valproic acid, decrease of body weight by Topiramate). Psychotropic effects of several drugs should be avoided (Levetiracetam in ADHD) or used (anti-depressive effects of Lamotrigine) as appropriate. The extent of stress caused by severe and frequent seizures may influence the choice of drugs (e.g., only slow titration of Lamotrigine possible).	Levetiracetam 30–40 mg/kg/d	Combination with Lamotrigine	Valproic acid (if possible), Topiramate, Phenobarbital, Zonisamide	Levetiracetam + Lamotrigine If possible: Valproic acid + Lamotrigine Valproic acid + Levetiracetam			Structural aetiology, frontal lobe epilepsy?
			Valproic acid 20 mg/kg/d	Combination with Levetiracetam or Lamotrigine	Topiramate, Phenobarbital, Zonisamide	Valproic acid + Lamotrigine Valproic acid + Levetiracetam Levetiracetam + Lamotrigine	-	-	Structural aetiology, frontal lobe epilepsy?
Independent of age	Non idiopathic focal epilepsy with or without known structural aetiology (MRI lesion)	Sufficient time to establish treatment	Lamotrigine 1–5 mg/kg/d	Levetiracetam, Oxcarbazepine	Sulthiame, Topiramate, Zonisamide, Lacosamide, Valproic acid, Pregabalin, Retigabine, Perampanel, Tiagabine, Vigabatrin, Vagus nerve simulation, Ketogenic diet	-	-	-	Presurgical evaluation! See chapter E.10 Epilepsy surgery

E.09 Therapeutic strategies in different electroclinical epilepsy syndromes | PCS-Therapy 6/6

Some time to establish treatment	Oxcarbazepine 20 mg/kg/d	Levetiracetam, Lamotrigine	Sulthiame, Topiramate, Zonisamide, Lacosamide, Valproic acid, Pregabalin, Retigabine, Perampanel, Tiagabine, Vigabatrin, Vagus nerve simulation, Ketogenic diet	-	-	-	Presurgical evaluation! See chapter E.10 Epilepsy surgery
No time to establish treatment	Levetiracetam 40 mg/kg/d	Oxcarbazepine, Lamotrigine	Sulthiame, Topiramate, Zonisamide, Lacosamide, Valproic acid, Pregabalin, Retigabine, Perampanel, Tiagabine, Vigabatrin, Vagus nerve simulation, Ketogenic diet	-	-	-	Presurgical evaluation! See chapter E.10 Epilepsy surgery

E.10 Epilepsy surgery | PCS-Diagnosis/Therapy 1/4

Epilepsy

Indication	Basic diagnostic work-up		Further non-invasive diagnostic work-up		Invasive diagnostic work-up		Therapy
Potential epileptogenic lesion irrespective of seizure semiology Or Clear partial seizures irrespective of MRI findings Or MRI negative epilepsy in children under 2 years And Pharmacoresistance (= no seizure control after **two** treatment attempts with appropriately selected drugs and adequate dose regimens)	Medical history ▶ Epilepsy ▶ Seizure semiology ▶ Prior treatment/ drugs ▶ Development Long-term video EEG ▶ Non-invasive ▶ At least for 72 hours ▶ Ictal recording(s) ▶ Optional Sphenoidal electrodes High-resolution MRI with epilepsy-specific protocol (Neuro-)psychological examination with standardized tests	Clear apparent epileptogenic lesion And Clear evidence for epileptogenic zone and its extent And clear Delineation of eloquent cortical areas					Standard resection (standard temporal lobectomy with or without amygdalohippocampectomy, selective amygdalohippocampectomy, frontal lobe resection, multilobectomy, functional hemispherotomy) Or Lesionectomy, topectomy
		Clear apparent epileptogenic lesion And Clear evidence for epileptogenic zone and its extent But No delineation of eloquent cortical areas	*Language* fMRI *Motor function* fMRI, WADA, TMS, MEG[1], MRI-DTI (fiber tracking) *Somatosensory* fMRI, MEG[1], MRI-DTI *Visual cortex* fMRI, perimetry MRI-DTI (fiber tracking)	▶ Delineation of eloquent cortical areas			Standard resection Or Lesionectomy, topectomy possibly with intraoperative ECoG[1]
				▶ No delineation of eloquent cortical areas	Subdural grid and/or stripe electrodes/ depth electrodes stereo-EEG	▶ Resection possible	Tailored resection
						▶ Resection not possible	Consider (palliative) incomplete resection and/or multiple subpial transections Or No surgery
		Clearly apparent epileptogenic lesion But No evidence for epileptogenic zone and its extent	PET Ictal SPECT, SISCOM[1] MEG[1] 3T-MRI	Evidence for extent of epileptogenic zone and clear delineation of eloquent cortical areas			Standard resection Or Lesionectomy, topectomy possibly with intraoperative ECoG[1]

E.10 Epilepsy surgery | PCS-Diagnosis/Therapy 2/4

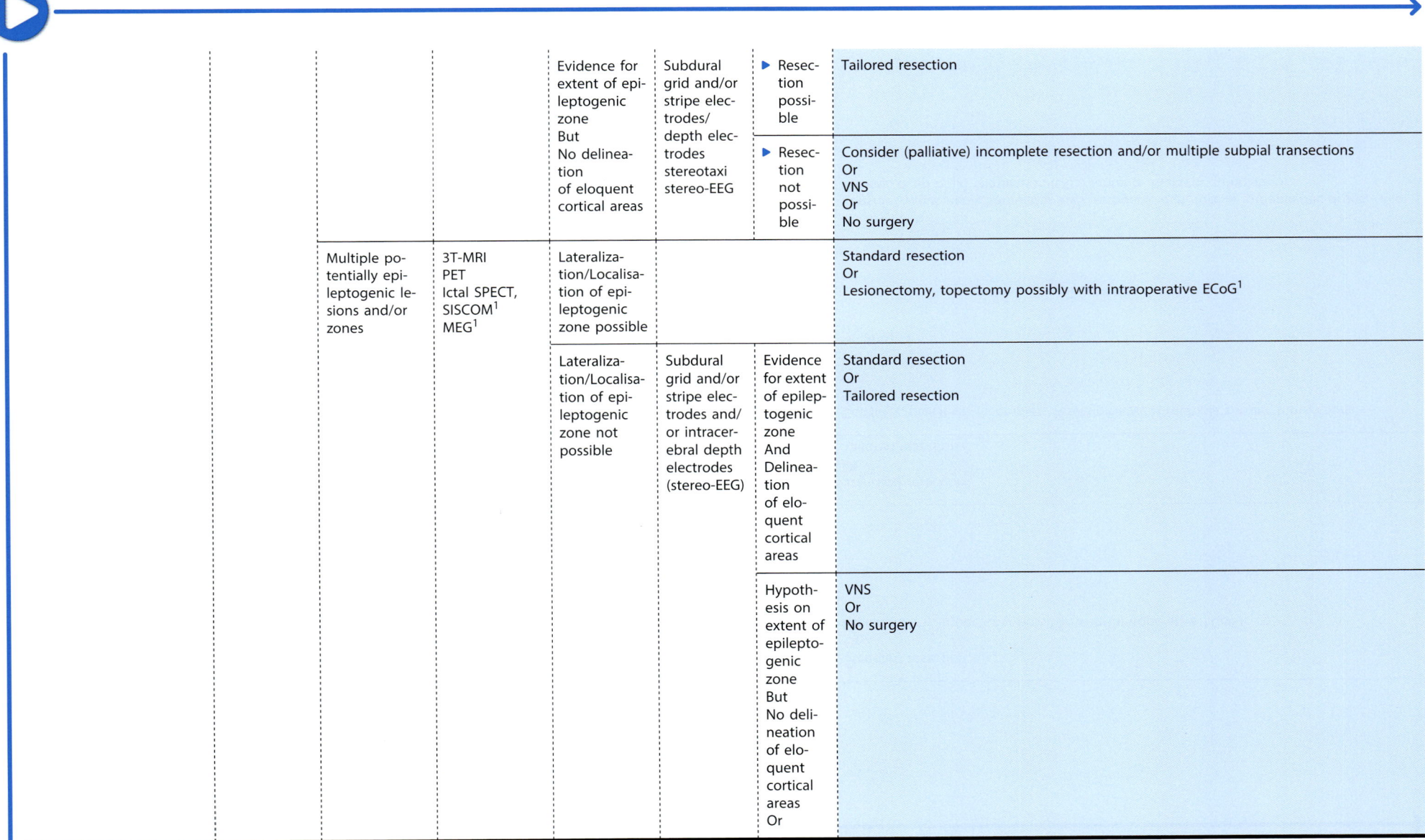

E.10 Epilepsy surgery | PCS-Diagnosis/Therapy 3/4

Epilepsy

				No evidence for epileptogenic zone	
Evidence for epileptogenic zone But No lesion	3T-MRI MRI post-processing PET Ictal SPECT, SISCOM[1] MEG[1]	Concordant results regarding extent of epileptogenic zone and delineation of eloquent cortical areas			Standard resection Or Lesionectomy, topectomy possibly with intraoperative ECoG[1]
		Concordant results regarding localization of epileptogenic zone But not regarding its extent Or No delineation of eloquent cortical areas	Subdural grid and/or stripe/ depths electrodes stereo-EEG electrodes and/or intracerebral depth electrodes (stereo-EEG)	Resection possible	Standard resection Or Tailored resection
				Resection not possible	Consider (palliative) incomplete resection and/or multiple subpial transections Or VNS Or No surgery
		Discordant or completely negative results			No resection Consider vagus nerve stimulator VNS, ketogenic diet, further antiepileptic drugs, callosotomy, deep brain stimulation (DBS) (anterior thalamic stimulation)
Epileptogenic zone But Resection not possible					
No epileptogenic lesion and no evi-					

E.10 Epilepsy surgery

E.10 Epilepsy surgery | PCS-Diagnosis/Therapy 4/4

dence for epileptogenic zone

Generalized Epilepsy
And
Palliative surgery considered

1 SISCOM: Substraction Ictal Spect Co-Registered to MRI
   MEG: Magnetoencephalogram
   ECoG: Electrocorticogram

Notes

Notes

F Vertigo

F.01 Vertigo and dizziness | PCS-Diagnosis 1/1

Medical history
- Acute/chronic
- Attacks/sustained
- Provoking factors
- Accompanying symptoms
- Migraine/family history

Clinical findings
- Peripheral vestibular deficit (head impulse test)
- Ocular motor deficits
- Auditory deficit
- Other neurological signs

Acute vertigo (< 4 weeks)	With auditory deficit ▶ Otoscopy ▶ Audiogram ▶ Nystagmogram	**Look for** ▶ Fever (labyrinthitis); *Note:* meningeal signs ▶ Trauma (CT, tests for Benign paroxysmal positional vertigo (BPPV) and perilymph fistula) ▶ Toxins (aminoglycosides, diuretics, ASA) ▶ Ear pressure (Menière's disease) ▶ Short attacks (sec: vestibular paroxysmia) ▶ Central ocular motor and neurological signs (→ MRI) ▶ Iritis/uveitis (autoimmune: e.g. Cogan's syndrome)		
	Without auditory deficit ▶ Otoscopy ▶ Nystagmogram	**Look for** ▶ Trauma ▶ BPPV, perilymph fistula ▶ Central ocular motor signs (MRI) ▶ Ataxia (→ MRI)	**Duration** ▶ Seconds – minutes	▶ Differential diagnosis – < 6y: Benign paroxysmal vertigo of childhood – On changing head position: BPPV – Orthostatic; vestibular paroxysmia – EEG: epileptic aura (rare)
			Duration ▶ Minutes – hours	▶ Differential diagnosis with headache: vestibular migraine with ear pressure: Menière's disease
			Duration ▶ Hours – days	▶ Differential diagnosis acute unilateral failure (vestibular neuritis)
Chronic Vertigo (> 4 weeks)	With auditory deficit ▶ Otoscopy ▶ Audiogram ▶ Nystagmogram ▶ CT/MRI	**Look for** ▶ Central ocular motor and neurological signs (e.g. brain stem/cerebellar tumor) ▶ Bilateral vestibulopathy (head impulse test; e.g. toxic: aminoglycoside) ▶ Inner ear malformation and inherited vestibular areflexia		
	Without auditory deficit ▶ Otoscopy ▶ Nystagmogram	**Look for** ▶ Psychopathology: anxiety, phobia, depression (somatoform vertigo) ▶ Bilateral vestibulopathy (head impulse test; e.g. idiopathic) ▶ Central ocular motor and neurological signs (→ MRI: e.g. brain stem/cerebellar tumor)		

F.01 Vertigo and dizziness | PCS-Therapy 1/2

Basic therapy	Syndrome	Standard therapy	Additional therapy
▶ Counseling about mechanisms, symptoms, course based on history, physical examination, and selected laboratory tests ▶ Use a diary to document attack frequency ▶ Nausea/vomiting: Dimenhydrinate 1–2 mg/kg (every 6 h if required) Suppositories Body weight 6–15 kg: 40 mg 1 × per day Body weight 15–25 kg: 40 mg 2–3 × per day Age 6–14 years. 70 mg 2–3 × per day Age > 14 years. 150 mg 1–2 × per day	**Migraine-associated vertigo** ▶ Benign paroxysmal vertigo of childhood (BPV) ▶ Vestibular migraine ▶ Basilar-type migraine	▶ Counseling about the favourable prognosis ▶ Non-pharmacological prophylaxis: – Avoid triggers – Relaxation techniques – Regular exercises/sports – Sufficient fluid intake	Pharmacological prophylaxis with > 3 attacks per month of sufficient severity: ▶ Magnesium aspartate 200–600 mg/d ▶ Propranolol 1–2 mg/kg/d ▶ Metoprolol succinate 1 mg/kg/d ▶ Topiramate 1–2 mg/kg/d ▶ Amitriptyline 1 mg/kg/d ▶ Valproic acid 10–45 mg/kg/d
	Benign paroxysmal positioning vertigo (BPPV) ▶ Posterior semicircular canal (> 90 %) ▶ Horizontal semicircular canal (< 10 %)	Specific liberatory maneuvers ▶ Posterior canal: – Semont/Epley ▶ Horizontal canal: – Lempert (Barbecue)/Gufari – Prolonged rest on unaffected side (> 12 h)	Symptomatic therapy for nausea if necessary
	Motion sickness/Kinetosis	▶ Non-pharmacological prophylaxis: – Sufficient visual control – Prevention of head movements distraction	Pharmacological prophylaxis: ▶ Dimenhydrinate 1–2 mg/kg, every 6 hours if required
	Acute unilateral vestibular failure ▶ Labyrinthitis – Viral – Bacterial (e.g. with meningitis) – Autoimmune (e.g. Cogan's syndrome) ▶ Trauma (e.g. with temporal bone fracture) ▶ Vestibular neuritis ▶ Menière's disease	In general: ▶ Symptomatic basic therapy ▶ Early mobilization (to support central compensation) ▶ Specific therapy of underlying disorder	**Viral:** in Zoster oticus: Aciclovir 5 mg/kg/d/SD × 3; otherwise symptomatic **Bacterial:** specific antibiotics **Autoimmune:** steroids, e.g. Prednisolone 1 mg/kg/d, tapering off over 5 to 10 days **Vestibular neuritis:** Prednisolone 1 mg/kg/d, every 3rd day reduce by 20 % **Menière's disease:** Betahistine 1–2 mg/kg/d (insufficient data for children)
	Vestibular paroxysmia	Carbamazepine – 2–6 mg/kg/d – 1–5 y: 100–200 mg/d – 6–10 y: 100–400 mg/d – 11–15 y: 100–600 mg/d – > 15 y: 200–800 mg/d	As an alternative: Oxcarbazepine 4–8 mg/kg/d

F.01 Vertigo and dizziness | PCS-Therapy 2/2

Perilymph fistula ▶ External fistula to the middle ear (after trauma, infection, cholesteatoma) ▶ Internal fistula to the middle intracranial fossa (superior canal dehiscence)	▶ Therapy of underlying disorder ▶ Avoid triggers ▶ Surgery is rarely necessary	
Bilateral vestibulopathy ▶ Congenital ▶ Infection (e.g. bacterial meningitis) ▶ Toxic (e.g. aminoglykoside) ▶ Malnutrition (e.g. Vitamin B_{12} deficiency) ▶ Autoimmune (e.g. Cogan's syndrome) ▶ Degenerative (e.g. spinocerebellar ataxia) ▶ Neoplastic (e.g. bilateral vestibular schwannoma) ▶ Idiopathic	In general: ▶ Training: balance, gait, visual, and somatosensory systems ▶ Specific therapy of underlying disorder if possible	
Central vestibular syndromes ▶ Neoplastic (e.g. brain stem/cerebellar tumor) ▶ Degenerative/hereditary (e.g. spinocerebellar ataxia, episodic ataxia type II) ▶ Inflammatory (e.g. brain stem encephalitis) ▶ Vascular (e.g. vascular malformation) ▶ Traumatic (e.g. brain stem contusion) ▶ Epileptic (e.g. vestibular aura)	Therapy depends on specific cause (see last column: additional therapy)	**Episodic ataxia type II** ▶ Acetazolamide 5–10 mg/kg/d ▶ 4-Aminopyridine 5 mg/d/SD × 1–3 (carefully consider each individual case, insufficient experience in children) **Downbeat/upbeat nystagmus** ▶ 4-Aminopyridine (see above)
Somatoform vertigo	▶ Counseling ▶ Psychotherapy	Specific therapy depends on psychopathology and psychodynamics

Notes

Notes

G Movement disorders

G.01 Cerebral palsy | PCS-Diagnosis 1/2

Movement disorders

**History
(Motor) Development?**
- Delayed developmental milestones
- Abnormal movement/movement patterns

Risk factors?
- Prenatal[1]
- Perinatal/Neonatal[2]
- Postnatal[3]

Type of muscle tone disorder?
- **Hypertonia**
- **Spasticity**
  - Resistance increases with increasing speed of passive stretch
  - "Catch" = sudden blocking on fast passive stretch or when reaching a certain joint angle.
  - Pathological reflexes
- **Dyskinesia**
  - Variable muscle tone
    - Dystonia: involuntary sustained or intermittent muscle contractions causing twisting and repetitive movements, abnormal postures or movements
  - Choreoathetosis: normal muscle tone during rest, hyperkinetic movements
- **Ataxia**
  - Ataxia during standing, walking
  - Ataxia of the trunk
  - Dysmetria, hypermetria, asynergy, dysdiadochokinesia
  - Generalized hypotonia

**Severity of motor disorder?
Mobility**
Gross Motor Function Classification System (GMFCS)

GMFCS Level[4]:
- I
- II
- III
- IV
- V

Hand-use in daily activities:
Manual Ability Classification System (MACS)

MACS Level[5]:
- I
- II
- III
- IV
- V

Not movement-related problems?
- Sensitivity
- Disorders of vision or hearing
- Mental retardation
- Speech and language disorders
- Behavioral disturbances
- Epilepsy
- Secondary muscular skeletal disturbances

Body regions?
- Bilateral
- Arms and legs
- Trunk
- Bulbar disturbances

Body regions?
- **Unilateral**

MRI:
- Cerebral malformation
- Cerebral lesion
  - Periventricular leukomalacia
  - Basal ganglia
  - Bilateral cortical/subcortical lesions

X-ray of hip joints (Rippstein I)
- Reimer's migration index
  - < 22 % right/left
  - 23–49 % right/left
  - > 50 % right/left

MRI:
- Cerebral malformation
- Cerebral lesion
  - Periventricular infarction
  - Parenchymal lesion after bleeding
  - Unilateral cortical/subcortical lesions
- **Diagnostic work-up thrombophilia[6]**

Cerebral Palsy[7]
- **Bilateral spastic CP**
- **Bilateral dyskinetic CP**
  - Dystonic
  - Choreoathetotic
- **Ataxic CP**
- **Hip joints**
  - Normal right/left
  - Subluxation right/left
  - Dislocation right/left

Cerebral Palsy[7]
- **Spastic unilateral CP**
- **Unilateral spastic dyskinetic CP**
  - Dystonic
  - Choreoathetotic

G.01 Cerebral palsy

G.01 Cerebral palsy | PCS-Diagnosis 2/2 — Movement disorders

▶ Progressive Disorder ▶ Deterioration of abilities or change of clinical symptoms ▶ Micro- or macrocephalus ▶ Neurological disorder other than CP present in family history **Clinical presentation** Signs of ▶ Elevated (distal) muscle tone ▶ Paresis ▶ Trunk hypotonia ▶ Reduced selective motor control e.g. extension of the foot ▶ Disturbed fine motor abilities ▶ Dysmorphic features ▶ Skin	▶ No anomaly of muscle tone	**DD guided by clinical symptoms** ▶ Paresis ▶ Hypotonia	Neuromuscular disorder (see chapter O.01 Neuromuscular disroders) Genetic syndrome (see chapter L.01 Genetics) Metabolic disorder (see chapter N.01 Neurometabolic disorders) Neurodegenerative diseases incl. leukodystrophy (see chapter N.02 Neurodegenerative disorders) Hereditary spastic paraplegia DD Dystonia (see chapter G.02 Dystonia) DD Choreoathetosis DD Ataxia (see chapter A.04 Acute Ataxia)
	▶ Pathologic muscle tone present	**DD guided by clinical symptoms** ▶ Spasticity ▶ Dystonia ▶ Choreoathetosis ▶ Ataxia	

1 Twin gestation, feto-fetal transfusion syndrome, fetal growth retardation, placental insufficiency, maternal infection, intrauterine infection, TORCH syndrome, chromosomal aberration with cerebral malformation.
2 Chorioamnionitis, placental separation with haemorrhage, infections (uterine and neonatal), thrombophilic disorders, neonatal encephalopathy (hypoxic ischaemic, check APGAR scores, evidence of metabolic acidosis in fetal umbilical arterial cord blood, pathological CTG, postpartal disturbance of liver and kidney function, neonatal ultrasound of the brain, icterus neonatorum)
3 Infections (e. g. meningitis, encephalitis), hypoxia due to near drowning events, traumatic brain injury, stroke. These events can cause a so called "post-neonatal cerebral palsy", although the authors question the usefulness of this term. Maybe in these "late" events a description of the brain lesion together with the clinical diagnosis is more accurate and informative compared to the umbrella term CP.
4 GMFCS: Illustration of the five levels for the age band 6 to 12 years. A detailed description can be found on the web: www.canchild.ca/en/measures/gmfcs.asp. We recommend to use the GMFCS expanded and revised version (2007). Description and illustrations can be found on the following web page: www.motorgrowth.canchild.ca/en/gmfcs/descriptors_and_illustrations.asp. Please note the copyright for the illustrations by Kerr Graham, The Royal Children's Hospital, Melbourne.

GMFCS Level I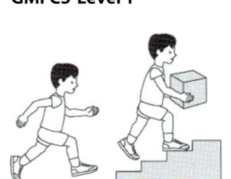

GMFCS Level II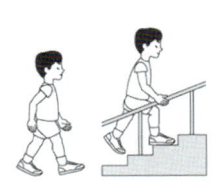

GMFCS Level III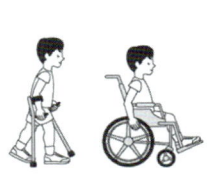

GMFCS Level IV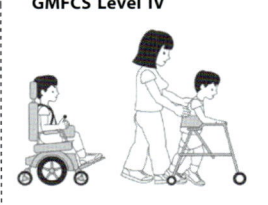

GMFCS Level V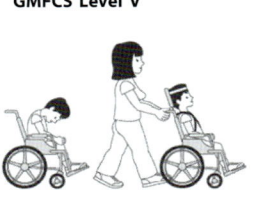

5 MACS describes how children with cerebral palsy use their hands to handle objects in daily activities. MACS I: handles objects easily and successfully. MACS II: handles most objects but with somewhat reduced quality and/or speed of achievement. MACS III: handles objects with difficulty; needs help to prepare and/or modify activities. MACS IV: handles a limited selection of easily managed objects. MACS V: does not handle objects and has severely limited ability to perform even simple tasks. For comprehensive information please visit www.macs.nu.
6 If an event suggests that the patient may have suffered a stroke: Look into the patient's history including family history with respect to thromboembolic events. Check for thrombophilia including factor V Leiden mutation, MTHFR polymorphism and prothrombin variation (genetic background) as well as functional tests like protein C activity.
7 In many children there will be signs of spasticity and possibly also dystonia. In such cases, classify according to the most prominent feature. Avoid terms like "mixed spastic dystonic cerebral palsy". Instead write down e. g. "bilateral spastic cerebral palsy with additional clinical signs of dystonia".

G.01 Cerebral palsy | PCS-Therapy 1/5

Basic therapy

Corrective exercises (physiotherapy, occupational therapy, oral motor therapy, speech therapy, and others)	▶ Goal setting: SMART (specific, measurable, action oriented, achievable, realistic and relevant, time-bound) ▶ Principles: stimulate and increase activity; keep in mind well known principles of motor learning; goal directed; include environmental factors; check and adapt intensity to the child's motivation and the clinical situation (e. g. post-operative); promote (motor) development; adapt to maturation and development of the individual child; educate caregivers; motivate the child and educate the parents to do and how to do activities and practice on their own; evaluate with adequate and standardized tests; test, recommend and adapt orthoses and aids; apply specific therapies, e. g. Constraint Induced Movement Therapy, treadmill training, robotic medicine, COOP) ▶ Framework: International Classification of Functioning, Disability and Health (ICF) ▶ Overall goal: As one important component of the multi-modal therapy, the aim is to support participation, independence, autonomy and increase quality of life.
Orthotics, aids, mobility-aids etc.	▶ Goal: increase function (e. g. compensate muscle weakness) or inhibit dysfunction (e. g. spastic pes equinus), promote activity and participation, improve biomechanical preconditions, prevent muscle shortening and malalignement of joints ▶ The GMFCS system is useful for goal setting and pre-selection of measures.

Muscle-tone modifying therapy

Muscle tone disturbance	Therapy		Note!
Spasticity, generalized	First choice	▶ Baclofen p.o. Start: 0,5 mg/kg as 3 SD, weekly increments of 0,5 mg/kg Maintenance: 2–5 mg/kg in 3–4 SD ▶ Diazepam Start: 0,25–0,5 mg/kg/d Maintenance: up to 1 mg/kg/d in 2–3 SD or ▶ Lorazepam Start: 0,05 mg/kg/d Maintenance: up to 0,2 mg/kg/d in 2–3 SD	▶ Limitations are increasing muscle weakness, trunk hypotonia, sedation, deterioration of swallowing or respiratory function. ▶ Benzodiazepines not useful for prolonged treatment (tachyphylaxis).
		▶ Baclofen intrathecal Dosage 150–2 000 mcg/24 h	▶ Side effects: obstipation, retention of urine, weakness ▶ Severe side effects: rarely overdose, acute withdrawal in case of malfunction of the system. Monitoring and treatment on an intensive care unit necessary for these cases. ▶ Good effect on proximal muscle groups, may be used in conjunction with Botulinum toxins for distal muscles.
	Second choice	▶ Tolperisone[1] Dosage for Mydocalm®: 6 months to 2 y. (5–12 kg) 25–50 mg/d; 3–5 y. (13–19 kg) 50–75 mg/d; 6–9 y. (20–29 kg) 75–100 mg/d; 10–12 y. (30–43 kg) 100–125 mg;	▶ Tolperisone: less sedation compared to benzodiazepines (and less effective?); side effects such as vertigo, dry mouth, arterial hypertonia, muscle weakness ▶ Dantrolene: regular laboratory tests for liver function

G.01 Cerebral palsy | PCS-Therapy 2/5

		13–14 y. (44–52 kg) 150 mg/d;
		Adolescents > 14 y. 150–450 mg/d;
		Dose recommendations (from Japan), preparation Muscalm®: 3–5 y. 20–60 mg 2–3 × daily;
		6–9 y. 30–90 mg 2–3 × daily;
		10–15 y. 100–200 mg 2–3 × daily.
		▶ Dantrolene
		  Start: 0,5 mg/kg/d, weekly increment 0,5 mg/kg/d
		  Maintenance: 2–8 mg/kg/d as 3–4 SD (max. 400 mg/d)
		▶ Tizanidine
		  Start: 1 mg/d
		  Maintenance: 0,3–0,5 mg/kg/d, max. 36 mg/d	

Spasticity (multi-)focal		▶ Botulinum toxins A intramuscular
		  – Anatomical guidance by ultrasound or electrical stimulation extremely helpful
		  – Get familiar with dosages and be aware of the botulinum toxin license in your home country
		Should be embedded in a multi-modal therapy and not applied as a stand alone treatment.	

Dystonia	First choice	▶ Trihexyphenidyl
		  Start: 0,5 mg, weekly increments of 0,5 mg (> 5 years: 1 mg), 3–4 SD
		  Maintenance: 10–20(–60) mg/d
		▶ L-DOPA
		  Start: 25 mg Levodopa, weekly increments of 25 mg
		  Maintenance: up to 10 mg/kg/d as 3 SD
		▶ Baclofen p.o.
		  see spasticity, generalized
		▶ Benzodiazepine p.o.
		  see spasticity, generalized
			▶ Trihexyphenidyl: dry mouth, anhidrosis, tachycardia, obstipation, retention of urine, dizziness, hallucinations, agitation.
			▶ L-DOPA: sedation, gastrointestinal problems, autonomic dysfunction with arterial hypotension.

		▶ Baclofen intrathecal ▶ see spasticity generalized	
		▶ Botulinum toxins ▶ see spasticity (multi-)focal	
	Individual decision	▶ Deep brain stimulation: Very successful for idiopathic torsion dystonia. Limited experience with secondary dystonic movement disorders; evidence suggests that the treatment effect is not as good as with idiopathic cases.	Treatment of choice in severely affected patients without structural lesions in basal ganglia (especially globus pallidus).

Choreoathetosis		▶ Tetrabenazine
		  Start: 12,5 mg/d, weekly increments of 12,5 mg/d
		  Maintenance: 100–200 mg/d as 3–4 SD
			Depression, akinetic syndrome

G.01 Cerebral palsy | PCS-Therapy 3/5

Movement disorders

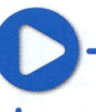

Therapy of concomitant disorders

Paresis	Muscle activity/muscle training does not increase spasticity. Paresis is present in the spastic muscles but especially in the antagonistic muscles. In combination with spasticity treatment, antagonistic muscles should be strengthened. Treadmill training, robot-supported trainings and specific sport programs could be worthwhile to include.		
Trunk hypotonia	Hippotherapy, sitting devices, corset, standing device or standing shell		
Disturbances of sensation	**Disorder of hearing**	Speech therapy Hearing aids Sign language If available, specialized school	
	Disorders of vision ▶ Retinopathia prematurorum ▶ Atrophy of nervus opticus primary or secondary ▶ Lesion within the visual pathway ▶ Cortical lesion ▶ Strabismus	Special therapy for children with poor vision Occupational therapy in children with visuomotor or visuoperceptual disturbances Conservative or surgical interventions to treat strabismus in consultation with ophthalmologist	
Mental retardation	Standardized testing of mental function, especially in children with dyskinetic form of cerebral palsy and impaired speech function is necessary. Individual support or specialized schools according to clinical need and the structure of health care and educational system.		

Disturbance of communication	**Speech comprehension**
	▶ Disturbance of vision or hearing may interfere with speech comprehension
	▶ May or may not correspond to level of mental retardation
	
	Communication (as a sender)
	▶ (Pseudo-)bulbar disturbance
	▶ Gestures and facial expression may be reduced by motor disorder
	▶ Mental retardation may affect communication skills
	
	Classification
	▶ Communication Function Classification System (CFCS)
	  – A tool used to classify the everyday communication of an individual with cerebral palsy
	  – Consists of five descriptive levels for everyday communication performance
	  – Source: http://cfcs.us
		▶ Promote nonverbal communication skills
		▶ Technical means to support communication
		▶ Input device according to the patient's needs
			Children with dyskinetic CP might be misclassified as mentally retarded

G.01 Cerebral palsy

G.01 Cerebral palsy | PCS-Therapy 4/5

Movement disorders

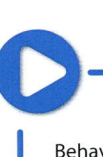

Behavioral disorder	Most important are interventions by behavioural psychologists. In rare cases, additional pharmacological treatment with neuroleptics is necessary.	Keep in mind the side effects of neuroleptics ▶ Early and late dyskinesia ▶ Parkinson-like effects ▶ Akathisia ▶ Provocation of epileptic seizures ▶ Malignant neuroleptic syndrome	

Disturbance of feeding and swallowing	**For many patients the time need for feeding is high**	Promote education and sympathy by care givers in kindergarten, school, etc.	▶ Insufficient weight gain
			  – Dietary supplements
			▶ Insufficient weight gain even with dietary supplements, or with clinical signs of aspiration
			  – Tube feeding via gastric tube
			▶ Gastroesophageal reflux disease with recurrent aspiration
			  – (Laparoscopic) Fundoplication
			▶ Visceral hypersensitivity or pain
			  – Gabapentin

	Undernourishment ▶ Check percentiles specific for CP children: http://www.lifeexpectancy.org/articles/NewGrowthCharts.shtml ▶ Feeding protocol	Dietary supplements	
	Aspiration ▶ Check frequency of pneumonia, check disturbance of swallowing with food of low viscosity, e.g. water and pay attention to coughing after swallowing.	▶ Slightly Thicken the food ▶ Correct sitting position and apply aids or devices within occupational therapist or oro-motor therapist. ▶ Reduce amount of saliva through injection of Botulinum toxin A into the salivary glands (see chapter M.01 Hypersalivation and dysphagia) ▶ Reduce saliva through application of scopolamine patches	

	Gastroesophageal reflux, Sandifer syndrome
	▶ Regurgitation of food, vomiting, typical posture of the child, signs of pain, increasing muscular hypertonia
		▶ Explore possible improvement through use of hypoallergenic food
		▶ Change dietary fiber with the aim to optimize stomach emptying
		▶ If evidence of esophagitis or gastritis
		  – Omeprazol or
		  – Esomeprazol (may be easier to apply through a gastric tube)	

Obstipation	▶ Check amount of daily liquids, change/increase dietary fibers (only in combination with increased amount of liquid, otherwise not helpful); add macrogol preparations; some children need enemas on a regular basis. ▶ Be aware that in severely affected patients visceral hyperalgesia or visceral hypersensitivity may be present and affect wellbeing and quality of life		
Pain	Reasons ▶ Gastroesophageal reflux ▶ Increased muscle tone ▶ Subluxation, luxation or dislocation of joints ▶ Vicious circle: pain → increased muscle tone → increased pain ▶ Neuropathic pain ▶ Visceral pain	Appropriate treatment according to the underlying cause	
Sleep disturbances	Circadian sleep disturbance ▶ Melatonin 5–15 mg ▶ Chloral hydrate 30–50 mg/kg	Chloral hydrate: Note liver toxicity when used for long time periods	

G.01 Cerebral palsy | PCS-Therapy 5/5

Movement disorders

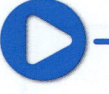

"Comple-
mentary
treatments"

So called "complementary therapies" are numerous, within the world wide web often described without any objective evidence, and sometimes they are quite expensive. However, cerebral palsy cannot be cured and service providers should be open-minded to the hopes and wishes of the affected families. Discussion of complementary treatments should be undertaken with a mutual understanding between the parents and the service provider. Before beginning with any alternative treatment however, the following issues should be settled (SMART).
- ▶ What is the treatment goal? Define clearly.
- ▶ What is the time frame for attaining the goal? (e. g. three months)
- ▶ How should the effect be evaluated and who should be involved?
- ▶ How stressful will the treatment be for the child and for the care givers? Consider time, financial strain, participation, and cooperation. Is financial compensation or "financial load" arguable?

1 bear in mind national child related licensing and/or contraindications

G.02 Dystonia | PCS-Diagnosis 1/2

Movement disorders

Medical history
- Initial symptoms: Which part of the body is affected; age at onset?
- Positive family history?
- Do symptoms occur only during certain tasks or sudden voluntary movements?
- Do symptoms vary during the day (increasing disability towards evening, at mealtime, food intake, after exercise etc.)?
- Aggravation of dystonia during agitation?
- Static or progressive course of symptoms?
- Pregnancy, birth, and neonatal history
- Psychomotor development?
- Medication history?

Symptoms
- Isolated dystonic movement disorder
- Additional symptoms (e.g. spasticity, ataxia, myoclonus, hyperkinesia, tre-

---

- Clinical grading, e.g. using Burke-Fahn-Marsden dystonia rating scale[1]
- Laboratory investigation
  - Blood smear (acanthocytosis?)
  - Calcium, phosphate
  - Copper, ceruloplasmin, uric acid
  - Transaminases, ammonia
  - Carnitine
  - Thyroid (TSH, T3)
  - Lactate
  - Antistreptolysin O titer, anti-DNase titer
  - Amino acids
  - Genetic testing
- Urine
  - Organic acids
  - Lactate, creatine metabolism
  - Copper in 24-h urine collection
  - Oligosaccharides, muco-polysaccharides
- Neurophysiology
  - EMG (co-contractures?)
  - EEG (spikes?)
- Liquor: lactate, biogenic amines
- Dopamine exposure test
- MRI
- MR-spectroscopy (lactate peak inside the basal ganglia or creatine deficiency?)

- Indicators for primary dystonia
  - Normal cranial MRI
  - Normal laboratory investigations
  - Normal mental development according to age

| | | | ▶ Primary dystonia |

- Indicators for idiopathic torsion dystonia (DYT-1)
  - Usually starts with minor symptoms in one of the lower limbs
  - Symptoms spread to trunk and upper limb
  - No mental impairment
  - Positive family history

- Molecular genetic testing: DYT-1 locus (< 50 %)
- Other genetic loci for generalized dystonias are DYT-4, DYT-6, DYT-17

▶ Idiopathic torsion dystonia

- Indicators for dopa-responsive dystonia
  - Aggravation of symptoms during the course of the day
  - Typical toe walking

- Treatment with Levodopa (L-dopa in combination with dopa decarboxylase-inhibitor carbidopa):
  - 1 mg/kg/d/single dose × 4 p. o, increase by 1 mg/kg/week
- Molecular genetic testing: DYT-5 locus

- Rapid response to low doses (rarely up to 10 mg/kg and delayed response after 4 months)

▶ Dopa-responsive dystonia (DRD), e.g. Segawa syndrome)

- Indicators for dyskinetic cerebral palsy
  - Additional symptoms of spasticity and impaired selective control
  - MRI findings: signs of alterations within the basal ganglia

▶ Dyskinetic cerebral palsy

- Indicators for paroxysmal dyskinesia
  - Hyperkinetic movements triggered by sudden voluntary movements (paroxysmal kinesigenic dyskinesia)

Versus
- Hyperkinetic movements with spontaneous onset (paroxysmal non-kinesigenic dyskinesia)

- Suspected paroxysmal kinesigenic dyskinesia
- Carbamazepine
- Usually very good response

▶ Paroxysmal kinesigenic dyskinesia

- Suspected paroxysmal non kinesigenic dyskinesia
- Clonazepam
- Usually moderate response

▶ Paroxysmal non-kinesigenic dyskinesia

- Calcification of basal ganglia (MRI, CT)

- Check differential diagnoses, e.g.
  - Mitochondriopathy (e.g. MELAS)
  - Fahr's syndrome (idiopathic basal ganglia calcification)
  - Posthypoxic, postinfectious
  - Hyperparathyroidism
  - Tuberous sclerosis, astrocytoma

Go to specific chapter

- Indicators for heredodegenerative dystonia
  - Progressive course of symptoms
  - Frequently associated with mental impairment
  - Morphologic alterations in MRI

- Signs of neuroacanthocytosis
  - Acanthocytes in blood smear
  - MRI: atrophy of the caudate nuclei, "eye of the tiger sign"

▶ Neuroacanthocytosis

- Symptoms of Wilson's disease
- Liver biopsy: Accumulation of copper

▶ Wilson's disease

G.02 Dystonia

200

G.02 Dystonia | PCS-Diagnosis 2/2 — Movement disorders

mor, mental retardation, etc.)?	▶ CT (calcifications?) ▶ Ophthalmologic examination (slit lamp: Kayser-Fleischer rings) ▶ Skin, muscle, liver and/or nerve tissue biopsies may be useful in selected patients ▶ Depending on the findings of above tests, additional genetic testing may be required		– Combination with other movement disorders possible, e.g. parkinsonism, tremor – Often neuropsychiatric comorbidity – Low serum ceruloplasmin level – Elevated copper secretion in 24-hour urine – Kayser-Fleischer corneal ring – Onset between the age of 10 and 40 years – MRI: basal ganglia and mesencephalic lesions, "face of the giant panda"	
		▶ Signs of aminoacidopathy – Pathologic elevation of metabolites in plasma	▶ Specific diagnostics, depending of the metabolic findings (Enzyme or genetic testing)	▶ Aminoacidopathy
		▶ Carnitine deficiency	Quantification of carnitine and acylcarnitine in serum sample	▶ Primary carnitine deficiency: isolated decreased carnitine level in serum ▶ Secondary carnitin deficiency: elevated acylcarnitine	▶ Carnitine deficiency
		▶ Signs of glutaric aciduria – Secondary carnitine deficiency – MRI: brain atrophy especially of the temporal lobes – Organic acids in urine sample: increased excretion of glutaric acid		▶ Glutaric aciduria
		▶ Signs of Lesch-Nyhan syndrome – Elevated uric acid in serum – Autoaggressive behaviour	▶ Serum hypoxanthine	▶ Hypoxanthine elevated	▶ Lesch-Nyhan syndrome
		▶ Associated deafness		▶ Dystonia deafness syndrome
	▶ Indicators for secondary dystonia – Asphyxia at birth – Encephalitis – Icterus gravis – Medication intake – Repeated streptococcal infections (throat infections: Sydenham's chorea, acute rheumatic fever) – MRI findings: cystic alterations of predominantly basal ganglia following, e.g., perinatal asphyxia			▶ Secondary dystonia of different genesis

1 The Barry Albright Scale is validated for children with dystonia, but it has been rarely used in studies (Burke et al. 1985, Barry et al. 1999).

G.02 Dystonia | PCS-Therapy 1/2

Movement disorders

Primary generalized dystonia	▶ Supportive measures – Orthoses, posturing aids, corset – Functional therapy – Communication aids (speech-/writing computers)	▶ L-Dopa (initial dose 1 mg/kg/d) increase in weekly steps by 1 mg/kg ▶ Lack of response: Trihexyphenidyl (initial dose 0,5 mg), increase by 0.5–1 mg/d	▶ Failure of conservative therapy	▶ Consider deep brain stimulation early (DBS) of internal pallidum[1,2]	▶ Persistent focal postureal problems	▶ Focal individualized therapy with Botulinum toxin A
Paroxysmal dystonia	▶ Paroxysmal kinesigenic dyskinesia (PKD)	▶ Carbamazepine (usually very good response, initial dose 10 mg/kg/d, max 200 mg/d)				
	▶ Paroxysmale non-kinesigenic dyskinesia (PNKD)	▶ Clonazepam (usually moderate response, infants 1,5–3 mg/d, school children 3–6 mg/d, adolescents 4–8 mg/d, 3 doses/day t.i.d)				
Dopa-responsive dystonia (DRD), e.g. Segawa-syndrome)	▶ L-Dopa in combination with dopa decarboxylase inhibitor carbidopa (initial dose 1 mg/kg/d, max. 50 mg initially); increase weekly by 25 mg/day to a maximum of 10 mg/day, divided in 3 doses/day)					
Heredodegenerative/secondary dystonia	▶ Supportive measures – Orthoses, posturing aids, corset – Functional therapy – Communication aids (computer with speech/writing processor)	▶ If possible specific therapy of underlying cause	Refer to specific chapter			
		▶ No specific therapy possible	▶ Individual trials of	▶ L-Dopa (initial dose 1 mg/kg) ▶ Trihexyphenidyl (initial dose 0,5 mg) ▶ Tetrabenazine (initial dose 12.5 mg) ▶ Baclofen p.o. (in severe dystonia consider intrathecal application (IT)), oral initial dose 0.75 mg/kg p.o. ▶ Focal use of Botulinum toxins	▶ Lack of response[4]	▶ Consider deep brain stimulation (DBS) of internal pallidum[3]

G.02 Dystonia

G.02 Dystonia | PCS-Therapy 2/2 — Movement disorders

Focal dystonia	▶ Focal injection of Botulinum toxin A	▶ Insufficient response: Trihexyphenidyl (dosing refer to primary dystonia) (initial dose 0,5 mg) or Tetrabenazine (initial dose 12.5 mg/d; increase every 3–7 days according to individual acceptance. Not more than 200 mg/d divided into 3 doses/day.)		▶ Consider DBS of internal pallidum
Dystonic state	▶ Basic care – Intensive care unit, ABC monitoring ▶ High-dose administration of benzodiazepines (e. g. Clonazepam initial dose 0,05 mg/kg IV, titrate slowly)	▶ Lack of response	▶ Initiation of intrathecal Baclofen by specialized neurosurgeon	▶ Lack of response[4]
Medication induced acute dystonic reaction	▶ Biperiden (First year: 1 mg/d, yrs. 2–6: 2 mg/d, yrs. 6–10: 3 mg/d, > year 10: 4–5 mg/d). If symptoms persist for more than 3 minutes after first Biperiden repeat dosage once. If symptoms persist for more than 60 minutes, change medication in an ICU setting.			

1 Level of evidence in primary generalized dystonia: Ib (Kupsch et al. 2006, Alterman und Tagliati 2007). Predictors of good outcome: early intervention (Holloway et al. 2006). Safety in childhood established (Lenders et al. 2006).
2 DBS: deep brain stimulation. Ultima ratio, LoE IV (Zhang et al. 2006). Significant clinical improvement in patients with pantothenate-kinase-associated neurodegeneration (PKAN, LoE III, Castelnau et al. 2005).
3 Fitz Gerald JJ et al. (2014). Long-term outcome of deep brain stimulation in generalised dystonia in series of 60 cases. J Neurol Neurosurg Psychiatry 85 (12): 1371-6.
4 Interdisciplinary decision involving paediatricians, neurologists, paediatric neurologists, rehabilitation specialists, and neurosurgeons in a specialized center.

Notes

Notes

H Cranial nerves

H.01 Facial palsy | PCS-Diagnosis 1/2

Cranial nerves

Medical history and clinical findings
▶ Unilateral or rarely bilateral facial palsy

▶ Evidence of **central palsy**
  – Lower half of the face is affected
  – Forehead can be wrinkled
  – The eye can be closed

▶ Search for contralateral CNS pathology
  – MRI

▶ Evidence of **peripheral/nuclear palsy**
  – Complete facial palsy with
  – Incomplete eye closure ("signe de cils")
  – Upward and outward movement of the eye, when an attempt is made to close the eyes (Bell phenomenon)
▶ Evidence of **lesion in the temporal bone section**
  – Dysgeusia
  – Hyperacusis
  – Reduced lacrimation
  – Reduced canalicular excitability
  – (Investigation only in cooperative adolescents and adults reliable)

▶ No general symptoms

▶ Evidence of **herpes zoster oticus**
  – Herpes zoster vesicles in ear and mouth
▶ Consider ENT/consult and ear microscopy

▶ Varicella-zoster serological examination
▶ Consider CSF examination

▶ Evidence of **Melkersson-Rosenthal syndrome**
  – Recurrent facial palsy
  – Facial swelling
  – Lingua plicata

▶ Acute peripheral facial palsy
▶ No specific other symptoms

▶ Serological screening
▶ CSF examination (cell count, proteins, borrelia serology)

Possible diagnoses
▶ Neuroborreliosis
▶ Idiopathic facial palsy
▶ Other infections

▶ Evidence of **rhabdomyosarcoma, malignant parotid tumor**
  – Ear ache
  – Secretion from the ear (possibly bloody)
  – Hearing loss
  – Periauricular swelling

▶ Blood count
▶ Bone marrow examination
▶ Histology

▶ Evidence of **brain stem lesion, Miller-Fisher syndrome, Tuberculosis**
  – Multiple cranial nerve palsies

▶ MRI
▶ CSF examination

▶ With general symptoms

▶ Evidence of **traumatic lesion**
  – History of traumatic brain injury
  – Haematotympaneum
  – Impaired hearing

▶ X-ray of petrous bone
Or
▶ CT of petrous bone

▶ Evidence of **otitis media, mastoiditis, parotitis**

▶ Evidence of **sarcoidosis**
  – Uveitis
  – Arthritis

▶ Rx thorax
▶ ACE (blood and CSE)
▶ Histological examination

▶ Clinical evidence of an infection with **EBV, CMV, HIV, myocoplasma or bastonella infection**

▶ Serological examination

H.01 Facial palsy

H.01 Facial palsy | PCS-Diagnosis 2/2

Cranial nerves

- ▶ Evidence of **leukemia**
  - Loss of appetite
  - Pallor
  - Lymphadenopathy
  - Haematoma

- ▶ Blood count
- ▶ Bone marrow examination
- ▶ Histology

H.01 Facial palsy │ PCS-Therapy 1/1

Cranial nerves

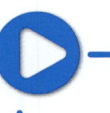

- ▶ Basic therapy
- ▶ Moisture chamber (watch glass bandage) during the day
- ▶ Eye ointment
- ▶ Physical therapy

▶ Neuroborreliosis	▶ Doxycycline p.o. (> 8 years of age) ▶ 3rd-generation cephalosporins (Cefotaxime or Ceftriaxone) Or ▶ Benzylpenicillin (Penicillin G)
▶ Varicella-Zoster-Virus infection	▶ Aciclovir IV
▶ Idiopathic facial palsy	▶ If presentation is less than 3(–7) days since onset, consider: Prednisolone 1 mg/kg/d as 2 SD for 7–10 days, taper over 7 days
▶ Traumatic	▶ Surgical decompression and nerve readaptation (depending on severity and course)

H.02 Optic neuritis | PCS-Diagnosis 1/1

Cranial nerves

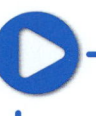

Medical history
- Headache
- Transient visual problems
- Transient/persistent problems
  - Motor: ataxia, paresis, tonus dysregulation
  - Sensory dysfunction
  - Cranial nerves: dizziness/vertigo, double vision, dysarthria, tinnitus
- Preceding infections
- Preceding vaccinations
- Preceding bee, wasp or tic bite
- Medication
  - Barbiturates
  - Cytotoxic drugs
- Toxins, alcohol

- Clinical signs suggesting optic neuritis
  - Impaired vision, mono- or bilateral
  - Pain aggravated by eye movement
  - Sensitivity to slight pressure on the bulb
  - Afferent pupillary defect
  - Fundoscopy abnormal in 1/3: acute disc swelling (papillitis), fine haemorrhages radiating from disc, perivenous shedding
  - Often central scotoma
  - Colour vision disturbed
  - Stereo vision disturbed

And
- No other neurologic symptoms

- Blood
  - Complete blood count, ESR, CRP
  - Electrolytes, glucose,
  - Liver enyzmes, transaminases
  - Creatinine, uric acid, LDH, CK
  - Serum electrophoresis
  - Serology: EBV, Borrelia, VZV, HSV, others (see DD)
  - ANA, ds-DNA-AB, ENA, cardiolipin-AB, ACE, anti-MOG antibodies (Myelin Oligodendrocyte Glycoprotein) tested in a live-cell-based assay
- CSF
  - Status with cell count, glucose, protein, lactate
  - Oligoclonal bands
  - Antibodies against measles, rubella, VZV, HSV
  - Serology/PCR Chlamydia pneum., EBV, Borrelia
- Visually evoked potentials
- MRI with thin slices of orbital region

- **Optic neuritis**

- Clinical signs suggesting optic neuritis

And
- Additional neurologic symptoms

- Spinal symptoms	- Signs for neuromyelitis optica
	  - Severe visual loss/poor recovery sometimes bilateral and simultaneous
	  - Myelitis (severe, bilateral motor, sensory, sphincter dysfunction)
		- MRI
		  - Brain
		  - Spinal cord
		- Possibly NMO-antibodies positive

- **Neuromyelitis optica**
- **(Devics disease)**

- Cerebral +/- spinal symptoms	DD: ADEM/Multiple sclerosis	See chapter J.01 Multiple sclerosis/ADEM

- Clinical signs suggesting optic neuritis

And
- Lymphadenopathy

Or
- Hepatosplenomegaly

Or
- Positive family history

Or
- Drug abuse

Or
- Signs of Vitamin deficiency (e.g. blood count, peripheral neuropathy)

- Signs for infectious mononucleosis
  - Flu-like symptoms
  - Fever
  - Pharyngitis, tonsillitis
  - Antibodies against EBV present in blood

- **Infectious mononucleosis**

- Signs for cat scratch disease
  - Contact to cats
  - Antibodies against B. henselae present in blood

- **Cat scratch disease**

- Analysis of LHON-mutation (Leber's hereditary optic neuropathy)

- **LHON**

- Toxicology in urine

- **Drug abuse (see chapter A.13 Intoxication)**

- Serum levels of Vitamin B_1, B_2, B_6, B_{12}, folic acid reduced

- **Vitamin deficiency**

H.02 Optic neuritis

H.02 Optic neuritis | PCS-Therapy 1/1

Cranial nerves

▶ Idiopathic optic neuritis	▶ IV Methylprednisolone 20–30 mg/kg/d, max. 1 g for 3 days[1] ▶ Check blood sugar, electrolytes, CRP, consider prophylactic measures against gastric ulcer	▶ Good recovery	No further therapy		
		▶ Insufficient recovery	▶ Continue therapy for 5 days	▶ Re-evaluation after 2 weeks with eye examination	▶ Still insufficient recovery – Repeat therapy with IV Methylprednisolone 20–30 mg/kg/d for 3 days – Further option: plasmapheresis
▶ Secondary causes of optic neuritis – Therapy of underlying disease	▶ Infections (e.g. Borreliosis)	▶ Antibiotic therapy		▶ Re-evaluation after completion of treatment	
	▶ Tumor	▶ Neurosurgery			
	▶ Medication	▶ Stop medication			
	▶ Posttraumatic	▶ Wait and watch			

[1] Therapy of childhood optic neuritis follows the published guidelines for adults (Dale et al. 2009 Paediatric central nervous system inflammatory demyelination: acute disseminated encephalomyelitis, clinically isolated syndromes, neuromyelitis optica, and multiple sclerosis. Curent Opin Neurol. 22(3) 233–40

Notes

Notes

I Rehabilitation

I.01 Rehabilitation (inpatient) | PCS-Diagnosis/Therapy

▶ Congenital disease E.g. cerebral palsy (see chapter G.01 Cerebral palsy)	▶ Reference system: International Classification of Functioning, Disability and Health (ICF)	▶ Intensified therapy ▶ Specialized therapy (e.g. comprehensive therapeutic approach to address special problems, e.g. hemiparesis, aphasia) ▶ Complex neurological disorder involving several issues that have to be addressed in parallel ▶ Combination of medical issues and psychosocial problems that are interdependent and only can be resolved together	▶ Access to rehabilitation medicine depends on the health care system and varies between different countries.	▶ Therapy according to treatment goals ▶ Consultations with neighbouring disciplines, e.g. paediatric orthopaedics ▶ Orthoses, splints, aids to support biomechanics or to prevent secondary deformities ▶ Long-term treatment plan based on prognosis and strategies considered most useful for the patient ▶ Adaptations of the environment if useful for activity, participation, independence and autonomy of the child ▶ Education and reinforcement of parents/caregivers	▶ Preservation or improvement of health status ▶ Improvement of wellbeing and quality of life

▶ Secondary brain lesion E.g. traumatic brain injury, infection of the central nervous system		▶ Because of his medical condition the patient will not be able to return to a "normal" life
		▶ Patient requires intensified treatment due to
		  – Medical problems, e.g. seizures
		  – Reduced consciousness
		  – Sensorimotor problems, e.g. paresis
		  – Reduced cognitive abilities
		  – Feeding and/or swallowing difficulties
		  – Speech and communication problems, e.g. aphasia
		  – Behavioral issues
		▶ The persistent neurological condition may require environmental adaptations.
			▶ Admission in most cases directly from the emergency unit after first aid treatment (intensive care unit) and stabilization of the patient.
			▶ The optimal time point for referring the patient to the inpatient rehabilitation unit depends on the facilities available at the rehabilitation unit.
			▶ In general, early referral is recommended to initiate rehabilitation without delay.
				▶ Comprehensive, patient centered care addressing the
				  – Medical
				  – Neuropsychological
				  – Therapeutic and
				  – Social issues
					▶ Back to former life after thorough investigation
					▶ Back home with minor adaptations (e.g. repeating one school term, support for traveling long distances, treatment as outpatient for a limited time period)
					▶ Back home with major adaptations including adaptation of the environment according to the patient's special needs. This includes recommendations for frequency and content of outpatient therapy, supply with a wheelchair, adaptations at home, support in transferring to an appropriate school environment.

Notes

Notes

J Inflammation and infection

J.01 Multiple sclerosis/ADEM | PCS-Diagnosis 1/1

Inflammation and infection

Medical history
- Age
- (Preceding) infection
- Fever
- Headache
- Encepahlopathy
  - Disturbed consciousness
  - Behavioral problems
- Concentration/difficulties in school
- Seizures

Clinial features
- Visual signs and symptoms (impaired vision, colour vision disturbed, visual field defects, ocular motor palsies, internuclear ophthalmoplegia, nystagmus)
- Sensory symptoms (numbness, paresthesia)
- Motor symptoms (weakness, paresis, ataxia)
- Tremor
- Bladder/bowel dysfunction
- Cognitive deficits

- MRI (brain and spinal chord)
- Laboratory
  - Blood count
  - BSG
  - CRP
  - ANA
  - Antiphospholipid antibodies
  - Lupus anticoagulants
  - Borrelia serology
  - Lactate, glucose
  - Vitamin B12, D
  - ACE, anti-MOG antibodies (Myelin Oligodendrocyte Glycoprotein) tested in a live-cell-based assay
- Urine status
- CSF (+ Serum)
  - Cell count
  - Protein, albumin
  - Glucose, lactate
  - Oligoclonal IgG bands, IgG, IgA, IgM index
  - AB indices (measles, mumps, rubeola, VCV, HSV)
- Neurophysiology (VEP, AEP, SSEP, MEP)

- **McDonald-criteria** (revised version, 2010; see chapter J.01 McDonald criteria)
- Clinical symptoms suggesting MS
  - Plus: dissemination in space
  - Plus: dissemination in time
- MRI
  - Periventricular, juxtacortical, infratentorial and spinal lesions
  - Dawson fingers (corpus callosum)
  - Black holes
- CSF
  - OKB positive, possibly marginal pleocytosis (< 60 cells/mm^3) and protein elevation)

▶ Multiple sclerosis

Signs indicating ADEM
- Often preceding infection
- Encephalopathy mandatory
- Polyfocal neurologic deficits
- CSF: OKB usually negative, pleocytosis/protein elevation not uncommon
- MRT
  - Bilateral, diffuse lesions

▶ ADEM[1]

- Results not appropriate for ADEM or MS
- Further work-up
  - Optic neuritis
  - Transverse myelitis
  - Neuromyelitis optica (NMO)
  - Infection-induced CNS disease: neuroborreliosis, HIV encephalomyelitis, whipple disease
  - Inflammatory autoimmune diseases with CNS component: lupus erythematodes, Behçet disease, vasculitis, neurosarcoidosis, Sjögren syndrome
  - Tumor
  - Neurometabolic diseases: adrenoleukodystrophy (ALD), metachromatic leukodystrophy (MLD), Krabbe's, Wilson's, Alexander's disease, mitochondrial disorder (e.g. Leigh, MELAS, LHON), disorders of vitamin metabolism
  - Angiopathy: Moyamoya, CADASIL
  - Lymphoproliferative diseases: Langerhans' cells histiocytosis, hemophagocytic lymphohistiocytosis (HLH)

---

1 Krupp LB, Tardien M, Amato MP et al. (2013) International Paediatric Multiple Sclerosis Study Group criteria for paediatric multiple sclerosis and immune-mediated central nervous system demyelinating disorders: revisions to the 2007 definitions. Mult Scler 19: 1261-1267.

J.01 Multiple sclerosis/ADEM | PCS-McDonald Criteria 1/1

Inflammation and infection

▶ ≥ 2 Attacks	▶ Objective clinical evidence of ≥ 2 lesions	
	▶ Objective clinical evidence of 1 lesion	▶ Dissemination in space (DIS), indicated by – MRI: ≥ 1 T2 lesion in at least 2 of 4 MS-typical regions of the CNS (periventricular, juxtacortical, infratentorial, or spinal cord), gadolinium-enhancing lesions not required. Or Wait for a further clinical attack involving a different CNS site
▶ 1 Attack	▶ Objective clinical evidence of ≥ 2 lesions	▶ Dissemination in time (DIT), indicated by – MRI: a) simultaneous presence of asymptomatic gadolinium-enhancing and non-enhancing lesions at any time or b) new T2 and/or gadolinium-enhancing lesion(s) on follow-up MRI irrespective of its timing with reference to a baseline scan Or Wait for a second clinical attack

	▶ Objective clinical evidence of 1 lesion (clinically isolated syndrome)	▶ Dissemination in space (DIS) and time (DIT), indicated by
		  – DIS: MRI: ≥1 T2 lesion in at least 2 of 4 MS-typical regions of the CNS (periventricular, juxtacortical, infratentorial, or spinal cord), gadolinium-enhancing lesions not required.
		Or
		Wait for a further clinical attack involving a different CNS site
		  – DIT MRI: a) simultaneous presence of asymptomatic gadolinium-enhancing and non-enhancing lesions at any time or b) new T2 and/or gadolinium-enhancing lesion(s) on follow-up MRI irrespective of its timing with reference to a baseline scan
		Or
		Wait for a second clinical attack involving a different CNS site

▶ Insidious neurological progression suggesting primary progressive MS (PPMS)	1 year of disease progression (retrospectively or prospectively determined) plus 2 of 3 of the following criteria: 1. Evidence for DIS in the brain based on 1 T2 lesions in the MS-typical (periventricular, juxtacortical, or infratentorial) regions 2. Evidence for DIS in the spinal cord based on ≥ 2 T2 lesions in the cord 3. Positive CSF (isoelectric focusing evidence of oligoclonal bands and/or elevated IgG index)	

Multiple sclerosis:
If the criteria are fulfilled and there is no better explanation for the clinical presentation, the diagnosis is "MS".
If MS is suspected, but the criteria are not completely met, the diagnosis is "possible MS"
If another diagnosis arises during the evaluation that better explains the clinical presentation, then the diagnosis is "not MS."

J.01 Multiple sclerosis/ADEM | PCS-Acute therapy

Inflammation and infection

- ▶ MS relapse
  - New or reactivated symptoms
  - Persisting > 24 hours
  - Interval of > 30 days prior to former relapse
  - Not related to increased body temperature (Uhthoff phenomenon or infections)

- ▶ IV Methylprednisolone 20–30 mg/kg/d, max. 1 g for 3 days[1]
- ▶ Check blood sugar, electrolytes, CRP, gastric protection
- ▶ Symptomatic therapy if required

- ▶ Good recovery
  - No relevant deficit

No further therapy

- ▶ Insufficient recovery
  - Persisting relevant deficits

- ▶ Continue therapy for 5 days (+/- oral taper)

- ▶ Reevaluation after 2 weeks

- ▶ Still insufficient recovery

- Repeat IV Methylprednisolone therapy 20–30 mg/kg/d for 3–5 days

- ▶ Still insufficient recovery and relevant deficit

- ▶ Further option in severe cases: plasmapheresis

- ▶ Profound relapse (e.g. brain stem, transverse myelitis)
- ▶ And/or worsening under steroids

- ▶ Plasmapheresis in severe cases

---

1 Therapy of acute demyelinating event follows the published guidelines for adults (Dale et al. 2009 Paediatric central nervous system inflammatory demyelination: acute disseminated encephalomyelitis, clinically isolated syndromes, neuromyelitis optica, and multiple sclerosis. Current Opin Neurol. 22(3) 233–40)

J.01 Multiple sclerosis/ADEM | PCS-Disease modifying drugs (DMD) 1/1

Inflammation and infection

▶ Confirmed diagnosis of MS ▶ No contraindication against Interferon beta or Glatiramer acetate	Interferon beta-1a or Interferon beta-1b (start with 1/4 of adult dose, titrate to full adult dose in 4 weeks)[1] – Consider lower than full dose in very young children – Preparation Rebif®: 44 mcg sc; 3 times/week – Preparation Betaferon®: 250 mcg every other day – Preparation Avonex®: 30 mcg/week Or ▶ Glatiramer acetate[2] – 20 mg/d	▶ Clinical re-evaluation every 3–6 months – Annual MRI – VEP – SSEP – Eye examination – EDSS[3]	▶ Good therapeutic response – With relapse rate reduction – With stable clinical course – MRI shows no signs of active disease	▶ Continue medication
			▶ Serious local or systemic side-effects Or ▶ Inadequate response to treatment, defined as follows – Minimum of 6 months full-dose therapy with full patient compliance and at least one of the following – Increase or no reduction in relapse rate, or new T2 or contrast enhancing lesions on MRI Or ▶ ≥ Two confirmed relapses (clinical or MRI) within 12 months or less	▶ Changing between first line therapies (see colum 2) Or ▶ Consider therapy escalation with – Natalizumab (Tysabri®) 300 mg every 4 weeks – Fingolimod (Gilenya®) – Cyclophosphamide
▶ Confirmed diagnosis of MS ▶ Contraindication against Interferon beta or Glatiramer acetate	▶ Consider alternative treatment options – Fumerate (Tecfidera®) – Fingolimod (Gilenya®) – Azathioprine 1–3 mg/kg/d (monitor WBC) Or – IVIG 2 g/kg/month			

1 Interferon beta. Absolute contraindication: history of hypersensitivity to natural or recombinant interferon beta, or any other component of the formulation, pregnancy. Relative contraindication: e.g. depression, suicidal tendencies (product information guidelines)

2 Glatiramer acetate. Absolute contraindication: history of hypersensitivity to Glatiramer acetate or mannitol.

3 EDSS – expanded disability status scale (based on J.F. Kurzke). Based on a standard neurological examination, the 7 functional systems (plus "other") are rated. EDSS is an ordinal clinical rating scale ranging from 0 (normal neurological findings) to 10 (death due to MS) in half-point increments.

J.01 Multiple sclerosis/ADEM

J.02 Cerebral vasculitis | PCS-Diagnosis 1/4

Inflammation and infection

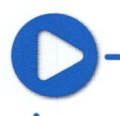

Medical history
Extracerebral involvement
Past medical history
Medication, including immunosuppressive drugs
Recent foreign travel
Family history

Presentation
Neurological deficits
Psychiatric symptoms
Headache, other pain
Malaise

Examination
Cranial MRI
– Diffusion
– Heme sequence (T2*)
– Contrast medium application
– MRA
Digital subtraction angiography DSA
Colour Doppler sonography
– Intra-/extracranial
– Temporal artery
EEG, ENG, if appropriate EMG
ECG, Echo (TEE)
Laboratory
– ESR, CRP
– Blood count and differentiation
– Haptoglobin
– Ferritin
– Creatine kinase, LDH
– ACE
– Transaminases, liver and renal function tests (incl. GFR)
– Coagulation tests
– TSH, thyroid antibodies
– Serum electrophoresis
– Complement
– Rheumatoid factor, ANA, c- and p-ANCA, SS-A, SS-B, anti-phospholipid Ab, lupus anticoagulant, immunoelectrophoresis, anti-histone Ab, anti-endothelial Ab

---

Findings suggest **PACNS (Primary angiitis of the central nervous system)**
Acquired neurological deficit unexplained after complete evaluation

MRI-findings
– Multifocal intracerebral lesions affecting both white and grey matter
– Hyperintense lesions in T2 und FLAIR
– Contrast medium enhancement
– Multiple vascular territories, uni- or bilateral
– MRA: irregular lesions of cerebral vessels

Digital subtraction angiography (DSA) findings in case of angiography-positive PACNS
– Occlusions, stenosis, beading, tortuosity of proximal large- and medium-sized vessels in the CNS
– Most commonly affected is the middle cerebral artery
– Typically multiple vascular territories

Laboratory findings
– CRP and ESR elevated or normal
– Possibly low-level ANA titers

CSF
– Protein elevation
– Mild lymphomonocytic pleocytosis

Angiography negative, multifocal inflammatory lesions in small-vessel distribution: brain biopsy

---

Lymphocytic, non-granulomatous small-vessel vasculitis, predominantly small muscular arteries: small-vessel vasculitis in childhood (SV-PACNS)

J.02 Cerebral vasculitis

J.02 Cerebral vasculitis | PCS-Diagnosis 2/4

Inflammation and infection

- Drug screening
- Serologic tests: syphilis, borreliosis, hepatitis B, C, HIV

Urine examination incl. electrophoresis
Fecal occult blood
Chest x-ray (if appropriate chest CT)
Abdominal sonography
CSF: cell differentiation, isoelectric focusing, cultures, antigens, PCR, oligoclonal bands

---

Findings suggesting Henoch-Schonlein purpura (HSP)
Focal neurologic deficits or seizures within two weeks after onset of purpura or petechiae (mandatory) with lower limb predominance, no thrombocytopenia and at least one of the four following criteria
- ▶ Abdominal pain
- ▶ Matching histopathology
- ▶ Arthritis or arthralgia
- ▶ Renal involvement

MRI
- Multifocal ischaemic or haemorrhagic lesions
- Subdural, subarachnoidal or parenchymal haemorrhage, possibly cerebellar

DSA
- Irregularities of medium-sized cerebral vessels

Laboratory
- CRP, ESR slightly elevated
- ANCA IgA elevated, IgG normal

Findings suggest Kawasaki syndrome (KS)
Fever for 5 days or more, plus 4 out of the 5 symptoms below
- ▶ Polymorphous rash
- ▶ Bilateral (non-purulent) conjunctival infection
- ▶ Skin changes of the extremities, e.g. peripheral erythema, periungual or generalized desquamation
- ▶ Cervical lymphadenopathy (> 1.5 cm)
- ▶ Affection of the mucous membranes of the upper respiratory tract

and exclusion of diseases with a similar presentation

MRI
- Rarely intracerebral lesions

Laboratory
- Marked elevation of ESR and CRP

KS with cerebral involvement

J.02 Cerebral vasculitis | PCS-Diagnosis 3/4

Inflammation and infection

– After five days of fever: hypoalbuminemia < 3 g/dl, anemia, ALT elevation; after seven days: thrombocytosis, leukocytosis
– Leukocyturia

Findings suggest Takayasu's arteritis (TA) Presentation as stroke or TIA, headache, malaise accompanying the following findings: Angiographic abnormalities of the aorta or its main branches and pulmonary arteries showing aneurysm/dilatation (mandatory criterion) plus one of the five following criteria ▶ Pulse deficit or claudication ▶ Four limbs BP discrepancy ▶ Bruits ▶ Hypertension ▶ Acute phase reaction (ESR > 20 mm/first hour, CRP elevated) **MRI** – Multifocal ischaemic or haemorrhagic lesions **Cranial DSA** – Affection of intracerebral vessels possible		TA with cerebral involvement
Findings suggest Wegener's granulomatosis (WG) Cranial nerve lesions, diabetes insipidus, possibly hydrocephalus, focal neurologic deficits and affection of the peripheral nervous system Criteria for the diagnosis of WG: at least three of the six following criteria ▶ Matching histopathology ▶ Upper airway involvement ▶ Laryngotracheobronchial stenosis ▶ Pulmonary involvement (nodules, cavities or fixed infiltrates on chest X-ray) ▶ ANCA positive (sensitivity 93 %, specificity 90 %) ▶ Renal involvement **MRI** – Multifocal ischaemic or haemorrhagic lesions – Meningeal or intracerebral granulomas, meningeal enhancement – Atypical CNS manifestation: intracranial haemorrhage	Biopsy, if necessary to establish diagnosis based on the listed criteria	WG with cerebral involvement
Findings discouraging the diagnosis of a CNS vasculitis Congenital neurologic deficit Thunderclap headache (Reversible cerebral vasoconstriction syndrome (RCVS)) Signs of encephalitis or cerebritis Conditions predisposing for stroke		

J.02 Cerebral vasculitis

J.02 Cerebral vasculitis | PCS-Diagnosis 4/4

MRI
- No pathological findings
- Space-occupying lesion
- Arteriovenous malformations
- Aneurysm
- Demyelinating lesions
- Diffuse inflammation

DSA
- Affection of the distal internal carotid artery with evidence of a collateral circulation (Moyamoya syndrome)
- Aneurysm, arteriovenous malformations

Laboratory
- Acute-phase reactants within normal range (discouraging systemic vasculitis)

CSF
- No pathological findings: discouraging the diagnosis of a cPACNS

J.02 Cerebral vasculitis | PCS-Therapy 1/2

Inflammation and infection

cPACNS	Progressive medium-to-large-vessel CNS vasculitis (P-cPACNS)	▶ Cyclophosphamide 500–750 mg/m² bsa IV monthly for 6 months ▶ Followed by oral maintenance therapy using Mycophenolate mofetil or Azathioprine for 18 months ▶ Prednisone 2 mg/kg/d, slow tapering off over 12 months ▶ Low-dose Acetylsalicylic acid (ASA)
	Non-progressive medium-to-large-vessel CNS vasculitis (NP-cPACNS)	Treatment controversial. May include ▶ Anticoagulation with Heparin, switch to oral antiplatelet agents ▶ Adjunctive corticosteroids
	Small-vessel CNS vasculitis (SV-cPACNS)	As in progressive medium-to-large-vessel CNS vasculitis (P-cPACNS)
HSP	Self-limiting course	No therapy required
	Recurrent episodes	Dapsone (1–2 mg/kg/d) for 1–2 weeks
	Severe recurrent episodes	Steroids, Methotrexate
	Cerebral manifestations	Prompt treatment as some of the cerebral manifestations may be reversible ▶ High-dose corticosteroids ▶ Intravenous Ig (IVIG) or plasmapheresis
	Abdominal symptoms	Paracetamol (Acetaminophen) Prednisolone 1–2 mg/kg/d for a few days
	Nephritis	Cyclosporine A – 4–8 mg/kg/d, aiming for a serum level of 150–200 mcg/l – Tapering off after six months	Proteinuria, arterial hypertension: – ACE-Inhibitors, e.g. Enalapril – Prednisone + Azathioprine
Kawasaki syndrome	All patients	▶ Intravenous immunoglobulin (IVIG) 2g/kg ▶ Acetylsalicylic acid – 30–40(–100) mg/kg/d in four doses per day as long as fever persists – followed by 3–5 mg/kg/d for 6–8 weeks – continued treatment in case of coronary aneurysms
		▶ IVIG-resistance – second dose IVIG 2 g/kg – If no improvement after two or more IVIG administrations: corticosteroids

J.02 Cerebral vasculitis

J.02 Cerebral vasculitis | PCS-Therapy 2/2

Takayasu's arteritis	Immunosuppressive therapy – Prednisolone – Consider immunosuppressive agent (Azathioprine, Methotrexate, Cyclophosphamide, Infliximab)
	Antiplatelet agents
	Interventional or surgical treatment of stenotic vessels
Wegener's granulomatosis	Remission induction – Fauci scheme: Cyclophosphamide + high-dose Prednisolone
	Post-remission therapy – Methotrexate + corticosteroids

J.03 Lyme disease | PCS-Diagnosis 1/1

Inflammation and infection

Medical history
- Outdoor activities
- Tick bite
- Previous erythema migrans
- Typically early summer or autumn

Clinical Findings
- Peripheral facial palsy (uni- or bilateral)
- Headache
- Meningism
- Stiffness of the spine
- Arthralgias
- Fever
- Other neurological symptoms (i.e. palsy of other cerebral nerves)
- Non-specific signs (e.g. malaise, fatigue)

▶ Cerebrospinal fluid (CSF)	▶ Pleocytosis with lymphocytes	▶ Suspected lyme disease	▶ Start antibiotic therapy ▶ Borrelia Ab tests are required for complete diagnostic work-up		▶ Neuroborreliosis (lyme disease)
	▶ No pleocytosis	▶ Lyme disease unlikely	▶ Take Borrelia serology	▶ If IgM-Ab positive	▶ Lyme disease cannot be excluded – antibiotic treatment
▶ Check for Borrelia antibodies in serum and CSF (ELISA, immunoblot)	▶ Serum positive for IgM Ab And/or ▶ CSF positive for IgM Ab (with or w/o IgG titers)	▶ Suspected lyme disease	▶ Start antibiotic therapy		
	▶ Serum and CSF negative for IgM Ab And ▶ CSF positive for IgG Ab (with or w/o IgG Ab positive in serum)	▶ Intrathecal antibody synthesis suspected	▶ CSF-serum index required	▶ CSF-serum index positive	▶ Lyme disease — ▶ Antibiotic therapy
				▶ CSF-serum index negative	▶ Lyme disease very unlikely — ▶ No antibiotic therapy ▶ Other diagnoses? ▶ Idiopathic facial palsy?
	▶ Serum and CSF negative for IgM Ab And ▶ IgG Ab positive only in serum	▶ Earlier infection without correlation to the acute symptoms	▶ No antibiotic treatment, control tests for antibodies after 2–3 weeks	▶ If no change in Borrelia titers	▶ No signs of acute infection
	▶ Serum negative for IgM and IgG Ab And ▶ CSF negative for IgM and IgG Ab	▶ Lyme disease excluded ▶ *But:* Lyme disease possible with very short incubation period		▶ Seroconversion points to acute infection	▶ Antibiotic therapy
▶ Check for Borrelia DNA in CSF (PCR; only done in special cases)	▶ Positive	▶ Lyme disease is suspected	▶ Antibiotic treatment		
	▶ Negative	▶ Lime disease cannot be excluded by negative PCR	▶ Look at other laboratory findings		

J.03 Lyme disease

J.03 Lyme disease | PCS-Therapy 1/1

Inflammation and infection

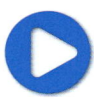

First line medication	Symptoms persist > 4–6 weeks[3,5]	Check for chronic neuroborreliosis: lumbar puncture	Lymphocytic pleocytosis in the CSF	Repeat antibiotic therapy
– Ceftriaxone (50 mg/kg/d in 1 single dose (SD) (max. 2 g/d); for 2 weeks)[1]		Differential diagnosis: chronic fatigue-syndrome		Reassess diagnosis
– Cefotaxime (200 mg/kg/d in 3 SD (max 6 g/d); for 2 weeks)			Oligoclonal bands in the CSF And/or	No active infection
Second line medication			Intrathecal synthesis of borrelia-specific antibodies (IgG and/or IgM) in the CSF	
– Penicillin (200 000–400 000 IU/kg/d in 4 SD (max. 12 Mega/d); for 2 weeks)[4]			Without lymphocytic pleocytosis	
In case of cephalosporin allergy				
– Imipenem (60 mg/kg/d in 4 SD (max. 4 g/d); for 2 weeks)				
Alternatively in children older than 8 years and over 50 kg body weight:				
– oral Doxycycline (200 mg/d in 1–2 SD for 4 weeks)[2]				

1 Ceftriaxone: risk of allergic rash (differential diagnosis: Jarisch-Herxheimer reaction), elevated risk of gallbladder sludge if dose is > 50 mg/kg/d.
2 Note: doxycycline may be phototoxic (treatment often during the summer months!); UV protection recommended.
3 Patients usually respond very reliably to intravenous antibiotic therapy with cephalosporins of class III. Non-responders are extremely rare.
4 High dosage is necesary due to poor penetration into the CSF
5 Antibody control tests are pointless unless clinical symptoms persist!

J.04 Meningitis and encephalitis | PCS-Diagnosis 1/1

Inflammation and infection

▶ Newborns and infants	**Medical history**
	▶ Pregnancy and delivery
	▶ Haemorrhage
	▶ Feeding difficulties
	
	Clinical signs[1]
	▶ Change of skin colour (pale, bluish or livid), petechiae
	▶ Bulging fontanelle
	▶ Opisthotonus
	▶ Impaired consciousness/lethargy
	▶ Shrill crying
	▶ Irritability
	▶ Fever
	▶ Vomiting and distended abdomen
	▶ Feeding problems
	▶ Hyperexcitability
	▶ Photophobia
	▶ Apnea
	▶ Seizures
		▶ Laboratory diagnostic work-up
		  – Complete blood count with differential
		  – C-reactive protein and/or procalcitonin
		  – Evaluation of clotting function
		  – Blood culture, urine culture
		▶ If increased intracranial pressure is suspected
		  – Funduscopy
		  – Imaging studies (sonography, CT, MRI)
			All	▶ Lab results suggest presence of inflammation
				And
				▶ No indication of increased ICP
					▶ Spinal tap[2]
					  – Opening pressure (normal < 28 cm H_2O)
					  – Cell count
					  – Culture results
					  – Virological tests
					  – If negative culture results, consider eubacterial PCR (16S-rDNA)
					  – Gram's stain
					  – Ratio of liquor to serum glucose levels
					  – Protein levels
						▶ Cloudy liquor
						▶ Cell count: > 1000/mm³
						▶ Predominance of granulocytes
						▶ Protein > 1 g/dl
						▶ Liquor glucose < 2,5 mmol/l
						▶ Gram-positive or gram-negative bacteria (cocci or rods)
							▶ Bacterial origin

▶ Toddler, children, and adolescents	**Medical history**
	▶ Headache
	▶ Development and time course of complaints
	▶ Prior medication
	▶ Seizures
	▶ Travel history, animal contact
	
	Clinical signs
	▶ Fever
	▶ Nuchal rigidity, Kernig-, Lasègue- and Brudzinski sign
	▶ Altered consciousness
	▶ Vomiting
	▶ Petechiae, purpura
		▶ Laboratory diagnostic work-up
		  – Complete blood count with differential
		  – C-reactive protein and/or procalcitonin
		  – Evaluation of clotting function
		  – Blood culture, urine culture
		▶ If increased intracranial pressure is suspected
		  – Funduscopy
		  – Imagining studies (sonography, CT, MRI)
		▶ Neurological examination with quantification of level of consciousness (Glasgow Coma Scale)
		▶ EEG
				▶ Signs of increased ICP	See chapter A.05 Acute increased intracranial pressure (ICP)		▶ Clear liquor
							▶ Cell count < 500 mm³
							▶ Primarily monocytic cells
							▶ Protein < 0,4 g/dl
							▶ Liquor glucose > 2,5 mmol/l
							▶ No bacteria in Gram's stain
								▶ Viral origin

1 Bacteremia is often associated with meningitis in newborns and infants.

2 NOTE: Laboratory results depend on the time course of the disease. Cell counts and protein content can be low in the early course of disease. A repeated spinal tap is usually not necessary unless there is no response to treatment. Some liquor should be stored for further analyses (e.g. specific viral or bacterial diagnostic work-up including PCR).

J.04 Meningitis and encephalitis | PCS-Therapy

Inflammation and infection

Basic interventions
- Monitor cardiovascular functions
- Monitor respiration
- Intensive care (if necessary)
- Medical treatment of seizures
- Laboratory analyses (pH, glucose, oxygenation etc.)

▶ Meningitis	▶ < 6th week	**Initial empiric therapy if causative pathogen unknown** ▶ Cefotaxime + Ampicillin IV for 14–21 days: – Cefotaxime 100–150 mg/kg/d q8h – Ampicillin 200 mg/kg/d q8h	▶ Adjust after identification of pathogen
	▶ > 6th week	**Initial empiric therapy if causative pathogen unknown** ▶ Dexamethasone before or with first application of antibiotics, 0,4 mg/kg/SD × 2 for 2 days ▶ Cefotaxime 200 mg/kg/d q8 h IV for 14 days	▶ Adjust after identification of pathogen
▶ Viral encephalitis	▶ HSV[1]	▶ Aciclovir[1] 3 × 15–20 mg/kg/d (for neonatal infection 3 × 20 mg/kg) for 21 days	
	▶ VZV		
	▶ CMV	▶ Ganciclovir (few case reports) 3 × 5 mg/kg/d	
	▶ Influenza	▶ Oseltamivir (4 mg/kg/2 SD/d)	
▶ Fungal meningoencephalitis	▶ Cryptococcus	▶ Liposomal Amphotericin B 3–5 mg/kg/d for 4 weeks, then consolidation with Fluconazole 3–6 mg/kg/d for 8 weeks	
	▶ Aspergillus	▶ Voriconazole 14 mg/kg/d as 2 separate SD	
	▶ Candida	▶ Fluconazole p.o. 3–6 mg/kg/d ▶ Caspofungin 50 mg/m²/d as single dose IV (day 1: 70 mg/m²; maximum daily dose: 70 mg)	

1 Start empiric therapy for herpes encephalitis immediately when suspected; discontinue Aciclovir if virology results negative (e.g. negative PCR)

Notes

Notes

K Oncology

K.01 Neoplasm of the CNS | PCS-Diagnosis Brain 1/1

Oncology

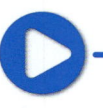

Medical history
- Genetic conditions with impaired tumor suppression
  - Neurofibromatosis type 1
  - Neurofibromatosis type 2
  - Tuberous sclerosis complex
  - Von Hippel-Lindau disease
  - Turcot syndrome
  - Li-Fraumeni family cancer syndrome
  - Gorlin Goltz syndrome
- Radiotherapy

Clinical Presentation
- Signs and symptoms (depending on the child's age and tumor location)
  - Skin abnormalities suggestive of phakomatosis
  - Increased head size (infancy)
  - Headaches
  - Vomiting, esp. in the morning
  - Progressive visual impairment
  - Papilloedema
  - Epileptic seizures
  - Behavioral change
  - Focal neurological deficit
  - Torticollis
  - Endocrine dysfunction (growth retardation, hypothyroidism, diabetes insipidus)
  - Dysphagia
  - Ataxia
  - Hemiplegia
  - Speech apraxia
  - Memory disorder
  - Neglect
  - Sleep-wake disorder
  - Cranial nerve dysfunctions
  - Strabism
  - Nystagmus, dancing eyes
  - Hearing loss
  - Other cranial nerve disorders
  - Sensory loss

- Cranial MRI[1]
  - Space-occupying lesion
  - Localization
  - Cysts
  - MRI intensity
  - Contrast enhancement
  - Demarcation
  - Surrounding oedema
  - Hydrocephalus
- Cranial CT
  - Calcifications (e. g. craniopharyngioma)
- Laboratory tests (suspected germ-cell tumor)
  - AFP
  - ß-HCG
- Lumbar puncture[2]
- Ophthalmologic investigation
  - Vision
  - Refraction
  - Visual field
  - Fundoscopy

- MRI: CNS neoplasm with high diagnostic certainty of tumor entity

- MRI: CNS neoplasm with unclear tumor entity

- Final diagnosis of tumor entity and dignity based on histology (stereotactic biopsy or tumor resection)

- Brain tumor clearly defined by WHO classification (see chapter K.01 WHO classification tumors)

---

1 T2-weighted spin echo sequence, axial T1-weighted sequence pre- and post-contrast, post-contrast fluid attenuated inversion recovery (FLAIR) sequence, and T1-weighted spin echo sequence at a further plane. Diffusion-weighted scans for differentiation of neoplasm from abscess or stroke. Consider positron emission tomography (PET), single photon emission computed tomography (SPECT), MR spectroscopy, functional MRI, and fiber tracking for surgery planning, follow-up control or diagnosis of relapse.

2 Tumor cells in cerebrospinal fluid determine prognosis and therapy (especially with medulloblastoma, supratentorial primitive neuroectodermal tumors, and germ-cell tumors). NOTE: Use pre-operative lumbar puncture **only if this is possible without risk of brain herniation. Obligatory lumbar puncture on post-operative day 14.**

K.01 Neoplasm of the CNS | PCS-Diagnosis Spine

Oncology

Medical history
- Genetic conditions with impaired tumor suppression
  - Neurofibromatosis type 1
  - Neurofibromatosis type 2
  - Tuberous sclerosis complex
  - Von Hippel-Lindau disease
  - Turcot syndrome
  - Li-Fraumeni family cancer syndrome
  - Gorlin Goltz syndrome
- Radiotherapy

Clinical presentation
- Signs and symptoms
  - Skin abnormalities suggestive of phakomatosis
  - Spinal pain
  - Spinal stiffness
  - Torticollis
  - Motor disturbances
  - Ataxia
  - Paresis
  - Sensory loss

- MRI[1]
  - Space-occupying lesion
  - Localization
  - Cysts
  - MRI intensity
  - Contrast enhancement
  - Demarcation
  - Surrounding oedema
- CT
  - Looking for calcifications
  - Bone lesions
- Laboratory tests (suspected neuroblastoma)
  - Neuron-specific enolase
  - Catecholamines in urine
- Laboratory tests (suspected germ-cell tumour)
  - AFP
  - ß-HCG
- Lumbar puncture[2]

- MRI: Spinal tumor with high diagnostic certainty of tumor entity

- MRI: Spinal tumor with unclear tumor entity

- Final diagnosis of tumour entity and dignity based on histology (stereotactic biopsy or tumour resection)

- Spinal tumour clearly defined by WHO classification (see chapter K.01 WHO classification of tumors)

---

1 T2-weighted spin echo sequence, axial T1-weighted sequence pre- and post-contrast, post-contrast fluid attenuated inversion recovery (FLAIR) sequence and T1-weighted spin echo sequence at a further plane. Diffusion-weighted scans for differentiation of an abscess or stroke. Consider: positron emission tomography (PET), single photon emission computed tomography (SPECT), MR spectoscopy, functional MRI, and fibre tracking for surgery planning, follow-up control or diagnosis of relapse.
2 Tumour cells in cerebrospinal fluid determine prognosis and therapy (especially with medulloblastoma, supratentorial primitive neuroectodermal tumours, and germ-cell tumours). NOTE: Pre-operative lumbar puncture **only if possible without risk of brain herniation, obligatory lumbar puncture on post-operative day 14.**

K.01 Neoplasm of the CNS | WHO classification of tumors 1/4

Oncology

	Grades			
	I	II	III	IV
Astrocytic tumours (40–50 %)				
Pilocytic astrocytoma (30–35 %)	x			
Subependymal giant cell astrocytoma	x			
Pilomyxoid astrocytoma		x		
Diffuse astrocytoma		x		
Pleomorphic astrocytoma		x		
Anaplastic astrocytoma			x	
Glioblastoma				x
Giant cell astrocytoma				x
Gliosarcoma				x
Oligondendroglial tumours (< 1 %)				
Oligodendroglioma		x		
Anaplastic oligodendroglioma			x	
Oligoastrocytic tumours				
Oligoastrocytoma		x		
Anaplastic oligoastrocytoma			x	
Ependymal tumours (10 %)				
Subependymoma	x			
Myxopapillary ependymoma	x			
Ependymoma		x		
Anaplastic Ependymoma			x	

K.01 Neoplasm of the CNS

K.01 Neoplasm of the CNS | WHO classification of tumors

	I	II	III	IV
Choroid plexus tumours (2–3 %)				
Choroid plexus papilloma	x			
Atypical choroid plexus papilloma		x		
Choroid plexus carcinoma			x	
Angiocentric glioma	x			
Choroid glioma of the third ventricle		x		
Neuronal and mixed neuronal-glial tumours				
Gangliocytoma	x			
Ganglioglioma	x			
Dysembryoplastic neuroepithelial tumour (DNT)	x			
Desmoplastic infantile astrocytoma/ ganglioglioma	x			
Paraganglioma	x			
Papillary glioneuronal tumour	x			
Rosette-forming glioneuronal tumour of the fourth ventricle	x			
Central neurocytoma		x		
Extraventricular neurocytoma		x		
Cerebellar liponeurocytoma		x		
Anaplastic Ganglioglioma			x	
Tumours of the pineal region (2–3 %)				
Pineocytoma	x			
Pineal parenchymal tumour of intermediate differentiation		x	x	

K.01 Neoplasm of the CNS | WHO classification of tumors 3/4

Oncology

	I	II	III	IV
Papillary tumour of the pineal region		x	x	
Pineoblastoma				x
Embryonal tumours (20 %)				
Medulloblastoma				x
CNS primitive neuroectodermal tumour				x
Ependymoblastoma				x
Atypical teratoid / rhabdoid tumour				x

	Grades			
	I	II	III	IV
Tumours of cranial and paraspinal nerves				
Schwannoma	x			
Neurofibroma	x			
Perineurinoma	x	x	x	
Malignant peripheral nerve sheat tumour		x	x	x
Tumours of the meninges (< 1 %)				
Meningeoma	x			
Atypical meningeoma		x		
Anaplastic/(malignant) meningeoma			x	
Haemangiopericytoma		x		
Anaplastic haemangiopericytoma			x	
Haemangioblastoma	x			

K.01 Neoplasm of the CNS | WHO classification of tumors 4/4

Oncology

Tumours of the sellar region (10 %)					
Craniopharyngeoma	x				
Granula cell tumour	x				
Pituicytoma	x				
Spindle cell oncocytoma of the adeno-hypophysis	x				
Pituitary adenoma					
Pituitary carcinoma					
Germ cell tumours (3–5 %)					
Germinoma					
Embryonal carcinoma					
Yolk sac tumour					
Teratoma (mature, immature, with malignant transformation)					
Mixed germ cell tumour					
Malignant CNS lymphomas					
Langerhans-cell histiocytosis					
Metastatic tumours					

Notes

Notes

L Genetics

L.01 Genetics | PCS-Orientation 1/2

Genetics

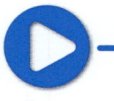

Medical history
- Pregnancy
  - Abortions
  - Preventive examinations (sonography, amniocentesis)
  - Infections
  - Complications, medication
  - Preeclampsia/HELLP syndrome
- Peripartal period
- Asphyxia
- Size, bodyweight and head circumference (percentiles)
- Statomotor and psychomotor development (milestones)
- Seizures
- Time of manifestation and development of clinical findings

Family history
- Malformations
- Sudden infant death syndrome SIDS/Apparent life threatening event ALTE ("near-missed SIDS")
- Pedigree
- Consanguinity

Physical examination
- Size, body weight, head circumference
- Dysmorphias:
  - Hypertelorism
  - Epicantus
  - Microstomia
  - Hairline/ears approach
  - Blepharophimosis
  - Microphthalmia
  - Skull shape
  - Pigmentations
  - Lumbar sacral dysmorphia
  - Genital dysmorphia
  - Contractures
  - Hexadactyly/clinodactyly
  - Palmar and plantar relief

Create a differential diagnosis profile based on leading symptoms
For example:
- Grew small
- Grew large
- Obesity
- Macrocephaly
- Facial dysmorphias
- Brain malformation
- Vitium organicum cordis (VOC)
- Mental retardation
- Skin lesions

Use the following tools:
- OMIM[1]
- OrphaNet[2]
- GeneReviews[3]
- BVDH-Guidelines[4]

Extended malformation diagnosis
- Ophthalmologic examination
- Echocardiography
- Abdominal sonography
- Cerebral sonography

Optional:
- Cranial MRI
- Spinal MRI
- Bone, spine, skull x-ray
- EEG
- Evoked potentials
- Neurography
- ENT examination

Genetic diagnosis
- Chromosome analysis
- Array CGH

Optional laboratory investigations
- Creatine kinase
- Lactate
- Blood count
- Liver function tests

See chapter N.01 Neurometabolic disorders, N.02 Neurodegenerative disorders and N.03 Mitochondrial disorders

Confirmation of diagnosis and classification according to the OMIM database, based on
- Specified molecular genetic investigations
- Cytogenetic investigations
- Multigene panel investigations/Whole genome sequencing
- Laboratory investigations
  (for example enzyme activity in fibroblasts)
- Analysis of biopsies
  (for example histology, enzyme histochemistry, electron microscopy)
- Constellation of clinical findings only

Genetic counselling
Specialized genetic consultation
(For German speaking countries: according the BVDH guidelines)

L.01 Genetics

L.01 Genetics | PCS-Orientation 2/2

- Neurological examination
- Diagnostic assessment of the patient's development
- Neuropsychological examination

1 OMIM: Online Mendelian Inheritance in Man (www.ncbi.nlm.nih.gov)
2 OrphaNet: European information service for rare diseases (www.orpha.net)
3 GeneReviews: Overview genetic diseases (www.geneclinics.org)
4 BVDH: Bundesverband Deutscher Humangenetiker (www.bvdh.de)

L.02 Neurocutaneous syndromes | PCS-Diagnosis Neurofibromatosis 1 (NF1) 1/1

Genetics

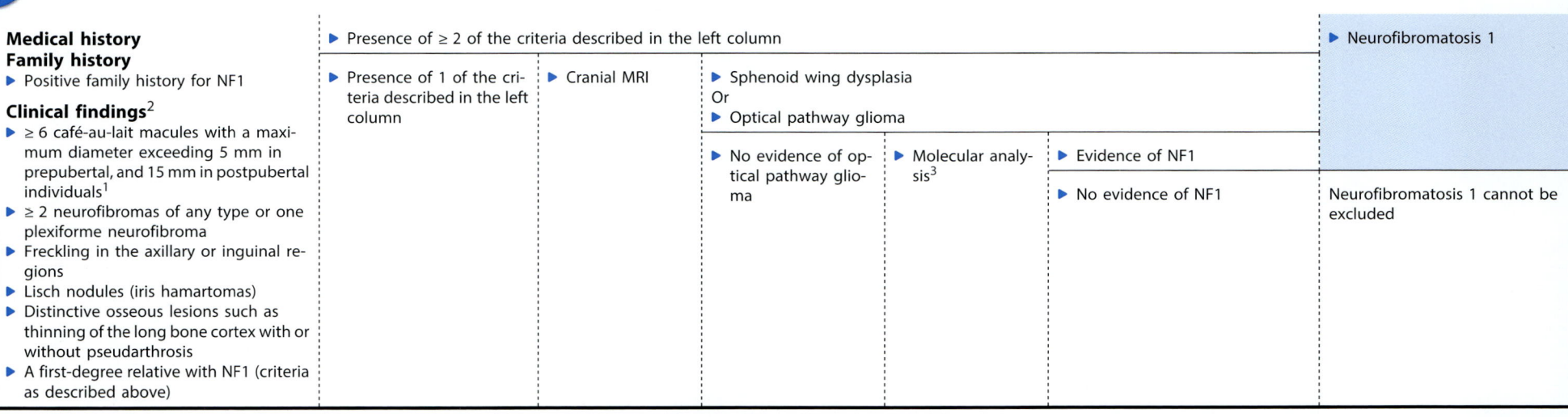

Medical history
Family history
- Positive family history for NF1

Clinical findings[2]
- ≥ 6 café-au-lait macules with a maximum diameter exceeding 5 mm in prepubertal, and 15 mm in postpubertal individuals[1]
- ≥ 2 neurofibromas of any type or one plexiforme neurofibroma
- Freckling in the axillary or inguinal regions
- Lisch nodules (iris hamartomas)
- Distinctive osseous lesions such as thinning of the long bone cortex with or without pseudarthrosis
- A first-degree relative with NF1 (criteria as described above)

- Presence of ≥ 2 of the criteria described in the left column
  - Neurofibromatosis 1

- Presence of 1 of the criteria described in the left column
  - Cranial MRI
    - Sphenoid wing dysplasia
      Or
    - Optical pathway glioma
      - Neurofibromatosis 1
    - No evidence of optical pathway glioma
      - Molecular analysis[3]
        - Evidence of NF1
          - Neurofibromatosis 1
        - No evidence of NF1
          - Neurofibromatosis 1 cannot be excluded

1 Café-au-lait macules may appear during the first weeks of life and tend to progress rapidly in size and number.
2 Based on these criteria the diagnosis of NF1 can be established in 60–80 % of all patients by the age of 6 years.
3 Molecular testing for NF1 mutations (in blood or mouth epithelial cells) is feasible but still challenging, tedious and expensive. Current molecular methodology will detect the presence of NF1 mutations in about 90 %. While evidence of a NF1 mutation will thus confirm the clinical diagnosis it is not possible to exclude NF1 if a mutation of the NF1 gene cannot be identified. For the vast majority of NF1 mutations identified up to date there is no clear genotype-phenotype correlation so that the further course of the disease cannot be predicted even if the mutation is known.

L.02 Neurocutaneous syndromes | PCS-Therapy Neurofibromatosis 1 (NF1)

Genetics

			Follow-up
Café-au-lait macules	No therapy necessary		▶ Annual visit at a specialized centre for clinical/physical evaluation
Axillary/inguinal freckling			▶ Bi-annual/annual ophthalmological examination including fundoscopy for all children from 0 to 8 years of age to detect symptomatic optical pathway gliomas
Dermal neurofibromas	▶ Painfulness Or ▶ (Functional) impairment Or ▶ Mechanical irritation	▶ (Laser-)surgical excision	▶ Additional diagnostic work-up depending on clinical symptoms and findings
Plexiform neurofibromas[1]	▶ Painfulness Or ▶ (Functional) impairment Or ▶ Mechanical Irritation	▶ Surgical excision[2]	
Iris hamartomas (Lisch nodules)	No therapy necessary		
Optical pathway gliomas (see chapter K.01 Neoplasm of the CNS)	▶ Radiologically proven tumor progress Or ▶ Clinical symptoms[3]	▶ Chemotherapy according to GPOH-Study (HIT-LGG) (additional operation[4], if applicable)	
Bone dysplasias (tibial pseudarthrosis, scoliosis etc.)	▶ Depending on the extent of the dysplasia, therapy may be necessary	▶ Operation by specialized orthopedic surgeon	
Specific motor, language and learning disabilities	▶ Specific therapy according to the results of a detailed psychological assessment		

1 Malignant transformation risk approximately 10%
2 Clinical studies investigating various drug treatment strategies are ongoing
3 In approx. 10% of NF1-associated optical pathway gliomas
4 Due to high risk of secondary tumors and other complications use of radiotherapy is discouraged

L.02 Neurocutaneous syndromes | PCS-Diagnosis Neurofibromatosis 2 (NF2) 1/1

Genetics

Medical history
Family history
▶ Positive family history for NF2

Clinical findings
▶ Neurofibromas
▶ Impaired hearing
▶ Impaired vision
▶ Vertebral pain
▶ Impaired motor function/ pareses
▶ Sensory failures
▶ Impaired sphincter function
▶ Torticollis
▶ Ataxia

▶ MRI
Brain and spinal cord
And
▶ Ophthalmologic examination

▶ Bilateral vestibular schwannomas (acoustic neuroma), consider molecular analysis

▶ Neurofibromatosis 2

▶ Family history of NF2
And
▶ Unilateral vestibular schwannoma before 30 years of age.
Or
▶ ≥ 2 of the following:
 – Meningeoma
 – Glioma
 – Ependymoma
 – Other schwannoma
 – Juvenile posterior cataract

Probable neurofibromatosis: Molecular analysis[1]

▶ Unilateral vestibular schwannoma before 30 years of age
And
▶ One of the following:
 – Meningeoma
 – Glioma
 – Ependymoma
 – Other schwannoma
 – Juvenile posterior cataract

Further evaluation, consider molecular analysis

▶ Family history positive

▶ Annual cranial MRI beginning at 10 years of life

▶ Evidence of tumor in MRI

▶ ≥ 2 Meningeomas
And
▶ Unilateral vestibular schwannoma before 30 years of age
Or
▶ One of the following:
 – Ependymoma
 – Other schwannoma
 – Juvenile posterior cataract
 – Glioma

▶ Family history negative

▶ Neurofibromas
And
▶ Ocular complications

▶ Passed 35 years of age

No further diagnostic work-up

▶ No neurofibromas
Or
▶ No ocular complications

No further diagnostic work-up

1 Sensitivity with positive family history approx. 90 %, with negative family history approx. 60 %

L.02 Neurocutaneous syndromes

258

L.02 Neurocutaneous syndromes | PCS-Therapy Neurofibromatosis 2 (NF2)

Vestibular schwannomas (acoustic neuroma)[1,3]	▶ Surgery with preservation of hearing feasible	▶ Surgery with preservation of hearing	▶ Annual follow-up with MRI		
	▶ Surgery with preservation of hearing not feasible	▶ Follow-up. Surgery may be indicated if other tumors are found	▶ Nerve preservation feasible	▶ Cochlear Implantation	▶ Audiological rehabilitation
			▶ Nerve preservation not feasible	▶ Auditory brain stem implant (ABI) if applicable	
Schwannomas of other cranial nerves	▶ Clinical follow-up ▶ Surgery only as a "last resort"				
Spinal schwannomas	▶ Clinical follow-up ▶ Surgery only as a "last resort"				
Cutaneous schwannomas	▶ Not painful	No therapy			
	▶ Painful	▶ Surgery	▶ Annual follow-up by MRI		
Meningeomas	▶ Symptomatic Or ▶ Progressive	▶ Operable	▶ Surgery	▶ Incomplete resection	▶ (Postoperative) Radiotherapy
		▶ Not operable			
	▶ Not symptomatic, not progressive	▶ Follow-up by MRI			
Ependymomas	▶ Surgery	▶ Incomplete resection	▶ Postoperative radiotherapy[2]		

1 Restrictive use of radiotherapy is recommended in NF2-associated tumors due to possible secondary malignant transformation
2 Especially in low-grade tumors
3 Early learning of sign language and lip reading applies to all patients

L.02 Neurocutaneous syndromes | PCS-Diagnosis Tuberous sclerosis complex (TSC) 1/1

Genetics

Medical history
- Cerebral seizures (especially infantile spasms)
- Congenital, cardiac rhabdomyoma
- Positive family history for TSC

Clinical findings
- Facial angiofibromas
- Periungual fibroma
- Hypomelanotic cutaneous macules (> 3 spots)
- Shagreen patch (connective tissue nevus)
- Multiple dental enamel pits
- Hamartomatous rectal polyps
- Gingival fibromas
- Non-renal hamartoma
- "Confetti skin lesions"[1]

Baseline diagnostic work-up
- Developmental assessment
- Ophthalmologic examination
- EEG
- ECG, echocardiography
- Renal ultrasound
- Cranial MRI

Major features
- Facial angiofibromas
- Periungual fibroma
- Hypomelanotic cutaneous macules (> 3)
- Shagreen patch (connective tissue nevus)
- Cortical tubera
- Subependymal nodules
- Subependymal giant cell astrocytoma
- Multiple retinal nodular hamartomas
- Cardiac rhabdomyoma
- Lymphangiomyomatosis
- Renal angiomyolipoma

Minor features
- Multiple dental enamel pits
- Hamartomatous rectal polyps
- Bone cysts
- Cerebral white matter "migration tracts"
- Gingival fibromas
- Non-renal hamartoma
- Retinal achromic patch
- "Confetti skin lesions"
- Multiple renal cysts

- 2 major features

Or

- 1 major feature and 2 minor features

- 1 major feature and 1 minor feature

Or

- 1 minor feature

Or

- Positive family history for TSC

- Molecular testing[2]: evidence of a mutation of
  - TSC 1 (9q34; coding for hamartin)

  Or
  - TSC 2 (16p13.3; coding for tuberin)

- Evidence of TSC1 or TSC2 mutation

- No evidence of mutation

- Tuberous sclerosis complex

Tuberous sclerosis complex cannot be excluded

---

1 "Confetti skin lesions" refers to multiple hypopigmented macules of 1–2 mm diameter, that typically appear on both lower arms or lower legs in a symmetric fashion.

2 Similar to NF, molecular testing for TSC mutations is feasible but still challenging, tedious and expensive. Evidence of a TSC mutation would confirm the clinical diagnosis. This might be crucial for diagnosis since very discrete phenotypes can occur which makes it difficult to come to a clear clinical diagnosis. Lack of evidence for the presence of a mutation, however, does not exclude TSC since the probability to find a given TSC mutation is well below 100 %. In any case, it is not possible to predict the further clinical course of the disease.

L.02 Neurocutaneous syndromes | PCS-Therapy Tuberous sclerosis complex (TSC)

Hypomelanotic macules ("white spots")	No therapy necessary		**Follow-up:** ▶ Annual visit at a specialized centre for clinical/physical examination ▶ Renal ultrasound, cranial MRI (children and adolescents only): every 1–3 years ▶ Developmental assessment, ophthalmological examination, EEG, ECG, echocardiography ▶ Thorax-CT, if suggested by clinical findings
Epilepsy	▶ Therapy with antiepileptic drugs according to seizure type (high efficacy of vigabatrin in TSC-associated infantile spasms!) ▶ Ketogenic diet if applicable	See chapter E Epilepsy, consider everolimus	
Facial angiofibromas Shagreen patches Periungual fibromas	▶ Depending on the extent of the lesion and subjective disturbance	▶ Surgical (excision, abrasion, laser therapy)	
Retinal hamartomas	▶ Growth Or ▶ Secondary complications	▶ Photocoagulation	
Renal angiomyolipomas	▶ Rapid growth And/or ▶ Bleeding	▶ Arterial embolisation ▶ Surgical resection if applicable ▶ Medical treatment with everolimus	
Renal cysts	▶ Large cysts Or ▶ Secondary complications (e.g. hypertonia)	▶ Surgical resection	
Cardiac rhabdomyomas[1]	▶ Outflow tract obstruction Or ▶ Arrhythmia	▶ Interventional or surgical	
Pulmonary lymphangioleiomyomatosis	▶ Lung transplantation		
Subependymal nodules Subependymal giant cell astrocytomas (SEGA)	▶ Continuous/rapid growth And/or ▶ Localization within the foramen Monroi and consecutive block of cerebrospinal fluid passage	▶ Medical treatment with Everolimus ▶ Surgical resection ▶ Consider hydrocephalus shunting	
Cortical tubers	▶ If epileptogenic And ▶ Failure of antiepileptic drug treatment ("drug failure")	Epilepsy surgery (see chapter E.10 Epilepsy surgery)	

[1] high rate of spontaneous remission

L.03 Craniosynostosis | PCS-Diagnosis 1/1

Genetics

Medical history
- Course of head growth
- Time of manifestation
- Milestones of development
- Cephalgia
- Seizures
- Pre-existing diseases
- Intrauterine medication

Family history
- Head shape and head size of parents, grandparents and siblings
- Malformations/syndromes
- Metabolic bone diseases

Physical examination
- Head shape, head size
- Palpation of skull sutures (bony rail?)
- Form, size and consistence of fontanelle
- Neurological examination (incl. ophthalmoscopy, hearing and vision assessment)
- Neurodevelopmental examination
- Dysmorphias

Diagnostic work-up
- Cerebral sonography
- Skull x-ray
- Ophthalmologic examination
- Optional
  - MRI
  - SEP, AEP, VEP
  - Detailed hearing assessment
  - Sonography for possible internal malformations (abdominal system, urinary tract, heart)
  - Laboratory (calcium, phosphate, AP, TSH, parathyroid hormone, Vit D, calcitonin)
  - EEG
  - Cranial CT/3D-CT: usually not necessary

Cranial deformity and radiological verification of premature craniosynostosis **without** any further malformations/dysmorphias

▶ Diagnosis: non-syndromic craniosynostosis

Hypotelorism, flat orbital edges, prominent sutura metopica	▶ Trigonocephaly (approx. 4 %)
Anterioposterior elongated head shape with prominent sutura sagittalis	▶ Scaphocephaly (approx. 40 %, m : f = 4 : 1)
Prominent forehead, hypertelorism, flat orbital edges, unilateral prominent sutura coronaria	▶ Brachycephaly (approx. 20 %)
Asymmetric forehead and midface area with lateral orbital flattening	▶ Frontal plagiocephaly (approx. 15 %)
Asymmetric occipital region with radiologically proven unilateral premature synostosis of the sutura lambdoidea *Caution:* Differential diagnosis of positional plagiocephaly without bony synostosis of the lambdoid suture.	▶ Occipital plagiocephaly (approx. 1 %)

Cranial deformity and radiological verification of premature craniosynostosis **with** further malformations/dysmorphias (e.g. midface hypoplasia, polydactyly, syndactyly)

▶ Diagnosis: complex/syndromic craniosynostosis

▶ Genetic analysis (chromosome analysis, molecular genetic analysis, e.g. FGFR 1–3)
▶ Genetic consultation

▶ Syndrome diagnosis, e.g. Crouzon-, Pfeiffer-, Apert syndrome

---

Asymmetric head shape (mainly posterior plagiocephaly) **without** radiological verification of premature craniosynostosis (and history of positional aetiology)

▶ Positional plagiocephaly

L.03 Craniosynostosis

L.03 Craniosynostosis | PCS-Therapy

Genetics

Indications for surgical approach
- Generalized or localized increased intracranial pressure (ICP) with evident or imminent functional deficits
- Risk of disturbed psychosocial development due to the misshaped head

Surgical intervention
Aims
- Enlargement of intracranial volume
- Improvement or prevention of functional deficits
- Aesthetic improvement

Possible techniques
- Parasutural craniectomy
- Craniotomy
- Fragmentation and reconstruction
- Fronto-orbital advancement

Follow-up (after surgery)
- Shape and size of the head
- Visual function test
- Neurodevelopmental assessment
- Optional EEG
- Optional hearing assessment
- Optional skull x-ray
- Optional genetic consultation

Caution:
- Re-synostosis
- ICP increase
- Functional deficits
- Aesthetic result

Indications for conservative treatment
- Positional plagiocephaly

Conservative treatment
- (Cranial remolding orthosis)
- Positional therapy
- Physiotherapy

Follow up (conservative treatment)
- Shape and size of the head
- Visual function test
- Neurodevelopmental assessment
- Optional procedures (see above)

Indications for conservative treatment
- Singular premature craniosynostisis (without syndrome diagnosis and without clinical or radiological signs of increased intracranial pressure)

Follow up (conservative treatment) in regular intervals
- Skull X-ray
- Visual function test
- Neurodevelopmental assessment
- Psychological development

L.04 Rett syndrome | PCS-Diagnosis 1/1

Genetics

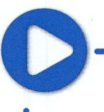

Medical history and clinical findings
- Necessary diagnostic criteria:
  - Normal pregnancy and birth
  - Normal or almost normal development during the first 6–18 months
  - Normal head circumference at birth
  - Deceleration of head growth
  - Loss of hand function between 6 and 30 months
  - Hand stereotypies
  - Loss of communication including speech, mental retardation
  - Gait apraxia
- Supporting diagnostic criteria:
  - Breathing abnormalities including hyperventilation, forced expiration and apnea
  - Bruxism
  - Abnormal sleep patterns
  - Increased muscle tone, atrophy and dystonia
  - Peripheral vasomotor disturbances
  - Scoliosis/kyphosis
  - Small stature
  - Small cold feet and hands

Checklist

Normal pre-/perinatal period	1
Normal development during the first 6 months	1
Normal head circumference at birth	1
Deceleration of head growth	1
Never had good hand function	1
Lost hand function	2
Stereotypic hand movements	1
Impaired communication	1
Never acquired the ability to speak	1
Lost the ability to speak	2
Severe mental retardation	1
Gait abnormalities	1
Maximum score	12 points

- \> 8 points
  - Molecular analysis of the *MECP 2* gene
    - Positive finding of *MECP 2* mutation

      Diagnosis Rett syndrome
      - Point mutations, insertions or deletions detectable in > 90 % of cases

    - Negative finding of *MECP 2* mutation
      - Send to specialist
      - Atypical Rett syndromes

- \< 8 points
  - Molecular analysis of *MECP2* gene is unlikely to detect any mutations

    Look for other diagnoses

L.04 Rett syndrome | PCS-Therapy

Therapy of epilepsy	▶ First line: Carbamazepine, Sulthiame ▶ See chapter E Epilepsy
	Only patients with epileptic seizures should be treated. Breathing abnormalities in Rett syndrome are not of epileptic nature.
Therapy of scoliosis	▶ Corset ▶ Operation
	A corset often only prolongs the time until operation is indicated
Therapy of sleep disturbance	▶ Melatonin (0–3 years: 3(–5) mg, 4–6 years: 5(–10) mg, 7–10 years: 10(–12)mg, > 10 years: 5(–10) mg)

L.05 Microdeletion syndromes | PCS-Diagnosis Angelman syndrome 1/1

Genetics

Medical history
- Normal prenatal and birth history
- Normal head circumference at birth
- Developmental delays evident at 6th–12th month of age
- No evident developmental stagnation or regression
- Delayed speech development

Cardinal clinical signs
- Persistent oral exploration
- Hypotonia in early infancy, myoclonic-atactic movement disorder
- Divergent strabismus
- Broad oral opening, prognathism
- Delayed growth of head circumference
- Brachymicrocephaly during 2nd year of life
- Severe mental disability
- Impaired movement and postural control, mainly gait ataxia/apraxia and/or jerking, and rapid, unsteady movements of limbs and trunk
- No speach acquisition
- Some receptive language skills and nonverbal communication skills
- Seizures (commonly evident < 3 years of age)
- Sleep disturbances

Investigations
- EEG
- Molecular genetics[1]
- (cranial MRI)

EEG findings typical
(96 % of patients show one or more of the findings listed below)
EEG pattern with anterior predominant theta-(delta) activity, showing the following characteristics:
- Rhythmic theta-(delta) bursts
- "Hypsarrhythmic-multi-focal" spikes
- Superposed spikes, leading to "slow spike wave-pattern"
- Triphasic morphology, provoked by closing the eyes, often not correlating with clinically obvious seizures

EEG findings not typical
Does not exclude diagnosis of Angelman

Molecular genetics

With causal mutation

Without causal mutation

Diagnosis: Angelman syndrome

Clarification differential diagnosis e.g.
- Disorders of purine metabolism
- Congenital disorders of glycosylation (CDG syndromes)
- Disorders of GABA metabolism
- Rett syndrome
- Autism spectrum disorders

Presumptive clinical diagnosis of Angelman syndrome without verifiable causal mutation (11 % of patients)

Still unknown cause(s) (Correct clinical diagnosis? Other gene(s) than UBE3A? Mutations in unknown regulatory elements?)

---

1 DNA methylation analysis at SNRPN (detection of microdeletion, uniparental disomy and imprinting defect without specification):– if normal, *UBE3A sequencing*– if methylation testing abnormal: - *FISH for microdeletion*– *DNA polymorphism analysis (including samples of the parents) for paternal uniparental disomy*– *if both normal: Imprinting Center (IC) analysis for deletions*– *if normal: IC epimutation*

L.05 Microdeletion syndromes

L.05 Microdeletion syndromes | PCS-Therapy Angelman syndrome

Anticonvulsive treatment	See chapter E.10 Epilepsy surgery Valproic acid 20–30(–60) mg/kg/d Ethosuximide 20 mg/kg/d divided in 2(–3) doses Benzodiazepine (e.g. Lorazepam (Tavor®) 0.05 mg/kg/d or Clobazam (Frisium®) 10–20 mg/d)
Severe distal myoclonic jerks	Piracetam 30–40 mg/kg/d divided in 3 doses PO
Disturbed sleep-wake cycle	Melatonin dose: 0–3 years: 3(–5) mg, 4–6 years: 5(–10) mg, 7–10 years: 10(–12) mg, > 10 years: 5(–10) mg; individualized dosing
Diminished rate of swallowing, drooling	According to PCS Sialorrhea (see chapter M.01 Hypersalivation and dysphagia)
Excessive oral exploration behaviour and hand biting	Positive behaviour support If indicated, apply arm splints that limit elbow flexion to 90°
	Prognathism due to jaw movements — Orthodontic provisions
At the age of about 3 years	Facilitate communication (sign language, picture boards) as far as the patient's attention and comprehension allow

L.05 Microdeletion syndromes | PCS-Diagnosis Prader-Willi syndrome 1/1

Genetics

Medical history:
- Decreased fetal movements
- Postpartum distress (APGAR)
- Weak suck and poor feeding
  (commonly tube feeding necessary during the first weeks)

Cardinal clinical signs:
- Marked muscular hypotonia and weakness in early infancy
- Poor head control
- Reduced motor activity
- Facial weakness
- Weak cry
- Feeding problems
- Growth delay

Investigations:
- Molecular genetics

Associated features:
- Delayed reaction to external stimuli
- Daytime sleepiness
- Early failure to thrive, later (> 2 years) hyperphagia
- Hypogonadism, cryptorchism
- Small hands and feet
- Short stature
- Slim head

Molecular genetics:[1]
- Paternal microdeletion 15q11–13 (70 %), maternal UPD (29 %)

Diagnosis: Prader-Willi syndrome

Associated features:
- Alert gaze
- Bell-shaped thorax
- Diaphragmatic breathing
- Ulnar deviation of hands
- Fibrillations of hands and tongue

EMG:
- Large polyphasic MUAPs
- PSW and fibrillation
- Normal NCV

Molecular genetics:
- Deletion in SMN1 gene (commonly homozygous deletion on exon 7 and 8), rarely point mutations

Spinal muscular atrophy (SMA)
Type 1 (severe): Werdnig-Hoffmann-Disease
(see chapter O.05 Spinal muscular atrophy SMA)

Associated features:
- Delayed reaction to external stimuli
- Mainly normal weight
- Congenital talipes equinovarus (in 50 %)

Maternal EMG:
- Myotonic discharges

Molecular genetics:
- CTG-Expansion in the DMPK-Gene (19q13.2-q13.3)

Congenital myotonic dystrophy
(see chapter O.02 Muscle dystrophies)

---

1 DNA methylation analysis at SNRPN (detection of microdeletion, uniparental disomy and imprinting defect without specification):
if abnormal: – FISH for microdeletion
DNA polymorphism analysis (including samples of the parents) for maternal uniparental disomy
if both normal: imprinting Center (IC) analysis for deletions
if normal: IC epimutation
(conventional cytogenetics for rare chromosomal structural aberrations)

L.05 Microdeletion syndromes

L.05 Microdeletion syndromes | PCS-Therapy Prader-Willi syndrome

Obesity, hyperphagia Compulsive eaters	▶ Dieting; dietary counseling ▶ Early preventive weight and behaviour management ▶ Encourage motor activity and exercise
Short stature	Growth hormone therapy
Learning and speech problems Facilitate speech comprehension	Early intervention; motor/speech therapy Be sure to speak slowly and articulate clearly – adjust to the child's slower processing abilities
Consider special, psychologically assisted residential groups for adolescents with Prader-Willi syndrome	Protective surroundings help to ensure a structured daily routine, appropriate nutritional monitoring, and physical activity
Preventive medical needs	▶ Audiology, Ophthalmology (strabismus; myopia) ▶ Orthopedics (feet; scoliosis) ▶ Dental intervention (reduced saliva viscosity and production; enamel hypoplasia; increased caries) ▶ Monitoring sleep apnea

L.06 Trisomy 21 | PCS-Overview 1 1/1

Genetics

	Medical Counseling	Psychosocial Counseling
Neonatal/infancy	▶ Clinical Diagnosis[1] ▶ FISH plus karyotyping ▶ Genetic counseling ▶ Heart echography: cardiac malformations (50 %) ▶ Icterus neonatorum ▶ Failure to thrive/dystrophy ▶ Gastrointestinal: stenosis, obstipation (12 %) ▶ Hip dislocation (6 %) ▶ West syndrome/infantile spasms ▶ Transient myeloproliferative disorder (4–10 %)	▶ Contact to support group ▶ Evaluation of family resources (psychosocial, financial)
Childhood	▶ Vaccinations ▶ Sinusitis/otitis/pneumonia ▶ Blepharitis ▶ Obesity (from 4 years of age onwards)	▶ Supporting therapies (speech therapy, occupational therapy, physiotherapy) ▶ Nutritional consultant ▶ Establish physical training ▶ Degree of cognitive impairment ▶ Ask for obstructive sleep apnea syndrome
Adolescence	▶ Psychiatric comorbidities (depression) ▶ Sexually transmitted diseases/contraception ▶ Obesity	▶ Preparation for working life ▶ Re-evaluation of family resources (continued financial dependency in adulthood) ▶ Prevent social withdrawal/depression/obesity
All ages	▶ Regular contact with paediatrician ▶ Infections/immune deficiency ▶ Thyroid disease (4–18 %) ▶ Celiac disease (5 %) ▶ Eye disease (60 %) ▶ Hearing loss (75 %) ▶ Acute leukemia (1 %) ▶ Obstructive sleep apnea syndrome (50–79 %) ▶ Atlanto-occipital instability ▶ Dental anomalies ▶ Cryptorchidism ▶ Autoimmune diseases ▶ Epilepsy	▶ Anticipating patient care: Do not explain to much at once, but call attention to later problems in due course. ▶ Warning parents of miracle healers ▶ Special situations of conflict: school start, puberty, work start ▶ Avoid doctor's language ("mongolism", "Down-Baby")

1 Hypotonia, small mouth and ears, epicanthal folds, upward-slanting palpebral fissures, single transverse palmar crease, short fifth finger with clinodactyly, sandal gap deformity, brachycephalic head, excessive neck skin, Brushfield spots

L.06 Trisomy 21 | PCS-Overview 2

		Assessment of Development[1]	Assessment of Growth[1]	Audiological Evaluation	Ophthalmologic Evaluation	Complete Blood Count	Thyroid Screening (free T4, TSH)	Echocardiography
Infant	Postnatal	S/○	○	○	S/○	○	○	○
	2 Months	S/○	○	S/○	S/○[§]		○	
	4 Months	S/○	○	S/○	S/○			
	6 Months	S/○	○	S/○	S/○			
	9 Months	S/○	○	S/○	S/○[§]			
Early childhood	12 Months	S/○	○	S/○[§]	S/○		○	
	15 Months	S/○	○					
	18 Months	S/○	○					
	24 Months	S/○	○	S/○[§]	S/○[§]		○	
	3 Years	S/○	○	S/○	S/○		○	
	4 Years	S/○	○	S/○	S/○		○	
Late childhood	Annual	S/○	○	S/○[#]	S/○[Δ]		○	
Adolescence 13–21 Years	Annual	S/○	○	S/○	S/○	○	○	

1 Committee on Genetics American Academy of Paediatric: Health supervision for children with Down syndrome, Paediatrics 2011

○ = standardized; S = subjective; § discuss referral to specialist; # once in this age group; Δ objective if necessary

Notes

Notes

M Autonomic nerve system

M.01 Hypersalivation and dysphagia | PCS-Diagnosis 1/1

Autonomic nerve system

Medical history
- Association with certain activities of daily life
- Perioral skin lesions
- Foetor ex ore
- Number of towels needed per day
- Frequency of clothes needed to be changed
- Exsiccosis (constipation, concentrated urine)
- Signs of gastroesophageal reflux disease (cough, choking, hoarseness)
- Aspiration during meal intake
- Infection of upper airways, aspiration pneumonia
- Social stigmatization
- Medication intake

Symptoms
- Lack of head control
- Perioral skin lesions
- Tongue size and movement (voluntary and involuntary)
- Palatine tonsils, adenoid vegetations
- Gingiva, dental state, occlusion
- Enoral sensitivity
- Gag reflex, swallowing act
- Nose/mouth breathing, nasal occlusions

- Score for clinical estimation of hypersalivation[1]:

Severity (1–5)
1. Dry (never drools)
2. Mild (only the lips are wet)
3. Moderate (lips and chin wet)
4. Severe (moist clothing)
5. Profuse drooling (wet clothing, hands, and objects)

Frequency (1–4)
1. Never drools
2. Occasional drooling (e.g. once a day)
3. Frequent drooling (multiple times per day)
4. Constant drooling

Total score (2–9)
- 3–4: mild
- 5: moderate
- 6–9: severe

- Reasons for hypersalivation
  - Medication intake: cholinergics[2], psychotropics, clozapine, antiepileptics
  - Intoxication (mercury, parathion/paraoxon)
  - Central autonomic dysregulation

- Possible causes of dysphagia
  - Movement disorder[3]
  - Mental retardation[4]
  - Neuroimmunologic diseases[5]
  - Neurodegenerative diseases, bulbar palsy, pseudobulbar palsy
  - Traumatic brain injury
  - Stroke
  - Cranial nerve lesions[6]
  - Macroglossia (e.g. symptom of storage disease)
  - Pharynx-, larynx-, esophageal anomalies (e. g. Zenker diverticulum)
  - Gastroesophageal reflux disease

- Improvement of hyper-salivation after withdrawal of agent

- No improvement after removal

- Medication- or intoxication-induced hypersalivation

- Quantification of saliva production per time (e.g. salivary gland scintigraphy or weighing of bibs/cotton balls)

- Increased saliva production

- Normal saliva production

Potential differential diagnoses
- Neuroimmunological diseases[5]
- Central dysautonomia

- Dysphagia

- Diagnostic work-up of dysphagia
  - Radiocontrast test (barium)
  - Video endoscopy (rarely used in paediatrics)
  - Work-up of aetiology
  - Audiography (adenoids)

- Dysphagia of neurologic origin

- Dysphagia caused by pharyngeal, laryngeal or esophageal anomalies

---

1 According to Thomas-Stonell, 1988
2 Muscarine, bethanechol, pilocarpine, nicotine, neostigmine, physostigmine, pyridostigmine, donepezil, rivastigmine, galantamine, malathion, pralidoxime
3 E.g. Cerebral palsy, dystonia and others
4 Rett Syndrome, Angelman syndrome, VACTERL association, mental retardation of unknown origin.
5 ADEM, MS, meningoencephalitis
6 E.g. hypoglossus, vagus, or facial nerve palsy

M.01 Hypersalivation and dysphagia | PCS-Therapy 1/1

Autonomic nerve system

Hypersalivation as a consequence of dysphagia or dysautonomia	**Basic therapy** ▶ Preparation of food (milling, pureeing of food, adding pudding, thickening of liquids) ▶ In case of malnutrition, enrich food or add industrially produced nutritionally complete, high energy, ready-to-use drinks ▶ In case of severe dysphagia and aspiration, discuss early different types of feeding tubes, gastric tubes ▶ Include speech-language therapists to improve oral motor control (e.g. Castillo Morales) ▶ Improve seating position, trunk and head alignment, neck extension before meals ▶ Discuss supply with a palatal plate to induce swallowing more easily[1] ▶ Practice of special swallowing maneuvers	▶ Total drooling score ≥ 6[1]	▶ Intraglandular injection of Botulinum toxins[2] – Usually in intervals of (2–)4–6 months	▶ If treatment outcome is unsatisfactory or if efficacy decreases in time – Follow-up evaluation to decide on additional needs – Objectively assess efficacy using the Thomas-Stonell rating scale[2]	▶ Anticholinergics[3] – Trihexyphenidyl (5 mg, up to 3 × 1/d) – Glykopyrrolate (120–400 mcg/kg/d/ SD × 3–4, max. 3 × 1–2 mg/d) – Scopolamine (1,5 mg/72 h) – Atropine (0,5 mg up to 3 × 0,5–2/d) – Amitriptyline (50 mg, up to 3 × ¼–½/d)	▶ After 6–12 months without success and persistent psychological strain	▶ Consider combination of anticholingergics and Botulinum toxins ▶ Re-consider Botulinum toxins, e.g. different preparation ▶ Consider surgical therapy by experienced ENT specialist[4] – Relocation of gland ducts (best option) – (Partial) excision of glands – Ligation of gland ducts
		▶ In case of muscular hypertension of cricopharyngeus muscle	▶ Consider endoscopic injection of Botulinum toxins[5]				
Medication-induced hypersalivation	▶ Reduce dosage, withdraw or change medication						
Intoxication-induced hypersalivation	▶ Stop exposition and withdraw toxic agent if possible						

1 To improve on closing the mouth, to passively stimulate the tongue, lips and cheek
2 Off-label therapy, requires written consent of the patient; dosage, dilution, and distribution is not interchangeable between different preparations; needs to be determined individually by an experienced user.
3 Reduced saliva production by blocking the activation of muscarinic receptors; side effects: reduced concentration, drowsiness, agitation, disturbed temperature regulation, disturbed gastrointestinal mobility, constipation, urine retention. Comment: due to the high rate of systemic side effects, not well established in paediatric care; possibly low dose combination with Botulinum toxin may be effective in increasing reinjection intervals.
4 Very rare indication in paediatric care due to irreversibility. Should only be performed in an experienced center.

M.02 Bladder dysfunction | PCS-Diagnosis 1/1

Autonomic nerve system

Basic investigations
- Bladder function
  - Capacity
  - Frequency of micturition
  - Urge
  - Incontinence
    - Primary/secondary?
    - Day/night?
- Exclusion of urinary tract infection
- Ultrasound
- Micturition protocol (2 days)

Clues for enuresis (monosymptomatic)
- Regular, strong nocturnal bed wetting without awakening
- Normal micturition during the day
- No repetitive urinary tract infections
- Emptying of the bladder
  - Functionally normal
  - Almost completely (< 10 % urine left)
  - "Wrong place, wrong time"
- Doctor's examination including neurological examination without findings
- Normal defecation

Enuresis
- The diagnosis shouldn't be given before 5 years of age
- Requires only few, non-invasive steps
- *Pitfalls:* Possible combination of enuresis and bladder dysfunction!
- Therapeutic options
  - Conditioning therapy (alarm therapy)
  - Drug therapy (Desmopressin)
  - Combined therapy (urotherapy, anticholinergic agents, biofeedback, psychology)
  - No go's: awakening at night-time, reward and punishment, restriction of fluid intake in the evening

Clues for bladder dysfunction (non-monosymptomatic)
- Structural anomalies seen on ultrasound
- Unintentional urination not caused by a normal emptying of the bladder
- Imperative urge to urinate
- Pollakisuria
- Obvious maneuvers prevent urine release
- Weak urinary stream
- Repetitive urinary tract infections

Clues for neurogenic bladder dysfunction
- Hints from medical history (myelomeningocele, cerebral palsy, tethered cord)
- Hints from physical examination (malformation syndrome or sequence (VACTERL), neurologic deficit particularly of the lower extremity)

- Urodynamic evaluation including cystometric studies and combined uroflowmetry and electromyography of the pelvic muscles
- MRI
- Consider voiding cysturethrography (Reflux?)

Neurogenic detrusor-sphincter dysfunction (NDSD)
- D+/U+ (34 %)
- D–/U– (32 %)
- D–/U+ (13 %)
- D+/U– (11 %)

D: M. detrusor vesicae
U: M. sphinkter urethrae ext.

- Clues for dysfunctional or structural causes of incontinence
- Check-up by a specialist (paediatrician, paediatric surgeon, paediatric urologist)

M.03 Sleep disorders │ PCS-Diagnosis 1/1

Autonomic nerve system

Medical History
- Sleep-wake behaviour
- Child development (milestones)
- Vaccination status
- Family structure
- Parent-child interaction
- For proper evaluation it is important to obtain complete information on complaints. Therefore, both child *and* parents should be interviewed.
- Sleep questionnaires

Sleep-wake diary
- Recording of sleep-wake patterns over a period of 3 weeks
  - Analysis of sleep disorders
  - Verification of anamnestic data

Physical examination
- Internal and neurological medical examination including developmental status

---

Resistant behavioural insomnia and long lasting frequent nightmares
- Referral to child psychiatric/psychological diagnosis

Suspected pulmonary causes
- Chest x-ray
- Pulmonary function tests

Sleep related breathing disorders
- Cardiorespiratory polygraphy (basic diagnostic work-up)
- According to clinical findings, consultations of ENT (adenotonsillar hypertrophy), orthodontist/oral surgeon (orthodontic anomalies/midface hypoplasia)

Suspected cardiac arrhythmias and symptoms of cardiac disorders
- ECG and, if indicated, long-term ECG
- If indicated, echocardiography

Suspected hypersomnias
- Home actigraphy for quantification of sleep-wake times
- Epworth Sleepiness Scale (ESS-K)

Suspected sleepwalking and sleep terrors and suspected sleep related movement disorders
- Home video recording of suspected events

Suspected restless-legs syndrome: in addition analysis of
- Ferritin
- Magnesium

Suspected sleep related epileptic seizures
- EEG
- Sleep EEG
- Sleep-deprived EEG

If above measures do not sufficiently clarify the symptoms
- Cardiorespiratory polysomnography
- If indicated, in addition Multiple Sleep Latency Test (MSLT) or Maintenance of Wakefullness Test (MWT) for diagnosing daytime sleepiness

In cases of severe and acute symptoms, especially sleep related cyanosis, immediate polysomnographic examination

---

Scientific hypothesis/differential diagnosis:
- Insomnia (inadequate sleep hygiene, behavioural insomnia of childhood)
- Sleep related breathing disorders (obstructive sleep apnea)
- Hypersomnias of central origin (narcolepsy)
- Circadian rhythm sleep disorders
- Parasomnias (sleepwalking, sleep terrors, nightmare disorder)
- Sleep related movement disorders (restless legs syndrome)
- Normal variants
- Isolated symptoms
- Other sleep disorders

M.03 Sleep disorders

M.03 Sleep disorders | PCS-Therapy

Functional sleep disruption	**General measures** ▶ Behavioral therapy including guidance on sleep hygiene and sleep environment ▶ Psychotherapy as indicated ▶ Infants/small children: primarily parental education; older children need to be included (e.g. using conditioning methods) ▶ If parent-child interaction is severely disturbed (e.g. due to psychiatric problems of the parents), psychotherapeutic support or treatment of the parents is necessary ▶ Relaxing techniques such as autogenic training or progressive muscle relaxation are recommended	
	Drug therapy ▶ Concomitant drug therapy should be understood as an acute intervention over a short period of time only ▶ Substances with respiratory suppressive effects can acutely worsen preexisting breathing disorders ▶ Phytotherapeutics, especially highly concentrated extracts of Valerian and St John's wort for school children with chronic sleep disorders ▶ Melatonin therapy (preschool ages: 3–5 mg; children up to 12 y: 6–10 mg; a little less for adolescents, e.g. 6 mg)	
Central breathing disturbance with hypoxemia	**Treatment with drugs that stimulate breathing** ▶ Theophylline/Aminophylline (3–4 mg/kg/d) Or ▶ Caffeine (initially 10 mg/kg, maintenance 3 mg/kg/d)	If no response and undisturbed central chemosensibility: Trial with Acetazolamide (5–10 mg/kg/d; *NOTE: possible metabolic deterioration*)
Obstructive sleep apnea syndrome	▶ In addition to sleep medicine diagnosis: ENT and orthodontist	If unsatisfying response to surgical intervention (e.g. adenotonsillectomy or intraoral orthodontic intervention: **CPAP, BiPAP or IPPV therapy**
Narcolepsy	▶ Good sleep hygiene with regular sleep-wake cycles and regular naps during daytime ▶ Central stimulating drugs (e.g. Methylphenidate) ▶ For pronounced sleep disruption during nighttime: gamma hydroxybutyrate ▶ For pronounced cataplexy, sleep paralysis and hypnagogic hallucinations: trial with tricyclic antidepressants	
Parasomnias: pavor nocturnus (night terror), somnambulism und night mares	**Parent counseling** (usually no need for further actions) ▶ Do not wake children from sleep (aggressive reactions) ▶ Somnambulism: protect the child's environment ▶ If nightmares persist: psychological counselling, treatment ▶ If child awakes from nightmare: provide feeling of security (physically close) ▶ Possible external causes: TV/video games ▶ Night-light or stuffed animal can reduce fear ▶ Recurring dreams or dreams that keep troubling the child also during daytimes: deal with the subject matter of the dreams ▶ Symptomatic therapeutic concept for nightmares: painting therapy (imagery rehearsal)	
Sleep-related movement disorders: extreme restlessness and tossing in bed (jactatio capitis and corporis), bruxism, restless legs syndrome (RLS)	▶ Parental counseling for rhythmic movement disorders (jactatio capitis and corporis), padding of the bed if necessary ▶ Referral to orthodontist for bruxism ▶ Treatment for RLS caused by iron or magnesium deficiency ▶ Idiopathic RLS: possible treatment with L-Dopa (adult neurology)	

Notes

Notes

N Neurometabolic and neurodegenerative disorders

N.01 Neurometabolic disorders | PCS-Diagnostic approach 1/1

Neurometabolic and neurodegenerative disorders

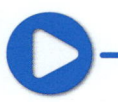

Basic work-up	Advanced diagnostic work-up	Cerebrospinal diagnostic work-up and biopsies

Medical history
▶ Present illness
▶ Past medical history
▶ Prenatal and birth history
▶ Mental development
▶ Developmental milestones
▶ Family history
▶ Social history
▶ Was newborn screening done?
 	
Physical examination
▶ Neurologic, general paediatric
 	
Laboratory tests
▶ Complete blood count, blood gas analysis, electrolytes (including anion gap), glucose, lactate, ammonia, liver function tests (transaminases, γGT, ALP, bilirubin), liver synthesis parameters (albumin, cholinesterase, coagulation tests), creatinine, urea, creatine phosphokinase, cholesterol, triglyceride, uric acid.
▶ Urine test strips: ketones, glucose, protein
	▶ **Diagnostic procedures**
	  – Imaging studies (ultrasound, MRI)
	  – ECG, echocardiography
	  – Electrophysiological investigations (EEG, EMG, NCV)
	  – VEP/ABEP
	  – Funduscopy, slit-lamp examination
	▶ **Biochemical analyses (metabolites)**
	▶ **Enzyme analyses**
	▶ **Molecular genetic analyses**
		Lumbar puncture
		Biopsy
		▶ Skin (fibroblast culture)
		▶ Muscle
		▶ Liver

N.01 Neurometabolic disorders | PCS-Symptoms, specific laboratory tests 1/3

Neurometabolic and neurodegenerative disorders

Clinical symptoms		Plasma	Urine	Additional	Possible diagnosis
Isolated mental retardation		Always exclude hypothyroidism!!			
	Basic metabolic tests	Amino acids Acylcarnitines	Organic acids		Organic acidurias Aminoacidopathies Disorders of the carnitine cycle and fatty acid oxidation Urea cycle defects
Mental retardation plus additional clinical features					
	+ Neurological abnormalities		Glycosaminoglycans, oligosaccharides, sialic acid	Lymphocyte vacuoles (blood smear), enzyme studies	Lysosomal storage diseases
		Isoelectric focusing (transferrin)			Congenital disorders of glycosylation (CDG)
		Total homocysteine, amino acids			Homocystinuria
		Creatine, creatinine, guanidinoacetate	Creatine, creatinine, guanidinoacetate		Disorders of creatine biosynthesis
			Purines/pyrimidines		Disorders of purine and pyrimidine metabolism
				Biogenic amines, pterins (CSF)	Neurotransmitter deficiencies
				Glucose ratio CSF/blood	GLUT1 deficiency
	+ Psychiatric abnormalities	Amino acids	Orotic acid		Urea cycle defects (late-onset)
	+ Morphological abnormalities	Sterols (e. g. 7-/8-Dehydrocholesterol)			Disorders of sterol biosynthesis (e. g. Smith-Lemli-Opitz syndrome)
			Glycosaminoglycans, oligosaccharides, sialic acid	Lymphocyte vacuoles (blood smear), enzyme studies	Lysosomal storage diseases
		Isoelectric focusing (transferrin)			Congenital disorders of glycosylation (CDG)
	+ Skin/hair alterations		Organic acids	Biotinidase activity	Biotinidase deficiency

N.01 Neurometabolic disorders | PCS-Symptoms, specific laboratory tests 2/3

Neurometabolic and neurodegenerative disorders

		Copper, Ceruloplasmin	Molecular genetic analysis	Menkes disease
	+ Cardiac abnormalities	Acylcarnitines		Disorders of the carnitine cycle and long-chain-fatty acid oxidation
		Acylcarnitines	Organic acids	Organic acidurias (PA)
			Oligosaccharides (Pompe disease)	Lymphocyte vacuoles (blood smear; Pompe disease), enzyme studies, molecular genetic analyses	Glycogen storage diseases (type II [Pompe disease]; type III; type IV)
			Glycosaminoglycans, oligosaccharides, sialic acid	Lymphocyte vacuoles (blood smear), enzyme studies	Lysosomal storage diseases
		Isoelectric focussing (transferrin)			Congenital disorders of glycosylation (CDG)
	+ Ocular abnormalities	Galactose, Galactose-1-phosphate		Enzyme studies, molecular genetic analyses	Galactosemia
		Total homocysteine, amino acids			Homocystinuria
		Very-long-chain fatty acids			Peroxisomal disorders (Zellweger syndrome)
			Glycosaminoglycans, oligosaccharides, sialic acid	Lymphocyte vacuoles (blood smear), enzyme studies	Lysosomal storage diseases
				Cystine in leukocytes	Cystinosis
	+ Organomegalies			Enzyme studies, molecular genetic analyses	Glycogen storage diseases
			Glycosaminoglycans, oligosaccharides, sialic acid	Lymphocyte vacuoles (blood smear), enzyme studies	Lysosomal storage diseases
	+ Hepatopathy	Galactose, Galactose-1-phosphate		Enzyme studies, molecular genetic analyses	Galactosemia
		Amino acids	Succinylacetone (urine, blood)	Porphobilinogen synthase activity	Hypertyrosinemia type I
			Bile acids		Disorders of bile acid synthesis
				Molecular genetic analyses	Hereditary fructose intolerance

N.01 Neurometabolic disorders

N.01 Neurometabolic disorders | PCS-Symptoms, specific laboratory tests 3/3

				Mitochondrial DNA	Mitochondrial DNA depletion syndrome
		Very-long-chain fatty acids			Peroxisomal disorders (Zellweger syndrome)
	+ Macrocephaly	Acylcarnitines	Organic acids (3-OH-glutaric acid, glutaric acid)		Glutaric aciduria type I
			Organic acids (N-acetylaspartic acid)		Canavan disease
			Glycosaminoglycans, oligosaccharides	Lymphocyte vacuoles (blood smear), enzyme studies	Lysosomal storage diseases (in particular Tay-Sachs disease, Sandhoff disease)
	+ Haematological abnormalities	Acylcarnitines	Organic acids		Organic acidurias (PA, MMA)
		Total homocysteine	Methylmalonic acid	Transcobalamin II (if applicable)	Disorders of cobalamin metabolism
	+ Nephrological abnormalities		Purines		Disorders of purine metabolism
	+ Multisystem involvement		Organic acids	Lactate (CSF), enzyme studies (liver, muscle), molecular genetic analyses (mitochondrial/nuclear DNA)	Mitochondrial disorders
		Very-long-chain fatty acids			Peroxisomal disorders (Zellweger syndrome)
			Glycosaminoglycans, oligosaccharides, sialic acid	Lymphocyte vacuoles (blood smear), enzyme studies	Lysosomal storage diseases
		Isoelectric focusing (transferrin)			Congenital disorders of glycosylation (CDG)

N.01 Neurometabolic disorders | PCS-Cerebrospinal fluid (CSF) diagnostic work-up 1/1

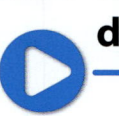

Neurometabolic and neurodegenerative disorders

Detectable diseases
- Aminoacidopathies
  (e.g. non-ketotic hyperglycinemia, serine deficiency disorders)
- Neurotransmitter defects
  (e.g. tetrahydrobiopterin (BH_4) deficiency, aromatic L-amino acid decarboxylase (AADC) deficiency)
- Folinic acid-responsive seizures
- Vitamin B_6 (pyridoxal phosphate)-responsive seizures
- Glucose transport protein deficiency (GLUT1 deficiency, glucose ratio CSF/blood < 0.35)

General approach
- CSF investigations to be performed in the morning (fasting; last meal in the evening). For infants: at least 4 hours fasting.
- Important: CSF and serum samples to be taken at the same time.
- Preparation and labeling of 6 (7) chronologically marked tubes.
- Tubes no. 3–6 (7) to be pre-cooled, immediately frozen (-80°C) and shipped on dry ice.

Specific approach

▶ Step 1	*Blood sampling* ▶ Sodium fluoride tubes → glucose, lactate ▶ EDTA plasma tubes → amino acids
▶ Step 2	*Lumbar puncture* **Infants** (each tube should contain 0.3–0.5 ml CSF); children > 1 year (each tube should contain 0.5–1 ml (SF) ▶ Tube 1: CSF status, glucose, lactate ▶ Tube 2: amino acids, pyridoxal phosphate (protected from light!) ▶ Tube 3–6: neurotransmitters (pre-cooled, immediately frozen)

N.01 Neurometabolic disorders | PCS-Specific therapies 1/3

Neurometabolic and neurodegenerative disorders

	Dietetic therapy		Medical therapy						Organ transplantation
	Substrate restriction	Alternative energy sources	Conjugating agents	Substrate reduction through the inhibition of enzymes in the metabolic pathway proximal to the metabolic block	Enzyme cofactors or chaperones	Correction of product deficiencies	Enzyme replacement therapy	Gene therapy	
Organic acidurias	Dietary restriction of protein and supplementation of unaffected amino acids (e.g. PA, MMA, IVA)		L-Carnitine, L-Glycine		Hydroxocobalamin (Vit B_{12}-responsive MMA)				Liver transplantation, combined liver-kidney transplantation (MMA, if applicable)
Aminoacidopathies	Dietary restriction of protein and supplementation of unaffected amino acids (e.g. PKU, Homocystinuria)			NTBC (Hypertyrosinemia type I)	BH_4 (BH_4-sensitive PKU) Pyridoxine (Homocystinuria)				
Urea cycle defects	Dietary restriction of protein and supplementation of essential amino acids (Late-onset forms)		Na-benzoate, Na-phenylbutyrate			Arginine (CPS, OCT, ASS, ASL deficiency)			Liver transplantation, hepatocyte transplantation (if applicable)
Disorders of the carnitine cycle and fatty acid oxidation	Avoid fasting	MCT (Disorders of the carnitine cycle and oxidation of long-chain fatty acids)	L-Carnitine in carnitine deficiency (controversially discussed; avoid in disorders of long-chain fatty acid oxidation or the carnitine cycle)			L-Carnitine (Systemic carnitine deficiency; carnitine transporter deficiency)			
Mitochondrial disorders	Carbohydrate restriction	Ketogenic diet (PDH deficiency)			Riboflavin, coenzyme Q10 (mitochondrial respiratory chain diseases) Dichloroacetate (PDH deficiency)				

N.01 Neurometabolic disorders | PCS-Specific therapies 2/3

Lysosomal storage diseases				Miglustat (Gaucher disease)	Galactose IV (Fabry disease, atypical form)		Gaucher disease, Fabry disease, MPS type I, MPS type II, MPS type VI, Pompe disease	Bone marrow transplantation
Peroxisomal disorders	Phytanic acid restriction (Refsum disease)						
Congenital disorders of glycosylation (CDG)						Mannose (CDG Ib), Fucose (CDG IIc)	
Disorders of creatine biosynthesis						Creatine	
Disorders of purine and pyrimidine metabolism							Adenosine deaminase deficiency (SCID)
Neurotransmitter deficiencies		Ketogenic diet (GLUT1 deficiency)			Pyridoxine (Vitamin-B_6-responsive seizures) Pyridoxal phosphate (Pyridoxal-phosphate-responsive seizures) Folinic acid (Folinic-acid-responsive seizures)	BH_4, 5-Hydroxytryptophan (BH_4-deficiency) L-Dopa (Dopa-responsive dystonia, Tyrosine hydroxylase deficiency)	
Galactosemia	Lactose-free, galactose-restricted diet						
Hereditary fructose intolerance	Fructose-restricted diet						
Glycogen storage diseases						Carbohydrate intake	

N.01 Neurometabolic disorders | PCS-Specific therapies 3/3

Disorders of sterol biosynthesis						Cholesterol	
Menkes disease						Copper	
Biotinidase deficiency					Biotin		

N.02 Neurodegenerative disorders | PCS-Orientation 1/1

Neurometabolic and neurodegenerative disorders

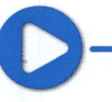

Medical history/ physical examination
- Sudden infant death syndrome (SIDS) in the family
- Neurodegenerative diseases/genetic conditions in the family (pedigree)
- Consanguinity
- Signs of global brain dysfunction
- Duration: > 3 months
- Typical: intellectual and neurological degeneration
- Often preceded by years of normal development (*NOTE:* early onset disease)
- Loss of acquired abilities (children < 4: stagnation)
- Focal neurological signs

Basic Investigations
- MRI of the brain +/- spinal cord
- Ophthalmologist
  - ERG (electroretinography)
  - VEP (visually evoked potentials)
- Neurophysiology:
  - EEG
  - MEP (motorically EP)/Transcranial magnetic stimulation (TMS)
  - SEP (somatosensory EP)
  - ABR (auditory brain stem response)
  - EMG (electromyography)
  - NCV (nerve conduction velocity)

Clues to diagnosis

Clues due to age of onset
- First year of life: infantile neuronal ceroid lipofuscinosis (NCL1), M. Krabbe (infantile globoid cell dystrophy), M. Tay-Sachs (GM2 gangliosidosis), M. Pelizaeus-Merzbacher, M. Niemann-Pick type IA (earlier: type A)
- 5–24(-36) months: late-infantile metachromatic leukodystrophy, Rett's syndrome, infantile neuroaxonal dystrophy (M. Seitelberger), progressive neuronal degeneration of childhood (PNDC, Alpers' syndrome, Huttenlocher syndrome, infantile poliodystrophy), M. Gaucher type 3 (neuronopathic)
- (1-)2–5(-7) years: late-infantile neuronal ceroid lipofuscinosis (NCL2), mucopolysaccharidosis type 3 (Sanfilippo), hereditary spastic paraparesis, pantothenate kinase-associated neurodegeneration (PKAN)
- 4–10 years: juvenile neuronal ceroid lipofuscinosis (NCL3), adrenoleukodystrophy (ALD), Rasmussen encephalitis
- 6–16 years: M. Niemann-Pick IS (earlier: type B), progressive myoclonic epilepsy of type Unverricht-Lundborg (EPM1), subacute sclerosing panencephalitis (SSPE)
- 10–20 years: juvenile M. Huntington, M. Wilson, Friedreich ataxia, progressive myoclonic epilepsy type 2 Lafora

Clues from medical history
- Myoclonus: gangliosidosis, Neuronal Ceroid Lipofuscinosis (NCL), M. Gaucher type 3, Leigh's syndrome, subacute sclerosing panencephalitis, Lafora's disease, Creutzfeld-Jakob-disease variant (vCJD), Unverricht-Lundborg disease
- Early visual impairment: neuronal ceroid lipofuscinosis, Adrenoleukodystrophy, GM2 gangliosidosis
- Behavioral disturbances: adrenoleukodystrophy, Sanfilippo, M. Wilson, juvenile M. Huntington, juvenile Neuronal Neroid Lipofuscinosis (NCL)
- Stroke-like episodes/episodic encephalopathy: mitochondrial disease (Leigh, MELAS), homocystinuria, Moyamoya disease
- Gastrointestinal symptoms (dystrophy, vomiting, diarrhea): abetalipoteinemia, Leigh's syndrome, M. Gaucher type 2, Sanfilippo's syndrome
- Rapid regression: gangliosidosis, PKAN, M. Krabbe, adrenoleukodystrophie (ALD), Alpers-syndrome, Leigh-syndrome
- Positive family history: recessive or X-bound heredity (M. Pelizaeus-Merzbacher, Adrenoleukodystrophie (ALD, M. Hunter)
- Grey versus white matter
  - Predominating seizures, personality changes, dementia (grey matter)
  - Predominating spasticity, ataxia, hearing/visual impairment (white matter)

Clues from physical examination
- Dysmorphic facial features: mucopolysaccharidosis, GM1 gangliosidosis, mucolipidosis
- Macrocephalus: M. Canavan, M. Alexander, M. Krabbe, metachromatic leukodystrophy
- Microcephalus: Rett's syndrome, infantile neuronal ceroid lipofuscinosis
- Skeletal changes: mucopolysaccharidosis, GM1 gangliosidosis, M. Gaucher
- Hepatosplenomegaly: M. Gaucher, M. Niemann-Pick, Mucopolysaccharidosis, gangliosidosis, M. Wilson
- Neuropathy: metachromatic leukodystrophy, mucosulfatidosis, M. Krabbe, Refsum's disease, adrenoleukodystrophy, M. Fabry, Leigh's syndrome, Friedreich ataxia, infantile neuroaxonal dystrophy
- Pyramidal tract signs: Leukoencephalopathies (metachromatic leukodystrophy, M. Krabbe, adrenoleukodystrophy etc.)
- Extrapyramidal signs: Leigh's syndrome, juvenile M. Huntington, PKAN, M. Wilson, vCJD
- Ataxia: Ataxia telangiectasia, Friedreich ataxia, Leigh's syndrome, M. Niemann-Pick, cerebrotendinous xanthomatosis, metachromatic leukodystrophy, vCJD, Refsum's disease
- Cataract: cerebrotendinous xanthomatosis, lysosomal disorders

N.02 Neurodegenerative disorders | PCS-Differential diagnosis of psychomotor regression – non-neurometabolic

All ages	0–2 years	2–5 years	School age	Adolescence
▶ Epileptic encephalopathy ▶ Deprivation/neglect ▶ Cerebrovascular disease ▶ Increased intracranial pressure ▶ Intoxication (lead) ▶ Endocrinologic (thyroid) ▶ Fetal alcohol syndrome ▶ Para-neoplastic ▶ Celiac disease ▶ Munchhausen by proxy	▶ West syndrome ▶ Autistic regression ▶ Static encephalopathy (hypoxic ischaemic encephalopathy)	▶ Lennox-Gastaut syndrome ▶ Brain/spinal tumor ▶ (DOPA-responsive dystonia)	▶ Landau-Kleffner syndrome ▶ Continuous spikes and slow waves during sleep (CSWS)/Electric status epilepticus during sleep (ESES) ▶ Autoimmune disorder (multiple sclerosis) ▶ Idiopathic torsion dystonia	▶ Autoimmune disease/vasculitis (SLE, sarkoidosis, autoimmune limbic encephalitis) ▶ Psychiatric disorders, somatoform disorders ▶ Chronic fatigue syndrome ▶ Substance abuse

N.03 Mitochondrial disorders | PCS-Diagnosis 1/3

Neurometabolic and neurodegenerative disorders

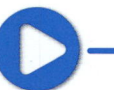

Medical history
- Positive family history
- Primary/secondary developmental delay, developmental arrest, infection-associated regression or crises, seizures, muscular exercise intolerance, muscle weakness
- Evidence for involvement of other organ systems (growth retardation, deafness; visual, cardiac, gastrointestinal, endocrine disorders)

Physical Examination
- Specific findings (selection)
  - Migraine-like headache
  - Stroke-like events
  - Ptosis, external ophthalmoplegia
  - Muscular exercise intolerance
  - Retinal visual disturbances
  - Deafness
- Non-specific findings (selection)
  - Mental retardation
  - Cognitive Regression
  - Seizures (focal, myoclonic)
  - Muscle hypotonia
  - Ataxia
  - Pyramidal symptoms (spasticity)
  - Extrapyramidal symptoms (dystonia, rigidity, akinesia)
- Organ-specific findings (selection)
  - Heart: bradycardia, heart failure
  - GI: dysphagia, gastroparesis, intestinal pseudo-obstruction, non-infectious diarrhea
  - Endocrine system: short stature, delayed puberty, signs of hypothyroidism, hypoparathyroidism, diabetes

Clinical chemistry of body fluids
- Basic diagnostic workup (blood)
- Specific analyses: blood (lactate, pyruvate, alanine), CSF (lactate, pyruvate, alanine, protein), urine (organic acids, amino acids, thymidine)
- Organ-specific diagnosis (selection)
  - Blood count (cytopenias)
  - Endocrine parameters (T4, TSH, parathyroid hormone, gonadotropins, HbA1c)
  - Liver parameters (transaminases, ammonia, synthesis parameters)
  - Muscle parameters: creatine kinase
  - Cardiac parameters: CK-MB, troponin T
  - Kidney parameters: creatinine, urea, uric acid, cystatin C
  - Urine: amino acids, electrolytes, protein

Technical diagnostic procedures
- MRI, MR spectroscopy
  - Malformations
  - Acute changes (ischaemia, symmetrical lesions in basal ganglia, midbrain, brain stem)
  - Chronic neurodegeneration (supra-infratentorial atrophy)
  - Focal/diffuse white matter changes (leukodystrophy, leukencephalopathy)
  - Local/generalized lactate accumulation
- Neurophysiological studies
  - EEG (general changes, focal slowing, epileptic discharges)
  - VEP, AEP, SSEP and neurography (NCV)
- Organ-specific diagnosis (selection)
  - ECG, echocardiography
  - Neuro-ophthalmology, funduscopy, ERG
  - Audiometry, brain stem evoked response audiometry (BERA)
  - Endocrine function tests
  - Oral glucose tolerance test
  - Sonography (brain, muscle, liver, kidney, pancreas)

Studies of muscle tissue (muscle biopsy)
- Muscle morphology
  - Standard stains ("ragged red fiber", fat deposits, cytochrome c – oxidase-negative fibers in a mosaic/diffuse pattern)
  - Electron microscopy (abnormal mitochondria, paracrystalline inclusions)
- Muscle biochemistry (native/frozen material)
  - ATP synthesis rate (only non-frozen material, immediate processing necessary)
  - Activity of pyruvate dehydrogenase, respiratory chain complexes I-V (V only vital material)
- Studies on cultured fibroblasts
  - Only on specific issues (e.g. verification of muscle biochemical findings or in preparation for a biochemically-based prenatal diagnosis)
- Genetic diagnosis
  - Mitochondrial DNA (mtDNA) from blood, urine sediment cells, muscle tissue
  - Specific disease-related mutations
  - Sequencing of genes or the entire genome (preferentially from muscle tissue)
  - Nuclear genes (nDNA) potentially relating to the disorder

N.03 Mitochondrial disorders

N.03 Mitochondrial disorders | PCS-Diagnosis 2/3

Diagnostic procedure in specific mitochondrial disorders (mitochondrial syndromes)
▶ Pearson's syndrome
Symptoms: congenital lactic acidosis, anemia, thrombocytopenia, pancytopenia, exocrine pancreatic insufficiency
– → mtDNA analysis: deletions/duplications in blood

▶ Kearns-Sayre syndrom/chronic progressive external ophthalmoplegia (CPEO) (plus)
Symptoms: ptosis, external ophthalmoplegia, retinitis pigmentosa (onset before 20 years); in some cases heart block, cerebellar signs, CSF protein > 100 mg/dl
– mtDNA analysis: deletions/duplications, 3 243A>G in blood/urine cell sediment
– If negative: muscle biopsy for morphology, biochemistry, mtDNA analysis in muscle tissue (deletions/duplications, 3 243A>G, other rare mutations)

▶ MELAS
Symptoms: occipitoparietal ischaemia; in some cases migraine headaches, stroke-like episodes, growth retardation, hearing loss, dementia, gastrointestinal pseudo-obstruction
– mtDNA analysis: 3 243A>G, deletions/duplications, rare mutations in blood/urine cell sediment
– If negative: muscle biopsy for morphology, biochemistry, mtDNA analysis in muscle tissue (3 243A>G, deletions/duplications, other rare mutations)

▶ MERRF
Symptoms: myoclonus, myoclonic and other seizures, ataxia, sensorineural hearing loss, impaired vision (optic atrophy), neuropathy, dementia
– mtDNA analysis: 8 344A>G, 3, 243A>G, deletions/duplications, rare mutations in blood/urine cell sediment
– If negative: muscle biopsy for morphology, biochemistry, mtDNA analysis in muscle tissue (8 344A>G, 3, 243A>G, deletions/duplications, other rare mutations)

▶ Neuropathy, ataxie, and retinitis pigmentosa (NARP)
Symptoms: NARP/MILS variations in maternal line, retinitis pigmentosa, neurogenic muscle atrophy, ataxia, neurogenic clubfoot
– mtDNA analysis: 8 993T>G, C

▶ Leigh's syndrome, variant maternally inherited Leigh's syndrome (MILS)
Symptoms: NARP/MILS variations in maternal line, progressive encephaloneuropathy; MRI: symmetrical lesions in the basal ganglia, midbrain, brain stem
– mtDNA analysis: 8 993T>G, C

▶ Alpers syndrome
Symptoms: acute onset of partial seizures, epileptic status, hepatopathy (progressive liver failure); EEG: occipital slowing or epileptic discharges
– nDNA analysis (polymerase γ, POLG1)

▶ Mitochondrial neurogastrointestinal encephalopathy (MNGIE)
Symptoms: variable neuromuscular symptoms associated with developmental disorders, neuropathy, gastrointestinal symptoms (gastroparesis, intestinal pseudo-obstruction, cachexia)
– Thymidine in urine, nDNA analysis (thymidine phosphorylase, platelet derived endothelial cell grouth factor (PD-ECGF); polymerase γ, POLG1)

Diagnostic procedure in specific mitochondrial disorders (mitochondrial syndromes) without primary mutation detection
– Muscle biopsy: morphology, biochemistry
– If "ragged red fibers" and/or individual cytochrome c oxidase-negative fibers are present: mtDNA analysis (sequencing of all tRNA genes)
– In the absence of "ragged red fibers" and normal cytochrome c oxidase staining: mtDNA and nDNA analysis depending on biochemical results (sequencing of known genes that are associated with the identified biochemical defect)

Diagnostic procedure in non-specific mitochondrial diseases
▶ Non-specific (non-syndromic) encephalomyopathies, MRI with characteristic lesions (symmetrical basal ganglia, midbrain, brain stem, focal/diffuse white matter changes; Leigh's syndrome):
– Muscle biopsy: morphology, biochemistry
– In case of negative cytochrome c oxidase staining (including MTCOX1–3, SURF1, SCO1+2): nDNA analysis
– When "ragged red fibers" and/or individual cytochrome c oxidase-negative fibers: mtDNA analysis (sequencing of all tRNA genes)
– In the absence of "ragged red fibers" and normal cytochrome c oxidase staining: mtDNA and nDNA analysis, depending on biochemical results (sequencing of known genes that are associated with the identified biochemical defect)

N.03 Mitochondrial disorders │ PCS-Diagnosis 3/3

Neurometabolic and neurodegenerative disorders

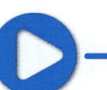

▶ **Non-specific (non-syndromic) encephalomyopathies, MRI without characteristic lesions**
  – Muscle biopsy: morphology, biochemistry
  – If "ragged red fibers" and/or individual cytochrome c oxidase-negative fibers are present: mtDNA analysis (sequencing of all tRNA genes)
  – In the absence of "ragged red fibers" and normal cytochrome c oxidase staining: mtDNA and nDNA analysis, depending on biochemical results (sequencing of known genes that are associated with the identified biochemical defect)

N.03 Mitochondrial disorders | PCS-Therapy 1/2

Neurometabolic and neurodegenerative disorders

Metabolic therapy	▶ Biochemically and/or genetically confirmed defect of pyruvate dehydrogenase	▶ Ketogenic diet (treatment of 1st choice) ▶ Supplement thiamine, α-lipoic acid
	▶ Biochemically and/or genetically confirmed defect of the respiratory chain complexes I and II	▶ Supplement Riboflavin (experimental therapy for 3–6 months, and during crisis) ▶ Ketogenic diet (in complex I defect as tentative treatment)
	▶ Biochemically and/or genetically confirmed defect of the respiratory chain complexes III, IV, V	▶ Supplement Coenzyme Q10, ascorbic acid, Menadione (tentative treatment for 3–6 months, and during crises)
	▶ Mitochondrial syndromes with mtDNA defects in tRNA genes Or ▶ Biochemically and/or genetically confirmed combined defects of the respiratory chain complexes I and IV	▶ Supplementation of Riboflavin and Coenzyme Q10 (tentative treatment for 3–6 months, and during crises)
	▶ Kearns-Sayre syndrome	▶ Substitution of Folic acid
	▶ "Stroke-like" episodes in MELAS	▶ Stereoids, arginine infusions (long-term oral therapy as prophylaxis)
	▶ Defects of the SCO1,2 gene	▶ Supplementation of copper-histidine
	▶ Ragged red fibers with/without defect respiratory chain complex I and/or IV	▶ Supplementation of Riboflavin and Creatine monohydrate, aerobic endurance training
	▶ Primary coenzyme Q10 deficiency	▶ Substitution of Coenzyme Q10
	▶ Thymidine excess in MNGIE	▶ Hemodialysis (temporary reduction of Thymidine) ▶ Platelet transfusion (temporary enzyme replacement) ▶ Stem cell transplantation
Symptomatic therapy	▶ Impending or overt secondary carnitine deficiency	▶ Supplementation or substitution of L-carnitine
	▶ Severe chronic lactic acidosis, persistent buffer requirement	▶ Therapy with Dichloroacetate
	▶ Metabolic crisis	▶ Parenteral rehydration, peritoneal dialysis
	▶ Bradycardia (Kearns-Sayre syndrome)	▶ Implantation of a pacemaker
	▶ Ptosis, cataract	▶ Surgical M. frontalis suspension, cataract surgery
	▶ Epileptic seizure	▶ Anticonvulsants
	▶ Acute stroke-like event ("MELAS stroke") (see chapter A.09 Paediatric stroke)	▶ Steroids, arginine hydrochloride, parenteral lipids
	▶ Hyperglycemia	▶ Dietary measures ▶ Therapy with Insulin

N.03 Mitochondrial disorders | PCS-Therapy 2/2

▶ Progressive cardiomyopathy	▶ Heart transplantation
▶ Neural deafness	▶ Hearing aids, cochlear implant, avoid aminoglycosides
▶ Chronic liver failure	▶ Liver transplantation
▶ Psychiatric symptoms	▶ Psychotropic drugs
▶ Spasticity	▶ Antispastic drugs ▶ Botulinum toxins
▶ Extrapyramidal movement disorders	▶ See chapter G Movement disorders
▶ Anemia Or ▶ Thrombocytopenia	▶ Transfusions
▶ Tubulopathy	▶ Substitution of electrolytes
▶ Endocrine disorders	▶ Substitution of hormones, vitamin D3 and others
▶ Poor weight gain (dystrophy, cachexia)	▶ High-calorie dietary supplements, early percutaneous endoscopic gastrostomy (PEG)

Notes

O Neuromuscular disorders

O.01 Neuromuscular disorders | PCS-Orientation 1/2

When should we think of a neuro-muscular disorder?

If a child presents with
▶ Muscle atrophy or (pseudo)hyper-trophy
▶ Delayed motor development with/without possibly delayed mental development
▶ Reduced muscle strength
▶ Reduced exercise tolerance
▶ Muscle weakness, spontaneous or after exercise
▶ Myalgia, muscle cramps, sponta-neous or after exercise
▶ Abnormal gait (waddling gait caused by proximal weakness or steppage gait caused by distal weakness or a mixed form)
▶ Reduced or absent tendon reflexes
▶ Contractures, clubfeet, scoliosis
▶ Problems with swallowing and sucking
▶ Elevated creatine kinase (CK)

Which important questions should be asked about the patient's history?

Pregnancy
▶ Abnormalities during pregnancy
▶ Oligo- or polyhydramnios (prob-lems with swallowing, renal failure)
▶ Reduced fetal movements
▶ Spontaneous delivery, caesarean section

Neonatal period
▶ Hypotonia
▶ Bulbar symptoms (problems with swallowing and sucking)
▶ Respiratory problems (from apnea to respiratory insufficiency)
▶ Arthrogryposis multiplex congeni-tal (AMC)

Later clinical course
▶ Age at manifestation

Clinical signs suggesting a neuromuscular disorder

(while each sign may be non-specific on its own, the pre-sence of several of the symptoms listed below and/or additional clues in the patient's medical history point to a neuromuscular disorder)
▶ Muscle hypotonia ("floppy infant", abnormal posture, hypermobility of joints)
▶ Muscle stiffness (e.g. Myo-tonia)
▶ Muscle atrophy (e.g. distal in neuropathies, proximal or general in myopathies)
▶ Muscle (pseudo-)hypertro-phy (e.g. in muscular dys-trophies, myotonia conge-nita)
▶ Abnormal reflexes, most often reduced tendon re-flexes
▶ Muscle weakness ("floppy infant", Gowers' phenom-enon)
▶ Gait abnormalities (wad-dling gait caused by proxi-mal muscle weakness of the lower limbs, steppage gait caused by distal weakness of the lower limbs)
▶ Bulbar symptoms (difficul-ties in swallowing and/or sucking)
▶ Respiratory symptoms (from apnea to respiratory insufficiency)
▶ Cardiac involvement (cardiomyopathy, cardiac arrhythmias)
▶ Contractures, scoliosis

The patients medical history, physical examination and CK findings provide the first clues for a possible diagnosis.

The following important points should be considered:
Is there any evidence of a neuromuscular disorder? Or do we have to think of other reasons, e.g. orthopaedic problems, primary central nervous system disorder?
If the available data suggest a neuromuscular disorder, can the affected system be determined, e.g. lower motor neuron, peripheral nerve, neuromuscular junction, skeletal muscle?
Is any other system affected (e.g. heart, liver, CNS, eyes, ears)?
Make a plan for diagnostic work-up for each individual patient to ensure that you obtain all important information from history and physical examination.
Observe carefully and formulate good questions for each investigation, otherwise you may not get very useful answers . Analyze the results carefully, are the methods used appropriate?
A normal CK does not exclude a neuromuscular disorder!

Possible clinical clues
▶ **Manifestation**
  – **Congenital:** often in congenital muscular dystrophies and myopathies, spinal muscular atrophy type I, less in congenital myasthenic syndromes and rarely in congenital hereditary neuropathies
  – **Infancy:** spinal muscular atrophy type Ib and II, milder forms of congenital disorders become obvious
  – **Childhood:** different muscular dystrophies with an early manifestation, Duchenne muscular dystrophy, spinal muscular dystrophy type II or III
▶ **Clinical course**
  – **Static:** congenital myopathies with structural abnormalities, the clinical course may even improve
  – **Slowly progressive:** muscular dystrophies, hereditary neuropathies, spinal muscular atrophy type II or III
  – **Rapidly progressive:** inflammatory disorders (neuritis, myositis), toxic disorders
▶ **Muscle trophic factor**
  – **Severe generalized muscular atrophy with mild muscle weakness:** congenital myopathies with structural abnormalities
  – **Severe generalized muscular atrophy with severe muscle weakness:** congenital muscular dystrophies and myopathies
  – **Severe generalized muscle hypertrophy:** hereditary myotonia congenita
  – **Localized muscular atrophy:** distal muscular atrophy in neuropathies
  – **Localized muscular hypertrophy (often of the calves), but may be non-specific:** Duchenne or Becker muscular dystrophy, but also in other limb-girdle or congenital muscular dystrophies
▶ **Exercise-induced symptoms**
  – **Severe impairment, up to crises:** disorders of the neuromuscular junction (Myasthenia gravis, congenital myasthenic syndromes) and mitochondrial disorders, less severe in metabolic myopathies
  – **Mild exercise intolerance** can be seen in every neuromuscular disorder
  – **Exercise-induced improvement of symptoms:** hereditary myotonia congenita, **exercise-induced impairment of symptoms** in hereditary paramyotonia congenita
▶ **Myalgia:** often in metabolic myopathies and mitochondrial disorders, malignant hyperthermia, may be a symptom in muscular dystrophies
▶ **Sensory involvement:** peripheral neuropathy, most often starting in the lower limbs, localized impairment in traumata (limb swelling or bone fractures), lesions of nerve roots
▶ **Respiratory problems:** apnea in congenital myasthenic syndromes, respiratory insufficiency caused by respiratory muscle weakness in myopathies or muscular dystrophies; these symptoms can appear neonatally or later in the clinical course
▶ **Cardiac involvement:** cardiomyopathies or cardiac arrhythmias appear in different muscular dystrophies or congenital myopathies, sometimes as the leading symptom (e.g. laminopathies, Becker muscular dystrophy, carrier for dystrophinopathies) or appear later in the

O.01 Neuromuscular disorders | PCS-Orientation 2/2

- Motor and mental development
- Time course of symptoms (slow or rapid progression, e.g. slow in Duchenne muscular dystrophy, rapid in juvenile autoimmune dermatomyositis)
- Episodic occurrence, e.g. episodic paralytic paresis
- Severe deterioration during crises (e.g. congenital myasthenic syndromes, mitochondrial disorders)
- Rhabdomyolysis (e.g. metabolic myopathies, muscular dystrophies, malignant hyperthermia)

Family history
- Other affected family members
- Clinical symptoms of elder family members

- Facial hypomimia
- Ptosis, ophthalmoparesis

Possible investigations for further diagnostic work-up
- Serum parameters (especially CK, AST, ALT, LDH)
- Neurophysiology (nerve conduction velocity, repetitive stimulation test, electromyography)
- Muscle ultrasound
- Muscle MRI
- Cranial MRI
- Electrocardiogram, echocardiography
- Vital capacity measurement
- Hearing investigation
- Ophthalmologic investigation
- Muscle biopsy (light and electron microscopy, metabolic analyses)
- Genetic analyses

clinical course (e.g. Emery Dreifuss muscular dystrophy, Duchenne muscular dystrophy, other limb-girdle muscular dystrophies, less in congenital muscular dystrophy (e.g. CMD with Merosin deficiency)
- **Contractures, scoliosis, AMC:** may be manifest at birth or caused later by an ongoing muscular degeneration, non-specific, can occur in different neuromuscular disorders
- **Involvement of external eye muscles:** mitochondrial disorder (CPEO), myasthenia gravis, congenital myasthenic syndromes, congenital myopathies with structural abnormalities
- **Involvement of mimic muscles:** myotonic dystrophy (DM1), congenital myopathies with structural abnormalities, myasthenia gravis, congenital myasthenic syndromes
- **CK level**
  - **Clearly increased** in progressive muscular dystrophies (e.g. Duchenne muscular dystrophy, limb-girdle muscular dystrophies), infectious myositis
  - **Intermittently increased** in metabolic myopathies, rhabdomyolysis, malignant hyperthermia
  - **Mildly increased or normal:** non-specific, a normal CK does exclude a Duchenne muscular dystrophy and is unlikely in other Limb-girdle dystrophies, but may occur in congenital muscular dystrophies
  - **A normal CK does not exclude a neuromuscular disorder!**

O.02 Muscle dystrophies

- See chapter O.02.1 Duchenne-Becker muscular dystrophy (DMD, BMD)
- See chapter O.02.2 Limb-girdle muscular dystrophy (LGMD)
- See chapter O.02.3 Emery-Dreifuss Syndrome
- See chapter O.02.4 Myotonic dystrophy, Dystrophia myotonica (DM)
- See chapter O.02.5 Facio-scapulo-humeral muscular dystrophy (FSHD)
- See chapter O.02.6 Distal muscular dystrophy
- See chapter O.02.7 Congenital muscular dystrophy (CMD))

O.02.1 Duchenne-Becker muscular dystrophy (DMD, BMD) | PCS-Diagnosis 1/1

Neuromuscular disorders

Medical history and clinical findings

- Early symptoms
  - Toe gait
  - Weakness of hip extensors
  - Problems at climbing stairs
  - Abnormal rising from floor (hands propped up on thighs = Gowers sign)
- Late symptoms
  - Spreading of weakness to trunk (scapular winging) and arms
  - Contractures of foot-, knee-, and hip joints
  - Scoliosis

Basic diagnostic work-up
- Serum CK

► Serum CK greatly elevated (> 10-times upper limit of normal)[1]	► Onset before 6th birthday **And** ► Loss of walking before 13th birthday	► Molecular genetics[2]	► Molecular genetic evidence of DYS[3] mutation (deletion, duplication or point mutation) breaking the open reading-frame		► Duchenne muscular dystrophy
			► No molecular genetic evidence of DYS mutation	1) NGS 2) Muscle biopsy	► Demonstration of progressive MD and lack of dystrophin with – Immunohistology **And/or** – Western blot
	► Onset after 6th birthday **And** ► Loss of walking after 13th birthday	► Molecular genetics[2]	► Molecular genetic evidence of DYS mutation (deletion, duplication or point mutation) without breaking the open reading-frame		► Becker muscular dystrophy
			► Molecular genetic demonstration of DYS[3] mutation not successful	1) NGS 2) Muscle biopsy	► Demonstration of dystrophin with – Immunohistology **And** – Western blot
► Serum-CK slightly elevated or not elevated	► Differential diagnosis work-up – Emery-Dreifuss syndrome (see chapter O.02.3 Emery-Dreifuss syndrome) – Congenital myopathies (see chapter O.03.1 Congenital myopathies) – Spinal muscular atrophy (see chapter O.05 Spinal muscular atrophy (SMA)) – Myasthenias (see chapter O.06 Neuromuscular transmission) – Limb-girdle muscular dystrophy (see chapter O.02.2 Limb-girdle muscular dystrophy(LGMD))			

---

1 In late stages of the disease, however, CK levels decrease considerably due to loss of muscle mass.

2 Molecular genetics: usually, MLPA searching for deletions and duplications should be done first. If negative complete sequence of dystrophin gene follows. If negative next generation sequencing (NGS) should be considered to look for other forms of Limb girdle muscular dystrophies. When genetic findings are positive a muscle biopsy is not necessary. In rare case all molecular genetics are negative muscle biopsy should be considered.

3 DYS = dystrophin gene

O.02.1 Duchenne-Becker muscular dystrophy (DMD, BMD) | PCS-Therapy

Basic measures ▶ Emergency health card (re. complications of anesthesia, malignant hyperthermia) **Technical aids to prevent contractures and to compensate for functional deficits in every-day life** ▶ Wheel chair (to enable participation in recreational activities) ▶ Electrically powered wheel chair (to enable independent mobility after definitive loss of walking; individual adaptation necessary; possibly with integrated device for standing and lying) ▶ Nursing bed, special mattress, patient lifter, aids for bathing and showers ▶ Consider night-time leg splints as prevention of contractures; short calf splints are less effective, but long splints are usually not accepted ▶ Light-weight femoral orthoses to enable therapeutic standing and walking (often not accepted) **Drug therapy[1]** ▶ Corticosteroids[2] – Prednisone 0,75 mg/kg/day Or – Deflazacort 0,9 mg/kg/day Either of these drugs to be administered as a single dose at breakfast (continuously or intermittently) ▶ Ataluren (Translarna®) has been approved in some countries for DMD boys with proven stop-codon mutations in the DYS gene. Approval is limited to patients still able to walk. ▶ Creatine monohydrate[3] – 100 mg/kg/day; treatment trial for 4–6 weeks, then decide for each individual patient whether to continue treatment ▶ L-Carnitine – 50 mg/kg/d (especially if muscle cramps are present)	▶ Appearance of functional limitations	▶ Physiotherapy	Depending on age ▶ Promotion of dexterity and motor skills ▶ Prophylaxis of contractures and scoliosis ▶ Respiratory treatment, thoracic mobilization ▶ Cardiovascular training, strengthening of muscles	
	▶ Duchenne-specific contractures with functional limitations	▶ Surgical release of contractures[4]	▶ Achilles tendon release or lengthening, knee- and hip-flexor release, resection of lateral femoral aponeurosis (combined or partial)	
	▶ Progressive scoliosis	▶ Cobb angle of > 20–30 degrees And ▶ Respiratory function: fVC still > 25 %	▶ Surgical stabilization of spine	
	▶ Cardiomyopathy	▶ Pathological SF and EF on echocardiography		▶ ACE-inhibitors and beta-blocking drugs in usual dosage[5]
		▶ Clinically manifest cardiac failure		▶ In addition to ACE-inhibitors, diuretics und digoxin
		▶ Cardiac dysrhythmias		▶ Antiarrhythmics
	▶ Decrease of respiratory strength and vital capacity And ▶ Night-time hypoventilation syndrome with daytime sleepiness and periodic oxygen desaturation during sleep	▶ Non-invasive home ventilation (NIHV) during night sleep[6]	▶ If considered necessary by the patient during the course of illness	▶ Daytime NIHV during daytime naps or for more extended periods of the day
			▶ Acute respiratory infection And/or ▶ NIHV not sufficiently effective	▶ Intubation and – Transitory invasive mechanical ventilation ▶ Tracheotomy and – permanent ventilation (if the fully informed patient agrees)

1 Attempt to relieve disease progression or to increase strength and function, up to now not curative. Metabolites, vitamins, hormones, growth factors: experimental, no proven efficacy, mostly shown to be not effective.
2 Efficacy shown in multiple trials and confirmed by Cochrane Review; intermittent dosage schedules with the aim to reduce side-effects have to be regarded as experimental.
3 Increase of strength and endurance by 5–10 % shown in healthy athletes and muscular dystrophy-patients with well-preserved function; effect in weak patients very questionable.
4 Prophylactic surgery according to Rideau: early surgery (age 6–7 years) to enable fast postoperative rehabilitation with still well-preserved strength.
5 Experimental prophylactic treatment starting from the age of 10 years.
6 After clarification of the economic, nursing and psychosocial condition and the consequences of a long time ventilator treatment.

O.02.2 Limb-girdle muscular dystrophy (LGMD) | PCS-Diagnosis 1/1

Neuromuscular disorders

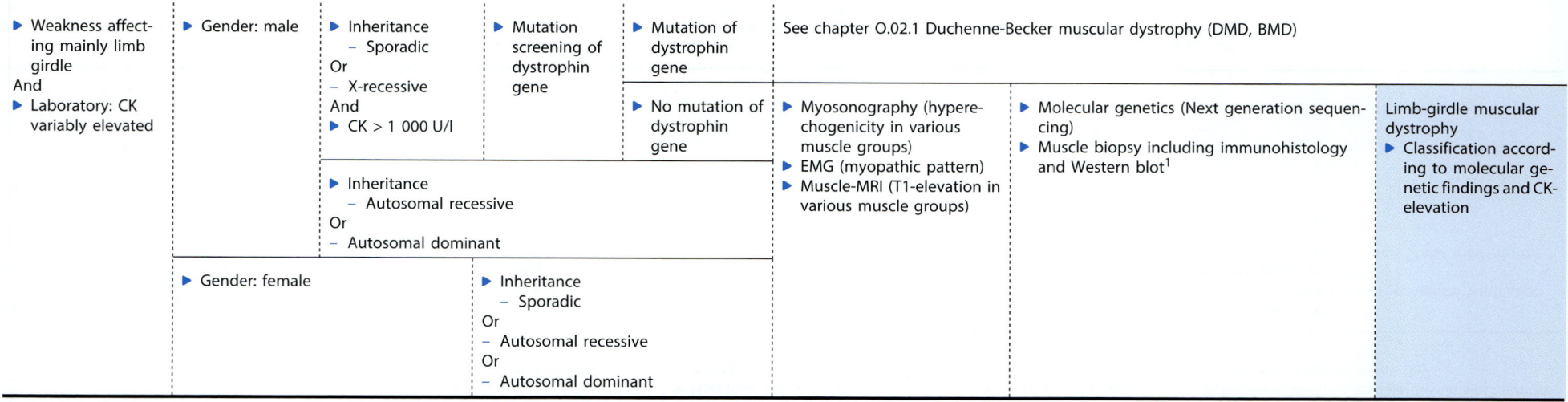

- Weakness affecting mainly limb girdle

  And
- Laboratory: CK variably elevated

→ Gender: male

- Inheritance
  - Sporadic

  Or
  - X-recessive

  And
- CK > 1 000 U/l

→ Mutation screening of dystrophin gene

→ Mutation of dystrophin gene → See chapter O.02.1 Duchenne-Becker muscular dystrophy (DMD, BMD)

→ No mutation of dystrophin gene

- Inheritance
  - Autosomal recessive

  Or
  - Autosomal dominant

→ Gender: female

- Inheritance
  - Sporadic

  Or
  - Autosomal recessive

  Or
  - Autosomal dominant

- Myosonography (hyperechogenicity in various muscle groups)
- EMG (myopathic pattern)
- Muscle-MRI (T1-elevation in various muscle groups)

- Molecular genetics (Next generation sequencing)
- Muscle biopsy including immunohistology and Western blot[1]

Limb-girdle muscular dystrophy
- Classification according to molecular genetic findings and CK-elevation

1 In a laboratory experienced with the differential diagnosis

O.02.2 Limb-girdle muscular dystrophy (LGMD) | PCS-Therapy 1/1

Neuromuscular disorders

Basic measures
- Emergency health card (re. complications of anesthesia, malignant hyperthermia)

Technical aids to prevent contractures and to compensate for functional deficits in every-day life
- Consider night-time leg splints as prevention of contractures; short calf splints are less effective, but long splints are usually not accepted
- Light-weight femoral orthoses to enable therapeutic standing and walking (frequently not accepted)
- Wheel chair (to enable participation in recreational activities)
- Electrically powered wheel chair (to enable independent mobility after definitive loss of walking; individual adaptation necessary; possibly with integrated device for standing and lying)
- Nursing bed, special mattress, patient lifter, aids for bathing and showers
- Height-adjustable chair and furniture
- Gripping pliers, special writing equipment, hair brush etc.

Drug therapy[1]
- Corticosteroids[2]
  - Prednisone 0,75 mg/kg/day
  Or
  - Deflazacort 0,9 mg/kg/day
  Either of these drugs to be administered as a single dose at breakfast (continuously or intermittently)
- Creatine monohydrate[3]
  - 100 mg/kg/day; treatment trial for 4–6 weeks, then decide for each individual patient whether to continue treatment
- Carnitine
  - 50 mg/kg/d (especially if muscle cramps are present)

▶ Appearance of functional limitations	▶ Physiotherapy	Depending on age ▶ Promotion of dexterity and motor skills ▶ Prophylaxis of contractures and scoliosis ▶ Respiratory treatment, thoracic mobilization ▶ Cardiovascular training, strengthening of muscles ▶ Assistance with technical aids
▶ Contractures	▶ Surgical release of contractures	▶ Operative lengthening of Achilles tendon, possibly knee- and hip-flexors – In the presence of functional limitations, only if improvement of walking ability and posture can be expected
▶ Cardiomyopathy (with variable frequency)	▶ Cardiac treatment	▶ Pathological SF and EF on echocardiography ▶ ACE-inhibitors and beta-blocking drugs
		▶ Clinically manifest cardiac failure ▶ In addition to ACE inhibitors, as per cardiologist decision diuretics und digoxin
		▶ Cardiac arrhythmias ▶ Antiarrhythmics
▶ Decrease of respiratory strength and vital capacity	▶ Ventilation treatment – After careful clarification of economical, nursing and psychosocial conditions and consequences – Permanent ventilation treatment via tracheotomy only in special individual cases	▶ Nighttime hypoventilation syndrome with daytime sleepiness and periodic oxygen desaturation during sleep ▶ Non-invasive home ventilation (NIHV)
		▶ If considered necessary by the patient during the course of illness ▶ Daytime NIHV during daytime naps or for more extended periods of the day
		▶ Acute respiratory infection And ▶ NIHV not sufficiently effective ▶ Intubation and transitory invasive mechanical ventilation

1 Attempt to relieve disease progression or to increase strength and function, up to now not curative. Metabolites, vitamins, hormones, growth factors: experimental, no proven efficacy, mostly shown to be not effective.
2 Corticosteroids have been shown to be useful in single patients with LGMD and a Duchenne-like clinical course; however, systematic trials are lacking so far.
3 Increase of strength and endurance by 5–10 % shown in healthy athletes and muscular dystrophy-patients with well-preserved function; effect in weak patients very questionable.

O.02.3 Emery-Dreifuss Syndrome | PCS-Diagnosis 1/1

Neuromuscular disorders

Medical history and clinical signs
- Early symptoms
  - Pes equinus due to achilles tendon contracture
  - Contracture of elbow flexors
  - Contracture of neck extensors
- Late symptoms
  - Weakness
  - Muscular atrophy
  - Rigidity of spine

Basic diagnostic work-up
- Serum-CK
- EMG
- ECG
- Echocardiography

- CK
  - Normal
  - Or
  - Slightly elevated
- EMG: myopathic
- Echocardiography: dilated cardiomyopathy
- ECG: arrhythmia

- Molecular genetics
  - Mutations of Emerin gene
  - FHL1
  - Mutations of Lamin A/C-gene
  - Syne1 gene
  - Syne2 gene

- Emery-Dreifuss syndrome X-recessive (Emerin, FHL1) or autosomal dominant (Lamin A/C, Syne1, Syne2)

- Diagnosis XR or AD Emery-Dreifuss syndrome not confirmed

- Muscle biopsy: further histological and immunohistological differential diagnostic work-up

Possible differential diagnoses
- Limb girdle muscular dystrophies
- Metabolic myopathies (mitochondrial myopathies, defects of ß-oxidation, glycogenosis)

O.02.3 Emery-Dreifuss Syndrome

O.02.3 Emery-Dreifuss Syndrome | PCS-Therapy

Neuromuscular disorders

▶ Weakness	▶ If functionally relevant		▶ Physiotherapy ▶ Possibly orthoses
▶ Contractures	▶ If functionally relevant		▶ Night splints, orthoses ▶ Achillotenotomy ▶ Surgical release of elbow contractures without functional benefit ▶ Surgical release of neck extensors not possible
▶ Cardiac arrhythmia	▶ If severe		▶ Antiarrhythmic drugs ▶ Cardiac pacemaker (with defibrillator)
▶ Dilated cardiomyopathy	▶ Regular screening	▶ At relevant severity	▶ ACE inhibitors ▶ Beta blockers ▶ Diuretics ▶ Digoxin ▶ Consider heart transplantation

O.02.4 Myotonic dystrophy, Dystrophia myotonica (DM) | PCS-Diagnosis 1/1

Neuromuscular disorders

▶ Neonatal age	▶ Clues for congenital myotonic dystrophy
	  – Polyhydramnios
	  – Congenital hypotonia and weakness
	  – Myopathic face
	  – Swallowing and respiratory insufficiency
	  – Contractures of lower extremity (especially "club foot")
	  – Intellectual deficiency
		▶ Mother shows symptoms of DM1
		Or
		▶ DM1 has been diagnosed in the mother
		Or
		▶ Clinical evidence for DM1
			▶ Molecular genetics: DM1-gene	Congenital myotonic dystrophy (DM1)

▶ School age or adolescence	▶ Clues to myotonic dystrophy
	  – Unspecific weakness with or without myotony
	  – Elevated CK
	  – EMG: myotonic bursts
		Further signs of myotonic dystrophy Curschmann-Steinert (DM1):
		▶ Muscular symptoms predominantly distal rather than proximal
		▶ Involvement of face and neck muscles
			▶ Molecular genetics: DM1-gene	Myotonic dystrophy Curschmann-Steinert (DM1)

		Further signs of proxymal myotonic myopathy PROMM (DM2) (very rare in children and adolescents): ▶ Muscular symptoms predominantly proximal rather than distal ▶ Myalgia	▶ Molecular genetics: DM2-gene	PROMM (DM2)

O.02.4 Myotonic dystrophy, Dystrophia myotonica (DM)

O.02.4 Myotonic dystrophy, Dystrophia myotonica (DM) | PCS-Therapy

Neuromuscular disorders

▶ Muscular weakness ▶ Contractures, joint malpositions	▶ If functionally relevant		▶ Physiotherapy ▶ Technical aids (walker, wheel chair) ▶ Serial casting (newborn age) ▶ Orthoses
▶ Myotonia	▶ If functionally relevant (rarely necessary)		▶ Sodium channel blockers (*CAUTION:* in DM2 deterioration possible!) – Mexiletine – Phenytoin – Carbamazepine – Gabapentin
▶ Cardiac arrhythmia	▶ Prospective screening at regular intervals ▶ *CAUTION:* Possible arrhythmia during anesthesia	▶ If deterioration	▶ Antiarrhythmics ▶ Cardiac pace maker
▶ Endocrine disorder	▶ Prospective screening at regular intervals		▶ Substitution therapy as needed
▶ Neuropsychological dysfunction	▶ If functionally relevant		▶ Cognitive training, rehabilitation
▶ Mental retardation	▶ Occupational therapy, special education		
▶ Increased daytime sleepiness	▶ Psychostimulants ▶ Consider treatment of sleep apnea syndrome		
▶ Cataract	▶ If functionally relevant (unlikely in children)		▶ Cataract surgery

O.02.5 Facio-scapulo-humeral muscular dystrophy (FSHD) │ PCS-Diagnosis 1/1

Neuromuscular disorders

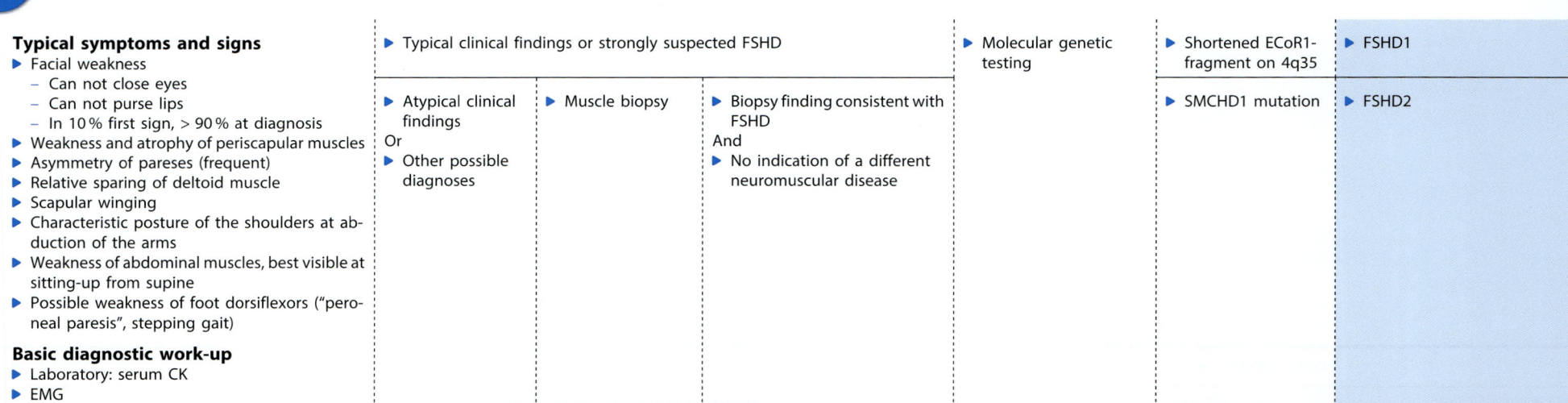

Typical symptoms and signs
- Facial weakness
  - Can not close eyes
  - Can not purse lips
  - In 10 % first sign, > 90 % at diagnosis
- Weakness and atrophy of periscapular muscles
- Asymmetry of pareses (frequent)
- Relative sparing of deltoid muscle
- Scapular winging
- Characteristic posture of the shoulders at abduction of the arms
- Weakness of abdominal muscles, best visible at sitting-up from supine
- Possible weakness of foot dorsiflexors ("peroneal paresis", stepping gait)

Basic diagnostic work-up
- Laboratory: serum CK
- EMG

- Typical clinical findings or strongly suspected FSHD

- Atypical clinical findings
  Or
- Other possible diagnoses

- Muscle biopsy

- Biopsy finding consistent with FSHD
  And
- No indication of a different neuromuscular disease

- Molecular genetic testing

- Shortened ECoR1-fragment on 4q35

- SMCHD1 mutation

- FSHD1

- FSHD2

O.02.5 Facio-scapulo-humeral muscular dystrophy (FSHD) | PCS-Therapy

Neuromuscular disorders

▶ Weakness	▶ With functional limitations	▶ Physiotherapy
		▶ Strengthening
		▶ Functional training
			All	Trial for a limited time, it strength improved continous administration
				▶ Creatine monohydrate
				  – Initially 0,2 g/kg
				  – Later 0,1 g/kg[1]
				▶ Albuterol[2]

▶ Limited shoulder abduction	▶ With functional limitations	▶ Surgical fixation of the scapulae to the rib-cage enables better abduction if deltoid muscle has sufficient strength		
▶ Peroneal paresis	▶ With functional limitations	▶ Peroneal orthosis	Severe progression	▶ Prednisone[3] – 0,75 mg/kg/d
▶ Neck and shoulder pain due to abnormal posture		▶ Physiotherapy ▶ Manual therapy ▶ Non-steroidal analgesics		

1 Limited efficacy in some controlled trials.
2 A pilot study and one controlled study showed an improvement of lean body mass and grip-strength.
3 In one study without effect, but partial efficacy has been observed in a few individual cases with "Duchenne-like" progression.

O.02.6 Distal muscular dystrophy | PCS-Diagnosis 1/1

Neuromuscular disorders

History and clinical findings
- Distal weakness and muscular atrophy of the lower and/or upper limbs
- Possible myalgia

Basic diagnostic work-up
- Serum CK
  (elevated or normal)
- Electrophysiology
  - Exclusion of polyneuropathy
  - EMG

- Serum CK raised or normal
  And
- Neuropathy excluded

- Muscle MRI
  Or
- Myosonography
  Both for definition of distribution patterns and selecting appropriate sites for biopsy

- Muscle biopsy
  - Histology
  - Immunohistology is only eligible for dysferlin deficiency
- Next generation sequencing

Diagnostically relevant results from
- Family history
- Clinical findings
- MRI
- Biopsy[1]

- Distal muscular dystrophy

- Signs of neuropathy at electrophysiological testing

See chapter O.08 Neuropathies

---

1 Molecular genetic analysis not routinely possible.

O.02.6 Distal muscular dystrophy

O.02.6 Distal muscular dystrophy | PCS-Therapy

Neuromuscular disorders

- ▶ Weakness
- ▶ Pain

- ▶ With functional limitations

- ▶ Physiotherapy
- ▶ Occupational therapy (upper limbs)
- ▶ Orthoses
- ▶ Other technical aids

O.02.7 Congenital muscular dystrophy (CMD) | PCS-Diagnosis 1/1

Neuromuscular disorders

Medical history and clinical findings
- Congenital hypotonia and weakness
- Possible congenital contractures

Basic diagnostic work-up
- Serum CK
  - CK variably elevated, in some types of CMD normal
  - In some patients only transient elevation of CK
- Cranial MRI

			Muscle biopsy[1]				
Normal cognitive function	MRI normal	Clues for Ulrich CMD (UCMD) – Distal hypermobility	Immunohistological analysis, poss. Western blot for laminin-alpha2, integrin, alpha-dystroglycan, collagen VI	Abnormal collagen VI	Molecular genetics available for some types	Mutation in one of three COLVI-genes	UCMD
		Clues for rigid spine with muscular dystrophy (RSMD) – Neck and spinal contracture (stiff neck)		Normal immunohistology		Mutation in SEPN1 gene, FHL1 gene	RSMD
		Clues for integrin alpha7 – Mild symptoms		Integrin alpha diminished		Mutation in integrin alpha7 gene	MCD with Integrin alpha7-deficiency
	T2 MRI: abnormal signal of white matter	Clues for Laminin a2-deficient CMD (MCD1A) – slowing of nerve conduction – epilepsy		Laminin a2 absent		Mutation in laminin a2 gene	MCD1A
				Laminin a2 diminished		No mutation in laminin a2 gene	MCD1B
Mental retardation	MRI: – Lissencephaly Typ II – Pachygyria – Brainstem- and cerebellar malformation	Clues for Fukuyama CMD (FCMD) – Epilepsy – Japanese ancestry		Alpha-dystroglycan diminished or absent	Molecular genetics of[2] – LARGE – Fukutin – POMGnT1 – POMT1 – POMT2 – FKRP – GTDC2 – ISPD	Fukutin	FCMD
		Clues for muscle-eye-brain disease (MEB) – Myopia – Visual loss – Large head				– POMGnT1 – ISPD – FKRP – GTDC2 – POMT2	MEB
		Clues for Walker-Warburg syndrome (WWS) – Hydrocephalus – Severe visual and neurologic disability				– FKTN – POMT1/2 – FKRP	WWS
	T2-MRI: abnormal signal of white matter	Clues for LARGE-related CMD (LARGE-CMD) – Severe symptoms				– LARGE	LARGE-CMD

1 Muscle biopsy usually necessary for reliable differential diagnostic work-up.

2 Lack of alpha-dystroglycan in immunohistology is an indication for a disorder of glycosylation; in these cases, all possible genes should be investigated because, in contrast to the gene involvement described in the early publications, there is a broad overlap of genotypes and phenotypes in this group of diseases.

O.02.7 Congenital muscular dystrophy (CMD) | PCS-Therapy

Neuromuscular disorders

- Drug therapy (symptomatic, no curative treatment available)
  - In mild cases creatine monohydrate can be considered
  - With epilepsy, anticonvulsive drugs
- Prophylaxis and treatment of contractures
  - Stretching
  - Positioning, standing frame, orthoses
  - Surgery of tendons if functional benefits can be expected (Achilles tendon lengthening)

▶ Hypotonia and weakness	▶ If clinically considerable	▶ Physiotherapy ▶ Strengthening ▶ Appropriate technical aids (for example powered wheel chair)
▶ Motor retardation	▶ If clinically considerable	▶ Physiotherapy ▶ Functional training
▶ Mental retardation	▶ If clinically considerable	▶ Educational center for children with special needs ▶ Occupational therapy to improve hand function
▶ Scoliosis	▶ Treatment and prophylaxis of progression – Physiotherapy – Corset – Surgery (difficult in the growth phase of the spine, possible from 6th–7th year onwards)	
▶ Ventilatory insufficiency (in some cases very early, possibly during the period of walking)	▶ Regular clinical and technical monitoring of lung function ▶ Poss. NIHV (see chapter O.02.1 Duchenne-Becker muscular dystrophy (DMD, BMD))	

O.03 Myopathies | PCS-Diagnosis congenital myopathy 1/1

Neuromuscular disorders

Medical history and clinical findings
Early onset of weakness,
Frequently slender muscles,
Dysmorphic stigmata
Hypo-/areflexia

Laboratory investigation
CK

▶ CK significantly increased

Differential diagnosis
▶ Duchenne muscular dystrophy (see chapter O.02.1 Duchenne-Becker muscular dystrophy (DMD, BMD))
▶ Limb-girdle muscular dystrophy (see chapter O.02.2 Limb-girdle muscular dystrophy (LGMD))
▶ Congenital muscular dystrophy (see chapter O.02.7 Congenital muscular dystrophy (CMD))

See the relevant chapter (see chapter O.02.1 Duchenne-Becker muscular dystrophy (DMD, BMD)), Limb girdle muscular dystrophy, (see chapter O.02.2 Limb-girdle muscular dystrophy (LGMD))

▶ CK normal or slightly increased	▶ NCV ▶ Muscle sonography ▶ EMG	▶ NCV pathological	▶ Neuropathy?	See chapter O.08 Neuropathies
		▶ EMG: neurogenic And ▶ NCV: normal	▶ SMA?	See chapter O.05 Spinal muscular atrophy (SMA)
		▶ EMG – Normal Or – Mixed pattern Or – Myopathic ▶ NCV: normal ▶ Muscle sonography: abnormal	▶ Muscle biopsy (including electron microscopy) ▶ Important: often normal at young age	▶ Molecular genetic testing

O.03 Myopathies

O.03 Myopathies | PCS-Therapy congenital myopathy

Basic measures
- Physiotherapy
- Adequate supply of aids

▶ Depending on the severity, additionally
  – Respiratory therapy
  – Non-invasive mask ventilation/invasive ventilation

O.03 Myopathies | PCS-Diagnosis metabolic myopathy 1/2

Neuromuscular disorders

Due to the complexity of the topic, the following table is incomplete and shall only be used as a first introductory approach to the topic.

Symptoms						
▸ Exercise-dependent weakness ▸ Basic diagnostic work-up ▸ Laboratory – CK – TSH, JT4, JT3 – Acylcarnitine, carnitine lactate – Acid maltase (enzymology) – Where indicated, ergometry with lactate and NH3 determination	▸ Myalgia – Muscle cramps during exercise – With or without recurrent rhabdomyolysis	▸ Pathological thyroid hormones		▸ Endocrine myopathy in hypo-/hyperthyroidism		If no clues to diagnosis ▸ Histochemistry for – Glykogen – Fat – Mitochondrial enzymes – Abnormal filaments und aggregates ▸ Mitochondrial enyzmes ▸ Mitochondrial genetics Further differential diagnoses: ▸ Rare congenital or myofibrillar myopathies
		▸ Lack of lactate increase during exercise	▸ Mc Ardle?	▸ Molecular genetic analysis (blood) – Mutation in the Myophosporylase gene	▸ McArdle	
		▸ Lack of NH3 increase during exercise	▸ Myoadenylate deaminase (MAD) deficiency?	▸ Genetic analysis	▸ Myoadenylate deaminase deficiency	
		▸ Serum lactate increased	▸ Mitochondriopathy?	▸ Molecular genetic analysis (blood) – mutations in mitochondrial and some nuclear genes (refer to respective publications or consult a specialized laboratory)[1] And/or ▸ Biopsy for enzymology and genetic analysis – Reduced activity of mitochondrial respiratory chain enzymes or depletion – Genetics above	▸ Mitochondriopathy	
		▸ Long-chain acylcarnitines increased	▸ CPT II deficiency	▸ CPT II gene analysis	▸ CPT II deficiency	
		▸ Carnitine decreased	▸ Primary or secondary carnitine deficiency	▸ Find the cause (disorder of the kidney, liver, organoacidopathies) – Chemistry: organic acids	▸ Carnitine deficiency of various origins	
		▸ Acid maltase deficiency	Pompe's disease?	Genetic analysis (blood) – Mutation in the GAA gene	▸ Pompe's disease	
	▸ Myasthenia? – Painless exercise-induced weakness			Exclusion myasthenia – See Chapter O.06 Neuromuscular transmission		
Symptoms ▸ Progressive weakness ▸ Myalgia Basic diagnostic work-up ▸ CK ▸ Myo-sonography	▸ Suspected metabolic myopathy – CK moderately increased	▸ Laboratory – lactate – acylcarnitine, carnitine – acid maltase (enzymology)	▸ Serum-Lactate increased	▸ Mitochondriopathy?	▸ Molecular genetic analysis (blood) – mutations in mitochondrial and some nuclear genes (refer to respective publications or consult a specialized laboratory)[1] And/or	▸ Mitochondriopathy

O.03 Myopathies | PCS-Diagnosis metabolic myopathy 2/2

Neuromuscular disorders

▶ EMG/NCV ▶ Echocardiography	▶ Hyperechogenic muscles ▶ EMG myopathic ▶ Cardiomyopathy	▶ NH3 ▶ Where indicated, ergometry with lactate and NH3 determination			▶ Biopsy for enzymology and genetic analysis – Reduced activity of mitochondrial respiratory chain enzymes or depletion – Genetics above	
			▶ Increased levels of acylcarnitines	▶ Disorder of ß-oxidation?	▶ Enzyme chemistry or genetic analysis – Reduction of MCAD activity in fibroblasts Or – Mutation in the ACADM gene Possibly – LCAD, LCHAD, VLCAD (see chapter N.01 Neurometabolic disorders)	▶ Defective beta-oxidation of various origins
			▶ Carnitine decreased	▶ Primary or secondary carnitine deficiency?	▶ Find the cause (disorder of the kidney, liver, organoacidopathies) – Chemistry: organic acids	▶ Carnitine deficiency of various origins
			▶ Acid maltase deficiency	▶ Pompe's disease?	Genetic analysis (blood) – Mutation in the GAA gene	▶ Pompe's disease
▶ CK greatly increased ▶ Myosonography: hyperechogenic muscles ▶ EMG: myopathic or neurogenic ▶ +/- Cardiomyopathy					▶ Other neuromuscular disorders	See chapter O.02.1–7 Muscle dystrophies

1 If there is clinical suspicion of mitochondrial disease to consult the website mitoNET and related policies is recommended. For differentiated genetic diagnosis consult specialist laboratories.

O.03 Myopathies | PCS-Therapy metabolic myopathy 1/1

Neuromuscular disorders

▶ Acute severe myalgia	▶ Determination of creatine kinase CK	▶ Highly elevated – > 20 000 U/l	▶ ICU – Monitor serum potassium and diuresis, forced diuresis, dialysis, if necessary	▶ Check whether dietary therapy is possible
		▶ Moderately elevated – < 20 000 U/l	▶ Analgesics ▶ Close monitoring	
▶ Chronic muscle weakness	▶ Causal therapy not possible	▶ Symptomatic therapy		▶ Respiratory failure
	▶ Causal therapy possible	▶ Pompe's disease	▶ Enzyme replacement therapy	▶ Respiratory therapy Or Ventilation
		▶ Carnitine deficiency	▶ Carnitine substitution	
▶ Chron. exercise intolerance/ muscle cramps	▶ Causal therapy possible	▶ Beta-oxidation defect	▶ Diet	
		▶ CPT deficiency	▶ Avoid fasting periods	
	▶ Causal therapy not possible	▶ Symptomatic treatment		

O.03 Myopathies

O.04 Myositis | PCS-Diagnosis 1/2

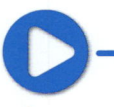

Neuromuscular disorders

Medical history
- Previously healthy child
- Progressive symmetrical muscle weakness
- Reduced exercise tolerance
- Loss of motor functions
- Muscle pain
- Poor general condition

Clinical symptoms
- Progressive symmetrical muscle weakness affecting proximal limb girdle, neck and back muscles
- Muscle and joint swelling
- Muscle pain

Diagnostic work-up
- Blood sample
  - Complete blood count
  - CRP
  - BSG
  - Muscle enzymes: CK[1], AST, LDH, aldolase[2]
  - Creatinine, urea
  - Von Willebrand factor
  - Myositis-specific antibodies
  - Additional antibodies to differentiate from other rheumatic diseases
- Muscle sonography: non-specific results with possibly increased intensity of affected muscles
  - Muscle MRI with increased signal intensity in T2 slides identifying muscle oedema
- Muscle biopsy with perivascular and perifascicular atrophy, inflammatory infiltrates and muscle fiber necrosis
- Electrocardiogram, echocardiography
- Vital capacity measurement
- Sonography of kidneys and liver
- **Optional diagnostic work-up**
- Nailfold capillary microscopy, if possible
- EMG: non-specific myopathic changes
- Tests for relevant infections
  - Viruses, e.g. Coxsackie-, Echo-, Influenza-virus

- **Historical clues for a juvenile dermatomyositis (JDM)**
  - Previous history normal
  - Sudden onset over days to weeks with muscle pain, often affecting proximal leg, neck and paravertebral muscles
  - Skin rashes (face, neck, extensor surfaces of joints)
  - Fatigue and unhappy mood
  - Previous infection possible, fever optional
- **Clinical clues for a juvenile dermatomyositis (JDM)**
  - Skin rashes
    - Heliotrope purple rash on face
    - Nailfold and eye lid capillary loops
    - Extensor surfaces of joints, especially elbows, fingers and knees, can be red, atrophic and scaly
  - Sudden onset over days to weeks with progressive muscle weakness, starting most often in the legs, later extending to upper extremities, abdominal and back muscles, as well as pharynx and larynx muscles causing dysphagia and dysphonia
  - Myalgia

Associated symptoms in case of an untreated ongoing clinical course:
- Arthritides, contractures
- Affection of other organ systems (see complications)

- **Clues for a juvenile dermatomyositis (JDM) as part of a systemic rheumatic disease**
  - Arthritis of peripheral joints, tendovaginitis, bursitis
  - Spondylitis
  - Rheumatic nodules, nailbed capillary loops
  - Pleuritis, interstitial pneumonia
  - Pericarditis, myocarditis
  - Renal affection, often initial proteinuria
  - Gastrointestinal involvement
  - Keratitis, iritis

- **Historical clues for a juvenile polymyositis (JPM)**

Sudden/slow onset without muscle pain or with only mild muscle pain, muscle weakness, reduced exercise tolerance, loss of motor functions
  - No skin rashes
  - Previous infection possible
  - Maybe history of cancer or other systemic diseases
- **Clinical clues for a juvenile polymyositis (JPM)**
  - Pronounced proximal muscle weakness, possibly also affecting paravertebral, abdominal and neck muscles
  - Rarely myalgia
  - Tenderness
  - Dysphagia

- **Further clues for juvenile dermatomyositis:**
  - Diagnostic criteria of Bohan and Peter
  - Symmetrical proximal muscle weakness
  - Typical skin rashes
  - Elevated muscle enzymes
  - Periorbital oedema
  - Muscle MRI: increased signal intensity in T2 slides identifying oedema
- Muscle biopsy: perivascular and perifascicular atrophy, inflammatory infiltrates and muscle fiber necrosis
- EMG: possibly myopathic changes, but non-specific
  - Capillary microscopy: Capillary loops, especially of eye lids and nail beds

---

- **Further diagnostic work-up to identify or rule out other multisystemic rheumatic diseases, especially**
- Systemic lupus erythematosus
- Sharp syndrome (mixed connective tissue disease)

- **Further clues for juvenile polymyositis:**
  - In the absence of skin rashes, JPM should be considered
  - Muscle enzymes are more often increased than in JDM

- Juvenile dermato-myositis

- Juvenile polymyositis

O.04 Myositis

330

O.04 Myositis | PCS-Diagnosis 2/2

Neuromuscular disorders

– Bacteria, e.g. Streptococci, Staphylococci, Mycoplasma – Parasites, e.g. Cestodes, Nematodes, Protozoa	▶ **Clues for other diseases (e.g. celiac disease, Morbus Werlhof, infection) associated to juvenile polymyositis** ▶ Initial symptoms without skin rashes ▶ Further symptoms associated with the suspected systemic disease	▶ **Further diagnostic work-up, e.g. virology, bacteriology, cold agglutinins**
	Clues for primary degenerative disorders (e.g. Becker muscular dystrophy or Limb-girdle muscular dystrophy; see chapter O.02.1 Duchenne-Becker muscular dystrophy (DMD, BMD) and O.02.2 Limb-girdle muscular dystrophy (LGMD) – Slow progression, even at the beginning	See chapter O.02 Muscle dystrophies
	▶ **Clues for a medication-induced juvenile polymyositis** – D-Penicillamine – Anti-malaria agents – Colchicines – Antithyroid drugs (thionamides) – Lipid-lowering agents – Steroids	▶ Discontinuation of medication

1 Often increased, normal values do not exclude a neuromuscular disorder
2 Increased values in some cases of dermatomyositis

O.04 Myositis | PCS-Therapy 1/1

Neuromuscular disorders

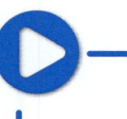

Basic therapy
- ▶ Symptomatic pain medication according to WHO recommendations (step-by-step plan)
- ▶ Physiotherapy important during rehabilitation
- ▶ Vitamin D 500 IU/d and calcium (2 × 500 mg ionized calcium/d) for osteoporosis-prophylaxis

▶ Mild manifestation	▶ Prednisone orally – Start with 2 mg/kg/d in two single doses – After improvement of symptoms within 6–12 weeks slow reduction, e.g. every 2 months reduction of 0,5 mg/kg/d – From 0,5 mg/kg/d on, reduction of 0,1 mg/kg/d every 2 months or medication of 0.5 mg/kg/d every other day			▶ In case of inadequate improvement	▶ Prednisone orally (see foregoing recommendations) And ▶ Methotrexate (MTX) orally/subcutaneously, 15 mg/m^2 BSA
▶ Moderate or severe manifestation	*1. Step* ▶ Start with a pulse of Methylprednisolone intravenously (20–30 mg/kg every day for 3 days) over 3–5 hours followed by oral Prednisone And ▶ Methotrexate (MTX) orally or subcutaneously 15 mg/m^2 body surface area (BSA) as a steroid reducing medication Recommendations for Methylprednisolone pulse therapy: after diagnosis, then after 1, 2, 4, 7 weeks, then every month for 1 year and every 3 months during the 2nd year.	▶ No adequate improvement with steroid and MTX therapy	*2. Step* ▶ Additionally Intravenous Immunoglobulins (IVIG) 2 g/kg	▶ Very severe manifestation And ▶ Inadequate improvement with medications of step 1 and 2	*3. Step (opportunities)* ▶ Cyclosporine A to max. 5 mg/kg/d, check serum level, aim for 100–200 mcg/ml ▶ Cyclophosphamide intravenously 0,7–1 mg/m^2 BSA monthly[1] ▶ Azathioprine: start with 1,5–2 mg/kg/d, sometimes 3 mg/kg/d is necessary to reach an adequate immuno-suppression[2] ▶ Mycophenolate mofetil: up to 2 g/d; positive effects are reported in single cases ▶ Rituximab: 4 intravenous doses on days 1, 8, 15 and 22, 100 mg/m^2 BSA each or 375 mg/m^2 BSA/week ▶ Etanercept, Infliximab: positive effects are reported in isolated cases ▶ Tacrolimus locally: positive effects are reported in single cases with ongoing skin rashes but good muscle function, apply 2 x/d for 4–6 weeks

1 Consider sufficient hydrogenation and application of antiemetics.
2 Onset of effects with 6 months latency.

O.05 Spinal muscular atrophy (SMA) | PCS-Diagnosis

Neuromuscular disorders

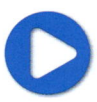

Clinical presentation	CK normal or mildly elevated	Molecular analysis of SMN1 gene	Homozygous deletion exon 7 (and 8) of SMN (SMN2 copy number correlates with severity but is not prognostic for individual patient)			SMA (5q)

• Muscle weakness
  – Proximal
  – Symmetric
  – Legs > arms
• No cerebral involvement
• Normal sensory system
• No facial weakness
• Reflexes reduced or absent
• Fasciculation of tongue or skeletal muscles
 	
Basic laboratory
• Creatine kinase (CK-)level
			No homozygous deletion exon 7 (and 8) of SMN1 gene	Confirm motor neuron disease through neurophysiology and muscle biopsy	Heterozygous deletion and point mutation of SMN1	

					Other types of SMA with additional symptoms	• SMARD (with respiratory distress, diaphragmatic palsy) • SMA + pontocerebellar atrophy • x-linked SMA (with congenital fractures)
				Motor neuron disease not confirmed	Evaluation for other neuromuscular diseases, e.g. – Congenital myotonic dystrophy (see chapter O.02.4 Myotonic dystrophy, Dystrophia myotonica (DM)) – Congenital myopathy (see chapter O.03 Myopathies) – Dermatomyositis (see chapter O.04 Myositis) – Myasthenia (see chapter O.06 Neuromuscular transmission) – Hereditary neuropathies (see chapter O.08 Neuropathies)	See corresponding chapters O.02.7 Congenital muscular dystrophy (CMD), O.03 Myopathies, O.04 Myositis, O.06 Neuromuscular transmission, O.08 Neuropathies
	CK > 5 fold of normal	Differential diagnosis • Muscular dystrophies (see chapter O.02 Muscle dystrophies) • Dermatomyositis (see chapter O.04 Myositis)				

O.05 Spinal muscular atrophy (SMA) | PCS-Therapy 1/2

Neuromuscular disorders

Basic therapy
- Regularly attending neuromuscular centre with expertise for children
  - Infants (3(–6) monthly)
  - School age (6(–12) monthly)
- In addition, local care as much as possible
- New: antisense-oligonucleotide Nusinersen ongoing trials, orphan drug status (FDA, EMA)

▶ Respiration

▶ Normal pulmonary function	No specific treatment needed		
▶ Clinical signs of ineffective coughing – Insufficient airway clearance during infections – Weak voice/crying – Tachypnea/dyspnea	▶ Peak cough flow > 160 l/min	▶ Physiotherapy for airway clearance	
	▶ Peak cough flow < 160 l/min or with infants clinical signs of insufficient coughing Or ▶ Oxygen saturation < 94 %	▶ Intensify airway clearance ▶ Consider mechanical cough assistance (cough assist) ▶ Consider (intermittent) pulse oximetry at home ▶ Consider starting (nocturnal) non-invasive ventilation ▶ Close monitoring during respiratory infections ▶ In infants consider RSV vaccination ▶ Gastrointestinal management (see below)	During acute respiratory infection ▶ Intensify airway clearance/cough assist ▶ Intensify non-invasive ventilation ▶ Intermittent invasive ventilation if needed During stable condition ▶ Discuss emergency care and CPR in advance
▶ Signs and symptoms of (nocturnal) hypoventilation – Restless sleep, nightmares – Tiredness during the day – Morning headache – Loss of appetite	▶ Polysomnography with CO_2-monitoring ▶ Pulmonary function test	▶ Normal	▶ Repeat during course of disease
		▶ Abnormal	▶ Non-invasive (nocturnal) ventilation in combination with airway clearance

▶ Nutrition

▶ Normal nutrition and development	No specific treatment		
▶ Swallowing problems ▶ Bulbar symptoms with severe weakness ▶ Fatigue with oral feeding ▶ Aspiration/recurrent pulmonary infections ▶ Gastroesophageal reflux	▶ Functional evaluation of swallowing	▶ Adaptation of alimentation ▶ Nasogastric tube (temporary) ▶ Gastrostomy tube ▶ Treatment of gastroesophageal reflux ▶ Fundoplication	
▶ Overnutrition Or ▶ Undernutrition	▶ Reduced mobility ▶ Increased respiratory work	▶ Evaluate growth charts; body weight in lower percentile range often appropriate (reduced muscle mass), early intervention when crossing percentiles ▶ Dietary record to assess intake ▶ Avoid prolonged fasting during acute illness and interventions (substitute full caloric need within 4–6 h after admission for acute illness) ▶ Effect of low-fat or protein-rich diet not evidence based	

O.05 Spinal muscular atrophy (SMA) | PCS-Therapy 2/2

Neuromuscular disorders

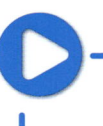

▶ Orthopaedic care	▶ Ambulant patients	▶ Functional limitation ▶ Frequent falls ▶ Contractures	▶ Daily activities ▶ Prevention of contractures ▶ Adaptation of environment ▶ Orthosis if needed ▶ Surgery for contracture, if functionally relevant
	▶ Non-ambulant patients, able to sit	▶ Scoliosis And/or ▶ Contractures	▶ Prevention of contractures ▶ Standing frame ▶ (Power-)wheelchair from 2–3 years of age ▶ Orthosis, bracing ▶ Consider surgery for progressive scoliosis
	▶ Patients not able to sit	▶ Poor head control ▶ Reduced mobility	▶ Standing frame ▶ Orthosis, bracing

O.06 Neuromuscular transmission | PCS-Diagnosis 1/1

Neuromuscular disorders

Medical history and clinical signs	▶ Confirmation of neuromuscular transmission disorder	▶ Myasthenia? ▶ Myasthenic syndrome?	▶ Antibody determination	▶ Antibody negative And	▶ Congenital myasthenic syndrome?	▶ Improvement with Edrophonium	▶ Genetics
▶ Exercise induced weakness ▶ Intermittent diplopia ▶ Intermittent dysphagia	– Repetitive exercise test – Simpson test – Repetetive stimulation test – Pharmacological test with Edrophonium		– Acetylcholine receptor antibodies And – MUSK-antibodies	▶ No response to corticosteroids[1]			– ACH receptor defects (fast-channel) – Defects of ACH synthesis/release
						▶ Double MUAP ▶ Worsening caused by Edrophonium	▶ Genetics – ACH receptor defects (slow-channel syndrome) – Cholinesterase deficiency
				▶ Antibody positive	▶ Myasthenia gravis?	▶ Thoracic MRI Or ▶ Computed tomography (thorax)	
	▶ Exclusion of other neuromuscular disease – CK-determination – Myosonography – EMG/NCV	▶ See chapter O.03 Myopathies ▶ Work-up in neuromuscular speciality clinics					

1 In ocular myasthenia gravis (MG) and also in children with generalized MG, the AChR AB are increased only in 50 % of cases!

O.06 Neuromuscular transmission

336

O.06 Neuromuscular transmission | PCS-Therapy

Neuromuscular disorders

• Defects in the acetylcholine receptor • Cong. myasthenic syndrome with receptor defect • Cong. myasthenic syndrome with reduction of receptors	• Test on intensive care unit: – Edrophonium chloride (0,1 mg/kg IV within 1 min) Or • Neostigmine (0,04 mg/kg IM)	• Positive response to treatment	• Pyridostigmine (individual dose must be adjusted according to observed clinical effect)
		• No response to treatment	• Reconsider diagnosis
Cholinesterase deficiency	• Ephedrine (not all patients respond) • Avoid cholinesterase inhibitors		
Presynaptic failure of vesicle release	• 3,4-Diaminopyridine • Consider combination with cholinesterase inhibitor		
Kinetic disorder (slow channel syndrome)	• Fluoxetine • Quinidine sulfate • Avoid cholinesterase inhibitor		
Autoimmune myasthenia gravis[3]	• Myasthenic crisis	• Intravenous immunoglobulins (2 g/kg) • Plasma exchange	
	• Chronic treatment[1,3]	• Corticosteroids[3] • Azathioprine (2 mg/kg/SD × 1)[3] • Cyclosporine A (no recommended dosage for children available, max 1 mg/kg/d)[3] • Thymectomy[2,3]	

1 The extent of immunosuppression depends on the severity of symptoms
2 After consultation with a neuromuscular center.
3 Thymectomy is recommended in generalized autoimmune myasthenia after the age of 8 years. There is no general consent about thymectomy in children.

O.07 Peripheral nerve lesions | PCS-Overview Obstetric brachial palsy 1/1

Neuromuscular disorders

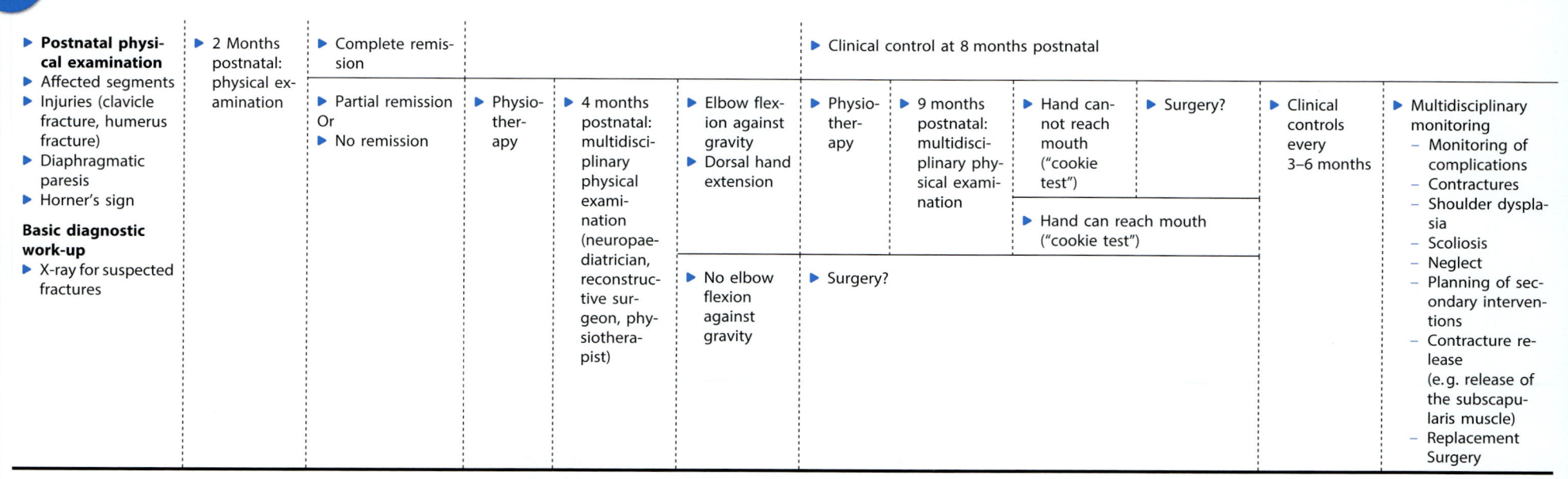

- **Postnatal physical examination**
- Affected segments
- Injuries (clavicle fracture, humerus fracture)
- Diaphragmatic paresis
- Horner's sign

Basic diagnostic work-up
- X-ray for suspected fractures

- 2 Months postnatal: physical examination

- Complete remission
- Partial remission Or
- No remission

- Physiotherapy

- 4 months postnatal: multidisciplinary physical examination (neuropaediatrician, reconstructive surgeon, physiotherapist)

- Elbow flexion against gravity
- Dorsal hand extension

- No elbow flexion against gravity

- Clinical control at 8 months postnatal

- Physiotherapy

- Surgery?

- 9 months postnatal: multidisciplinary physical examination

- Hand cannot reach mouth ("cookie test")

- Hand can reach mouth ("cookie test")

- Surgery?

- Clinical controls every 3–6 months

- Multidisciplinary monitoring
  – Monitoring of complications
  – Contractures
  – Shoulder dysplasia
  – Scoliosis
  – Neglect
  – Planning of secondary interventions
  – Contracture release (e.g. release of the subscapularis muscle)
  – Replacement Surgery

O.07 Peripheral nerve lesions

O.07 Peripheral nerve lesions | PCS-Therapy Obstetric brachial palsy

Neuromuscular disorders

- ▶ Pain management
  - Carbamazepine, Oxcarbazepine
  - Tricyclic antidepressants
  - Opioids
  - Transcutaneous electrical nerve stimulation (see chapter C Pain)

- Neurological examination and EMG after 4 months

- ▶ No functionally relevant reinnervation or electromyographically detectable reinnervation

- ▶ Surgery
  - Nerve transplantation
  - Neurolysis
  - In case of root avulsion, connect distal stump of the nerve root with the accessory nerve or other nerves
  - Muscle transfer

O.08 Neuropathies | PCS-Diagnosis 1/3

Neuromuscular disorders

Medical history	Obligatory diagnostic work-up	Differential diagnoses	Therapy
Medical history ▶ Manifestation can vary from the neonatal period to adolescence ▶ Progression often very slow, rarely within a few weeks ▶ Gait disturbances ▶ Reduced exercise tolerance ▶ Sensory impairment ▶ Muscle atrophy, often starting distally in lower extremities ▶ Loss of motor functions	**Obligatory diagnostic work-up** ▶ Blood sample – Complete blood count – CRP – ESR – Liver enzymes – Glucose – Urea – Thyroid hormones – Porphyria parameters – Phytanic acid – Vitamin B_1, B_6, B_{12}, E – Lumbar puncture (elevated protein)	**Differential diagnoses in neuropathies include hereditary motor and sensory neuropathies, hereditary sensor and autonomic neuropathies, neurometabolic/neurodegenerative neuropathies, infectious neuropathies, and medication – toxin – or malnutrition-induced neuropathies.** ▶ **Clues for a hereditary motor and sensory neuropathy (HMSN)** – Positive family history – Clinical symptoms as described – Usually a slowly progressive clinical course ▶ **Clues for a hereditary sensory and autonomic neuropathy (HSAN)** – Additional autonomic dysfunction such as alacrima, anhidrosis, mutilated arthropathy, sensory impairment, especially reduced sensation of pain ▶ **Clues for a hereditary neurometabolic/neurodegenerative neuropathy** – Additional symptoms and progressive clinical course – Often CNS involvement – CSF with elevated protein – Pertinent results from special metabolic investigations of serum, urine and cerebrospinal fluid (CSF)	**Therapy is symptomatic and depends on the underlying defect.** Therapy includes neuropaediatric and orthopaedic follow-up including physiotherapy, orthotics and surgery if necessary Ventilation, nasogastric tube feeding
Family history ▶ In hereditary neuropathies, other family members may be affected **Clinical symptoms** ▶ **Neonatal:** "floppy infant" with areflexia ▶ **Later manifestations** ▶ Delayed motor development ▶ Gait disturbances ▶ Often symmetrical distal	**Special diagnostic work-up** ▶ Lysosomal enzymes (M. Krabbe, metachromatic leukodystrophy) ▶ Serum protein electrophoresis (Abetalipoproteinemia)	▶ **Clues for an infectious neuropathy** – Gullain-Barré syndrome (GBS): disease progression up to 4 weeks; progressive, usually symmetrical motor weakness, areflexia, autonomic dysfunctions, elevated protein in CSF, respiratory involvement in 50 %, bulbar and ocular symptoms possible, slow nerve conduction with conduction block, enhanced nerve roots on MRI. See chapter A.06 Guillain-Barré syndrome (GBS). – Chronic demyelinating inflammatory polyneuropathy (CIDP): progression more subacute (> 4 weeks – 2 months), clinical course can be fluctuating	– **GBS:** IVIG 0.4 g/kg/d over 5 days or 1 g/kg/d over 2 days, plasmapheresis in severe cases, ventilation, nasogastric tube feeding – **CIDP:** Steroids (1–2 mg/kg alternate days), recurrent IVIG in individual intervals, plasmapheresis in severe cases, other immunosuppressive agents only if the first line treatment fails
	▶ Refsum's disease ▶ Toxins (arsenic, lead, mercury, thallium)	▶ **Clues for a medication-, toxine-, or malnutrition-induced neuropathy** – Vincristine, isoniacide – Arsenic, lead, mercury, thallium – History of malnutrition	Therapy includes neuropaediatric and orthopaedic follow-up incuding physiotherapy, orthotics and surgery if necessary – Withdraw toxins, optimize nutrition, substitution of vitamins may be necessary.

O.08 Neuropathies

O.08 Neuropathies | PCS-Diagnosis 2/3

Neuromuscular disorders

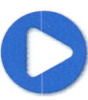

weakness and sensory disturbances of lower extremities, later possibly also affecting the upper extremities
- Muscle hypotonia
- Distal muscle atrophy
- Hypo- to areflexia
- Feet deformities, later atrophy of small hand muscles and hand deformities
- Contractures and scoliosis
- Autonomic dysfunction

Associated symptoms
- Hearing loss
- Cataracts, impaired vision, pupillary anomalies
- ZNS involvement (leukoencephalopathy)

- **Motor and sensor nerve conduction velocities** of the lower and upper extremities
- Upper extremities: e.g. N. ulnaris and N. medianus
- Lower extremities: e.g. N. suralis, N. tibialis, N. peroneus

Most often, values of the motor nerve conduction velocity of N. medianus is used to differentiate demyelinating neuropathy (value < 38 m/s) from axial neuropathy (value > 38 m/s), but even in young children and single subtypes of neuropathies motor nerve conduction velocity of N. medianus can be normal!

- Ophthalmological evaluation
- Audiological evaluation
- MRI
- **Genetic analyses:** Today,

O.08 Neuropathies | PCS-Diagnosis 3/3

Neuromuscular disorders

there is a growing list of disease causing genes. In demyelinating neuropathies most often *PMP22, MPZ* and *Cx32* are found. In clinical practice it is helpful to characterize the patient carefully clinically and neurophysiologically, maybe also with a special diagnostic work-up. Depending on these data a more directed genetic analysis can be discussed with the geneticist.

▶ **Nerve biopsy** is only recommended in cases which can not be diagnosed by clinical, neurophysiological, metabolic and genetic analyses.

Notes

Notes

P Hydrocephalus, Myelomeningocele (MMC), Chiari Malformations

P.01 Hydrocephalus in infants | PCS-Diagnosis 1/1

Hydrocephalus, MMC, Chiari Malformations

Medical history and symptoms ▶ Premature birth ▶ Maternal infection ▶ MMC/CM[1] ▶ Tense fontanelle ▶ Distended sutures ▶ Irritability ▶ Bradycardia ▶ Failure to thrive ▶ Vomiting ▶ Reduced muscular tone ▶ Sun-setting eyes **Basic examination** ▶ Head circumference (percentile) ▶ Transcranial ultrasound[2]	▶ No/moderate symptoms And ▶ Head growth above average		▶ Enlarged ventricles with abnormal configuration Or ▶ No enlarged ventricles but suspected lesion of the posterior fossa ▶ No enlarged ventricles, suspected slit ventricle syndrome	▶ MRI: exclusion of – Tumor – Vascular malformation – CM – Dandy-Walker malformation/ variant – Aqueductal stenosis – Ventricular cysts – Isolated ventricles	▶ Hydrocephalus of various aetiology
	▶ Severe symptoms Or ▶ Transcranial ultrasound impossible	▶ MRI or in an emergency situation CT			
			▶ No evidence for cerebral pathology	▶ Exclusion of intoxication	See chapter A.13 Intoxications

1 Myelomeningocele/Chiari-Malformation type II
2 Not suitable for assessing the posterior fossa

P.01 Hydrocephalus in infants | PCS-Therapy 1/1

Hydrocephalus, MMC, Chiari Malformations

Malresorptive hydrocephalus	▶ Ventricular puncture[1] – CSF examination	▶ < 2 000 g body weight	▶ Ventricular catheter with reservoir/ommaya reservoir
		▶ > 2 000 g body weight And ▶ CSF protein < 200 mg/dl	▶ Ventriculoperitoneal shunt
		▶ > 2 000 g body weight And ▶ CSF protein > 200 mg/dl	▶ Ventriculoperitoneal shunt[2]
		▶ < 2 000 g body weight And ▶ CSF protein > 200 mg/dl	▶ Ventriculosubgaleal shunt[3]
Occlusive hydrocephalus	▶ Ventricular puncture[1] – CSF examination	▶ < 2 000 g body weight	▶ Ventricular catheter with reservoir/ommaya reservoir
		▶ > 2 000 g body weight And ▶ CSF protein < 200 mg/dl	▶ Ventriculoperitoneal shunt
		▶ > 2 000 g body weight And ▶ CSF protein > 200 mg/dl	▶ Ventriculoperitoneal shunt[2] Or ▶ Ventriculosubgaleal shunt
		▶ Aqueductal stenosis	▶ Endoscopic third ventriculostomy[4] (ETV)
		▶ Tumor related	▶ Tumor resection (dependent on tumor type)

1 For temporary pressure release
2 With increased revision rate to detect and remove any occlusion
3 Hansasuta et al. 2007
4 High re-occlusion rate

P.02 Management of the shunted hydrocephalus PCS 1/1

Hydrocephalus, MMC, Chiari Malformations

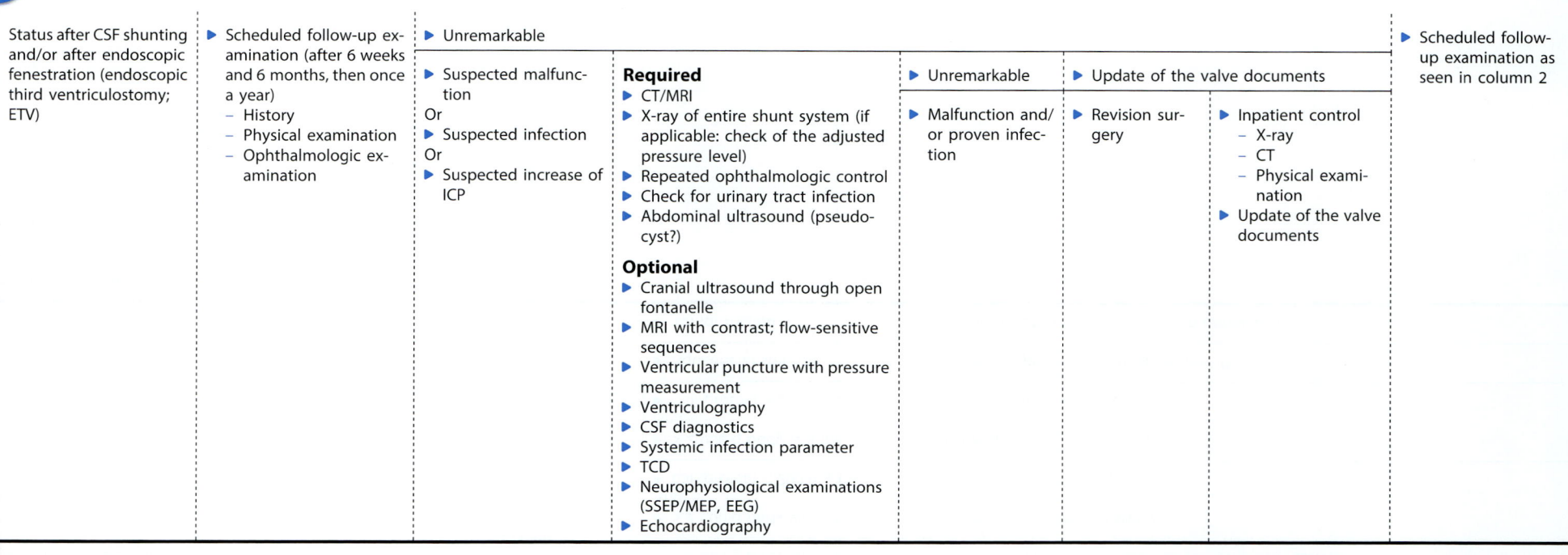

Status after CSF shunting and/or after endoscopic fenestration (endoscopic third ventriculostomy; ETV)

▶ Scheduled follow-up examination (after 6 weeks and 6 months, then once a year)
  – History
  – Physical examination
  – Ophthalmologic examination

▶ Unremarkable

▶ Suspected malfunction
Or
▶ Suspected infection
Or
▶ Suspected increase of ICP

Required
▶ CT/MRI
▶ X-ray of entire shunt system (if applicable: check of the adjusted pressure level)
▶ Repeated ophthalmologic control
▶ Check for urinary tract infection
▶ Abdominal ultrasound (pseudocyst?)

Optional
▶ Cranial ultrasound through open fontanelle
▶ MRI with contrast; flow-sensitive sequences
▶ Ventricular puncture with pressure measurement
▶ Ventriculography
▶ CSF diagnostics
▶ Systemic infection parameter
▶ TCD
▶ Neurophysiological examinations (SSEP/MEP, EEG)
▶ Echocardiography

▶ Unremarkable

▶ Malfunction and/or proven infection

▶ Update of the valve documents

▶ Revision surgery

▶ Inpatient control
  – X-ray
  – CT
  – Physical examination
▶ Update of the valve documents

▶ Scheduled follow-up examination as seen in column 2

P.03 Myelomeningocele (MMC) | PCS-Diagnosis 1/1

Hydrocephalus, MMC, Chiari Malformations

Prenatal diagnostic screening	▶ Cranial and spinal cord sonography, 16.–20. gestational week ▶ Alpha fetoprotein (AFP)1		Sonography ▶ Hydrocephalus ▶ Increased interpeduncular distance ▶ Posterior cystic mass AFP ▶ Increased[1]
MMC	▶ MRI of the complete spinal cord ▶ Sonography of spinal cord		▶ Spinal dysraphism and associated intraspinal malformations ▶ Low conus medullaris, decreased pulsations and mobility of spinal cord
Assessment of the level of neuro-segmental lesion[2]	Physical examination of ▶ Motor function ▶ Sensory function ▶ Sphincter function		See chapter R Neurological examinations
Hydrocephalus	▶ Symptoms see chapter P.01 Hydrocephalus in infants		
Chiari malformation type II (CM II)	▶ Symptoms see chapter P.04 Chiari malformations (CM)	▶ MRI, sMRI cervical ▶ Evoked potentials (ABEP, SSEP) ▶ Polysomnography	▶ Caudal herniation of cerebellum, associated intraspinal and intracranial malformations ▶ Increased latencies ▶ Central and obstructive sleep apneas
Tethered spinal cord (TC)	▶ Symptoms ▶ Reduced sensation, gait spasticity, bladder and bowel dysfunction, low back and leg pain, scoliosis	▶ Sonography ▶ sMRT ▶ Evoked potentials (SSEP) ▶ Myelo-CT ▶ See chapter M.02 Bladder dysfunction	▶ Low conus medullaris, decreased pulsations and mobility of spinal cord ▶ Spinal dysraphism and associated intraspinal malformations ▶ Increased latencies ▶ In special cases, imaging of osseous structures
Neurogenic bladder dysfunction	▶ Regular evaluation of bladder function	▶ Detailed analysis of neurogenic bladder dysfunction including sonography, MCU and urodynamic studies See chapter M.02 Bladder dysfunction	

1 Can be within normal range in membrane-covered MMC; also increased in gastroschisis or in multifetal pregnancy
2 The level of neurosegmental lesion is pivotal for ambulatory outcome. L5-S1: community ambulation; L3–4: walking in indoor environment, community ambulation possible, L2-T6: walking for therapeutic purposes; reciprocal gait orthosis.

P.03 Myelomeningocele (MMC)

P.03 Myelomeningocele (MMC) | PCS-Therapy

Hydrocephalus, MMC, Chiari Malformations

MMC	▶ Early closure of the defect using microsurgical techniques ▶ Preparation of the physiological tissue layers to reconstruct spinal cord and reduce the occurrence of inclusion tumors		
Hydrocephalus	▶ See chapter P.01 Hydrocephalus in infants ▶ See chapter P.02 Management of the shunted hydrocephalus		
Chiari malformation type II	▶ Surgical treatment in symptomatic CM II ▶ Craniocervical decompression by enlargement of foramen magnum, cervical laminectomy according to the extent of caudal herniation of the cerebellum, expansile duroplasty		
Tethered cord[1]	▶ Asymptomatic TC (secondary): no surgical treatment		
	▶ Symptomatic TC	▶ Presurgical MRI of the complete spinal cord to identify dysraphism and associated malformations ▶ Microsurgery for untethering and reconstruction of the spinal cord	
Neurogenic bladder dysfunction	▶ See chapter M.02 Bladder dysfunction		

Neurogenic bowel dysfunction	▶ High fibre diet, sufficient fluid balance
	▶ Nutrition diary
	▶ Daily bowel movements at regular times, < 30 min
	▶ Laxatives
	  – Oral: macrogol, lactulose, salinic laxatives
	  – Rectal: sorbitol, glycerin enema
	▶ Mechanical stimulation: irrigation, colon massage, enema, Malone stoma; artificial anus as last resort		

Contractures/scoliosis	Exclusion of symptomatic TC/CM II or shunt dysfunction	▶ Symptomatic TC or CM II, CSF shunt dysfunction	▶ Surgical treatment
		▶ No symptomatic TC/CM II or CSF shunt dysfunction	▶ Physiotherapy ▶ Orthosis ▶ Surgical treatment ▶ See chapter Q.02 Scoliosis
Paresis/spasticity	Paresis	▶ Physiotherapy ▶ Dynamic orthosis according to the level of neurosegmental lesion	
	Spasticity	▶ Exclusion of symptomatic TC/CM II or shunt dysfunction ▶ Botulinum toxins, surgical treatment, selective posterior rhizotomy as last resort ▶ See chapter G.01 Cerebral palsy	

[1] Secondary tethered cord (TC) persists in MMC patients after closure of the spinal defect.

P.04 Chiari malformations (CM) | PCS-Diagnosis 1/1

Hydrocephalus, MMC, Chiari Malformations

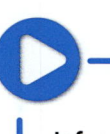

Infancy[1]

▶ Signs of brain stem dysfunction:
  – Stridor (vocal cord palsy)
  – Apnea/dyspnea
  – Weak cry
  – Absent/diminished gag reflex (aspiration pneumonia?)
  – Nystagmus
▶ Signs of impaired CSF flow
  – Opisthotonus, torticollis
▶ Failure to thrive
▶ Spasticity/hypertonicity of the upper limbs, paresis
▶ Scoliosis

Childhood

▶ Headache, neck pain (episodic or chronic, often occipital)
▶ Nystagmus, other eye motility disturbances
▶ Signs of cranial nerve dysfunction
▶ Spasticity/hypertonicity of the upper limbs, paresis
▶ Recurrent pneumonia (aspiration)
▶ Syncope
▶ Valsalva maneuver worsens/produces symptoms

Adolescence

▶ Chronic (maybe episodic) occipital headache/neck-pain
▶ Signs of caudal cranial nerve dysfunction
▶ Shooting pain of shoulder/arm (radicular signs)
▶ Vertigo, cerebellar ataxia
▶ Nystagmus (or other eye motility disturbances)
▶ Torticollis/opisthotonus
▶ Pollakisuria
▶ (Obstructive) sleep apnea
▶ Scoliosis
▶ Valsalva maneuver worsens/produces symptoms

MRI of the CNS, looking out for
▶ Anatomical changes
▶ Syrinx
▶ Signs of impaired CSF flow (detectable with cine-MRI)

Pitfalls
▶ Chiari malformation type I does not necessarily require any therapy if not symptomatic. Often, this malformation is discovered as incidental finding on MRI carried out for other diagnostic purposes.
▶ Almost all children with myelomeningocele (see chapter P.03 Myelomeningocele (MMC)) can be expected to have Chiari II
▶ Chiari III (occipitocervical encephalomyelocele) and Chiari IV (cerebellar hypoplasia, no longer considered to belong to the Chiari group) lack clinical significance and are not covered here.

▶ Herniation of cerebellar tonsils (diagnostic) ▶ Syrinx (typical), can be surrounded by compression oedema ▶ Kinking of the medulla oblongata (not in all cases) ▶ Hydrocephalus (uncommon), see chapter P.01 Hydrocephalus in infants	Chiari malformation type I
▶ Herniation of the cerebellar tonsils and the vermis cerebelli (diagnostic) ▶ Caudal displacement and deformation of medulla oblongata (diagnostic) ▶ Spina bifida/MMC (very typical) ▶ Hydrocephalus (common)[2]	Chiari malformation type II

---

1 Chiari II is usually symptomatic at birth; 30% develop signs of brain stem dysfunction within 5 years.

P.04 Chiari malformations (CM) | PCS-Therapy

CM type I	Cerebellar tonsils herniated > 10 mm below the foramen magnum (usually symptomatic)		▶ Suboccipital decompression with or without reconstruction of the CSF compartment of the posterior fossa with dura patch[1] ▶ If concomitant hydrocephalus: implant ventriculoperitoneal shunt
	Cerebellar tonsils herniated < 10 mm below the foramen magnum	Neurological deficit	
		No neurological deficit	▶ Regular controls[2] ▶ Headache therapy (see chapter C.02 Primary headache)
CM type II	▶ Management of the associated spinal dysraphism ▶ Suboccipital decompression with or without reconstruction of the CSF compartment of the posterior fossa with dura patch[1] ▶ If concomitant hydrocephalus: ventriculoperitoneal shunt		
Signs for syrinx/syringomyelia ▶ Paresthesias ▶ Disturbances of deep sensibility ▶ Loss of bladder/bowel control ▶ Paresis of the upper limps ▶ Muscular atrophy ▶ Palsies of cranial nerves	Multimodal therapeutic regimen ▶ Pain therapy (see chapter C.03 Secondary headache) ▶ Physical therapy ▶ Placement of ventriculoperitoneal shunt		
▶ Signs of elevated intracranial pressure	Ventriculoperitoneal shunt is already in place ▶ Exclude dysfunction, see chapter A.05 Acute increased intracranial pressure (ICP) and P.02 Management of the shunted hydrocephalus		
	No ventriculoperitoneal shunt in place ▶ See chapter P.01 Hydrocephalus in infants		

1 60–85 % of patients improve through the operation
2 Herniation of the cerebellar tonsils can improve over time as the posterior fossa grows

Notes

Notes

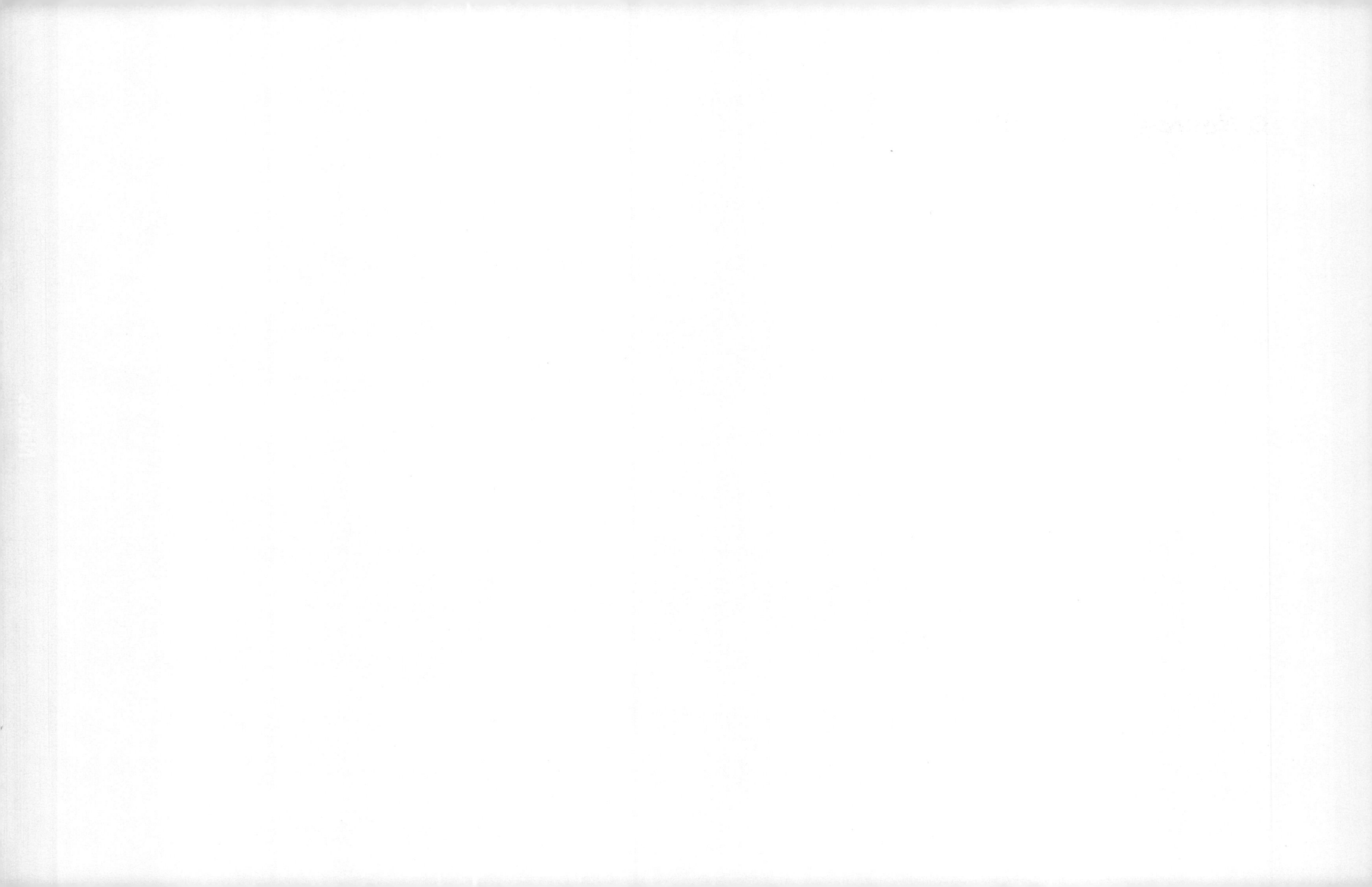

Q.02 Scoliosis | PCS-Diagnosis 1/1

Neuro-Orthopaedics

Medical history
- Increasing asymmetry
- Sitting and standing height
- Sitting ability

Physical examination
- Asymmetry

▸ Asymmetry
  – During sitting
  – During sitting/lying
  – Of waistline
  – Of shoulders
  – Of pelvis
	▸ X-ray in standing or sitting position of patient
	▸ If findings suggest scoliosis, X-ray of hips
		Positive X-ray findings	▸ Scoliosis

		Negative X-ray findings	Consider differential diagnosis
▸ Decreasing standing and sitting height ▸ Rib hump	▸ X-ray standing or sitting	Positive X-ray findings	▸ Scoliosis
		Negative X-ray findings	Consider differential diagnosis
	▸ Optional MRI to rule out intraspinal anomalies (e.g. Myelomeningocele)	In case of intraspinal anomalies refer to Neurology, Neurosurgery	
▸ Limited sitting ability ▸ Pelvic asymmetry ▸ Pseudo leg length discrepancy	▸ If clinical findings suggest scoliosis, X-ray of hips	Negative hip X-ray findings / Positive spine X-ray findings	▸ Scoliosis without hip pathology
		Positive hip X-ray findings / Positive spine X-ray findings report	▸ Scoliosis with hip pathology
		Positive hip X-ray findings / Negative spine X-ray findings	Consider differential diagnosis

Q.01 Hip joint | PCS-Therapy 1/1

Neuro-Orthopaedics

Spastic movement disorder (see chapter G.01 Cerebral palsy)	Step-by-step therapy aiming for centralized hip
	▶ Treatment of agonist weakness
	  – Training/strengthening abductors (virtualization, standing and walking, if necessary standing frame, NF-Walker etc.)
	▶ Reduction of antagonist spasticity
	  – Reducing adductor activity (muscle relaxants, orally, locally, intrathecally), see chapter G.01 Cerebral palsy.
	▶ Lengthening antagonist
	  – Surgical lengthening/weakening adductors (lengthening adductors, hamstrings, iliopsoas, rectus femoris)
	▶ Correction of femoral deformity
	  – Bony correction of antetorsion (DVO, supracondylar derotation)
	▶ Correction of acetabular deformity
	  – Bony correction of acetabular roof (Salter, Dega, Pemberton, Triple)
	▶ Reduction of hip dislocation
	  – Reduction of joint (closed reduction, open reduction)
	▶ Treatment of osteoarthritis due to long lasting failure load
	  – Endoprothesis

Hypotonic movement disorder (see chapter P.03 Myelomeningocele (MMC))	Step-by-step therapy for goal of mobile hip
	▶ Agonist weakness
	  – Positioning in neutral position, avoidance of contractures, functional orthotics, compensation of functional deficits, external stabilization
	▶ Antagonist shortening
	  – Weakening hip flexors and adductors, balanced muscle weakness
	▶ Joint deformity
	  – Only in case of enough residual muscle function: bony reconstruction
	▶ Joint dislocation
	  – Preservation of mobility despite dislocation

Q.01 Hip joint | PCS-Diagnosis 1/1

Neuro-Orthopaedics

Medical history
- Pre-existing conditions
- Pregnancy/delivery
- Sonography of hip joints
- Development/milestones
- Spasticity
- Epilepsy
- Pain
- Weight bearing
- Laxity of ligaments
- Medication
- Previous surgeries

Clinical findings
- Inspection
  - Sitting, stance, gait
  - Spontaneous position
  - Symmetry
  - Leg length
  - Muscle composition, soft tissue composition
- Palpation
  - Laxity of ligaments
  - Sensibility
  - Pain
- Motion tests
  - ROM[1]
  - Ashworth[2]
- Classification/functional tests
  - GMFCS, see chapter G.01 Cerebral palsy
  - Strength
  - Circumferences
  - GMFM

- Radiographs: pelvic overview, Rippstein I + II
  - Symmetry
  - Centering of hip
  - Articular cartilage angle
  - Reimers migration index
  - Shenton-Ménard line
  - Caput-collum-diaphyseal angle
  - Centre-edge angle
  - Anterior centre-edge angle
  - Pelvic balance/pelvic tilt
- CT hip joint
  - Measurement of torsion
  - 3-D-Reconstruction for investigation of spatial relationship and dislocation gap
- MRT hip joint
  - Effusion
  - Necrosis
- Instrumental gait analysis

Diagnosis
- Skeletal muscles
  - Weakness agonist/overactivity antagonist
  - Spasticity agonist/inhibition antagonist
  - Shortening agonist/overstretching antagonist
  - Paralysis, paresis
- Bone
  - Femoral deformity, acetabular deformity
  - Torsional deformity
- Joint
  - Instability, subluxation, luxation

---

1 Range of movement
2 Measuring of muscle tone (spasticity = velocity dependent increase of muscle tone)

Q Neuro-Orthopaedics

Q.02 Scoliosis | PCS-Therapy

Scoliosis postural		▶ Observation ▶ Sitting shell support ▶ Brace	
Scoliosis structural	< 40–50 %	▶ Observation ▶ Seating-shell support ▶ Brace ▶ In case of obvious progression, optional surgery – E.g. neuromuscular scoliosis	
	> 40–50 %	▶ Observation ▶ Seating-shell support ▶ Brace ▶ Potentially surgery[1]	In case of surgery, usually long fusion to L5 or to the sacrum In patients < 8–10 years, non-fusion techniques (e. g. VEPTR or growing rods) possible

1 Individual indication for surgery depends on age of patient, progression of scoliosis, underlying disease, cardiac function, pulmonary function, prospective rehabilitation.

Notes

Notes

R Neurological examinations

R.01 Neurological examinations (from 2 years of age*) 1/2

Neurological examinations

Name of patient:	Phenomenology I Status	Evaluation
		typical atypical

Name of patient:

Date of examination:

___ | ___ | _____

Time of examination:

___ | ___

Duration of examination:

_____ min

Name of examiner:

_____

Appearance
- ► Fully awake and typical responsiveness
- ► Tired
- ► Sleeping (see GCS)
- ► Coma (see GCS)
- ► Screaming/resisting
- ► Comments about atypical "first" observations/impressions:

Cranial nerves: Dimension I
- ► Meningism (YES/NO)
- ► I — Anamnestic, test: methyl salicylate = chewing gum, coffee e.g.)
- ► II — Visual acuity (vision chart), fundoscopy, field of vision, using glasses?
- ► III/IV/VI — Eye movements (slow and fast), nystagmus, diplopic images, pupils: size (mm), reactivity to light (right/left), symmetry, accommodation reflex (r/l), direct reaction to light (r/l), indirect reaction to light (r/l)
- ► V — Exit foramina / skin sensitivity $V_{1,2,3}$, jaw closure, lateral jaw movement and opening of the jaw, ICU: corneal reflex (piece of cotton wool rolled to a finely tapered thread)
- ► VII — Muscles of facial expression: frown, whistling, smiling (show teeth), eye squinting, blowing out cheeks. (Taste sensations on the anterior two-thirds of the tongue)
- ► VIII — Hearing: whispering, wrist watch ticking, rubbing of fingertips/Weber's test/Rinne's test
- ► IX/X — Anamnestic: Drinking/ eating – solid/ liquid. Watch swallowing act, watch soft palate ICU: testing for swallowing reflex
- ► XI — Against resistance: lift shoulders (trapezius m), turn head (sternocleidomastoid m), Anterior and posterior flexion of the head
- ► XII — Show tongue (stick tongue straight out), aberration?

I- - - - - - - - - - - - - - -I

Motor system: Dimension II
- ► Muscle stretch reflexes: (jaw jerk, without spinal pathway), biceps, triceps, brachioradialis, patellar tendon, Achilles tendon (Jendrassik's maneuver)[1]
- ► Superficial (skin muscle) reflexes: anal wink, cremasteric reflex, superficial abdominal reflexes
- ► Pathological reflexes: Babinski's sign
- ► Muscular strength (0-5)[2]
- ► Muscle tone: normotonia or hypotonia or hypertonia (dependent on speed of passive movement)

I- - - - - - - - - - - - - - -I

Somatosensory system: Dimension III
- ► Superficial: touch, pain, temperature (cold metal)
- ► Deep: vibration (tuning fork), movement, position

I- - - - - - - - - - - - - - -I

Coordination: Dimension IV
- ► Standing, walking, running, standing/jumping on one leg, raising from floor, walking a straight line, toe/heel walking, Fogs test, climbing stairs (up/down), Romberg's test
- ► Intentional movements: finger-nose, finger-finger, heel-knee
- ► Fine motor skills: diadochokinesis, hand/foot tapping

I- - - - - - - - - - - - - - -I

---

[1] 0 = absent reflex, 1 = sluggish, 2 = normal, 3 = brisk, 4 = clonus, 4+ = sustained clonus

R.01 Neurological examinations (from 2 years of age*) 2/2

	Mental state, neuropsychologic evaluation I Orientation I "Go by the eyes": Dimension V
	▶ Facility
	  ▶ Kindergarten: regular, integrative/inclusive
	  ▶ School: regular, integrative/inclusive, other
	▶ Speech comprehension
	▶ Spontaneous language
	▶ Drawing: drawing a human (developmental medicine/preschool ages)
	▶ Writing/reading
	Behavior during examination:
	▶ Activity/attention
	▶ Motivation
	▶ Cooperation/collaboration
	▶ Implementing and understanding of instructions
	▶ Orientation in space
	▶ Social competence I Interaction with caregiver/examiner
		I- - - - - - - - - - - - - - - -I

	Head general ▶ Dysmorphic features Head circumference (OFC _____ cm)/percentile (curves) _____ ▶ Hair (brittle/low/high hair line/alopecia) ▶ Shunt valve? (type, localization, filling pressure) ▶ Nuchal rigidity, Kernig, Lasegue	I- - - - - - - - - - - - - - - -I
	Skin ▶ Telangiectasias, café au lait spots, white spots, nevi	I- - - - - - - - - - - - - - - -I
	Vegetative function ▶ Sweating, bladder/bowel control, blood pressure, temperature, sleep, pains	I- - - - - - - - - - - - - - - -I
	Orthopedic status ▶ Spine bending, straining, bending restriction? (distance fingertips-floor, Schober's test), pain during palpation ▶ Joint mobility (contractures, hypermobility)	I- - - - - - - - - - - - - - - -I

Interpretation, working hypothesis, maximum three lines (typical/atypical):

* From 6 years of age, the neurological examination can be conducted formally as in adult neurology. The phenomenology is similar but not the same. Between the 3. and the 6. year of life, the neurological examination can pragmatically be described in terms of adult neurology. This must be taken as an orientation only and interpreted over time. Between birth and 2 years of age, other rules apply (see respective chapter)

… a masterful history and examination, conducted with competence and grace, leads to the physician's pleasure in discovery and to the patient's trust in the physician. No technologic procedure or computerized form can ever replace the mutual knowing process and bonding that occur during the clinical encounter. Mastery of the neurological examination provides a giant step in achieving the clinical competence that foster the maximum reward for you and the maximum benefit for your patients throughout your career …
(William E. DeMyer, M.D. Professor Emeritus of Pediatric Neurology, Indiana School of Medicine, Indianapolis, Indiana, see also: William E. DeMyer, Technique of the Neurological Examination, a programmed text, fifth edition McGraw-Hill Companies Inc. 2004)

R.02 6 minutes neurological examination 1/2

Neurological examinations

6-min 10-point screening neurological examination for schoolchildren without neurologic symptoms
(adapted from William E. DeMyer, Technique of the Neurologic Examination McGraw Hill Medical Publishing Division, Table 15-1)

Name: _____

Date: _____

Time of examination (in minutes): _____

Typical	Atypical	
☐	☐	**1. General appearance, mental and somatic status:** Age: _____ School grade: _____ School: _____ Behavior/Cooperation: _____ Affect: _____ Orientation: _____ Memory: _____
☐	☐	**2. Head** ▸ Normocephalic, head circumference (OFC), percentile rank, percentile curve ▸ Shape, (tenderness on) palpation ▸ Meningism, passive and active mobility of the cervical spine
☐	☐	**3. Visual system:** ▸ Acuity and visual field ▸ Pupils: mm in size, react to light (r/l), symmetry ▸ Eye movements, nystagmus ▸ Funduscopic examination
☐	☐	**4. Non-ocular cranial nerves:** ▸ Facial movements ▸ Tongue, jaw, masseter muscles and palate midline ▸ Word articulation, speech ▸ Swallowing (fluids and solid food)

R.02 6 minutes neurological examination

☐	☐	**5. Motor system:** ▸ Gait/station: free walking, toe/heel, balancing on an imaginary tightrope, deep knee bend ▸ Atrophy/hypertrophy/fasciculations ▸ Mirror movements, associated movements, diadochokinesia, tremor, ataxia (involuntary movements) ▸ Strength: lift arm over shoulder, extend/bend arm, handshake, hand/foot extension and flexion, hip flexion, knee extension/flexion ▸ Muscle tone (normal/hypotonia/hypertonia)
☐	☐	**6. Sensory system:** ▸ Hearing: voice, finger rustling ▸ Touch/temperature: face/hand/feet ▸ Recognition of numbers (on the back of the hand), joint positioning, vibration
☐	☐	**7. Skin:** ▸ Café au lait spots, white spots, nevi, dysmorphic features
☐	☐	**8. Overall developmental appearance:** ▸ According to age

9. Working hypothesis/provisional diagnosis/case summary (no more than three lines):

10. Next step/recommendations:

R.03 Developmental assessment – overview & orientation 1/2

Neurological examinations

Age	3 months	6 months	9 months	12 months	15 months	18 months	2 years	3 years	4 years	5 years	6 years
Gross motor function	Lifts head in prone. Pushes up on forearms	Pulls to sit: both arms in flexion, head and trunk in line.	Sits independently for unlimited time, keeps back upright and stable head control.	Supports weight while in standing. Holds on furniture and walls.	Walks with holding on adult's hands, or holding on furniture and walls.	Walks independently, displays stable balance.	Runs well-coordinated, bypasses barriers.	Jumps with both feet from bottom step.	Well coordinated pedaling of a tricycle or similar vehicle.	Walks stairs up and down easily by alternating feet, without holding on.	Stands on one foot for 10s without holding. Hops on either the right or the left foot about 8-10 times
Fine motor function	Moves and keeps hands at midline.	Transfers objects from one hand to the other. Uses whole hand/radial palmar grasp.	Transfers objects from one hand to the other. Keeps two objects in one or both hands. Manipulates intensively.	Uses pincer grasp (with thumb and index finger)	Copies on demand stacking two toy cubes (edge length 2–3 cm).	Hands objects on request, drops pellets into a vessel or takes them out.	Turns single pages of a book, unwraps sweeties in a skillful way.	Grasps little objects with fingertips, inserts or stacks them to another place.	Holds a crayon with thumb and 2 fingers.	Snips with scissors for children, sticks, makes simple handicrafts, colors picture neatly.	Paints recognizable objects (house, tree, little man, cars). Does handicrafts as folding, cutting out, sticking, using adhesive tapes. Holds pencil between middle, index finger and thumb
Cognition	Follows moving objects with eyes	Manipulation and oral exploration of objects. Observes surrounding activities attentively.	Intensive exploration of objects with hands-mouth-eyes.	Finds objects easily after visual displacement.	Manipulates objects, explores them for usability.	Constructs (after demonstration) a tower with 2–4 toy cubes, enjoys looking at an age-adequate picture book, points to familiar objects, exhibits representational plays with him-, herself.	Representational play with puppet, bear. Initiates constructive plays.	Draws a person with head and legs, explains the picture. Alters use of objects, exhibits intensively representational plays.	Asks questions, listens to readings and explanations. Demonstrates representational plays in a sophisticated way, e.g. with dollhouse, stores, vehicles, often on her/his own.	Intensive representational plays in a sophisticated way, also with other children, e.g. with dollhouse; plays on the ground, imitates situations. Constructs with or without models.	Recognizes and names shapes as circle, triangle, square. Constructs objects e.g. with Lego, understands and executes instructions. Draws a person with details (head, eyes, nose, mouth, upper trunk, arms and legs).

[1] adapted from„R. Michaelis, G. Niemann: Entwicklungsneurologie und Neuropädiatrie", 4th Edition, Thieme Verlag 2010, R. Michaelis et al. Validierte und teilvalidierte Grenzsteine der Entwicklung, Monatsschrift für Kinderheilkunde und Jugendmedizin, 2013)

R.03 Developmental assessment – overview & orientation

R. 3 Developmental assessment – overview & orientation 2/2

Language	Variable, meaningful sounds when crying (hunger, discomfort, pain)	Spontaneous, variable vocalizations; alone or in dialogue.	Spontaneous vocalizations such as a-a-a-a, wa-wa-wa-ra-ra-ra.	Produces consonant and vowel combinations with „a" (ma-ma, pa-pa, da-da)	Personal language, uses "mama", "papa" with purpose.	Uses verbal combinations with variable intonation for objects, animals, e.g. "wau-wau".	Produces one or two word combinations/ sentences	Produces combinations with three to five words, uses plural forms, talks to him-/herself when playing.	Connects sentences with „and, then" Reports daily experiences in a chronological and logical way.	Pronounces almost error free. Reports daily experiences in a chronological and logical way. Uses simple grammatical structures.	Uses 6-8 word sentences correctly, applies grammatical rules as subordinate clauses. Reports on something that had happened before in an understandable and chronological way, comments spontaneously. Has no obvious problems in articulation
Socialization	Keeps eye contact, changes head position to stay in contact. Smiles at known and unknown faces.	Initiates contact by vocalizing or touching. Enjoys playful, abrupt changes of body position. Enjoys nonverbal positive communications.	Distinguishes familiar from unfamiliar persons, with or without being scared.	Initiates, keeps, terminates social interactions.	Enjoys nursery and finger rhymes, imitates rhythmic plays.	Understands simple commands, objections, e.g. with or without compliance.	Plays alone in a room in the absence of the mother.	Helps at home and in the garden. Imitates actions of adults.	Can wait for her/his turn in collective plays. Shares with others.	Is cooperative in social plays. Understands emotional expressions of other children, reacts in a proper way, e.g. consoles, helps.	Plays with playmates, pretends role-playings as thieve and policeman or family, repeats what has happened earlier, replays a story. Enjoys and forces social plays, competition plays. Has a best friend for at least some weeks

R.04.1 Basic developmental assessment – up to 20 days

Name: _____ Age: _____ Date: _____ Examiner: _____

Item		Normal		Abnormal
Behavioral state	☐	awake, some spont. movements awake, lively spont. movements	☐	irritable, crying, drowsy, apathetic, seizures
Visual system	☐	pupils bilateral round coordinated eye movements optical blink reflex: prompt closure both lids	☐	pupils different, sunset sign strabismus conv (r/l), div (r/l), nystagmus absent/delayed/uncertain, asymm.
Auditory system	☐	acoustic blink reflex: prompt closure lids	☐	absent/delayed/uncertain, asymm.
Facial expression, mouth, swallowing	☐	variable facial expressions, symm. mouth: closed while in rest tongue: unrestricted movements in mid-pos vigorous rhythmic sucking, easy swallowing	☐	no/poor expressions, asymmetries mostly open, drooling restricted movements, asymm. no/poor suck, frequent choking, vomiting
Crying and vocalization	☐	vigorous, variable intonation	☐	no/rarely/weak/high pitched/monotonous
Spontaneous posture (supine, prone)	☐	head in supine: stable in mid-position head in prone: some head-lifting, able to turn head to both sides trunk: stable symmetrical posture arms: relaxed, symm. posture legs: relaxed, symm. posture hands, fingers: relaxed, half-open	☐	unstable/floppy/hyperextended, asymm. no/poor head lifting, unable to place head (r/l) unstable/floppy/hyperextended, asymm. persistently floppy (r/l)/flexed (r/l)/extended (r/l) persistently floppy (r/l)/flexed (r/l)/extended (r/l) persistently fisted (r/l)
Spontaneous movements (supine, prone)	☐	a few to vigorous spont. movements variable, smooth, symmetrical head and trunk rotation: unrestricted prone: some head lifting, head turning to both sides unrestricted arms: variable flexing and extending legs: variable flexing and extending hands: variable flexing and extending feet: variable flexing and extending	☐	hyperkinetic/hypokinetic invariable, clumsy, asymm. restricted, where? no/poor head lifting no head turning (r/l)/poor head turning (r/l) restricted, where? restricted, where? fisted (r/l)/restricted, where? restricted, where?
Passive muscle tone	☐	unrestricted joint range of motion: head, hand, elbow, shoulder, spine, hip, knee, ankle	☐	↑ hypertonic, where? ↓ hypotonic, where? change in tone, where?
Knee jerk	☐	bilateral, prompt	☐	absent (r/l)/weak (r/l)/exaggerated
Early motor reactions	☐	grasp reaction: prompt, vigorous Moro phase I: prompt, symmetrical Moro phase II: prompt, symmetrical ATNR: absent/incomplete	☐	absent (r/l)/poor (r/l)/persistent fisting (r/l) absent/exaggerated/spontan., asymm. absent /exaggerated, asymm. prompt (r/l)/persistent (r/l)
Provoked motor responses	☐	pulled up to half seat: arms bent, back straight, head quite stable in mid-position, hip and knee joints semiflexed; symmetrical prone suspension: head stable in mid-position, back straight, arms and legs slightly bent; symmetrical	☐	hyperflex.: head, elbow (r/l), hip (r/l), knee (r/l) hyperext.: head, trunk, hip (r/l), leg (r/l) floppy: head, elbow (r/l), trunk, leg (r/l) no/poor head lifting, rounded back, arms: floppy (r/l)/extended (r/l)/hyperflex (r/l) legs: floppy (r/l)/extended (r/l)/hyperflex (r/l)
Active muscle tone	☐	activation and exertion of muscular strength appropriate to function	☐	↑ hypertonic, where? ↓ hypotonic, where?
Sensorimotor development	☐	stable in supine position, symm. stable in prone position, symm. tolerates examination well	☐	supine unstable, asymm. prone unstable, asymm. clearly irritated by examination

Neurological examinations

R.04.1 Basic developmental assessment – up to 20 days 1/2

R.04. Basic developmental assessment – up to 20 days 2/2

Neurological examinations

Neurodevelopmental result:

Recommendations:

R.04.2 Basic developmental assessment – 4th to end of 8th week

Name: _____ Age: _____ Date: _____ Examiner: _____

Item	Normal	Abnormal	☐
Behavioral state	awake, some spont. movements; awake, lively spont. movements	irritable, crying, drowsy, apathetic, seizures	☐
Visual system	pupils bilateral round; coordinated eye movements; constant eye contact; optical blink reflex: prompt closure both lids	pupils different, sunset sign; strabismus conv (r/l)/div (r/l)/nystagmus; absent/poor/delayed/uncertain; absent/delayed/uncertain, asymm.	☐
Auditory system	acoustic orientation: reacts when verbally addressed; acoustic blink reflex: prompt closure lids	absent/poor/delayed/uncertain; absent/delayed/uncertain, asymm.	☐
Facial expression, mouth, swallowing	variable facial expressions, symmetrical; mouth: closed while in rest; tongue: unrestricted movements in mid-posit.; vigorous rhythmic sucking, easy swallowing	no/poor expressions, asymm.; mostly open, drooling; restricted movements, asymm.; no/poor suck, frequent choking, vomiting	☐
Crying and vocalization	vigorous with variable intonation; variable prosody	no/rarely/weak/high pitched/monotonous; monotonous prosody	☐
Spontaneous posture (supine, prone)	head in supine: stable in mid-position; head in prone: some head-lifting, able to turn head to both sides; trunk: stable symmetrical posture; arms: relaxed, symm. posture; legs: relaxed, symm. posture; hands, fingers: relaxed, half open	unstable/floppy/hyperextended, asymm.; no/poor head lifting, unable to place head (r/l); unstable/floppy/hyperextended, asymm.; persistently floppy (r/l)/flexed (r/l)/extended (r/l); persistently floppy (r/l)/flexed (r/l)/extended (r/l); persistently fisted (r/l)	☐
Spontaneous movements (supine, prone)	a few to vigorous spont. movements variable, smooth, symmetrical; head and trunk rotation: unrestricted; prone: some head lifting; head turning to both sides unrestricted; arms: variable flexing and extending; legs: variable flexing and extending; hands: variable flexing and extending; feet: variable flexing and extending	hyperkinetic/hypokinetic; invariable/clumsy, asymm.; restricted, where?; no/poor head lifting; no head turning (r/l)/poor head turning (r/l); restricted, where?; restricted, where?; persistently fisted (r/l), restricted, where?; restricted, where?	☐
Passive muscle tone	unrestricted joint range of motion: head, hand, elbow, shoulder, spine, hip, knee, ankle	↑ hypertonic, where?; ↓ hypotonic, where; change in tone, where?	☐
Knee jerk	bilateral, prompt	absent (r/l)/weak (r/l)/exaggerated (r/l)	☐
Early motor reactions	grasp reaction: prompt, vigorous; Moro phase I: present, symmetrical; Moro phase II: present, symmetrical; ATNR: absent/incomplete	absent (r/l)/poor (r/l)/persistent fisting (r/l); absent/exaggerated/spontan., asymm.; absent/exaggerated, asymm.; prompt (r/l)/persistent (r/l)	☐
Provoked motor responses	pulled up to half seat: arms bent, back straight, head stable in mid-position, hip and knee joints semiflexed; symmetrical; prone suspension: head stable in mid-position, back straight, arms and legs slightly bent, symmetrical	hyperflex.: head, elbow (r/l), hip (r/l), knee (r/l); hyperext.: head, trunk, hip (r/l), leg (r/l); floppy: head, elbow (r/l), trunk, leg (r/l); no/poor head lifting, rounded back, arms: floppy (r/l)/extended (r/l)/hyperflexed (r/l); legs: floppy (r/l)/extended (r/l)/hyperflexed (r/l)	☐
Active muscle tone	activation and exertion of muscular strength appropriate to function	↑ hypertonic, where?; ↓ hypotonic, where?	☐
Sensorimotor development	stable in supine and prone position; prone: starts taking weight on both arms; plays with its own fingers; intention to move both arms and hands to meet over midline	supine: unstable, prone: unstable, asymm.; no/poor attempts taking weight on arms (r/l); no/poor play with own fingers (r/l); no tendency (r/l)/poor tendency (r/l) to midline	☐

Neurological examinations

R.04.2 Basic developmental assessment – 4th to end of 8th week 1/2

R.04.2 Basic developmental assessment – 4th to end of 8th week

Neurological examinations

Neurodevelopmental results:

Recommendations:

R.04.3 Basic developmental assessment – 3rd to end of 4th months

Neurological examinations

Name: _____ Age: _____ Date: _____ Examiner: _____

Item	Normal	Abnormal
Behavioral state	☐ awake, moderate to vigorous spontan. moving interested in visual and verbal contacts	☐ irritable, crying, drowsy, apathetic, seizures no/poor interest in visual and verbal contacts
Visual system	☐ pupils bilateral round coordinated eye movements constant eye contact	☐ pupils different, sunset sign strabismus conv (r/l)/div (r/l)/nystagmus absent/poor/delayed/uncertain
Auditory system	☐ prompt acoustic orientation prompt reaction if addressed from behind	☐ absent/poor/delayed/uncertain absent/poor/delayed/uncertain
Facial expression, mouth, swallowing	☐ variable facial expressions, symmetrical mouth: closed while in rest tongue: unrestricted movements in mid-pos. vigorous rhythmic sucking, easy swallowing	☐ no/poor expressions, asymmetries. mostly open, drooling restricted movements, asymm no/poor suck, frequent choking, vomiting
Crying and Vocalization	☐ vigorous, variable intonation variable prosody	☐ no/rarely/weak/high pitched/monotonous monotonous prosody
Spontaneous posture (supine, prone)	☐ head in supine: stable in mid-position head in prone: good head and chest lifting, able to place head on both sides trunk: stable symmetrical posture arms: relaxed symmetrical posture legs: relaxed, symm. posture hands, fingers: relaxed half open	☐ unstable/floppy/hyperextended, asymm. no/poor head lifting, no/poor chest lifting unable to place head (r/l) unstable/floppy/hyperextended, asymm. persistently floppy (r/l)/flexed (r/l) extended (r/l) persistently floppy (r/l)/flexed (r/l)/ extended (r/l)/persistently fisted (r/l)
Spontaneous movements (supine, prone)	☐ moderate to vigorous variable, smooth, symmetrical head and trunk rotation: unrestricted prone: easy lifting head and chest, turning head (r/l), stable bearing of weight on extended fore-arms and open hands arms: variable flexing and extending legs: variable flexing and extending hands/fingers: variable flexing and extending	☐ hyperkinetic/hypokinetic invariable/clumsy, asymm. restricted, where? no/poor head lifting, no/poor head turning (r/l), no/poor bearing of weight on forearms (r/l), hands fisted (r/l) floppy (r/l)/hyperext. (r/l)/flexed (r/l)/add. (r/l) floppy (r/l)/hyperext. (r/l)/flexed (r/l)/add. (r/l) persistently fisted (r/l), restricted, where?
Passive muscle tone	☐ unrestricted joint range of motion: head, hand, elbow, shoulder, spine, hip, knee, ankle	☐ ↑ hypertonic, where? ↓ hypotonic, where? change in tone, where?
Knee jerk	☐ bilateral, prompt	☐ absent (r/l)/weak (r/l)/exaggerated (r/l)
Early motor reactions	☐ grasp reaction: prompt, vigorous Moro phase I : absent/weak Moro phase II: absent/weak ATNR: absent/incomplete	☐ absent (r/l)/weak (r/l)/constant fisting (r/l) present/exaggerated/spontan., asymm. present/exaggerated, asymm. present (r/l)/persistent (r/l)
Provoked motor responses	☐ pulled up to half seat: arms bent, back straight, head stable in mid-position, hip and knee joints semiflexed; symmetrical prone suspension: head stable in mid-position, back straight, arms and legs slightly bent, symmetrical standing position: taking over the weight fully plantar or with fore-feet, knees extended, hips semiflexed, symmetrical	☐ hyperflex.: head, elbow (r/l), hip (r/l), knee (r/l) hyperext.: head, trunk, hip (r/l), leg (r/l) floppy: head, elbow (r/l), trunk, leg (r/l) no/poor head lifting, back rounded, arms: floppy (r/l)/extended (r/l)/hyperflex (r/l) legs: floppy (r/l)/extended (r/l)/hyperflex (r/l) no taking weight (r/l)/poor taking weight (r/l) no/poor extension knee (r/l) hips: hyperflex (r/l)/hyperext (r/l)/adducted (r/l)
Active muscle tone	☐ activation and exertion of strength appropriate to function	☐ ↑ hypertonic, where? ↓ hypotonic, where?
Sensorimotor development	☐ supported sitting position: head well balanced; trunk straight, legs slightly bent grasping with whole hand and fingers keeps objects with hands and fingers hand-hand contact in body mid-line	☐ no supported sitting, no/poor head control, no/poor trunk control, legs hyperext. (r/l) no grasping (r/l)/poor grasping (r/l) no keeping obj. (r/l)/poor keeping obj. (r/l) no/poor hand-hand contact in mid-line

R.04. Basic developmental assessment – 3rd to end of 4th months 2/2

Neurological examinations

Neurodevelopmental results:

Recommendations:

R.04.4 Basic developmental assessment – 6th to end of 8th months

Neurological examinations

Name: _____ Age: _____ Date: _____ Examiner: _____

Item	Normal	Abnormal	☐
Behavioral state	awake, alert short visual and verbal dialogues	irritable, crying, drowsy, apathetic, seizures no/poor communication	☐
Visual system:	pupils bilateral round coordinated eye movements constant eye contact visual orientation	pupils different, sunset sign strabismus conv (r/l)/div (r/l)/nystagmus absent/poor/delayed/uncertain absent/poor/delayed/uncertain	☐
Auditory system:	prompt acoustic orientation prompt reaction if addressed from behind	absent/poor/delayed/uncertain absent/poor/delayed/uncertain	☐
Facial expression, mouth, swallowing	variable facial expressions, symmetrical mouth: closed while in rest tongue: unrestricted movements in mid-pos easy swallowing	no/poor expressions, asymm. mostly open, drooling restricted, where? frequent choking	☐
Vocalization and articulation	vigorous vocalization and articulation clearly articulated strings of syllables using closing consonants like b, d, m variable prosody	no/poor vocalization, no/poor articulation no/poor strings of syllables, no use of b, d, m/poor use of b, d, m monotonous prosody	☐
Spontaneous posture (supine, prone)	head: stable in mid-position trunk: stable symmetrical posture arms: relaxed, symm. posture legs: relaxed, symm. posture hands, fingers: relaxed, half open	unstable/floppy/hyperextended, asymm. unstable/floppy/hyperextended, asymm. persistently floppy (r/l)/flexed (r/l)/extended (r/l) persistently floppy (r/l)/flexed (r/l)/extended (r/l) persistently fisted (r/l)	☐
Spontaneous movements (supine, prone)	a few to vigorous spont. movements variable, smooth, symmetrical prone: easy lifting head and chest, turning head (r/l), stable bearing of weight on extended fore-arms and open hands head and trunk: straight, rotation unrestricted arms: variable flexing and extending legs: variable flexing and extending hands, fingers: relaxed flexing and extend.	hyperkinetic/hypokinetic invariable/clumsy, asymm. no/poor head lifting, no/poor chest lifting no turning head (r/l)/poor turning (r/l), no bearing weight (r/l)/poor bearing weight (r/l) head: floppy/hyperext, trunk: floppy/hyperext restricted, where? floppy (r/l)/hypertext. (r/l)/flexed (r/l), adducted (r/l) floppy (r/l)/hyperext. (r/l)/flexed (r/l)/adducted (r/l) no moving (r/l)/poor moving (r/l)/tremor (r/l) persistently fisted (r/l)/athetotic (r/l)/atactic (r/l)	☐
Passive muscle tone	unrestricted joint range of motion: head, hand, elbow, shoulder, spine, hip, knee, ankle	↑ hypertonic, where? ↓ hypotonic, where? change in tone, where?	☐
Knee jerk	bilateral prompt	absent (r/l)/weak (r/l)/exaggerated (r/l)	☐
Babinski	bilateral absent	present (r/l)/uncertain (r/l)	☐
Early mot reac	none	present: grasp reaction (r/l), ATNR (r/l), Moro (r/l)	☐
Provoked motor responses:	pulled up to half seat: arms bent, back straight, head stable in mid-position, hip and knee joints semiflexed; symmetrical passive turn-over (r/l) from supine to prone: smooth rotation of pelvis and shoulders, active forward movement with extended arm and open hand, symmetrical attain standing position: taking over the weight fully plantar or with fore-feet, head and back straight, symmetrical knees and hips extended, symmetrical	hyperflex.: elbow (r/l), head, hip (r/l), knee (r/l) hyperext.: head, trunk, hip (r/l), leg (r/l) floppy: elbow (r/l), head, trunk, leg (r/l) rotation: poor (r/l)/clumsy (r/l), restricted pelvis (r/l)/restricted shoulder (r/l) absent (r/l)/poor (r/l)/delayed (r/l)/clumsy (r/l) arm restricted (r/l), hand fisted (r/l) no/poor taking weight (r/l), pes equinus (r/l), head: floppy/hyperext., back: floppy/hyperext. hips: hyperflex. (r/l)/hyperext. (r/l)/adducted (r/l) knees: hyperflex. (r/l)/hyperext. (r/l)	☐
Active muscle tone:	activation and exertion of strength appropriate to function	↑ hypertonic, where? ↓ hypotonic, where?	☐
Sensorimotor development:	moves on floor by rolling/creeping/squirming precise scissors grasp (r/l) hands, fingers manipulate small toy precisely passing it from hand to hand, symmetrical	absent/poor/clumsy absent (r/l)/poor (r/l)/grasping with fist (r/l) no manipulation (r/l)/poor manipulation (r/l) no transfer (r/l)/clumsy transfer (r/l)	☐

R.04.4 Basic developmental assessment – 6th to end of 8th months 2/2

Neurological examinations

Neurodevelopmental result:

Recommendations:

R.04.5 Basic developmental assessment – 11th to end of 13th months

Name: _____ Age: _____ Date: _____ Examiner: _____

Item	Normal	Abnormal
Behavioral state	awake, alert; some visual and verbal dialogues	irritable, crying, drowsy, apathetic, seizures; no/poor communication
Visual system	pupils bilateral round; coordinated eye movements; constant eye contact; visual orientation	pupils different; strabismus conv (r/l)/div (r/l)/nystagmus; absent/poor/delayed/uncertain; absent/poor/delayed/uncertain
Auditory system	prompt acoustic orientation; prompt reaction if addressed from behind	absent/poor/delayed/uncertain; absent/poor/delayed/uncertain
Facial expression, mouth, swallowing	variable facial expressions, symmetrical; mouth: closed while in rest; tongue: unrestricted movements in mid-pos; easy swallowing	no/poor expressions, asymm.; mostly open, drooling; restricted, where?; frequent choking
Articulation	babbles vigorously and articulates some single words, articulation contains most vowels and consonants, variable prosody	no/poor babbling, no/poor articulation of single words, no/restricted use of vowels and consonants, monotone prosody
Spontaneous posture (supine, sitting, standing)	head: stable in mid-position; trunk: stable symmetrical posture; arms: relaxed, symm. posture; legs: relaxed, symm. posture; hands, fingers: relaxed, half open	unstable/floppy/hyperextended, asymm.; unstable/floppy/hyperextended, asymm.; persistently floppy (r/l)/flexed (r/l)/extended (r/l); persistently floppy (r/l)/flexed (r/l)/extended (r/l); persistently fisted (r/l)
Spontaneous movements (sitting, standing)	a few to vigorous spont. movements, variable, smooth, symmetrical; sitting: stable balanced; standing: balanced with or without support: hips and legs straight, weight on whole sole; head and trunk: straight, rotation unrestricted; arms: variable flexing and extending; legs: variable flexing and extending; hands, fingers: variable flexing and extending	hyperkinetic/hypokinetic; invariable/clumsy, asymm.; absent/poor balance/needs support; absent/poor balance/needs support; hips: hyperextended (r/l)/flexed (r/l)/adducted (r/l); knees: hyperextended (r/l)/flexed (r/l); weight on forefoot (r/l)/pes equinus (r/l); head: floppy/hyperext, trunk: floppy/hyperext restricted, where?; floppy (r/l)/hypertext. (r/l)/flexed (r/l), adducted (r/l); floppy (r/l)/hypertext. (r/l)/flexed (r/l), adducted (r/l); no moving (r/l)/poor moving (r/l)/tremor (r/l); persistently fisted (r/l)/athetotic (r/l)/atactic (r/l)
Passive muscle tone	unrestricted joint range of motion: head, hand, elbow, shoulder, spine, hip, knee, ankle	↑ hypertonic, where?; ↓ hypotonic, where?; change in tone, where?
Knee jerk	bilateral prompt	absent (r/l)/weak (r/l)/exaggerated (r/l)
Babinski	bilateral absent	present (r/l)/uncertain (r/l)
Early mot reac	none	present: grasp reaction (r/l), ATNR (r/l), Moro (r/l)
Provoked motor response:	standing position: taking over weight with full soles or with fore-feet, head and back straight, symmetrical knees and hips extended, symmetrical	no/poor taking weight (r/l), pes equinus (r/l); head: floppy/hyperext., back: floppy/hyperext.; hips: hyperflex. (r/l)/hyperext. (r/l)/adducted (r/l); knees: hyperflex. (r/l)/hyperext. (r/l)
Active muscle tone	activation and exertion of strength appropriate to function	↑ hypertonic, where?; ↓ hypotonic, where?
Sensorimotor development	sitting: well balanced without support pulls up to standing, precise scissors- and pincer-grasp (r/l); intensive visual and tactile exploration with fingertips and hands, symmetrical	absent/poorly balanced/needs support; absent/poor/clumsy; absent (r/l)/poor (r/l)/grasping with fist (r/l); no/poor visual exploration (r/l); no/poor tactile exploration (r/l)

R.04.5 Basic developmental assessment – 11th to end of 13th months 2/2

Neurodevelopmental result:

Recommendations:

R.04.6 Basic developmental assessment – 17th to end of 19th months

Neurological examinations

Name: _____ Age: _____ Date: _____ Examiner: _____

Item		Normal		Abnormal
Behavioral state	☐	awake, alert; fair to lively visual and verbal dialogues	☐	irritable, crying, drowsy, apathetic, seizures no/poor communication
Visual system	☐	pupils bilateral round coordinated eye movements constant eye contact visual orientation	☐	pupils different strabismus conv (r/l)/div (r/l)/nystagmus absent/poor/delayed/uncertain absent/poor/delayed/uncertain
Auditory system	☐	prompt acoustic orientation prompt reaction if addressed from behind	☐	absent/poor/delayed/uncertain absent/poor/delayed/uncertain
Facial expression, mouth, swallowing	☐	variable facial expressions, symmetrical mouth: closed while in rest tongue: unrestricted movem. in mid-pos. easy swallowing	☐	no/poor expressions, asymm. mostly open, drooling restricted where? frequent choking
Articulation	☐	lively dialogues with people, and monologues when playing; speaks most of vowels and consonants articulates about 20 words correctly; variable prosody	☐	no/poor articulation to people no/poor articulation in play missing closure consonants like b, g, d, t no/only few clearly articulated words monotonous prosody
Spontaneous posture (sitting, standing)	☐	head: stable in mid-position trunk: stable symmetrical posture arms: relaxed, symm. posture legs: relaxed, symm. posture hands, fingers: relaxed, half open	☐	unstable/floppy/hyperextended, asymm. unstable/floppy/hyperextended, asymm. persistently floppy (r/l)/flexed (r/l)/extended (r/l) persistently floppy (r/l)/flexed (r/l)/extended (r/l) persistently fisted (r/l)
Spontaneous movements (sitting, standing, walking)	☐	moderate to vigorous spont. movements, variable, smooth, symm. sitting: stable balanced standing: balanced, without support: hips and legs straight, weight on whole sole walking: well balanced, symmetrical, arms may still be slightly extended, legs straight, slightly apart, weight on full sole head and trunk: straight, rotation unrestricted arms: moving unrestricted, symm legs: moving unrestricted, symm. hands, fingers: variable flexing and extending	☐	hyperkinetic/hypokinetic invariable, clumsy, asymm. absent/poor balance/needs support absent/poor balance/needs support hips: hyperext. (r/l)/flexed (r/l)/adducted (r/l) knees: hyperextended (r/l)/flexed (r/l) weight on fore-foot (r/l)/pes equinus (r/l), absent, poor balance, needs support arms: hyperext. (r/l)/flexed (r/l)/adducted (r/l) hips: hyperext. (r/l)/flexed (r/l)/adducted (r/l) knees: hyperextended (r/l)/flexed (r/l) weight on fore-foot (r/l)/pes equinus (r/l) head: floppy/hyperext, trunk: floppy/hyperext restricted, where? floppy (r/l)/hyperext. (r/l)/flexed (r/l)/add. (r/l) floppy (r/l)/hyperext. (r/l)/flexed (r/l)/add. (r/l) no moving (r/l)/poor moving (r/l)/tremor (r/l) persistently fisted (r/l)/athetotic (r/l)/atactic (r/l)
Passive muscle tone	☐	unrestricted joint range of motion: head, hand, elbow, shoulder, spine, hip, knee, ankle	☐	↑ hypertonic, where? ↓ hypotonic, where? change in tone, where?
Knee jerk	☐	bilateral prompt	☐	absent (r/l)/weak (r/l)/exaggerated (r/l)
Babinski	☐	bilateral absent	☐	present (r/l)/uncertain (r/l)
Early mot reac	☐	none	☐	present: grasp reaction (r/l), ATNR (r/l), Moro (r/l)
Active muscle tone	☐	activation and exertion of strength appropriate to function	☐	↑ hypertonic, where? ↓ hypotonic, where?
Sensorimotor development	☐	manages to climb stairs step by step holding rail or hand of a person hands-fingers: precise pointing, grasping, holding, manipulating small toys, pencils, spoon, cups, symmetrical	☐	absent/clumsy/poorly balanced absent (r/l)/poor (r/l)/clumsy (r/l)

Neurological examinations

Neurodevelopmental result:

Recommendations:

R.04.7 Basic developmental assessment – 21st to end of 26th months

Name: _____ Age: _____ Date: _____ Examiner: _____

Item	Normal		Abnormal	
Behavioral state	awake, alert; fair to lively visual and verbal dialogues	☐	irritable, crying, drowsy, apathetic, seizures no/poor communication	☐
Visual system	pupils bilateral round coordinated eye movements constant eye contact visual orientation	☐	pupils different strabismus conv (r/l)/div (r/l)/nystagmus absent/poor/delayed/uncertain absent/poor/delayed/uncertain	☐
Auditory system	prompt acoustic orientation prompt reaction if addressed from behind	☐	absent/poor/delayed/uncertain absent/poor/delayed/uncertain	☐
Facial expression, mouth, swallowing:	variable facial expressions, symmetrical mouth: closed while in rest tongue: unrestricted movem. in mid-pos easy swallowing	☐	no/poor expressions, asymm. mostly open, drooling restricted, where? frequent choking	☐
Articulation	speaks with clear articulation to people and when playing, using closure consonants like b, p, d, t, g, k articulates about 30 words correctly 2-word sentences, variable prosody	☐	no/poor articulation to people no/poor articulation in play missing closure consonants, which? no/only some correctly articulated words no 2-word sentences, monotonous prosody	☐
Spontaneous posture (sitting, standing)	head: stable in mid-position trunk: stable symmetrical posture arms: relaxed, symm. posture legs: relaxed, symm. posture hands, fingers: relaxed, half open	☐	unstable/floppy/hyperextended, asymm. unstable/floppy/hyperextended, asymm. persistently floppy (r/l)/flexed (r/l)/extended (r/l) persistently floppy (r/l)/flexed (r/l)/extended (r/l) persistently fisted (r/l)	☐
Spontaneous movements (sitting, standing, walking)	moderate to vigorous spont. movements, variable, smooth, symm. sitting: stable balanced standing: balanced without support, hips and legs straight, weight on whole sole walking: well balanced, symmetrical arms may still be slightly extended, legs straight, slightly apart, weight on full solehead and trunk: straight, rotation unrestricted arms: moving unrestricted, symm legs: moving unrestricted, symm. hands, fingers: variable flexing and extending	☐	hyperkinetic/hypokinetic invariable, clumsy, asymm absent/poor balance/needs support absent/poor balance/needs support hips: hyperext. (r/l)/flexed (r/l)/adducted (r/l) knees: hyperextended (r/l)/flexed (r/l) weight on fore-foot (r/l)/pes equinus (r/l), absent, poor balance, needs support arms: hyperext. (r/l)/flexed (r/l)/adducted (r/l) hips: hyperext. (r/l)/flexed (r/l)/adducted (r/l) knees: hyperextended (r/l)/flexed (r/l) weight on fore-foot (r/l)/pes equinus (r/l) head: floppy/hyperext, trunk: floppy/hyperext restricted, where? floppy (r/l)/hyperext. (r/l)/flexed (r/l)/add. (r/l) floppy (r/l)/hyperext. (r/l)/flexed (r/l)/add. (r/l) no moving (r/l)/poor moving (r/l)/tremor (r/l) persistently fisted (r/l)/athetotic (r/l)/atactic (r/l)	☐
Passive muscle tone	unrestricted joint range of motion: head, hand, elbow, shoulder, spine, hip, knee, ankle	☐	↑ hypertonic, where? ↓ hypotonic, where? change in tone, where?	☐
Knee jerk	bilateral prompt	☐	absent (r/l)/weak (r/l)/exaggerated (r/l)	☐
Babinski	bilateral absent	☐	present (r/l)/doubtful (r/l)	☐
Early mot reac	none	☐	grasp reflex (r/l), ATNR (r/l), Moro I (r/l), Moro II	☐
Active muscle tone	activation and exertion of strength appropriate to function	☐	↑ hypertonic, where? ↓ hypotonic, where?	☐
Sensorimotor development	runs safely, on whole feet, avoiding obstacles easily manages to climb on chairs/sofas etc. gets down again scribbles circular and to and fro lines neatly removes wrapping from small sweets	☐	absent/unstable/clumsy/asymm not able to avoid obstacles absent/hardly/clumsy absent/hardly/clumsy no lines (r/l)/poor lines/(r/l) no/poor/clumsy/asymm.	☐

Neurological examinations

Neurological examinations

Neurodevelopmental result:

Recommendations:

Notes

Notes

Medication

A

Acetazolamide (AZA)

Dosage:

- ▶ epilepsy: 8–30 mg/kg/d (as stated in the Summary of Product Characteristics, SPC)
- ▶ type 2 episodic ataxia: 5–10 mg/kg/d (off-label)
- ▶ idiopathic intracranial hypertension/pseudotumor cerebri (off-label)
  - infants: initial dose 8 mg/kg/d as 3 separate doses, increase if required to a maximum of 100 mg/kg/d
  - children: start with 25 mg/kg/d, increase by 25 mg/kg/d if required (max. 100 mg/kg/d or 2 g/d)
  - adolescents: start with 25 mg/kg/d, increase by 25 mg/kg/d if required (max. 100 mg/kg/d or 2 g/d)
- ▶ central respiratory disorder with accompanying hypoxemia: 7.5–10.0 mg/kg/d (caution: metabolic decompensation)

Neuropaediatric indications:

- reduction of cerebrospinal fluid (CSF) production with increase of intracranial pressure (ICP) (including posthemorrhagic ventricular dilatation and idiopathic intracranial hypertension)
- alternative therapy for partial, generalized or absence epilepsy (short-term)
- type 2 episodic ataxia
- central respiratory disorder with accompanying hypoxemia

Mechanism of action:

- carbonic anhydrase inhibitor

Relevant contraindications:

- hypokalemia, hyponatremia

Relevant side effects and interactions:

- metabolic acidosis
- frequent urination
- skin rash
- paresthesia
- hypercalciuria/nephrolithiasis
- nephrotoxic in combination with NSAIDs
- increase of Carbamazepine level
- (rarely) Stevens-Johnson syndrome

Approval status: –

Sources:

- Germany – SPC: –
- USA – T:
  - epilepsy
    - oral
    - 4–16 mg/kg/d as 1–4 separate doses, not to exceed 30 mg/kg/d or 1 g/d; extended release capsule is not recommended for treatment of epilepsy
  - oedema
    - oral or IV
    - 5 mg/kg/d as a SD or 150 mg/m²/d as a SD
- United Kingdom – BNFC:
  - epilepsy
    - oral or by slow intravenous injection
      - **neonate:** initial dose 2.5 mg/kg 2–3 times daily; maintenance dose 5–7 mg/kg 2–3 times daily
      - **children 1 month–12 years:** initial dose 2.5 mg/kg 2–3 times daily, followed by 5–7 mg/kg 2–3 times daily, max. 750 mg/d (maintenance dose)
      - **children 12–18 years:** 250 mg 2–4 times daily
  - **raised intracranial pressure**
    - oral or by slow intravenous injection
      - **children 1 month–12 years:** initial dose 8 mg/kg 3 times daily, increasing as necessary to max. 100 mg/kg/d

Comment:

- careful use of long term administration
- frequent control of acid-base homeostasis as well as electrolytes

Acetylsalicylic acid (ASA)

Dosage:

- ▶ stroke prophylaxis: 1–3 mg/kg/d
  - initial dose for acute stroke treatment or in case of temporary symptoms: 3–5 mg/kg/d (information only for adults available, not for children)
  - after 3–6 months of LMWH therapy following the clinically acute phase, in a stable situation: 3–5 mg/kg/d (no information on dosage and tolerability of ASA available for newborns)
- ▶ acute tension-type headache treatment: 10–15 mg/kg p.o./IV
- ▶ acute migraine treatment: 10–15 mg/kg p.o./IV
- ▶ migraine prophylaxis: 2–3 mg/kg/d p.o.
- ▶ Kawasaki disease with fever: 50 mg/kg/d or 80–100 mg/kg/d as 4 separate doses over 48–72 h, followed by 3–5 mg/kg/d; discontinue treatment after 6–8 weeks

Neuropaediatric indications:

– primary and secondary stroke prevention/prophylaxis
– tension-type headache
– acute migraine treatment
– migraine prophylaxis
– Kawasaki disease

Mechanism of action:

– inhibition of platelet aggregation through inhibition of cyclo-oxygenase with consecutive reduction of thromboxane A2 and prostacyclin synthesis

Relevant contraindications:

– severe liver or renal failure
– children and adolescents with feverish illness

Relevant side effects and interactions:

– very rare at low dose
– nausea, heartburn, vomiting
– bronchoconstriction
– mucosal irritation, gastrointestinal bleeding and peptic ulcer
– relapse of (chronic) inflammatory bowel diseases
– Reye syndrome in children (and adolescents) with feverish illness (historical)

Approval status:

– varies depending on product (see SPC)

Sources:

– **Germany – SPC:**

Age:	Single dose (SD):
7–9 years	1 tablet, i.e. 250 mg
9–12 years	1–1½ tablet, i.e. 250–375 mg
> 12 years	2–3 tablets, i.e. 500–750 mg

– The SD can be given every 4–8 h, if necessary.
– **USA – T:**
  – **Kawasaki disease**
    – oral
      – 80–100 mg/kg/d divided into 4 doses, i.e. 20–25 mg/kg, administered every 6 h for up to 14 d (until fever resolves for at least 48 h); then decrease the dose to 3–5 mg/kg/d once daily. In patients without coronary artery abnormalities, continue with the low dose for 6–8 weeks. In patients with coronary artery abnormalities, maintain the low-dose treatment indefinitely (in addition to therapy with Warfarin).

– **analgesic**
  – oral, rectal, IV
    – 10–15 mg/kg every 4–6 h, max. dose: 4 g/d
– **anti-inflammatory**
  – oral
    – initially: 60–90 mg/kg/d divided into several doses
    – usual maintenance dose: 80–100 mg/kg/d given in appropriate doses every 6–8 h
    – monitor ASA serum concentration
– **antiplatelet effects**
  – adequate paediatric studies have not been performed; paediatric dosage is derived from adult studies and clinical experience and is not well established
  – Suggested doses have ranged from 1–5 mg/kg/d to 5–10 mg/kg/d as a SD. Doses are typically rounded to a convenient amount.
– **arterial ischemic stroke, recurrent:** 1–5 mg/kg/d as a SD after anticoagulation therapy has been discontinued.
– **United Kingdom – BNFC:**
  – **Kawasaki disease**
    – oral
      – **neonates:** initially 32 mg/kg/d as 4 separate doses for 2 weeks or until afebrile, followed by 5 mg/kg/d as a SD for 6–8 weeks; if no evidence of coronary lesions after 8 weeks, discontinue treatment or seek expert advice
      – **children 1 month–12 years:** initally 30–50 mg/kg/d as 4 separate daily doses for 2 weeks or until afebrile, then 2–5 mg/kg/d as a SD for 6–8 weeks; if no evidence of coronary lesions after 8 weeks, discontinue treatment or seek expert advice
  – **inhibition of platelet aggregation, prevention of thrombus formation after cardiac surgery**
    – oral
      – **neonates:** 1–5 mg/kg/d as a SD
      – **children 1 month–12 years:** 1–5 mg/kg/d (usual max. 75 mg) as a SD
      – **children 12–18 years:** 75 mg/d as a SD

IV comment:

– increased (potentially/historical) risk of developing Reye syndrome (< 12 years)
– should not be administered during acute febrile disease (especially varicella disease and influenza)
– optional monitoring of anticoagulation: platelet function testing

Aciclovir

Dosage:
- suspected HSV-1 or -2 encephalitis: 45 mg/kg/d as 3 separate doses (with neonatal infection: 60 mg/kg as 3 separate doses) over 21 d
- up to age 12 as IV therapy
- with confirmed HSV encephalitis or with immunosuppression, doses should be doubled and treatment continued for 14 d (newborns 21 d)

Neuropaediatric indications:
- confirmed or suspected herpes simplex or varicella zoster encephalitis
- varicella zoster virus with facial nerve paralysis

Mechanism of action:
- antimetabolite, inhibition of viral DNA polymerase
- phosphorylated by viral thymidine kinase and further phosphorylated to acyclo-GTP by cellular kinase
- by incorporating and using acyclo-GTP instead of GTP for DNA replication via DNA polymerase, no more deoxyribonucleotides (dNTP) can be attached as acyclo-GTP has no 3'-OH group and termination of DNA synthesis occurs

Relevant contraindications:
- none

Relevant side effects and interactions:
- reduced dose in renal disease to lower the risk of toxic encephalopathy

Approval status:
- varies depending on product (see SPC)

Sources:
- **Germany – SPC:**
  - **Herpes simplex infection**
    - **children > 2 years:** see dose recommendation for adults
    - **children < 2 years:** half dose of adults' dose
    - **adults:** 800 mg/d as 4 separate doses (alternatively as 2 separate doses). This is the recommended dose for prophylaxis in immunocompromised patients.
    - **note:** For severely immunocompromised patients (e.g. after organ transplantation) a dose of 1,600 mg/d as 4 separate doses may be indicated.
- **USA – T:**
  - **Herpes zoster in immunocompetent host**
    - oral
      - **children ≥ 12 years:** initiate treatment within 48 hours of rash onset using 4000 mg/d as 5 separate doses for 5–7 d
    - IV
      - **infants 1 month–< 1 year:** 30 mg/kg/d as 3 separate doses for 7–10 d
      - **children ≥ 1 year:** 30 mg/kg/d as 3 separate doses or 1500 mg/m²/d as 3 separate doses for 7–10 d
  - **Herpes zoster in immunocompromised host**
    - IV
      - 30 mg/kg/d as 3 separate doses for 7–10 d; note: the AIDS info guidelines recommended duration of therapy is 10–14 d
  - **HSV encephalitis**
    - IV
      - **infants 1–3 months:** 60 mg/kg/d as 3 separate doses for 14–21 d
      - **children 3 months–12 years:** 60 mg/kg/d as 3 separate doses for 14–21 d; some clinicians recommend 45 mg/kg/d or 1500 mg/m²/d as 3 separate doses for 14–21 d
      - **children ≥ 12 years:** 30 mg/kg/d as 3 separate doses for 14–21 d
  - **Varicella-zoster in immunocompromised host**
    - IV
      - **infants < 1 year:** 30 mg/kg/d as 3 separate doses for 7–10 d
      - **children 1–12 years:** 1500 mg/m²/d or 30 mg/kg/d as 3 separate doses for 7–10 d
      - **children ≥ 12 years:** 30–45 mg/kg/d as 3 separate doses for 7–10 d
  - **Varicella-zoster-virus in immunocompetent host** (initiate treatment within the first 24 h of rash onset)
    - oral
      - **children ≥ 2 years and ≤ 40 kg:** 80 mg/kg/d as 4 separate doses for 5 d, max. 3200 mg/d
      - **children > 40 kg:** 3200 mg/d as 4 separate doses for 5 d
- **United Kingdom – BNFC:**
  - **Herpes simplex treatment**
    - oral
      - **children 1 month–2 years:** 500 mg/d as 5 separate doses usually for 5 d (longer if new lesions appear during treatment or if healing incomplete); double the dose for immunocompromised patients or if absorption is impaired
      - **children 2–18 years:** 1000 mg/d as 5 separate doses usually for 5 d (longer if new lesions appear during treatment or incomplete healing); double the dose for immunocompromised patients or if absorption is impaired
  - by intravenous infusion
    - **neonate:** 60 mg/kg/d as 3 separate doses for 14 d (21 d if CNS involvement)
    - **children 1–3 months:** 60 mg/kg/d as 3 separate doses for 14 d (21 d if CNS involvement)
    - **children 3 months–12 years:** 750 mg/m²/d as 3 separate doses usually for 5 d; double the dose to 500 mg/m² given every 8 h if CNS involvement (given for up to 21 d) or if immunocompromised
    - **children 12–18 years:** 15 mg/kg/d as 3 separate doses usually for 5 d; double the dose to 30 mg/kg/d as 3 separate doses if CNS involvement (given for up to 21 d) or if immunocompromised

- **Herpes simplex prophylaxis in immunocompromised patients**
  - oral
    - **children 1 month–2 years:** 400–800 mg/d as 4 separate doses
    - **children 2–18 years:** 800–1600 mg/d as 4 separate doses
- **Herpes simplex suppression**
  - oral
    - **children 12–18 years:** 800 mg/d as 2 or 4 separate doses; increase to 1,200 mg/d as 3 separate doses if symptoms recur on standard suppressive therapy or for suppression of genital herpes during late pregnancy (from 36 weeks gestation); stop therapy every 6–12 months to reassess recurrence frequency – consider restarting after two or more recurrences
- **prophylaxis of chickenpox after delivery**
  - by intravenous infusion
    - **neonates:** 30 mg/kg/d as 3 separate doses; continued until serological tests confirm absence of virus
- **chickenpox and herpes zoster infection**
  - oral
    - **children 1 month–2 years:** 800 mg/d as 4 separate doses for 5 d
    - **children 2–6 years:** 1600 mg/d as 4 separate doses for 5 d
    - **children 6–12 years:** 3200 mg/d as 4 separate doses for 5 d
    - **children 12–18 years:** 4000 mg/d as 5 separate doses for 7d
  - by intravenous infusion
    - **neonates:** 30–60 mg/kg/d as 3 separate doses for at least 7 d
    - **children 1–3 months:** 30–60 mg/kg/d as 3 separate doses for at least 7 d
    - **children 3 months–12 years:** 750 mg/m²/d as 3 separate doses usually for 5 d, double the dose for immunocompromised patients
    - **children 12–18 years:** 15 mg/kg/d as 3 separate doses for 5 d, double the dose for immunocompromised patients
    - **note:** to avoid excessive dose in obese patients, parenteral dose should be calculated on the basis of ideal weight for the patient's height
- **attenuation of chickenpox if administration of anti-varicella-zoster immunoglobulin preparation contraindicated**
  - oral
    - **children 1 month–18 years:** 40 mg/kg/d as 4 separate doses for 7 d starting 1 week after exposure

IV comment:

- IV therapy over 60 min, as fast infusion/injection increases risk of kidney damage; ensure adequate hydration

ACTH

(Tetracosactide)

Dosage:
- ▶ 15–30 U/m² IM as a SD (maximum 60 U/d)
- ▶ duration of therapy has not yet been systematically examined in studies.
- ▶ ACTH is usually intramuscularly administered each day over a period of 2–3 weeks, after that the dosage is reduced and/or the administration interval increased over a period of 1–15 weeks to gradually discontinue the medication

Neuropaediatric indications:

- West syndrome, epileptic encephalopathy

Mechanism of action:

- as a glandotropic hormone, the drug controls synthesis and release of corticosteroids

Relevant contraindications:

- acute systemic infection
- do not use in newborns (depot preparation contains benzyl alcohol)

Relevant side effects and interactions:

- hypertonia, cardiomyopathy, nephrocalcinosis, hypokalemia
- anaphylaxis
- frequent hyperglycemia
- irritability
- increased appetite and weight gain
- increased risk of infection due to immunosuppression
- gastrointestinal bleeding
- osteoporosis
- iatrogenic Cushing's syndrome
- enhanced efficacy of cardiac glycosides
- increased potassium excretion due to diuretics
- decreased efficacy of anti-diabetic medications and coumarins
- decreased efficacy in patients on comedication with Rifampicin, barbiturates, Phenytoin
- increased risk of gastrointestinal bleeding in patients on comedication with salicylates
- increase of stereoidal efficacy by Theophylline and Propranolol
- attenuation of cortisol release by Omeprazole and Dexamethasone
- liver damage possible in patients on comedication with anticonvulsants

Approval status:

- explicit approval for West syndrome

Sources:

- Germany – SPC:
  - **West syndrome**
    - IM
      - **Depot ACTH (Tetracosactide):** 40 IE for two weeks in a SD every two days. Tapering after two weeks using Prednisolone (see Prednisolone).
- USA – T:
  - **infantile spasms**
    - IM
      - **children ≤ 2 years:**
      - **short-term treatment:** 5–40 U/d for 1–6 weeks
      - **long-term treatment:** 40–160 U/d for 3–12 months
      - **manufacturer recommendations:** 150 U/m²/d as 2 seperate doses for 2 weeks, followed by a 2-week taper: 30 U/m²/d as a SD in the morning for 3 d, followed by 15 U/m²/d as a SD in the morning for 3 d, followed by 10 U/m²/d as a SD in the morning for 3 d and 10 U/m²/d every other morning for 6 d
      - A prospective, single-blind study found no major differences in efficacy between high-dose long-duration versus low-dose short-duration ACTH therapy. Hypertension, however, occurred more frequently in the high-dose group. Further studies comparing long-term outcomes are needed. Low-dose regimen used in this study: initial dose 20 U/d for 2 weeks; if patient responds, taper off over a 1-week period and then discontinue; if patient does not respond, increase dose to 30 U/d for 4 weeks, then taper off over a 1-week period and discontinue.
      - **children > 2 years:** 40–80 U/dose every 24–72 h
- United Kingdom – BNFC:
  - **infantile spasms**
    - IM
      - **Depot ACTH (Tetracosactide):** 40 U for two weeks in a SD every two days. Tapering after two weeks using Prednisolone (see Prednisolone).

Comments:

- ACTH is partly seen as superior to oral Prednisolone, although the level of evidence is low and ACTH is less well tolerated by patients than Prednisolone.
- high infection-related risk of mortality (up to 5 %); has to be taken into consideration in the risk assessment of the treatment
- the rate of successful treatment outcome ranges between 42 and 87 % in prospective and randomized double-blinded trials
- indisputably the undesirable effects of ACTH depend on dose and dosage regimen and are more pronounced with synthetic ACTH
- dosages published in common paediatric sources may vary

Activated charcoal

Dosage:

▶ 1–2 g/kg/dose (SPC)

Neuropaediatric indications:

- acute oral intoxication and overdosing of medication

Mechanism of action:

- highly effective adsorption onto the extremely large surface area of the suspended microporous charcoal particles (inner surface: 300–2000 m²/g charcoal)

Relevant contraindications:

- intoxication with strong acids or bases

Relevant side effects and interactions:

- constipation, black colouring of the feces
- adsorption of orally administered medication in the gastrointestinal tract

Approval status:

- intoxication and diarrhea in children and adults

Sources:

- Germany – SPC:
  - **acute poisoning or overdosing of pharmaceutical products**
    - oral
      - **children < 4 years:** initially 12.5 g; may be repeated
      - **children ≤ 12 years:** 1 g/kg or 25 g SD
      - **adolescents > 12 years:** 50–100 g, followed by 20 g/dose every 4–6 h for some days
- USA – T:
  - **acute poisoning**
    - oral (single dose charcoal with sorbitol)
      - **infants < 1 year:** not recommended
      - **children 1–12 years:** 1–2 g/kg or 25–50 g or approximately 5–10 times the weight of the ingested poison on a gram-to-gram basis; 1 g adsorbs 100–1000 mg of poison
      - **adolescents:** 30–100 g
    - oral (charcoal in water; a cathartic such as sorbitol should be added in appropriate doses)
      - **infants < 1 year:** 1 g/kg
      - **children 1–12 years:** 1–2 g/kg or 25–50 g
      - **adolescents:** 30–100 g or 1–2 g/kg
    - oral (multiple dose, charcoal in water)
      - **infants < 1 year:** 1 g/kg/dose every 4–6 h
      - **children 1–12 years:** 1–2 g/kg/dose or 15–30 g/dose every 2–6 h
      - **adolescents:** 25–60 g/dose or 1–2 g/kg/dose every 2–6 h

- **note:** doses are repeated until clinical signs and symptoms of toxicity subside and serum drug concentrations have returned to a subtherapeutic range or until absence of bowel movement or intestinal obstruction develops; use only one dose of cathartic daily)
  - **United Kingdom – BNFC:**
    - **reduction of absorption of poisons**
      - oral
        - **neonates:** 1 g/kg
        - **children 1 month–12 years:** 1 g/kg (max. 50 g)
        - **children 12–18 years:** 50 g
    - **active elimination of poisons**
      - oral
        - **neonates:** 1 g/kg/dose every 4 h
        - **children 1 month–12 years:** 1 g/kg/dose (max. 50 g) every 4 h
        - **children 12–18 years:** 50 g/dose every 4 h

Comments:

- not effective in intoxication with organic or inorganic salts (e. g. Lithium, Thallium, cyanide, salts of iron) and solvents (methanol, ethanol, ethylene glycol)

Almotriptan

Dosage:

▶ acute migraine treatment if unsuccessful with NSAID(s): 12.5 mg as SD (off-label)

Neuropaediatric indications:

- reduction of acute migraine symptoms if unsuccessful with NSAID

Mechanism of action:

- acts as selective agonist at the serotonin receptors 5-HT 1B and 5-HT 1D, leading to vasoconstriction ofcerebral blood vessels and decrease of inflammatory mediator release

Relevant contraindications:

- vasospasm, former cerebrovascular problems or TIA
- peripheral vascular diseases, arterial hypertonia, ischaemic heart diseases
- simultaneous intake of MAOIs (contraindication for up to 2 weeks after discontinuation)
- severe liver dysfunction

- use special caution when using in basilar migraine, hemiplegic or ophthalmoplegic migraine, other serious neurological conditions, obesity, hypercholesterolemia, diabetes mellitus, children and young people < 18 years of age (lack of experience), severe renal failure

Relevant side effects and interactions:

- angina pectoris-like complaints, change in blood pressure
- dizziness, fatigue, sedation
- palpitation, tightness in throat and neck
- erythema
- in high doses green-blackish colour change of the blood (sulfhemoglobinemia)
- serotonin syndrome when given a triptan in combination with the SSRI and SNRI classes of antidepressants
  - nausea, vomiting and diarrhea
  - agitation, hallucinations, loss of coordination
  - tachycardia, fluctuation of blood pressure, elevated body temperature
  - overactive reflexes
- no simultaneous intake of Monoamine oxidase inhibitors (MAOIs)
- ergotamines or its derivates increase the risk of coronary artery spasm (administration not earlier than 6 h after Almotriptan or administration of Almotriptan 24 h after ergotamines)

Approval status:

- no approval for patients < 18 years

Sources:

- **Germany – SPC:**
  - **acute treatment of migraine with or without aura in adults**
    - **children and adolescents < 18 years:** no data available for use of Almotriptan in children and adolescents. Therefore, use in patients < 18 years is not recommended.
- **USA – T:**
  - **migraine with or without aura**
    - oral
      - **children 12–17 years:** initially 6.25–12.5 mg as a SD; if headache returns, give a second dose after 2 hours; do not give more than 2 doses (max. daily dose: 25 mg).
- **United Kingdom – BNFC:** –

Amantadine

Dosage:
- 5 mg/kg/d over 2–7 d

Neuropaediatric indications:
- influenza A encephalitis

Mechanism of action:
- interference with the viral M2 protein (proton-selective ion channel) while binding to its transmembrane region and sterically hindering the ion channel
- this consecutively inhibits the uncoating of the viral particle once endocytosis has taken place
- furthermore, Amantadine also acts as an antagonist at the NMDA receptors and is therefore used to treat Parkinson's syndrome

Relevant contraindications:
- severe non-compensated heart failure (stage NYHA IV)
- cardiomyopathy, myocarditis
- first and second degree AV block
- bradycardia < 55/min
- known long QT interval (QT by Bazett > 420 ms) or identifiable U waves or congenital (long) QT syndrome known from family history
- severe ventricular arrhythmias including torsade de pointes
- simultaneous treatment with budipine or other QT-prolonging drugs
- hypokalemia, hypomagnesemia
- p.o.: < 5 years of age
- take special caution when using in children, closed-angle glaucoma, renal insufficiency, episodes of arousal and confusion, acute confusional state/delirium as well as in patients with a medical history of exogenic psychosis, organic brain syndrome or cerebral palsy, risk groups for electrolyte imbalance, cardiovascular diseases, simultaneous treatment with memantine and the combination triamterene/hydrochlorothiazide, pregnancy

Relevant side effects and interactions:
- dizziness, headache, nausea, vomiting, diarrhea
- concentration disorders, depression, euphoria, states of confusion, hallucinations, nightmares
- blurred vision
- sleep disorder
- livedo reticularis, sometimes associated with oedemas in the lower leg and ankle
- epileptic seizures, myoclonus, symptoms of peripheral neuropathy
- voiding dysfunction
- leukopenia, thrombocytopenia
- orthostatic dysregulation
- ventricular tachycardia, ventricular fibrillation, torsade de pointes, QT prolongation, cardiac arrhythmia with tachycardia
- prolongation of QT interval in combination with class IA and III antiarrhythmic agents, antipsychotics, tri- and tetracylic antidepressants, antihistamines, macrolide antibiotics, gyrase inhibitor, azole antifungals, budipine, halofantrine, cotrimoxazole, pentamidine, cisapride, bepridil
- increased side effects of Amantadine in combination with antiparkinsonian drugs
- increase of side effects of anticholinergics
- increased efficacy of Amantadine when simultaneously taken with further NMDA antagonists, indirect centrally operating sympathomimetics, L-dopa
- combination of triamterene and hydrochlorothiazide leads to accumulation of Amantadine in the body

Approval status:
- varies depending on specific product (see SPC)

Sources:
- **Germany – SPC:**
  - **prophylaxis and treatment of influenza A viral infection**
    - Amantadine should be started before or after a known exposure and should be administered for the following 10 d. A 3 months prophylactic treatment is recommended in cases of repeated exposure.
    - usual dose:
      - **children ≥ 5 years:** 100 mg/d as a SD
      - **children ≥ 10 years or > 45 kg:** 200 mg/d as 2 separate doses
- **USA – T:**
  - **Influenza A treatment/prophylaxis**
- Note: Due to issues of resistance, Amantadine is no longer recommended for the prophylactic treatment of influenza A. Please refer to the current ACIP recommendations. The following is based on the manufacturer's labeling and earlier ACIP dosing recommendations:
- **Influenza A treatment**
  - **children 1–9 years:** 5 mg/kg/d as 2 separate doses (range: 4.4–8.8 mg/kg/d); max. 150 mg/d
  - **children ≥ 10 years and < 40 kg:** 5 mg/kg/d as 2 separate doses, i.e. 2 × 2.5 mg/kg
  - **children ≥ 10 years and ≥ 40 kg:** 200 mg/d as 2 separate doses, i.e. 2 × 100 mg
  - **note:** initiate within 24–48 h after onset of symptoms; continue for 24–48 h after symptom resolution (duration of therapy is generally 3–5 d)
- **Influenza A prophylaxis**
  For dose recommendations, refer to influenza A treatment
  Note: continue prophylaxis throughout the peak influenza activity in the community or throughout the entire influenza season in patients who cannot be vaccinated. Development of immunity following vaccination takes ~ 2 weeks; Amantadine therapy should be considered for high-risk patients from the

time of vaccination until immunity has developed. For ages < 9 years receiving influenza vaccine for the first time, Amantadine prophylaxis should continue for 6 weeks (4 weeks after the first vaccine dose and 2 weeks after the second).
- **United Kingdom – BNFC:** is licensed for prophylaxis and treatment of influenza A in children > 10 years, but it is no longer recommended.

4-Aminopyridine

Dosage (off-label):
▶ type 2 episodic ataxia: 3 × 5 mg/d (assess on a case by case basis, no sufficient experience in children)
▶ downbeat/upbeat nystagmus: 3 × 5 mg/d (evaluate on a case by case basis, no sufficient experience in children)

Neuropaediatric indications:
- type 2 episodic ataxia
- downbeat/upbeat nystagmus
- neurogenic pain
- symptomatic myasthenia in the context of malignant diseases (LEMS)

Mechanism of action:
- reversible inhibition of voltage-gated (axoplasmic) potassium channels due to/based on (an) interaction with the alpha-subunit of the channel protein
- leads to increased presynaptic release of acetylcholine (reason for treatment of LEMS)

Relevant contraindications:
- epilepsy

Relevant side effects and interactions:
- in the recommended dose range, no severe side effects are mentioned in the literature
- hypertonia, cardiac arrythmia
- headache, fatigue, paresthesia, sleep disorder
- epileptic seizures
- states of confusion
- opisthotonus, dystonia, tachycardia, tachypnea

Approval status:
- not approved pharmaceutical preparations

Sources:
- **Germany – SPC:** –
- **USA – T:** –

- **United Kingdom – BNFC:** –
- **Uptodate.com:** –

Comment:
- caution with long-term use

Amitriptyline

Dosage:
▶ prophylaxis of migraine and chronic tension-type headache: initially 0.1 mg/kg/d, maximum 0.5–1 (–1.5) mg/kg/d (maximum 75–100 mg/d); increase dose gradually, assess effect after 6–8 weeks; tentative withdrawal after approximately 6 months
▶ sialorrhea: maximum dose 3 × 50 mg/d, increase gradually
▶ neuropathic pain: starting dose 0.2 mg/kg/d p.o. at night; increase after 2–3 weeks to a final dose of 1 mg/kg/d or lowest effective dose
▶ gradually withdraw medication: give for 4 weeks half of the dose used so far, followed by 2 weeks with a quarter of the dose

Neuropaediatric indications:
- chronic headache (tension-type headache) or other chronic pain syndromes particularly in combination with sleep disorder (weak evidence)
- alternative treatment of patients with peripheral neuropathic pain
- migraine prophylaxis (not superior placebo)
- sialorrhea

Mechanism of action:
- non selective monoamine reuptake inhibitor (MRI), tricyclic antidepressant

Relevant contraindications:
- cardiac arrhythmias (therefore ECG before starting treatment)

Relevant side effects and interactions:
- do not administer in combination with MAOIs
- confusion, fatigue, sedation, postural hypotension, syncope
- anticholinergic effects (dry mouth, blurred vision, urinary retention, obstipation)
- exanthema, changes in blood count, cardiac conduction disorder
- ECG before and on a regular basis

Approval status:
- varies depending on the specific product (see SPC)

Sources:
- Germany – SPC:
  - **depressive disorders**
    - **children and adolescents < 18 years:** 25–150 mg or up to max. 4–5 mg/kg/d. But the risk-benefit-assessment should be considered carefully.
  - **chronic pain**
    - no published paediatric dosage
- USA – T:
  - **chronic pain management**
    - oral
      - initial dose 0.1 mg/kg at bedtime, may be increased as tolerated over 2–3 weeks to 0.5–2 mg/kg at bedtime
  - **depressive disorders**
    - oral
      - **children in study (n = 9, age 9–12 years):** initially 1 mg/kg/d as 3 separate doses; maintenance dose 1.5 mg/kg/d; clinically, doses up to 3 mg/kg/d (5 mg/kg/d if monitored closely) have been proposed
      - **note:** Not FDA approved for use in paediatric patients; controlled clinical trials **did not show the drug to be superior to placebo.**
      - **adolescents:** initially 25–50 mg/d; may be divided into several doses; increase gradually to 100 mg/d divided into several doses; max. dose 200 mg/d
  - **migraine prophylaxis**
    - oral
      - **note:** only a few studies available, did not show the drug to be superior to placebo
      - **children (n = 24; mean age 8 years, range: 6–12 years):** use of increasing doses over 5 d to reach a final dose of 1.5 mg/kg/d; was effective in 19 of 24 patients, but 5 children dropped out of the trial due to adverse effects (Sorge 1982)
      - **children (n = 192, mean age 12 ± 3, > 3 headaches/month):** initially 0.25 mg/kg/d given before bedtime; doses were increased every 2 weeks by 0.25 mg/kg/d to a final dose of 1 mg/kg/d
      - **note:** the mean number and duration of headaches significantly decreased, minimal adverse effects; mean final dose 0.99 ± 0.23 mg/kg, range 0.16–1.7 mg/kg/d; ECGs were obtained on children receiving > 1 mg/kg/d or in those experiencing cardiac side effects
- United Kingdom – BNFC:
  - **depression**
    - oral
      - **children 16–18 years:** 30–75 mg/d as 3 separate doses (alternatively, the total daily dose may be given as a SD at bedtime), increased gradually as necessary to 150–200 mg/d
  - **neuropathic pain**
    - oral
      - **children 2–12 years:** initially 200–500 mcg/kg/d as a SD (max. 10 mg) at night, increased if necessary; max. 2 mg/kg/d as 2 separate doses on specialist advice
      - **children 12–18 years:** initially 10 mg/d as a SD at night, increased gradually if necessary to the usual dose of 75 mg/d as a SD at night; higher doses on specialist advice

Comment:
- review duration of therapy frequently and critically!
- good option for combination with Carbamazepine for treatment of neuropathic pain

Amphotericin B

Dosage (liposomal):
- ▶ meningoencephalitis caused by Cryptococcus or Aspergillus: 1–1.5 mg/kg/d
- ▶ if Candida meningoencephalitis, combination therapy with Flucytosine 100–150 mg/kg/d + Amphotericin B 1–1.5 mg/kg/d

Neuropaediatric indications:
- meningoencephalitis caused by Cryptococcus, Aspergillus, Candida

Mechanism of action:
- through interaction with ergosterol in the fungal cell membrane, a channel is formed that increases potassium permeability of the membrane which leads to potassium influx and cell death
  - effective against nearly all fungal infections in humans such as trichomonas, leishmania, trypanosoma, entamoeba
- no effect against actinomyces and bacteria

Relevant contraindications:
- use special caution in liver or renal dysfunction and in comedication with anti-neoplastic agents

Relevant side effects and interactions:
- fever with chills, circulatory disorder
- exanthema, flush
- headache, nausea, vomiting, diarrhea
- severe myalgia and arthralgia
- renal dysfunction
- leukopenia, anemia, thrombopenia, hypokalemia/hyperkalemia
- phlebitis
- liver dysfunction, icterus
- angiooedema, paresthesia, impaired vision
- tinnitus, loss of hearing
- gastrointestinal bleeding
- seizures
- pulmonary oedema, difficulty breathing up to acute dyspnea

- acute liver, renal or heart failure
- when giving IV infusion avoid further agents with nephrotoxic activity
- concurrent treatment with Foscarnet or Ganciclovir can increase nephrotoxic activity and change in blood cell count
- intensified activity of cardiac glycosides, muscle relaxants and antiarrhythmic agents via hypokalemia
- concurrent treatment with diuretics and glucocorticoids can increase hypokalemia

Approval status:
- varies depending on specific product (see SPC)

Sources:
- **Germany – SPC:**
- **Preparation conventional Amphotericin B; AmBisome®**
    - **treatment of severe systemic and central nervous system infections caused by susceptible fungi such as Candida species, Histoplasma capsulatum, Cryptococcus neoformans, Aspergillus species, Blastomyces dermatitidis, Torulopsis glabrata, and Coccidioides immitis**
    - **treatment of severe systemic and central nervous system infections caused by susceptible fungi**
        - IV conventional Amphotericin B
            - **children:** total dose of 1–2 mg (i.e. < 0.25 mg/kg) is sufficient. Considering adverse effects, gradual titration to 0.25 mg/kg may be necessary.
        - IV liposomal Amphotericin B
            - **children:** initially 1.0 mg of AmBisome/kg, increase gradually to 3.0 mg/kg. A total dose of 1–3 g AmBisome® over 3–4 weeks is recommended; adjust according to response.
    - The use of Amphotericin B in children < 1 month of age is not recommended.
- **USA – T:**
- **Preparation conventional Amphotericin B (Fungizone®)**
    - **note:** medication errors, leading to adverse events including deaths, have resulted from confusion between lipid-based forms of Amphotericin and conventional Amphotericin B for injection; conventional Amphotericin B for injection doses should not exceed 1.5 mg/kg/d
- **Severe systemic infections**
    - IV
        - **neonates:** initially 0.5 mg/kg/d as a SD. The daily dose can then be gradually increased, usually in daily increments of 0.25 mg/kg until the desired daily dose is reached (max. dose: 1.5 mg/kg/d); in critically ill patients, more rapid dosage acceleration (up to daily increments of 0.5 mg/kg) may be warranted.
        - maintenance dose: 0.25–1 mg/kg/d as a SD; infuse over 2–6 h; rapidly progressing disease may require short-term use of doses up to 1.5 mg/kg/d; once therapy has been established, Amphotericin B can be administered on every other day at 1–1.5 mg/kg
        - **note:** maintaining a sodium intake of > 4 milliequivalent/kg/d in premature neonates may reduce Amphotericin B-associated nephrotoxicity
        - **infants and children**
        - trial dose: 0.1 mg/kg/dose, max. 1 mg; infuse over 20–60 min; an alternative method to the 0.1 mg/kg trial dose is an initiate therapy with 0.25 mg/kg Amphotericin administered over 6 h; frequent

observation of the patient and assessment of vital signs during the first several hours of the infusion is recommended.
- if the 0.1 mg/kg trial dose is tolerated without any serious adverse effects, a therapeutic dose of 0.4 mg/kg can be given the same day as the trial dose
- maintenance dose: 0.25–1 mg/kg/d as a SD, infuse over 2–6 h; rapidly progressing disease may require short-term use of doses to 1.5 mg/kg/d; once therapy has been established, Amphotericin B can be administered on every other day at 1–1.5 mg/kg
- **HIV-infected infants and children with invasive candidiasis**
    - IV
        - consider possible comedication with oral Flucytosine 100–150 mg/kg/d as 4 separate doses in addition to Amphotericin B therapy
- **cryptococcal meningitis in HIV-infected infants and children**
    - IV
        - consider comedication with oral Flucytosine 100 mg/kg/d as 4 separate doses in addition to Amphotericin B therapy
        - intrathecal, intraventricular, intracisternal: 25–100 mcg every 48–72 h, increase to 500 mcg as tolerated
- **Preparation liposomal Amphotericin B (AmBisome®)**
- **systemic fungal infections**
    - IV
        - **neonates:** 3–7 mg/kg/d as a SD has been used in a number of trials; in one trial treatment was initiated with 1 mg/kg/d and then increased by 1 mg/kg every day to a maximum of 5 mg/kg/d as a SD in 40 preterm and four term neonates for 1–7 weeks.
        - **infants ≥ 1 year and children:** empiric therapy with 3 mg/kg/d as a SD
- **systemic fungal infections**
    - IV
        - 3–5 mg/kg/d as a SD; doses as high as 10 mg/kg/d have been used in patients with confirmed Aspergillus infection; for HIV-infected patients with invasive candidiasis consider comedication with oral Flucytosine
- **cryptococcal meningitis in HIV-infected patients**
    - IV
        - 6 mg/kg/d as a SD (consider comedication with oral Flucytosine)
- **visceral leishmaniasis**
    - IV
        - **immunocompetent patients:** 3 mg/kg/d as a SD on days 1–5, day 14 and 21. The treatment course may be repeated in patients who did not respond with satisfactory parasite clearance.
        - **immunocompromised patients:** 4 mg/kg/d as a SD on days 1–5, day 10, 17, 24, 31, and 38
- **United Kingdom – BNFC:**
- **Preparation conventional Amphotericin B (Fungizone®)**
- **systemic fungal infection**
    - IV
        - **neonates:** 1 mg/kg/d as a SD, increased if necessary to 1.5 mg/kg/d; after 7 days, the dose may be reduced to 1–1.5 mg/kg given every other day

- **children 1 month–18 years:** initial trial with 100 mcg/kg (max. 1 mg) included as a part of 250 mcg/kg/d, increased over 2–4 d, if tolerated up to 1 mg/kg/d; in severe infection max. 1.5 mg/kg/d given every or every other day
- **note:** prolonged treatment usually necessary; if interrupted for longer than 7 d, recommence at 250 mcg/kg/d and increase gradually
- Preparation liposomal Amphotericin B (AmBisome®)
- Severe systemic or deep mycoses where toxicity (particularly nephrotoxicity) precludes use of conventional Amphotericin
  - IV
    - **neonates and children 1 month–18 years:** 100 mcg/kg as a SD (initial test dose) as a part of first SD of 1 mg/kg/d, increased if necessary to 3 mg/kg/d as a SD (increasing of the dose in steps of additional 1 mg/kg/d); max. 5 mg/kg/d as a SD
- Suspected or proven infection in febrile neutropenic patients unresponsive to broad-spectrum antibiotics
  - IV
    - **children 1 month–18 years:** initial test dose of 100 mcg/kg/d (max. 1 mg/kg/d) SD, followed by 3 mg/kg/d as a SD until free of fever three days in row; max. duration of treatment 42 d; max. 5 mg/kg/d as a SD

Comments:
- does not enter the circulatory system when administered orally, as it can not be absorbed and therefore only acts in the mouth and throat region as well as the gastrointestinal tract
- Amphotericin B-containing solutions should never be diluted with saline solutions

Ampicillin

Dosage:
▶ 200 mg/kg/d as 3 separate doses

Neuropaediatric indications:
- meningitis 0–6 weeks of life

Mechanism of action:
- β-lactam antibiotic
- bacteriostatic, because Ampicillin inhibits the cross-linking of peptidoglycans by opening and binding the β-lactam ring structure, thus preventing formation of new cell layers
- compared to penicillin G wider broad-spectrum efficacy, especially on Gram-negative bacteria
- effective against: streptococci, enterococci, Haemophilus species, Neisseria meningitidis, Neisseria gonorrhoeae, Proteus mirabilis, Listeria monocytogenes, corynebacteria, Clostridium, Bacillus anthracis, Erisypelothrix rusiopathiae, Salmonella, Shigella, Escherichia coli
- not effective against penicillinase-producing bacteria (e.g. most staphylococci), Klebsiella, Pseudomonas aeruginosa, Enterobacter, Serratia, Yersinia

Relevant contraindications:
- penicillin hypersensitivity
- use special caution when treating concomitant viral infections, especially infectious mononucleosis and lymphatic leukemia (increased risk of exanthema)

Relevant side effects and interactions:
- Ampicillin-related exanthema, urticaria, vasculitis, laryngeal oedema
- temporary change of taste, dry mouth
- nausea, vomiting, meteorism, diarrhea, pseudomembranous colitis
- leukopenia, thrombopenia, agranulocytosis
- interstitial nephritis
- IV: CNS agitation conditions, myoclonia, seizures, phlebitis
- prolonged bleeding and prothrombin time
- bleeding complications in combination with anticoagulants, inhibitors of thrombocyte aggregation
- decreased efficacy of oral contraceptives

Approval status:
- depends on the specific product (see SPC)

Sources:
- Germany – SPC:
  - meningitis
    - **children < 6 years:** 200–400 mg Ampicillin/kg/d; recommended dosing intervals:
      - twice daily; every 12 h
      - 3 times daily; every 8 h
      - 4 times daily; every 6 h
- USA – T:
  - meningitis
    - IM and IV
      - neonates
        - **postnatal ≤ 7 d, ≤ 2000 g:** 100 mg/kg/d as 2 separate doses given in 12-h intervals; **> 2000 g:** 150 mg/kg/d as 2 separate doses given in 8-h intervals; group B streptococcal meningitis: 200 mg/kg/d as 3 separate doses given in 8-h intervals
        - **postnatal > 7 d: < 1200 g:** 100 mg/kg/d as 2 separate doses given in 12-h intervals, i.e. 50 mg/kg per injection; **1200–2000 g:** 150 mg/kg/d as 3 separate doses given in 8-h intervals; **> 2000 g:** 200 mg/kg/d as 4 separate doses given in 6-h intervals; group B streptococcal meningitis: 300 mg/kg/d as 4 separate doses given in 6-h intervals
      - **children:** 200–400 mg/kg/d as 4 separate doses given in 6-h intervals, max. 12 g/d

- **United Kingdom – BNFC:**
  - **listerial meningitis, group B streptococcal infection**
    - IV
      - **neonates < 7 d:** 200 mg/kg/d as 2 separate doses
      - **neonates 7–21 d:** 300 mg/kg/d as 3 separate doses
      - **neonates 21–28 d:** 400 mg/kg/d as 4 separate doses
      - **children 1 month–18 years:** 50 mg/kg every 4–6 h (max. 2 g every 4 h)

Comment:

- broad-spectrum efficacy is almost identical to that of orally applicable amoxicillin

Atomoxetine

Dosage (as stated in SPC):

▶ no immediate effect, it develops over some weeks
▶ initial dose and escalation regimen: 500 mcg/kg/d once daily for 7 d (children > 6 years); increase in intervals of 4–6 weeks
▶ maintenance dose: 1.2 mg/kg/d as SD or 2 separate doses
▶ maximum dose: 1.8 mg/kg/d

Neuropaediatric indications:

- hyperkinetic disorders

Mechanism of action:

- selective inhibition of the presynaptic noradrenaline transport

Relevant contraindications:

- MAOI (allow at least 2 weeks of discontinuation)
- angle closure glaucoma
- < 6 years

Relevant side effects and interactions:

- weight loss, dry mouth, nausea, abdominal pain, vomiting
- drowsiness, irritability, emotional lability, vertigo, somnolence
- dermatitis, pruritus, rash
- rare liver function disorders

Approval status:

- ADHD from 6 years on

Sources:

- **Germany – SPC:**
- **Preparation Strattera®**
- **ADHD**
  - oral:
    - **children ≥ 6 years and adolescents ≤ 70 kg:** initial dose 0.5 mg/kg/d; increase after 7 d to 1.2 mg/kg/d (adjust according to response and patient's body weight). Note: Doses > 1.2 mg/kg/d have not been shown to provide any additional benefit.
    - **children ≥ 6 years and adolescents > 70 kg:** initial dose 40 mg/d; increase after 7 d to 80 mg/d (adjust according to response); consider increasing to 100 mg/d if required. Doses > 80 mg have not been shown to provide any additional benefit.
- **USA – T:**
  - **ADHD**
    - oral
      - **children ≥ 6 years and adolescents ≤ 70 kg:** initial dose 0.5 mg/kg/d; increase after a minimum of 3 d to approximately 1.2 mg/kg/d; may be administered once daily in the morning or divided into two doses and administered in the morning and late afternoon/early evening. Max. 1.4 mg/kg/d but not exceeding a total of 100 mg/d
      - **note:** doses > 1.2 mg/kg/d have not been shown to provide any additional benefit
      - In patients receiving strong CYP2D6 inhibitors (e. g. paroxetine, Fluoxetine, quinidine) or patients known to be poor CYP2D6 metabolizers, maintain the above listed initial dose for 4 weeks; increase dose to 1.2 mg/kg/d only if clinically needed and if the initial dose is well tolerated; do not exceed 1.2 mg/kg/d
      - **children ≥ 6 years and adolescents > 70 kg:** initial dose 40 mg/d; increase after a minimum of 3 d to approximately 80 mg/d; may be administered once daily in the morning or divided into two doses and administered in the morning and late afternoon/early evening. May be increased to 100 mg/d for 2–4 additional weeks if required.
      - **note:** In patients receiving strong CYP2D6 inhibitors (e. g. paroxetine, Fluoxetine, quinidine) or patients known to be poor CYP2D6 metabolizers, maintain the above listed initial dose for 4 weeks; increase dose to 80 mg/d only if clinically needed and if the initial dose is well tolerated; do not exceed 80 mg/d.
- **United Kingdom – BNFC:**
  - **attention deficit hyperactivity disorder**
    - oral
      - **children ≥ 6 years (body-weight ≤ 70 kg):** initial dose 0.5 mg/kg/d for 7 d, increased according to response; usual maintenance dose is 1.2 mg/kg/d, but this may be increased to 1.8 mg/kg/d (max. 120 mg/d) under specialist supervision
      - **children ≥ 6 years (body-weight > 70 kg):** initial dose 40 mg/d for 7 d, increased according to response; usual maintenance dose is 80 mg/d, but this may be increased to max. 120 mg/d under specialist supervision
      - **note:** the total daily dose may be given either as a single dose in the morning or in 2 separate doses with the last dose no later than early evening

Comments:
- use special caution for patients with cardiovascular or hepatic diseases
- onset of effect after 4–6 weeks
- may provoke epileptic seizures in patients affected with epilepsy (but is not contraindicated)
- recommended: monitor pulse and blood pressure
- interindividual differences in bioavailability

Atropine

Dosage:
- ▶ prophylaxis of reflectory laryngeal spasm in gastric lavage: 0.5 mg Atropine
- ▶ organophosphate poisoning: initial dose 0.05 mg/kg IV, followed by 0.02–0.05 mg/kg every 15–60 min until achieving Atropine effect (continue for 12–24 h)
- ▶ sialorrhea: 0.5 mg up to 3 mg/d as 3 separate doses

Neuropaediatric indications:
- prophylaxis of reflectory laryngeal spasm in gastric lavage
- intoxication with organic phosphoric acid esters and phosphonic acid esters: paraoxon, parathion (E605), malathion, tabun, soman, VX-gas
- sialorrhea

Mechanism of action:
- vagolytic drug
- competitive inhibition of the muscarinergic acetylcholine receptors (M_1-, M_2-, and M_3-receptors) at the postsynaptic membrane

Relevant contraindications:
- angle-closure glaucoma
- voiding dysfunction with development of post-void residual urine
- mechanic stenosis in the gastrointestinal tract
- tachyarrhythmia
- megacolon
- acute pulmonary oedema

Relevant side effects and interactions:
- tachycardia, mydriasis, accommodation impairment, dry red skin, dry mouth, hypotension, micturition problems
- disorders of muscle coordination
- glaucoma
- agitation, restlessness, illusions, delirium
- increased anticholinergic effect in combination with Amantadine, chinidin, tri- and tetracyclic antidepressants, neuroleptics
- mutually decreased efficacy on gastrointestinal motility in combination with dopamine antagonists

Approval status:
- depends on the specific product (see SPC)

Sources:
- Germany – SPC:
  - pre-anesthetic
    - children:
      - IV 0.01 mg/kg (max. 0.5 mg) 3–5 min preoperatively
      - IM 0.02 mg/kg (max. 0.5 mg) 30–60 min preoperatively
- USA – T:
  - neonates, infants, children
    - oral, IM, IV, or SC
      - **neonates < 5 kg:** a dose of 0.02 mg/kg 30–60 min preoperatively, then every 4–6 h as needed; there is no documented minimum dosage in this age group
      - **infants < 5 kg:** a dose of 0.02 mg/kg 30–60 min preoperatively, then every 4–6 h as needed; there is no documented minimum dosage in this age group
      - **infants and children > 5 kg:** a dose of 0.01–0.02 mg/kg not exceeding 0.4 mg, 30–60 min preoperatively; minimum dose 0.1 mg
  - organophosphate or carbamate poisoning:
    - IV
      - 0.02–0.05 mg/kg every 10–20 min until Atropine effect is observed then every 1–4 h for at least 24 h
    - IM (AtroPen®)
      - **neonates:** 0.25 mg; mild symptoms, 1 injection as soon as exposure is known or suspected; severe symptoms, 2 additional injections (a total of 3) given in rapid succession 10 min after the first injection. If patient is unconscious, immediately administer 3 AtroPen® injections into the patient's midlateral thigh in rapid succession.
      - **infants 1–6 months (< 6.8 kg):** 0.25 mg
      - **infants 6 months–4 years (6.8–18 kg):** 0.5 mg
      - **children 4–10 years (18–41 kg):** 1 mg
      - **children > 10 years (> 41 kg):** 2 mg
- United Kingdom – BNFC:
  - premedication
    - oral (1–2 h before inducing anesthesia)
      - **neonates:** 0.02–0.04 mg/kg
      - **children 1 month–18 years:** 0.02–0.04 mg/kg (max. 0.9 mg)
    - SC or IM injection (30–60 min before inducing anesthesia)
      - **neonates:** 0.01 mg/kg
      - **children 1 month–12 years:** 0.01–0.03 mg/kg (min. 0.1 mg, max. 0.6 mg)
      - **children 12–18 years:** 0.3–0.6 mg

- IV injection immediately before inducing anesthesia
  - **neonates:**0.01 mg/kg
  - **children 1 month-12 years:** 0.02 mg/kg (min. 0.1 mg, max. 0.6 mg)
  - **children 12–18 years:** 0.3–0.6 mg

Comment:

- small therapeutic range
- use especially cautious dosing in children < 12 years because children are particularly sensitive to other toxic effects of Atropine sulfate

Azathioprine

Dosage:

- ▸ MS: 1–3 mg/kg/d (dose adjustments according to lymphocyte counts)
- ▸ Takayasu's arthritis: 2–3 mg/kg/d
- ▸ myositis: start with 1.5–2 mg/kg/d; sometimes 3 mg/kg/d are required for sufficient immunosuppression
- ▸ autoimmune myasthenia: 1–3 mg/kg/d (dose adjustments according to lymphocyte counts)

Neuropaediatric indications:

- immunomodulating therapy in MS and contraindications for Interferon beta and Glatiramer acetate
- immunosuppressive therapy in sarcoidosis, Wegener's granulomatosis, Takayasu's arthritis, SLE, myasthenia and therapy-resistant severe myositis

Mechanism of action:

- the prodrug is converted to 6-mercaptopurine by xanthine oxidase
- as an atypical nucleoside, 6-mercaptopurine interferes with DNA-/RNA-synthesis

Relevant contraindications:

- pregnancy
- severe infections
- severe liver disorder or bone marrow dysfunction
- pancreatitis
- vaccination with viable attenuated vaccines (especially BCG, smallpox, yellow fever)
- use special caution in patients with thiopurine methyl transferase deficiency, Lesch-Nyhan syndrome

Relevant side effects and interactions:

- blood count changes, hair loss, increased risk of infection

- photosensitization
- nausea, vomiting, diarrhea, weight loss
- fever, arthralgia
- leukopenia, thrombocytopenia, anemia, agranulocytosis
- liver function disorder
- pancreatitis
- combination with allopurinol (xanthine oxidase inhibitor, interferes with the breakdown of Azathioprine) enhances the efficacy and the side effects of Azathioprine; therefore, dose reduction of Azathioprine
- no vaccination with "live" vaccines during therapy; "dead" vaccines can lose their efficacy
- decreased efficacy of Warfarin

Approval status:

- depends on the specific product (see SPC)

Sources:

- **Germany – SPC:**
  - oral
    - **children:** depending on the immunosuppressive regimen, the initial dose is up to 5 mg/kg/d; maintenance dose 1–4 mg/kg/d; adjust to clinical and haematological response
  - **juvenile idiopathic arthritis**
    - **children:** no data available regarding efficacy and safety in patients < 18 years of age
  - **other indications**
    - **children:** initially 1–3 mg/kg/d, adjust to clinical and haematological response. For treatment of chronic hepatitis, a range of 1–1.5 mg/kg/d is recommended. Reduce to lowest effective dose. If no improvement of condition is achieved after 3–6 months of treatment, consider stopping treatment. Usual maintenance dose 1–3 mg/kg/d
- **USA – T:**
  - **note:** Patients with intermediated TPMT (Thiopurinmethyltransferase) activity may be at risk for increased myelosuppression; those with low or absent TPMT activity are at risk for developing severe myelotoxicity. Dosage reductions are recommended for patients with reduced TPMT activity.
  - **lupus nephritis**
    - oral
      - **children:** 2–3 mg/kg/d as a SD
- **United Kingdom – BNFC:**
  - **systemic lupus erythematosus, vasculitis, auto-immune conditions (usually when corticosteroid therapy alone has proven inadequate)**
    - oral
      - **children 1 month-18 years:** initially 1 mg/kg/d, adjusted according to response to max. 3 mg/kg/d (consider withdrawal if no improvement within 3 months)

Comments:

- solar radiation, solarium and phototherapy have to be avoided

Baclofen

Dosage:
- ▶ spasmolysis as pain therapy: 10–40 mg/d as 3 separate doses
- ▶ generalized spasticity/dystonia in cerebral palsy:
  - p.o.: initially 0.5 mg/kg/d as 3 separate doses, increase weekly by 0.5 mg/kg/d; maintenance dose 2–5 mg/kg/d as 3–4 separate doses
  - intrathecal: 150–2000 mcg/d via implanted pumps/catheter system, telemetric management of electronic pumps
- ▶ heredodegenerative or secondary dystonia, p.o.: 0.75 mg/kg/d as 3 separate doses, increase up to 2(–5) mg/kg/d as 3 separate doses
- ▶ status dystonicus after relapse of benzodiazepines: intrathecal application (see above)

Neuropaediatric indications:
- generalized spasticity (e.g. in cerebral palsy)
- heredodegenerative or secondary dystonia (e.g. in cerebral palsy)
- therapy-resistant dystonic status

Mechanism of action:
- specific agonist for $GABA_B$-receptor

Relevant contraindications:
- peptic ulcers, myasthenia gravis

Relevant side effects and interactions:
- gastrointestinal disorders
- lethargy, sedation and bulbar symptoms often limit drug administration
- proconvulsive effect

Approval status:
- depends on the specific product (see SPC)

Sources:
- **Germany – SPC:**
  - **alleviation of signs and symptoms of spasticity resulting from multiple sclerosis, particularly for the relief of flexor spasms and concomitant pain, clonus, and muscular rigidity**
  - oral
    - **children (> 33 kg):** initial daily dose approximately 0.3 mg/kg/d as 2–4 separate doses. Titrate dose gradually over weekly intervals until obtaining optimum response.
    - maintenance dose: 0.75–2 mg/kg; children < 8 years max. 40 mg/d; children > 8 years max. 60 mg/d
    - Lioresal® is not recommended for children weighing < 33 kg
- **USA – T:**
  - **treatment of cerebral spasticity, reversible spasticity associated with MS or spinal cord lesions**
    - oral
      - **children < 2 years:** 10–20 mg/d as 3 separate doses; titrate dose every 3 days in increments of 5–15 mg/d to max. 40 mg/d
      - **children 2–7 years:** 20–30 mg/d as 3 separate doses; titrate dose every 3 days in increments of 5–15 mg/d to max. 60 mg/d
      - **children ≥ 8 years:** 30–40 mg/d as 3 separate doses; titrate dose to max. 120 mg/d
      - **note:** Lubsch (et al.) observed that higher daily dosages of Baclofen were needed with increasing time from onset of injury, increasing age, and number of concomitant antispasticity medications. Each of these variables may represent drug tolerance or progressive spasticity. Lubsch (et al.) used doses as high as 200 mg/d.
    - intrathecal
      - **children:**
      - trial dose: 50 mcg, observe for 4–8 h; very small children may receive 25 mcg; if ineffective, give a second dose increased by 50 % (e.g. 75 mcg) may be repeated in 24 h; if still suboptimal, a third dose increased by 33 % (e.g. 100 mcg) may be repeated after 24 h; patients who do not respond to intrathecally administered 100 mcg should not be considered for continuous chronic administration via implanted pump
      - maintenance dose: continuous infusion, initial dose depends on the effective trial dose and its administration rate
      - if the trial dose was administered for > 8 h: daily maintenance dose = effective screening dose
      - if the trial dose was administered for < 8 h: daily maintenance dose = 2 × effective screening dose
      - **note:** further adjustments of infusion rate may be done every 24 h as needed; for spinal cord-related spasticity, increase in 10 % to 30 % increments/24 h; for spasticity of cerebral origin, increase in 5 % to 10 % increments/24 h
    - average daily dose
      - **children ≤ 12 years:** 100–300 mcg/d (4.2–12.5 mcg/h); doses as high as 1000 mcg/d have been used
      - **children > 12 years:** 300–800 mcg/d (12.5–33 mcg/h); doses as high as 2000 mcg/d have been used
- **United Kingdom – BNFC:**
  - **chronic severe spasticity of voluntary muscle**
    - oral
      - **children 1–2 years:** initially 0.3 mg/kg/d as 4 separate doses, increased gradually to the usual maintenance dose of 0.75–2 mg/kg/d (max. 40 mg) as several separate doses (or 10–20 mg/d as several separate doses); review treatment if no benefit is apparent within weeks
      - **children 2–6 years:** initially 0.3 mg/kg/d as 4 separate doses, increased gradually to the usual maintenance dose of 0.75–2 mg/kg/d (max. 40 mg) as several separate doses (or 20–30 mg/d as several separate doses); review treatment if no benefit is apparent within weeks

- **children 6–8 years:** initially 0.3 mg/kg/d as 4 separate doses, increased gradually to the usual maintenance dose of 0.75–2 mg/kg/d (max. 40 mg) as several separate doses (or 30–40 mg/d as several separate doses); review treatment if no benefit is apparent within weeks
  - **children 8–10 years:** initially 0.3 mg/kg/d as 4 separate doses, increased gradually to the usual maintenance dose of 0.75–2 mg/kg/d (max. 60 mg) as several separate doses; review treatment if no benefit is apparent within weeks
  - **children 10–18 years:** initially 15 mg/d as 3 separate doses increased gradually; usual maintenance dose up to 60 mg/d as several separate doses (max. 100 mg/d); review treatment if no benefit is apparent within weeks
- **severe chronic spasticity of cerebral origin unresponsive to oral antispastic drugs (or oral therapy not tolerated), as alternative to ablative neurosurgical procedures–requires specialist skills**
  - intrathecal injection
    - **children 4–18 years:** initial trial dose 0.025 mg over at least 1 min via catheter or lumbar puncture. To determine appropriate dose, increase in 0.025-mg steps (not more than once every 24 h) to max. 0.1 mg. This is followed by a dose titration phase, usually involving an infusion pump (implanted into chest wall or abdominal wall tissues), to establish the maintenance dose (ranging from 0.024 mg/d to 1.2 mg/d for **children under 12 years** and up to 1.4 mg/d for those **over 12 years**), retaining some spasticity to avoid muscle paralysis.

Comments:

- avoid sudden discontinuation; note: DD withdrawal/overdosing
- for the treatment of spasticity of cerebral origin, continuous intrathecal infusion via implanted pump is possible (dose 100–1200 mcg/24 h)

Benzatropine

Dosage (off-label):

▶ children > 3 years: 20–100 mcg/kg (max. 2 mg) IV/IM, followed by p.o. (20 mcg/kg max. 1 mg) if necessary
▶ max. 6 mg/d or up to dilatation of pupils

Neuropaediatric indications:

- emergency treatment of acute dystonia

Mechanism of action:

- anticholinergic agent

Relevant contraindications:

- colitis ulcerosa, ileus, megacolon, pyloric stenosis
- angle closure glaucoma
- pulmonary oedema

- tachyarrhythmia
- severe cerebral palsy

Relevant side effects and interactions:

- interactions with other anticholinergic agents
- tachycardia
- constipation, nausea, dermal changes, loss of appetite, weight loss, vomiting, ileus, dry mouth
- urinary retention
- blurred vision, mydriasis
- psychic changes, slow reactions
- allergic reactions
- disorders of sweat production

Approval status:

- not approved for use in children

Sources:

- **Germany – SPC:** –
- **USA – T:** –
- **United Kingdom – BNFC:** –
- **Uptodate.com:**
- **Drug-induced extrapyramidal reaction**
  - oral, IM, IV
    - **children > 3 years:** 0.02–0.05 mg/kg/dose 1–2 times/d; use in children < 3 years should be reserved for life-threatening emergencies

Comment:

- parenteral administration enables the treatment of severe dystonia and status dystonicus

Benzhexol

(See Trihexyphenidyl)

Benzylpenicillin

(= Penicillin G)

> **Dosage:**
> ▸ chorea minor and PANDAS:
> - acute: Penicillin 100 000 U/kg/d, max. 1.2 Mio U/d for 10 d p.o.
> - prophylactic: Penicillin 200 000 U/d p.o.
> - duration of treatment: months to years
> ▸ neuroborreliosis: 200 000–400 000 U/kg/d as 4 separate doses; max. 12 Mio. U/d; duration: 2 weeks

Neuropaediatric indications:
- brief infusion in severe infections caused by sensitive pathogens (syphilis, Lyme borreliosis, gangrene, tetanus, diphtheria)
- chorea minor
- PANDAS

Mechanism of action:
- β-lactam antibiotic, is not produced synthetically but is obtained from mold cultures (Penicillium notatum) by a fermentation process
- penicillinase sensible
- broad spectrum efficacy:
  - gram-positive bacteria
  - gram-negative cocci
  - gram-negative anaerobic rod cells

Relevant contraindications:
- penicillin hypersensitivity (cross allergy with other β-lactam antibiotics are possible)
- careful use: treatment of concomitant infections of viral origin, especially infectious mononucleosis and lymphatic leukemia (increased risk of exanthema)

Relevant side effects and interactions:
- IV administration: CNS agitation conditions, myoclonia, seizures (in very high dosages)
- IM administration: tumescences and pain at the injection site
- nausea, vomiting, meteorism, diarrhea

Approval status:
- depends on the specific product (see SPC)

Sources:
- Germany – SPC:
  - treatment of bacterial infections caused by susceptible, usually Gram-positive, organisms
    - IM, IV
      - **children > 12 years:** 1–5 Mio. U/d (600–3000 mg Benzylpenicillin sodium) as 4–6 separate doses; for severe infections (i.e. meningitis): 20–60 Mio. U/d (12 000–36 000 mg Benzylpenicillin sodium)
      - **children 1–12 years:** 0.05–0.5 Mio. U (30–300 mg Benzylpenicillin sodium)/kg/d as 4–6 separate doses
      - **infants < 1 year:** 0.05–1.0 Mio. U (30–600 mg Benzylpenicillin sodium)/kg/d as 3–4 separate doses
      - CAUTION: fast infusion may trigger cerebral seizures
      - **neonates:** 0.05–0.1 (–0.5) Mio. U (30–60(–300) mg Benzylpenicillin sodium)/kg/d as 2 separate doses
    - **preterms and neonates:** do not fall below 12 h dosing intervals
- USA – T:
  - treatment of meningitis
    - IM, IV
      - neonates
      - **postnatal ≤ 7 d, ≤ 2000 g body weight:** 100 000 U/kg/d as 2 separate doses; **> 2000 g body weight:** 150 000 U/kg/d as 3 separate doses; group B streptococcal meningitis: 250 000–450 000 U/kg/d as 3 separate doses
      - **postnatal > 7 d, < 1200 g body weight:** 100 000 U/kg/d as 2 separate doses; **1200–2000 g body weight:** 150 000 U/kg/d as 3 separate doses; **> 2000 g body weight:** 200 000 U/kg/d as 4 separate doses; group B streptococcal meningitis: 450 000 U/kg/d as 4 separate doses
  - severe infections
    - IM, IV
      - **infants > 1 month and children:** 250 000–400 000 U/kg/d as separate doses every 4–6 h, max. 24 Mio. U/d
- United Kingdom – BNFC:
  - meningitis, meningococcal disease
    - by slow IV injection or infusion
      - **neonate:** 225 mg/kg/d as 3 separate doses
      - **children 1 month–18 years:** 50 mg/kg/dose every 4–6 h (max. 2.4 g/dose every 4 h)
      - note: if meningococcal disease is suspected, a SD should be given before transferring to a specialist: **infants < 1 year:** 300 mg; **children 1–9 years:** 600 mg; **children > 10 years:** 1.2 g
      - note: in penicillin allergy, Cefotaxime may be an alternative.
  - proven or suspected neonatal group B streptococcus infection
    - by slow IV injection or infusion
      - **neonates < 7 d:** 100 mg/kg/d as 2 separate doses
      - **neonates (7–28 d):** 150 mg/kg/d as 3 separate doses

Comments:
- not stable to acids, thus only insufficient uptake of active drug in the stomach, complete absorption in intramuscular injection, highest plasma level is achieved via intravenous injection

– in meningitis, the drug level in liquor is about 5 % of that in the plasma (in remission, the liquor level decreases dramatically due to the recovered blood-brain-barrier function)

Biperiden

Dosage:

▶ acute dystonic reaction: slow IV 0.05–0.1 mg/kg (max. 5 mg/6 h)
▶ in acute drug induced dystonic reaction: IV children aged 1 year: 1 mg, 2–6 years: 2 mg, 6–10 years: 3 mg, > 10 years: 4–5 mg (SPC)

Neuropaediatric indications:

– acute dystonic reaction
– drug induced and other extrapyramidal symptoms

Mechanism of action:

– anticholinergic agent
– competitive muscarinergic antagonist with mostly central efficacy (peripheral effects only in high dosages)

Relevant contraindications:

– angle closure glaucoma, mechanic stenosis of the gastrointestinal tract, megacolon
– careful use: urinary retention, myasthenia gravis, tachyarrhythmia, increased disposition of seizures
– hereditary galactose intolerance, lactase deficiency, glucose-galactose malabsorption

Relevant side effects and interactions:

– flush
– anxiety, hallucination, euphoria, fatigue, drowsiness, vertigo, headache
– accommodation impairment, glaucoma
– dry mouth, micturition problems, constipation
– dyskinesia, ataxia
– tachycardia
– IV: hypotension
– enhanced anticholinergic effect of antihistamines, spasmolytic agents
– increased efficacy of Meperidine (synonym Pethidine)
– enhanced L-dopa-dyskinesia and neuroleptics-induced tardive dyskinesia

Approval status:

– Extrapyramidal symptoms without age limitations

Sources:

– **Germany – SPC:** –
– **USA – T:** –
– **United Kingdom – BNFC:** –
– **Uptodate.com:** –

Botulinum toxins

Dosage:

▶ CAUTION: do not interchange preparations using a fixed calculation scheme!
  – sonography guidance!
  – dose calculations per kilogram bodyweight only applicable up to 25 kg bodyweight; thereafter adapt adult dosing – national guidelines
▶ (spastic) movement disorders:
  – Onabotulinumtoxin A (preparation: Botox®):
    – total dose per treatment, e.g. 10–20 U/kg and generally not exceeding 20–25 U/kg. Dose injected per single muscle, 3–6 U/kg for large muscles and 0.5–2 U/kg for small muscles.
    – published maximum dose: 30 U/kg (50 U per injection site; 100 U per muscle; 400–600 U per treatment)
  – Abotulinumtoxin A (preparation Dysport®):
    – total dose 20–30 U/kg. Dose injected per single muscle: 10–15 U/kg for large muscles and 5–10 U/kg for small muscles.
    – published maximum dose: 30 U/kg (125 U per injection site; 250 U per muscle; 1000 U per treatment)
  – Incobotulinumtoxin A (preaparation Xeomin®): (systemic data/studies in neurology, anecdotic and study data in paediatric neurology): equivalent dose recommendations to preaparation Botox®
  – (Botulinumtoxin type B [preparation Neurobloc®/Myobloc®]: [box warning: may not be used in children < 18 yrs.])
▶ sialorrhea (intraglandular injection):
  – note: to be injected in equal portions into the Gl. parotis (1–2 injection sites on each side) and the Gl. submandibularis (1 injection site on each side)
  – Preparation Botox®: 50–100(–150) U ad 2–4 ml of 0.9 % NaCl
  – Preparation Dysport®: 150–300 U ad 1–2 ml of 0.9 % NaCl
  – Preparation Xeomin®: 50–100(–150) U ad 2–4 ml of 0.9 % NaCl
  – (Preparation Neurobloc®/Myobloc®: [box warning: may not be used in children < 18 yrs.])

Neuropaediatric indications:

- spastic and dystonic movement disorders (cerebral palsy, focal/multifocal)
- sialorrhea, intraglandular injection
- neurogenic voiding disorder
- pain management (in muscular hypertonicity)
- primary and secondary dystonia (focal problem)
- velum (or palatal) tremor (with ear click)
- spasmodic dysphonia

Mechanism of action:

- specific binding to the presynaptic SV2 receptor (plus other membranous acceptors) of cholinergic axons and (clinically reversible) inhibition of acetylcholine release
- taken up by the synapses via endocytosis
- fusion of vesicles with the synaptic membrane and the subsequent release of acetylcholine is inhibited
- various serotypes of Botulinum toxin (only class A and B are approved) differently target the vesicle fusion system: serotype A proteolytically cleares the membranous protein SNAP25. Serotype B cleares the vesicle protein VAMP/synaptobrevin
- with the established dose, the muscle is reduced in volume by 15–30 % and "weakened"
- change of afferent information (via the neuromuscular spindles)
- (neuro-)modulation of sensory-motor-loops
- (neuro-)modulation via "protein release", "protein trafficing", "binding" and expression of specific binding sites
- clinical duration of action: 2–3(–6)(–9) months
- Clinical efficacy is modulated by the local paresis of the target muscle and the intramuscular and central plasticity as a reaction to the induced paralysis. Most of these adaptive interactions are not sufficiently understood. The resulting focal neurogenic atrophy lasts over a time period of several months to years. Neuroplastic changes can be observed with an onset of weeks to months.

Relevant contraindications:

- myasthenia, neuromuscular diseases, coagulation disorders, simultaneous treatment with aminoglycosides (potentiation theoretically)

Relevant side effects and interactions:

- local pain during the intramuscular injections
- note: distal effects like swallowing problems, voiding dysfunction etc., and procedural side effects of the analgosedation: use special caution/monitoring/planning for patients with GMFCS IV and V with current swallowing disorders and/or (anamnestic) aspiration pneumonia
- flu-like symptoms over a few days

Approval status:

- Onabotulinumtoxin A and Abotulinumtoxin A in pes equinus in cerebral palsy in children > 2 years of age

Sources:

- **Germany – SPC:**
- **preparation Botox®:** the safety and efficacy of Botox for treatment of dystonia, hemifacial spasms and blepharospasm (children < 12 years) have not yet been proven.
- **USA – T:**
- **Onabotulinumtoxin A (preparation Botox®)**
    - **spasticity associated with cerebral palsy**
        - IM
            - **children > 18 months–18 years:** small muscle, 1–2 U/kg; large muscle, 3–6 U/kg; max. dose per injection site, 50 U; max. total dose at any one visit, 12 U/kg, up to 400 U in total; do not exceed a total of 400 U during a 3-month period
    - **cervical dystonia**
        - IM
            - **adults:** initial and subsequent doses should be individualized according to the patient's head and neck position, localization of pain, muscle hypertrophy, and patient's response; mean dosage used in research trials, 236 U (range: 198–300 U) (max. ≤ 50 U/site) divided among affected muscles; limit total dose into sternocleidomastoid muscles to ≤ 100 U to reduce the risk of dysphagia
- **United Kingdom – BNFC:**
- **Botulinum toxin type A**
    - **cerebral palsy**
        - **note:** consult product literature (SPC) for dose recommendations (important: the information provided is specific for each individual preparation and not interchangeable between different preparations)

Comments:

- adequate setting with satisfactory pain- and anxiety-free procedure/safety/analgosedation/monitoring (see above), sonographic injection control, and evaluation
- safety: keep in mind national regulations, boxed warning
- for safe differentiation the following terminology is used (FDA):
    - Onabotulinumtoxin A (preparation Botox®)
        - see actual labeling (EMA)
    - Abotulinumtoxin A (preparation Dysport®)
        - see actual labeling (EMA, FDA)
    - Incobotulinumtoxin A (preparation Xeomin®)

Bromides

Dosage:
- children ½–3 years: 50(–70) mg/kg/d as 2–3 separate doses
- children 4–15 years: 40(–60) mg/kg/d as 2–3 separate doses
- adults: 30(–50)mg/kg/d as 2–3 separate doses

Neuropaediatric indications:
- primary and secondary generalized tonic-clonic seizures in early childhood and severe myoclonic syndrome in children (e.g. Dravet syndrome)

Mechanism of action:
- unknown

Relevant contraindications:
- hypersensitivity to potassium bromide or any other ingredients
- known bromide intolerance
- renal insufficiency
- pregnancy and lactation period
- relative: bronchial asthma, malnutrition or dystrophy

Relevant side effects and interactions:
- papulopustular skin irritations (bromide acne) in approximately 25 % of treated patients (partially dose unrelated)
- fatigue, prolonged response time, headache, concentration disorder
- rhinitis, increased secretion, bronchitis, and exacerbation of bronchial asthma
- bloating, stomach pain, vomiting, constipation, diarrhea, gastritis, ulcers, pancreatitis

Approval status:
- approved for the treatment of primary and secondary generalized tonic-clonic seizures in early childhood and severe myoclonic syndromes in children (e.g. Dravet syndrome)

Sources:
- Germany – SPC:
- Preparation Dibro-Be® 850 mg tablets
  - the following doses are recommended for the treatment of generalized tonic-clonic seizures:

- oral

Age	Bodyweight in kg	Daily maintenance dose		Number of tablets DIBRO-BE mono, given in 2–3 divided doses**
		Bodyweight in mg/kg	in mg*	
Children				
½–3 years	7–15	50–70	350–1050	½ up to 1½
4–8 years	16–28	40–60	640–1680	1–2
9–15 years	29–58	40–60	1160–3500	1½–4
Adults***		30–50	Up to 4000	Up to 4½

* The dose recommendations are intended for initial orientation only.

** The amount of intake is adjusted to individually calculated administration (ie. alternate intake of half a tablet).

*** Only if seizures are still present in patients > 18 years

- **USA – T:** –
- **United Kingdom – BNFC:** –

Comments:
- DIBRO-BE mono tablets are dividable, to be taken with sufficient fluid (about 100–150 ml) after meals
- soluble in warm water
- in potassium defined or potassium free diet consider that 1 tablet of 850 mg potassium bromide contains 278.6 mg potassium
- due to the narrow therapeutic range it is recommended to administer DIBRO-BE mono only under the control of a specialist with adequate experience in epilepsy and bromide therapy
- during infection: children are given 50 % of the normal dose to prevent accumulation and side effects
- do not exceed a total daily dose of 4000 mg, because frequent side effects can occur with higher dosages

Bromocriptine

Dosage:
- ▸ initially 0.05–0.075 mg/kg/d as 2–3 separate doses; max. 1.25 mg/d
- ▸ increase weekly up to 0.05–0.2 mg/kg/dose every 6–12 h; max. 2.5–10 mg/d

Neuropaediatric indications:
- prolactinoma (anterior pituitary)
- parkinson's disease

Mechanism of action:
- dopamine-D_2 agonist
- derivate of ergocryptine (ergoline)

Relevant contraindications:
- hypersensitivity to ergolines
- coronary heart diseases and vascular diseases
- severe psychic disorders
- pregnancy toxicosis
- uncontrolled hypertension
- especially careful use in children and adolescents, pregnancy and hepatic diseases
- in high dosages: medical history of psychic disorders, severe organic brain syndrome, severe cardiovascular diseases, gastrointestinal ulcers, gastrointestinal bleeding

Relevant side effects and interactions:
- headache, vertigo, fatigue, depressive mood
- psychomotor agitation, sleeping disorder, impaired vision, visual hallucination, psychoses, confusion, drowsiness, anxiety, nervousness, dyskinesia/ataxia
- allergic skin reactions
- lividity, sweating
- hyposmia
- nausea, vomiting, diarrhea, upper abdominal problems, cramps, dyspepsia, loss of appetite, obstipation
- dry mouth, gastrointestinal bleeding
- urinary retention, incontinence, pollakisuria
- abnormal liver function parameters: elevated urea, uric acid, alkaline phosphatase, SGOT, SGPT, gamma-GT, CK (reversible)
- muscle cramps
- seizures
- paresthesia, dysarthria
- somnolence, sudden stroke
- syncopes, angina pectoris episodes, orthostatic hypotension, arrhythmias, ventricular tachycardia, hypertension, heart attack, stroke
- long term treatment:
  - vasospastic blood circulation disorders in fingers and toes caused by cold
  - retroperitoneal fibrosis
  - pleural effusion and pleuropulmonal fibrosis
- galactorrhea after discontinuation
- possible interactions with blood pressure influencing medication
- decreased or failing efficacy of Bromocriptine due to interaction with dopamine antagonists
- loss of Bromocriptine efficacy due to interaction with Griseofulvin and Tamoxifen
- macrolide antibiotics and octreotides increase and prolong efficacy of Bromocriptine

Approval status:
- depends on specific product (see SPC)

Sources:
- **Germany – SPC:**
- No published paediatric dosage
- **USA – T:**
  - **hyperprolactinemia**
    - oral
      - **children 11–15 years:** initially 1.25–2.5 mg/d; dosage may be increased as tolerated to achieve a therapy response (range: 2.5–10 mg/d)
      - **children ≥ 16 years:** initially 1.25–2.5 mg/d; dosage may be increased as tolerated every 2–7 d by 2.5 mg/d until achieving optimal response (range: 2.5–15 mg/d)
  - **parkinson**
    - oral
      - no dose recommendations for children available
      - **adults:** 2.5 mg/d as 2 separate doses, increased in 2- to 4-week intervals by 2.5 mg/d (usual dose range is 30–90 mg/d as 3 separate doses), though elderly patients can usually be managed on lower doses
  - **neuroleptic malignant syndrome**
    - oral
      - no dose recommendations for children available
      - **adults:** 2.5–5 mg/dose 3 times daily
- **United Kingdom – BNFC:** –

Comments:
- variable dose recommendations in published common paediatric sources

Butylscopolamine

Dosage:

▶ 0.3–0.6 mg/kg/dose every 6 h IM or IV; max. 1.5 mg/kg/d (leaflet instruction)

Neuropaediatric indications:

– colics
– gastrointestinal spasms, biliary tract spasms

Mechanism of action:

– vagolytic drug due to its antagonistic effect at muscarinergic acetylcholine receptors

Relevant contraindications:

– angle closure glaucoma
– tachyarrhythmia
– myasthenia gravis
– voiding dysfunction with residual urine
– mechanic stenosis of gastrointestinal tract, megacolon

Relevant side effects and interactions:

– redness of the skin, bloating, constipation, decreased sweat production, dry mouth, tachycardia
– accommodation impairment, impaired vision
– increased anticholinergic effect of antihistamines, Amantadine, chinidin, tri- and tetracyclic antidepressants
– increased tachycardic effect of β-sympathomimetics, in combination with dopamine antagonists mutual decrease of the effect on gastrointestinal tract motility

Approval status:

– gastrointestinal, biliary and urinary tract spasms/colics without age limitation

Sources:

– **Germany – SPC:**
  – IM, SC, slow IV
    – **children and adolescents:** 0.3–0.6 mg/kg, max. 1.5 mg/kg/d
  – **preparation Buscopan® suppository (status 11/2011)**
    – **children ≥ 6 years:** 3–5 times daily 1–2 suppositories (10–20 mg); max. 100 mg/d
– **USA – T:**
  – **preoperatively and antiemetic**
    – IM, SC, IV
      – **children:** 6 mcg/kg/dose, max. 300 mcg/dose, may be repeated every 6–8 h

– **United Kingdom – BNFC:**
  – **symptomatic relief of gastro-intestinal or genitourinary disorders characterized by smooth muscle spasm**
    – oral
      – **children 6–12 years:** 30 mg/d as 3 separate doses
      – **children 12–18 years:** 80 mg/d as 4 separate doses
  – **excessive respiratory secretions and bowel in palliative care**
    – oral
      – **children 1 month – 2 years:** 0.3–0.5 mg/kg/dose (max. 5 mg) 3–4 times daily
      – **children 2–5 years:** 5 mg/dose 3–4 times daily
      – **children 5–12 years:** 10 mg/dose 3–4 times daily
      – **children 12–18 years:** 10–20 mg/dose 3–4 times daily
    – IM, IV injection
      – **children 1 month–4 years:** 0.3–0.5 mg/kg/dose (max. 5 mg) 3–4 times daily
      – **children 5–12 years:** 5–10 mg/dose 3–4 times daily
      – **children 12–18 years:** 10–20 mg/dose 3–4 times daily
  – **acute spasm, spasm in diagnostic procedure**
    – IM, IV injection
      – **children 2–6 years:** 5 mg, repeated after 30 minutes if necessary (may be repeated more frequently in endoscopy), max. 15 mg/d
      – **children 6–12 years:** 5–10 mg, repeated after 30 minutes if necessary (may be repeated more frequently in endoscopy), max. 30 mg/d
      – **children 12–18 years:** 20 mg, repeated after 30 minutes if necessary (may be repeated more frequently in endoscopy), max. 80 mg/d

Caffeine

Dosage:

▶ initially 10 mg/kg (as Caffeine base; not as Caffeine citrate)
▶ maintenance with 3 mg/kg/d (as Caffeine base; not as Caffeine citrate)

Neuropaediatric indications:

– central respiratory disorders with concomitant hypoxemia

Mechanism of action:

– competitive antagonist at the adenosine receptors → increased activity
– mild inhibition of the phosphodiesterase → cerebral vasoconstriction

Relevant contraindications:
- tachyarrhythmia
- liver cirrhosis
- hyperthyroidism
- anxiety syndrome

Relevant side effects and interactions:
- insomnia, headache
- irritability, inner anxiety, tremor
- tachycardia, tachyarrhythmia
- gastrointestinal problems
- increased tachycardia in combination with sympathomimetics, thyroid gland hormones
- reduced break down caused by oral contraceptives, cimetidine, disulfiram
- accelerated break down caused by barbiturates
- gyrase inhibitors delay elimination
- delayed elimination of Theophylline

Approval status:
- depends on the specific product (see SPC)

Sources:
- **Germany – SPC:**
  - **apnea of prematurity (Caffeine citrate)**
    - IV
      - **neonates:** loading dose of 20 mg/kg over 30 min (if no response, may be repeated with 10–20 mg/kg 24 h after loading dose); maintenance with 5 mg/kg/24 h over 10 min starting 24 h after loading dose. Maintenance dose may be increased to 10 mg/kg/24 h if no response (monitor carefully).
- **USA – T:**
  - **apnea of prematurity (Caffeine citrate)**
    - oral, IV
      - **neonates:** loading dose of 20 mg/kg as Caffeine citrate (10 mg/kg as Caffeine base); loading doses as high as 80 mg/kg of Caffeine citrate have been reported; in refractory patients, some centers repeat with a load of 20 mg/kg as Caffeine citrate to a max. cumulative dose load of 80 mg/kg as Caffeine citrate. Maintenance with 5–10 mg/kg/d Caffeine citrate once daily starting 24 h after the loading dose; in refractory patients, some centers increase maintenance dose in 5 mg/kg/d increments of Caffeine citrate to max. 20 mg/kg/d according to clinical response and serum Caffeine levels.
- **United Kingdom – BNFC:**
  - **neonatal apnea**
    - oral (expressed as Caffeine base)
      - **neonates:** initially 10 mg/kg, followed 24 hours later by 2.5–5 mg/kg/d as a SD
    - IV infusion (expressed as Caffeine base)
      - **neonates:** initially 10 mg/kg over 30 minutes, followed 24 hours later by 2.5–5 mg/kg/d as a SD over 10 minutes

Calcium and Vitamin D

Dosage:
▶ 500 U/d Vitamin D + 2 × 500 mg ionized Calcium/d

Neuropaediatric indications:
- prophylaxis of osteomalacia in long-term treatment with corticosteroids or Phenytoin

Mechanism of action:
- direct substitution

Relevant contraindications:
- hypercalcemia, nephrocalcinosis, intoxication with digitalis, severe renal insufficiency

Relevant side effects and interactions:
- feeling hot, sweating attacks, decreasing blood pressure, nausea, vomiting

Approval status:
- depends on the specific product (see SPC)

Sources:
- **Germany – SPC:**
  - **prophylaxis of rickets**
    - oral
      - usual dose: 0.02 mg/d or 800 U Vitamin D/d; dissolve tablets in water on a teaspoon and administer directly to the patient. Do not use this in bottle feeding for infants. If administration has to be with feeding, Vitamin D should be added only after cooking. Keep an eye on feeds containing Vitamin D and ensure correct dosing.
- **USA – T:** –
- **United Kingdom – BNFC:** –

Comments:
- long-term use (> 3 months) with corticosteroids: monitor bone density
- variable published dosage recommendations in common paediatric sources

Carbamazepine (CBZ)

Dosage:

▶ in epilepsy:
  – (5–)10–20(–30) mg/kg/d as 3 separate doses p.o.
  – can be increased over 2 weeks up to 15–25 mg/kg/d (SPC)
  – level: 20–50 mcmol/l or 4–12 mcg/ml
▶ vestibular paroxysmia: 2–6 mg/kg/d
  – 1–5 years 100–200 mg/d
  – 6–10 years 100–400 mg/d
  – 11–15 years 100–600 mg/d
  – > 15 years 200–800 mg/d
▶ paroxysmal kinesigenic dyskinesia: initially 10 mg/kg
  – chronic substance abuse (in overdosing or severe withdrawal symptoms): 200–1000 mg/d
  – myotonic dystrophy: 4–15 mg/kg/d as 2–3 separate doses; increase dose gradually
▶ neurogenic pain
  – initially 2 mg/kg every 12 h p.o.
  – target dose: max. 20 mg/kg/d as 2–3 separate doses

Neuropaediatric indications:

– focal epilepsy
– (neonatal seizures [small case numbers/some cases are reported] or West syndrome)
– startle epilepsy
– alternative therapy of Rolandic epilepsy
– benign hereditary chorea (conservative indication)
– neurogenic pain
– paroxysmal kinesigenic dystonia
– mood stabilizer (incl. bipolar disorder)
– myotonic dystrophy
– special paroxysmal disorders (e.g. vestibular paroxysmia)
– (chronic drug abuse)
– vestibular paroxysmia

Mechanism of action:

– reduction of the enhanced response to the stimulus after repeated stimuli of the afferences; presumably by blocking the axonal sodium channels

Relevant contraindications:

– possibly aggravates primary generalized epilepsies (especially JME), tonic, atonic and absence epilepsy

– AV block
– medical history of bone marrow depression
– acute intermittent porphyria
– combination with MAOIs (discontinue MAOI 14 d prior to start of the treatment)
– combination with Voriconazole (therapy failure)
– sustained release formulations: children < 6 years of age
– careful use: absence epilepsy, hematologic diseases, medical history of hematologic reactions to other medication, impaired sodium metabolism, severe cardiovascular diseases, liver and renal impairment, myotonic dystrophy (frequent cardiac conduction disorders), glaucoma, combination with lithium (CAUTION: Carbamazepine plasma concentration max. 8 mcg/ml, lithium level 0.3 up to 0.8 mval/l, finish treatment with neuroleptics at least 8 weeks prior to start with Carbamazepine), prevention of seizures in alcohol withdrawal syndrome, alcohol, pregnancy

Relevant side effects and interactions

– allergic exanthema
– delayed hypersensitivity reactions with fever, rash, vasculitis, swelling of lymph nodes, joint pain, leukopenia, eosinophilia, hepatosplenomegaly or changed liver function
– somnolence, sedation, drowsiness, vertigo, ataxia
– loss of appetite, dry mouth, nausea, vomitus, diarrhea, constipation
– jaundice, hepatitis
– headache, asterixis, tics
– hyponatremia, hypocalcemia
– hirsutism, gynecomastia, galactorrhea
– AV block, bradycardia, cardiac arrhythmias, deterioration of a present coronary heart disease (primarily patients with known heart function disorders), decrease in blood pressure (especially with high dosages of Carbamazepine)
– changes in blood count (leukocytosis, eosinophilia, leukopenia, thrombocytopenia); benign leukopenia (10 % temporary, 2 % persistent) is most frequent, especially in the first four months of treatment
– renal impairment, e.g. proteinuria, hematuria, oliguria and other symptoms of a kidney disease, very rarely up to an interstitial nephritis or renal failure, dysuria, pollakisuria, urinary retention
– activation of a latent psychosis, deterioration of multiple sclerosis symptoms
– recurring seizures, especially absence seizures
– septic meningitis
– alopecia, increased sweating, changes in skin pigmentation, acne
– rarely lupus-like symptoms, changes of blood count, osteomalacia, SIADH
– in patients with cerebral impairment, dyskinetic disorders like orofacial dyskinesia and choreoathetosis
– no combination with MAOIs

- decreased Carbamazepine plasma levels via CYP450-enzyme induction (primarily CYP3A4) by
    - anticonvulsants (Clonazepam, Ethosuximide, Felbamat, Primidone, Lamotrigine, Tiagabine, Topiramate, Valproic acid)
    - benzodiazepines (Alprazolam, Clobazam)
    - tricyclic antidepressants (e.g. Imipramine, Amitryptiline, Nortryptiline, Clomipramine)
    - typical neuroleptics (Haloperidol, Bromperidole)
    - atypical neuroleptics (Clozapine, Olanzapine, Risperidone, Quetiapine)
    - tetracyclics (e.g. Doxycycline)
    - corticosteroids (e.g. Prednisolone, Dexamethasone)
    - ciclosporin, Tacrolimus
    - Warfarin, Dicoumarin, Phenprocoumon
    - Praziquantel, Digoxin, Caspofungin, Indinavir, Fentanyl, Midazolam, Phenazone, Methadone, Methylphenidate, Theophylline, Chinidin, Propranolol, Felodipine, Flunarizine
- decreased plasma levels of azole-type antifungal agents (e.g. Voriconazole, Itraconazole) and hormonal contraceptives via CYP-450-enzyme induction; therapy failure is possible
- plasma levels of Phenytoin can be increased or decreased (confusion up to coma).
- decreased plasma levels of Trazodone, but partially increased antidepressive effect
- decreased plasma levels of Bupropion and increased levels of its metabolite hydroxy Bupropion (clinical efficacy and safety decreased)
- possible acceleration of zotepine-metabolism
- anticonvulsants (Phenobarbital, Phenytoin, Primidone, Valproic acid), Theophylline, Rifampicin, Doxorubicin, Cisplatin, Hypericum reduce the plasma level of Carbamazepine.
- Valproic acid, Primidone increase the plasma level of active Carbamazepinemetabolite.
- combination with Felbamat leads to reduced plasma levels of Carbamazepine and Felbamat and to increased plasma levels of Carbamazepine-10,11-epoxide
- increased plasma concentration of Carbamazepine:
    - macrolide antibiotics (e.g. Erythromycin, Troleandomycin, Josamycin, Clarithromycin)
    - antimycotics of azole-type (e.g. Itraconazole, Fluconazole, Ketoconazole)
    - Calcium antagonists (e.g. Verapamil, Diltiazem)
    - Isoniazid, Ritonavir, Acetazolamide, Dextropropoxyphene, Propoxyphene, Danazol, Viloxazine, Nicotinamide (high dosages in adults), Fluoxetine, Terfenadine, Loratadine, Cimetidine
    - Desipramine, Fluvoxamine
- increased neurologic side effects with concurrent administration of neuroleptics or metoclopramide
- concurrent administration of Lithium leads to increased neurotoxic effect of both drugs
- increased hepatotoxicity with concurrent intake of Isoniazid
- hyponatremia with concurrent administration of Hydrochlorothiazide and Furosemide
- fast removal of the neuromuscular block of muscle relaxants
- monitoring of Carbamazepine plasma levels is necessary with concurrent administration of Isoretinoin
- reduced bioavailability of Paracetamol
- accelerated elimination of thyroid gland hormones [especially with concurrent administration of other anticonvulsants (e.g. Phenobarbital), assess thyroid function, dose adjustments if necessary]
- in combination with SSRI, possible toxic serotonin syndrome
- significant reduction of Nefazodone plasma levels up to failing efficacy, increased plasma levels of Carbamazepine and reduced levels of Carbamazepine-10,11 epoxide (combination is not recommended)
- risk of cardiac conduction disorders with concurrent administration of antiarrhythmics, cyclic antidepressants and erythromycin
- increased risk of a malignant neuroleptic syndrome or Stevens-Johnson syndromes with concurrent administration of neuroleptics
- grapefruit juice increases Carbamazepine bioavailability and plasma levels.
- reduced alcohol tolerance

Approval status:
- patients with focal and secondary generalized seizures and mixed epilepsies
- no limitation in age, however, children < 6 years of age should not be given sustained release tablets of 400 mg or 600 mg

Sources:
- **Germany – SPC:**
    - **epilepsy**
        - oral
            - **children 1–5 years:** initially 100 mg 1–2 times daily; usual maintenance with 200 mg 1–2 times daily
            - **children 6–10 years:** initially 100 mg 2 times daily; usual maintenance with 200 mg 3 times daily
            - **children 11–15 years:** initially 100 mg 2–3 times daily; usual maintenance with 200–400 mg 3 times daily
            - **note:**

- **children < 4 years:** for this age group the 200 mg tablets are not recommended; use suppositories instead. Based on clinical experience the following dosage is recommended: initially 20–60 mg/d. Increase by 20–60 mg/d every other day until response is satisfactory. But do not exceed the aforementioned doses (see dosage).
- **children > 4 years:** Based on clinical experience the following dosage is recommended: initially 100 mg/d (immediate release formulation). Increase by 100 mg/d every other day or once weekly until response is satisfactory. But do not exceed the aforementioned doses (see dosage).
- USA – T:
  - **epilepsy**
    - **children < 6 years:** initially 10–20 mg/kg/d as 2–3 separate doses as tablets or 4 times/d as suspension; increase dose every week until achieving optimal response and therapeutic levels; maintenance dose: divide daily dose into 3–4 separate doses (tablets or suspension); max. 35 mg/kg/d
    - **children 6–12 years:** initially 200 mg/d as 2 separate doses (tablets or extended release tablets) or 50 mg of suspension 4 times/d (total of 200 mg/d); increase up to 100 mg/d at weekly intervals using a twice daily regimen of extended release tablets or a 3–4 times daily regimen of other formulations until achieving optimal response and therapeutic levels; usual maintenance with 400–800 mg/d; max. 1000 mg/d
    - **children> 12 years:** initially 400 mg/d as 2 separate doses (tablets, extended release tablets, or extended release capsules) or 400 mg/d as 4 separate doses of a suspension formulation; increase up to 200 mg/d at weekly intervals using a twice daily regimen of extended release tablets or capsules, or a 3–4 times/d regimen of other formulations until achieving optimal response and therapeutic levels; usual dose: 800–1200 mg/d
- **United Kingdom – BNFC:**
  - **focal and generalized tonic-clonic seizures, trigeminal neuralgia, prophylaxis of bipolar disorder**
    - oral
      - **children 1 month–12 years:** initially 5 mg/kg/d as a SD at night or as 2 separate doses during the day. Increase if necessary by 2.5–5 mg/kg every 3–7 d; usual maintenance with 5 mg/kg/dose 2–3 times daily, max. 20 mg/kg/d
      - **children 12–18 years:** initially 100–200 mg/dose 1–2 times daily. Increase slowly to usual maintenance with 200–400 mg/dose 2–3 times daily. In some cases doses up to 1.8 g/d may be needed
    - rectal
      - **children 1 month–18 years:** use approx. 25 % more than the oral dose (max. 250 mg) up to 4 times daily

Comments:
- rectal administration for up to one week is possible (dose should be increased by 25 %)
- in neurogenic pain: combination option with amitryptiline

Carglumic acid

> **Dosage:**
> ▶ 100 mg/kg/d as 3 separate doses p.o.

Neuropaediatric indications:
- neurometabolic lapse: hyperammonemia in propionic or methylmalonic acidemia

Mechanism of action:
- restores the urea cycle

Relevant contraindications:
- none

Relevant side effects and interactions:
- limited experience

Approval status:
- orphan drug status

Sources:
- **Germany – SPC:**
- **Preparation Carbaglu® 200 mg**
- No published paediatric dosage
- **USA – T: –**
- **United Kingdom – BNFC:**
  - **hyperammonemia due to N-acetyl glutamate synthase deficiency**
    - oral
      - **neonates:** initially 100–250 mg/kg/d as separate doses immediately before feeds, adjusted according to plasma ammonia concentration; maintenance with 10–100 mg/kg/d as 2 separate doses. Alternatively, total daily dose may be given as 3–4 separate doses.
      - **children 1 month–18 years:** initially 100–250 mg/kg/d as separate doses immediately before feeds, adjusted according to plasma ammonia concentration. maintenance with 10–100 mg/kg/d as 2 separate doses. Alternatively, total daily dose may be given as 3–4 separate doses.

Comments:
- early therapy: normal growth and normal intellectual development
- patients do not require special diet
- FDA approved since 2008
- various dosages were published in common paediatric sources

L-Carnitine

Dosage:
▶ 50 mg/kg/d

Neuropaediatric indications:
- Duchenne/Becker muscular dystrophy (add-on therapy)
- Limb-girdle muscular dystrophy (does not increase power, but partially reduces muscle pain)

Mechanism of action:
- L-carnitine serves as a carrier for long-chain activated fatty acids in the cytosol (acyl-CoA) across the mitochondrial membrane.
- Long-chain fatty acids can only pass the mitochondrial membrane when linked to L-carnitine. As acylcarnitine they can then be metabolized via β-oxidation to acetyl-CoA and thus support energy generation in the citric acid cycle.
- primarily taken up via food, but also endogenously synthesized from methionine and lysine in the liver and kidneys; essential cofactors (*Furosawa et al., Biol. Pharmaceut. Bull. 31, 1673–9*), Vitamin B_6, niacin and iron

Relevant contraindications:
- none

Relevant side effects and interactions:
- nausea, vomiting, diarrhea
- sweating

Approval status:
- not applicable

Sources:
- **Germany – SPC:**
  - **adjunctive treatment of muscular dystrophy (Duchenne)**
  - no published paediatric dosage
- **USA – T:**
- **Primary carnitine deficiency**
  - oral
    - **children:** 50–100 mg/kg/d as 2–3 separate doses, max. 3 g/d; dosage must be individually adjusted based on each patient's specific response; higher dosages have been used
  - IV
    - **children:** loading dose of 50 mg/kg, followed (in severe cases) by 50 mg/kg/d as up to 4–6 separate doses if needed
- **United Kingdom – BNFC:** –

Comments:
- level in body: about 20–25 g, particularly in tissues with a high turn-over of fatty acids (about 98 % in heart and skeletal muscles)
- plasma level: about 40–80 µmol/l (70–85 % as free carnitine)
- daily intake: 100–300 mg with a balanced mixed diet, 2–10 mg with a vegetarian diet
- highest content in read meat, less in poultry meat; vegetarian food contains less or no L-carnitine (highest amount in cheese, milk and avocado)
- renal elimination (about 20 mg/d)
- questionable hepatoprotective effect in combination with Valproic acid

Cefotaxime

Dosage:
▶ 200 mg/kg/d as 3 separate doses (max. 6 g/d); duration: 2 weeks
▶ in severe cases (> 12 years): 12 g/d (SPC)

Neuropaediatric indications:
- neuroborreliosis
- bacterial meningitis

Mechanism of action:
- third generation cephalosporin (β-lactam antibiotics)
- bacteriostatic, because Cefotaxime inhibits the crosslinking of peptidoglycans by opening and binding the β-lactam circle, thus preventing the formation of new cell layers
- effective against Gram-positive bacteria (group A streptococcus, pneumococci) and many Gram-negative bacteria (gonococci, meningococci, pseudomonas, enterobacteriaceae, haemophilus influenzae etc.)
- β-lactamase stable
- in the Gram-positive area: insufficient efficacy against staphylococci
- in severe infections: very poor efficacy against pseudomonas, enterococci, anaerobic bacteria

Relevant contraindications:
- hypersensitivity to cephalosporins
- careful use: medical history of distinct allergies or asthma, severely impaired renal function, risk factors that lead to Vitamin K deficiency or influence other coagulation mechanisms

Relevant side effects and interactions:

- urticaria, exanthema, pruritus
- loss of appetite, nausea, vomiting, stomach pain, diarrhea
- myoclonics, seizures (tonic/clonic), vertigo
- mild, temporary increase of bilirubin or liver enzymes (AST, ALT, gamma-GT, LDH, alkaline phosphatase)
- elevation of creatinine- and urea concentration in the serum
- pseudomembranous colitis
- severe cardiac arrhythmias
- hemolytic anemia, granulocytopenia, leukocytopenia, eosinophilia, thrombocytopenia, agranulocytosis
- acute interstitial nephritis
- anaphylaxis
- decreased efficacy with bacteriostatics (e.g. chloramphenicol, erythromycin, sulfonamides, tetracyclines)
- increased serum levels caused by probenecid
- enhanced nephrotoxic effect in combination with amino glycosides, polymyxin B, colistin, loop diuretics

Approval status:

- depends on product (see SPC)

Sources:

- Germany – SPC:
- **Preparation Cefotaxime Fresenius® IV**
  - **severe infections (e.g. Lyme disease)**
    - IV
      - **infants and children < 12 years:** 50–100(–150) mg/kg/d as 2–4 separate doses according to severity of infection; may be increased to 200 mg/kg/d in life-threatening situations
      - **neonates:** do not exceed 50 mg/kg/d. Treatment period for neuroborreliosis is at least 14 d
      - **children > 12 years:** 2–4 g/d as 2 separate doses. 12 g/d as 2 separate doses (for severe cases). Doses above 12 g/d must be given as 3–4 separate doses.
- **USA – T:**
  - **meningitis**
    - IM, IV
      - **neonates < 1200 g:** 100 mg/kg/d as 2 separate doses
      - **note:** for treatment of meningitis use IV route only, upper end of the dosage range, shortest dosage interval, and treat for a minimum of 21 d
      - **postnatal ≤ 7 d: 1200–2000 g:** 100 mg/kg/d as 2 separate doses; **> 2000 g:** 100–150 mg/kg/d as 2–3 separate doses
      - **postnatal > 7 d: 1200–2000 g:** 150 mg/kg/d as 3 separate doses; **> 2000 g:** 150–200 mg/kg/d as 3–4 separate doses

- **infants and Children < 12 years: < 50 kg:** 200 mg/kg/d as 4 separate doses, invasive pneumococcal meningitis: 225–300 mg/kg/d as 3–4 separate doses; **≥ 50 kg:** moderate to severe infection: 1–2 g/dose every 6–8 h; life-threatening infection: 2 g/dose every 4 h, max. 12 g/d
  - **children > 12 years:** 1–2 g/dose every 6–8 h, max. 12 g/d
- United Kingdom – BNFC:
  - **meningitis, infections due to sensitive Gram-positive and Gram-negative bacteria**
    - IM, IV injection, IV infusion
      - **neonates ≤ 7 d:** 100 mg/kg/d as 2 separate doses
      - **neonates 7–21 d:** 150 mg/kg/d as 3 separate doses
      - **neonates 21–28 d:** 50 mg/kg/dose every 6–8 h
      - **children 1 month-18 years:** 200 mg/kg/d as 4 separate doses; max. 12 g/d
      - **note:** if meningococcal disease is suspected and the child cannot be given Benzylpenicillin, a single dose of Cefotaxime before urgent transfer to hospital is recommended: children < 12 years: 50 mg/kg; child ≥ 12 years: 1 g

Ceftriaxone

Dosage:

▶ 50 mg/kg/d as a SD (max. 2 g/d); duration: 2 weeks

Neuropaediatric indications:

- neuroborreliosis
- bacterial meningitis

Mechanism of action:

- third generation cephalosporin (β-lactam antibiotics)
- bacteriostatic, because Ceftriaxone inhibits the crosslinking of peptidoglycans by opening and binding the β-lactam ring structure, thus preventing formation of new cell layers.
- β-lactamase stable
- gram-positive bacteria
- haemophilus, Neisseria
- enterobacteria:
  - very effective against E. coli, Klebsiella, Proteus mirabilis, P. vulgaris, Morganella morganii, Providencia rettgeri
  - moderately effective against Enterobacter cloacae, Citrobacter freandii, Serratia marcescens
- resistant are members of the Bacteroides-fragilis group, enterococci, Pseudomonas aeruginosa

Relevant contraindications:

- hypersensitivity to cephalosporins
- hyperbilirubinemic, especially premature neonates
- for IM injection:
  - neuroborreliosis
  - severe infections
  - < 2 years
- treatment with Lidocaine in cardial conduction disorders or acute decompensated heart failure
- careful use: known hypersensitivity to penicillins or other non-cephalosporins with a β-lactam structure, tendency for allergic reactions, severely reduced renal function, concurrent severe renal and liver damages

Relevant side effects and interactions:

- headache, vertigo
- stomatitis, glossitis
- loss of appetite, nausea, vomiting, stomach pain, diarrhea
- pseudomembranous colitis
- in children: Formation of Calcium salt deposits in the gall bladder or bile ducts
- elevated liver enzymes levels in serum (AST, ALT, alkaline phosphatase)
- increase of the serum creatinine, oliguria
- pancreatitis
- phlebitis, thrombophlebitis
- slightly increased prothrombin time, leukocytopenia, neutropenia, eosinophilia, thrombocytopenia, agranulocytosis, hemolytic anemia
- genital tract mycoses
- formation of renal Ceftriaxone deposits (mostly in children > 3 years)
- anaphylaxis
- in the treatment of spirochetoses, Herxheimer reactions may occur, such as fever, headache, shivering, joint pain, skin reactions, pruritus, leukopenia, elevation of the liver enzymes, respiratory problems
- dermatitis, urticaria, exanthema, pruritus, swelling of the skin and joints
- severe skin reactions, including erythema multiforme, Stevens-Johnson syndrome and Lyell's syndrome/toxic epidermal necrolysis
- impairs the efficacy of oral contraceptives

Approval status:

- depends on the specific product (see SPC)

Sources:

- Germany – SPC:
  - meningitis
    - IV, IM
      - initially 100 mg/kg/d as a SD (max. 4 g/d). Dose can be reduced once susceptibility of the pathogen is confirmed. Neonates 0–14 d: max. 50 mg/kg/24 h. Fatal reactions involving Calcium- Ceftriaxone participates in the lungs and kidneys of neonates have been reported, even when Calcium-containing solutions were administered through separate sites and/or at different times.
      - **preparation Rocephin®, 500 mg, 1 g IV, or 2 g for infusion**
      - **note: Do not reconstitute or mix Ceftriaxone with any Calcium -containing** product, because this can result in formation of poorly soluble particles. Do not mix or (simultaneously) administer Ceftriaxone with Calcium-containing IV-solutions (even not via different lines or sites) within 48 hours of each other.
    - **patients > 28 d of age:** Ceftriaxone and Calcium-containing products may be administered sequentially (at different locations), provided the infusion lines are thoroughly flushed between infusions with a compatible fluid.
  - **adolescents > 12 years:** 2 g/d as a SD for at least 14 d. Doses up to 4 mg/d in severe infections were reported.
  - **children ≤ 11 years:** 50–100 mg/kg/d as a SD (max. 2 g/d as a SD) for at least 14 d
- USA – T:
  - meningitis
    - IM, IV
      - **postnatal ≤ 7 d:** 50 mg/kg/d given every 24 h
      - **postnatal > 7 d:** ≤ 2000 g: 50 mg/kg/d given every 24 h; > 2000 g: 50–75 mg/kg/d given every 24 h
      - **infants and children:** 100 mg/kg/d as 1–2 separate doses. A loading dose of 100 mg/kg may be administered at the start of therapy; max. 4 g/d
  - lyme disease (meningitis, encephalitis)
    - **infants and children:** 75–100 mg/kg, max. 2 g, for 2–4 weeks
- United Kingdom – BNFC:
  - **infections due to susceptible Gram-positive and Gram-negative bacteria**
    - IV infusion over 60 minutes
      - **neonates:** 20–50 mg/kg/d as a SD
  - meningitis
    - IV or deep IM injection over 2–4 minutes, or by IV infusion
      - **children 1 month–12 years (body-weight < 50 kg):** 80 mg/kg/d as a SD
      - **children 12–18 years or body-weight > 50 kg:** 2–4 g/d; > 1 g IM divided to more than one site; SD > 1 g IV by IV infusion only.

Comments:

- different dosage recommendation published in common paediatric sources

Chloral hydrate

Dosage:
▶ sedation: 25–75 mg/kg/d as (1–)3–4 separate doses (doses of max. 1 g, max. 1.5 g/d) (SPC)
▶ circadian sleeping disorder in cerebral palsy: 30–50 mg/kg (off-label)

Neuropaediatric indications:
- therapy-resistant dystonic status, agitation and nonconvulsive epileptic status
- sedation for painless procedures (MRT, CT, EEG), sedation for the night
- circadian sleeping disorder in cerebral palsy
- stand-by medication in emergency therapy of tonic-clonic seizures or convulsive status

Mechanism of action:
- hypnotic without influence on REM sleep
- precise mechanism is not known

Relevant contraindications:
- severe liver insufficiency
- severe renal insufficiency
- heart failure (NYHA III and IV)
- pulmonary diseases (no absolute CI)

Relevant side effects and interactions:
- no combination with Triclofos
- stomach irritation, nausea, vomiting
- rare CNS disorders: fatigue, confusion
- rash
- mutually increased effect when combined with centrally depressant drugs such as alcohol, barbiturates, opioids
- enhanced efficacy of anticoagulants

Approval status:
- anxiety-, agitation-conditions and sleeping disorders in children, adolescents and adults

Sources:

Germany – SPC:
Preparation Chloraldurat® 250, 500 mg (status 08/2011)
- oral
- **children < 18 years:** not recommended

- USA – T:
  - **short-sedative and hypnotic (< 2 weeks)**
    - oral (rectal)
      - **neonates:** 25 mg/kg/dose for sedation prior to procedure; Caution: repeat doses should be used with great caution as drug and metabolites accumulate with repeated use; toxicity has been reported after 3 d in a preterm neonate and after 7 d in a term neonate receiving Chloral hydrate 40–50 mg/kg/dose every 6 h
  - **sedation, anxiety**
    - oral (rectal)
      - **infants and children:** 25–50 mg/kg/d as 3–4 separate doses, max. 500 mg/dose
  - **sedation prior to EEG**
    - oral (rectal)
      - **infants and children:** 25–50 mg/kg/dose 30–60 min prior to EEG; may be repeated after 30 min to a total of max. 100 mg/kg or a total of 1 g for infants and 2 g for children
  - **sedation, painless procedures**
    - oral (rectal)
      - **infants and children:** 50–75 mg/kg/dose 30–60 min prior to procedure, may be repeated 30 min after initial dose if needed, to a total of max. 120 mg/kg or a total of 1 g for infants and 2 g/d for children
  - **hypnotic**
    - oral (rectal)
      - **infants and children:** 50 mg/kg/dose at bedtime; total of max. 1 g/d for infants and 2 g/d for children
- United Kingdom – BNFC:
  - **short-term treatment of insomnia**
    - oral
      - **children 2–12 years:** 1–1.75 ml/kg (Chloral hydrate 30–50 mg/kg) with water or milk at bedtime; max. 35 ml/d (Chloral hydrate 1 g)
      - **children 12–18 years:** 15–45 ml (Chloral hydrate 0.4–1.3 g) with water or milk at bedtime; max. 70 ml/d (Chloral hydrate 2 g)
      - **children 12–18 years:** 1–2 tablets with water or milk at bedtime, max. 5 tablets/d (Chloral hydrate 5 g)
  - **sedation for painless procedures**
    - oral (rectal)
      - **neonates:** 30–50 mg/kg/dose 45–60 minutes before procedure; doses up to 100 mg/kg may be used with respiratory monitoring
      - **children 1 month–12 years:** 30–50 mg/kg/dose 45–60 minutes before procedure; higher doses up to 100 mg/kg/dose (max. 2 g) may be used
      - **children 12–18 years:** 1000–2000 mg/dose 45–60 minutes before procedure

Comments:
- p.o. administration: mix with milk, juice, or water
- CAVE: safety – rebound effects (hours after intake)

Ciclosporin A

> **Dosage:**
> - always monitor serum levels
> - nephritis in Henoch Schonlein purpura: 4–8 mg/kg/d (control serum levels to 150–200 mcg/l); reduce dose after 6 months
> - myositis: up to max. 5 mg/kg/d, control serum levels to 100–200 mcg/ml
> - autoimmune myasthenia: 3–5 mg/kg/d

Neuropaediatric indications:
- remission or salvage of nephritis in Henoch Schonlein purpura
- therapy-resistant severe myositis
- autoimmune myasthenia

Mechanism of action:
- calcineurin inhibitor
- Binds to calcineurin and thereby blocks binding of calcineurin to the nuclear factor of activated T-Cells in the cytoplasm (NFATc). This prevents dephosphorylation of NFATc, a necessary step for its activation and translocation into the nucleus where it would upregulate.
- the transcription of cytokines and cell surface receptors (including interleukin 2 and gamma-interferon) important in the T-cell response

Relevant contraindications:
- vaccination with live vaccines
- pregnancy
- severe infections
- severe hepatic diseases
- increased uric acid and potassium levels
- < 18 years
- patients with previous Methotrexate therapy
- combination with potassium-sparing diuretics or potassium-containing medication

Relevant side effects and interactions:
- gingiva hyperplasia (especially in combination with Nifedipine), hirsutism, oedema, weight gain
- hypertension, hyperlipidemia
- regular intake of high dosages increases the risk of malignancy
- increased risk of infection
- fibroadenoma, rash, acne
- renal impairment
- headache, fatigue, shiver
- peripheral neuropathy
- nausea, vomiting, diarrhea, gastrointestinal ulcers
- anemia
- epileptic seizures
- amenorrhea
- glucocorticoids increase the tendency for seizures
- increased risk of renal damages: antibiotics (gyrase inhibitors, aminoglycosides, cotrimoxazole), NSAR, fibrates, antiviral drugs, Tacrolimus
- Live vaccines should not be administered. Dead vaccines can lose their efficacy.
- increase of potassium levels by potassium-rich food, potassium-sparing diuretics
- increases the efficacy (and side effects) of oral contraceptives, glucocorticoids, digoxin, colchicines, CSE inhibitors
- ciclosporin is broken down via the cytochrom-P450 system:
  - enzyme induction (= decreased efficacy) is caused by Rifampicin, Isoniazid, Hypericum, Carbamazepine, Phenobarbital, Phenytoin, Efavirenz, Nevirapine
  - enzyme inhibition (= increased efficacy) is caused by Fluconazole, Ketoconazole, Itraconazole, Voriconazole, Clarithromycin, Erythromycin, Telithromycin, Amprenavir, Indinavir, Nelfinavir, Ritonavir, Diltiazem, Nicardipine, Verapamil, grapefruit juice

Approval status:
- depends on the specific product (see SPC)

Sources:
- **Germany – SPC:**
  - **nephrotic syndrome**
    - oral
      - **children:** Dose has to be established depending on efficacy (proteinuria) and safety (serum creatinine level); max. 6 mg/kg/d as 2 separate doses.
      - patients with reduced renal function (CAUTION: contraindicated in children with serum creatinine levels > 140 mmol/l): initial dose should not exceed 2.5 mg/kg/d. Monitor patients carefully and titrate to lowest effective dose. Control renal function continuously in the first three months (normal renal function: every two weeks, reduced renal function: once a week).
      - If serum creatinine levels remain constant, evaluate this parameter every 2 months. Reduce dose by 25–50 %, if serum creatinine levels increase by more than 30 % of the baseline value, even if within normal range.
      - Reduce dose by at least 50 %, if serum creatinine levels increase by more than 50 % of the baseline value.
      - If there is no response to the dose reduction within one month, discontinue ciclosporin treatment.
      - In patients with severe liver disorders, initial dose should be reduced by 25–50 %.
      - note: indication for nephrotic syndrome not specified in SPC

- **USA – T:**
  - **focal segmental glomerulosclerosis**
    - oral
      - **children:** initially 3 mg/kg/d as 2 separate doses
  - **autoimmune diseases**
    - oral
      - **children:** 1–3 mg/kg/d
- **United Kingdom – BNFC:**
  - **nephrotic syndrome**
    - oral
      - **children 1 month– 18 years:** 6 mg/kg/d as 2 separate doses, increase if necessary in corticosteroid-resistant disease; for maintenance, reduce to lowest effective dose according to whole blood ciclosporin concentrations, proteinuria, and renal function
        - note: indication for nephrotic syndrome not specified in SPC

Comments:

- small therapeutic range requires monitoring of blood levels
- Live vaccines should not be administered. Dead vaccines can lose their efficacy.
- combined posterior encephalopathies can occur (PRES – posterior reversible encephalopathy syndrome)

Clobazam (CLB)

Dosage:

- ▶ children between 3 and 15 years: start with 5 mg/d (maintenance dose 0.3–1 mg/kg/d); from 15 years on titrate gradually from 5–15 mg/d up to max. 80 mg/d (SPC)
- ▶ absence: second choice monotherapy with 0.2–1 mg/kg/d as 2 separate doses; target plasma level: 0.1–0.6 mg/l (off-label)
- ▶ hyperekplexia/primary Startle syndrome/congenital Stiff-Person syndrome: 0.5–1.0(–2) mg/kg/d (off-label)

Neuropaediatric indications:

- absence
- hyperekplexia/Startle syndrome/congenital Stiff-person syndrome
- radiation-therapy-associated epilepsy
- anticonvulsive therapy for Angelman syndrome

Mechanism of action:

- benzodiazepine
- opens chloride channels resulting in increased inhibitory function of GABA-ergic neurons especially in the limbic system

Relevant contraindications:

- known hypersensitivity to benzodiazepines
- medication-, drugs-, alcohol addiction
- acute angle-closure glaucoma
- myasthenia gravis
- careful use: severe hepatic damage, ataxia, acute poisoning with alcohol, sopophorics or analgesics, neuroleptics, antidepressants, Lithium, severe chronic respiratory insufficiency, sleep apnea syndrome, pregnancy

Relevant side effects and interactions:

- hypersensitivity reactions
- muscle weakness, dry mouth, gastrointestinal disorders
- temporary elevation of liver function parameters
- fatigue, drowsiness, weakness, vertigo
- headache, confusion, anterograde amnesia, depressive mood
- paradox reactions (e.g. acute agitation, temper tantrums)
- decreased libido
- decreased blood pressure, respiratory depression
- sedation (increased efficacy in combination with other medication, e.g. Phenobarbital)
- in high dosing and long-term treatment:
  - gait and other locomotor problems
  - articulation disorders
  - vertigo
  - addiction, withdrawal syndrome (sudden discontinuation after long term treatment): sleeping disorder and increased dreaming, anxiety, tension, agitation, inner anxiety, shivering, sweating, increased tendency for seizures, and/or symptomatic psychoses
  - impaired vision, double vision, nystagmus
- mutually increased effect when combined with centrally depressant drugs such as alcohol, barbiturates, opioids
- increased effect of muscle relaxants, analgesics and laughing gas
- reduced metabolic breakdown and thus increased effect and prolonged action of Clobazam when used in combination with Cimetidine
- in long-term treatment with centrally acting antihypertensives, beta blockers and anticoagulants, side effects are not predictable in combination with benzodiazepines

Approval status:

- add-on therapy of epilepsy, symptomatic treatment of tension, agitation and anxiety conditions in children aged ≥ 3 years

Sources:
- Germany – SPC:
  - adjunctive therapy for epilepsy, treatment of acute and chronic anxiety and agitation with one or more other anticonvulsive drugs
    - oral
      - **children 3–15 years:** initially 5 mg/d, maintenance with 0.3–1.0 mg/kg/d
      - **adolescents > 15 years:** initially 5–15 mg/d, titrate to max. 80 mg/d
      - **note:** interval therapy with a constant dosage (e.g. 20 mg/d) is recommended
- USA – T: –
- United Kingdom – BNFC:
  - adjunctive therapy for epilepsy, monotherapy under specialist supervision for catamenial (menstruation) seizures (usually for 7–10 d each month, just before and during menstruation), cluster seizures
    - oral
      - **children 1 month–12 years:** initially 0.25 mg/kg/d as 2 separate doses, increased every 5 d to the usual maintenance dose of 0.5 mg/kg/d as 2 separate doses; max. 1 mg/kg/d as 2 separate doses, not exceeding 30 mg/d as 2 separate doses
      - **children 12–18 years:** initially 20 mg/d as 2 separate doses, increased every 5 d to the usual maintenance dose of 20–30 mg/d as 2 separate doses; max. 60 mg/d as 2 separate doses

Comments:
- good add-on medication
- good rescue medication
- development of tolerance
- risk of seizures after sudden discontinuation
- less stable when dissolved in water

Clomethiazole

Dosage:
- 1–3 mg/kg p.o. every 4 h; if no response, increase administration to 2-h intervals (off-label)

Neuropaediatric indications:
- convulsive status epilepticus

Mechanism of action:
- presumably acts as a sedative at the cerebral cortex and the formatio reticularis, hypnotic and anticonvulsive

Relevant contraindications:
- respiratory insufficiency, obstructive respiratory diseases
- severe renal insufficiency, severe liver insufficiency

Relevant side effects and interactions:
- nausea, vomiting, sneezing attacks, allergic reactions
- respiratory depression, sedation, decrease in blood pressure, increased bronchial and salivary secretion
- do not concurrently administer analgesics, barbiturates, psychotropic drugs or other centrally depressant substances

Approval status:
- not approved for paediatric treatment

Sources:
- Germany – SPC:
- Not recommended for use in children
- USA – T: –
- United Kingdom – BNFC: –

Clonazepam

Dosage:
- West syndrome: 0.5–1 mg/kg as 2–4 separate doses p.o.
- paroxysmal non-kinesigenic dyskinesia: young children 1.5–3 mg/d as 3 separate doses, school children 3–6 mg/d as 3 separate doses, adolescents 4–8 mg/d as 3 separate doses p.o.
- essential myoclonus: medication on demand (rare); children > 30 kg: initially 1.5 mg/d as 3 separate doses p.o.; increase by 0.5 mg/d every third day to achieve the desired effect without side effects
- hyperekplexia/primary Startle syndrome/congenital Stiff-person syndrome: 0.1–0.2 mg/kg/d p.o.
- startle epilepsy: 0.1–0.2 mg/kg/d
- status epilepticus:
  - after 5–20 min, if Lorazepam is not available: 0.01–0.05 mg/kg over 1–5 min; max. 0.5 mg/min IV

Neuropaediatric indications:
- rescue medication in West syndrome
- paroxysmal non-kinesigenic dyskinesia
- essential myoclonus
- hyperekplexia/primary Startle syndrome/congenital Stiff-person syndrome
- startle epilepsy

- status epilepticus
- benign hereditary chorea

Mechanism of action:

- benzodiazepine
- opens chloride channels resulting in increased inhibitory function of GABAergic neurons especially in the limbic system

Relevant contraindications:

- known hypersensitivity to benzodiazepines
- medication, drugs, alcohol addiction
- acute angle-closure glaucoma
- myasthenia gravis
- careful use: severe hepatic damages, ataxia, acute poisoning with alcohol, sopophorics or analgesics, neuroleptics, antidepressants, Lithium, severe chronic respiratory insufficiency, sleep apnea syndrome, pregnancy

Relevant side effects and interactions:

- hypersensitivity reactions
- muscle weakness, dry mouth, gastrointestinal disorders
- temporary elevation of liver function parameters
- fatigue, drowsiness, weakness, vertigo, drowsiness
- headache, confusion, anterograde amnesia, depressive mood
- paradox reactions (e.g. acute agitation, temper tantrums)
- decreased libido
- decreased blood pressure, respiratory depression
- sedation (increased in combination with other medication, e.g. Phenobarbital)
- in high dosing and long-term treatment:
  - gait and other locomotor problems
  - articulation disorders
  - vertigo
  - addiction, withdrawal syndrome (sudden discontinuation after long-term treatment): sleeping disorder and increased dreaming, anxiety, tension, agitation, inner anxiety, shivering, sweating, increased tendency for seizures, and/or symptomatic psychoses
  - impaired vision, double vision, nystagmus
- mutually increased effect when combined with centrally depressant drugs such as alcohol, barbiturates, opioids
- increased effect of muscle relaxants, analgesics and laughing gas
- reduced metabolic breakdown and thus increased effect and prolonged action of Clonazepam when used in combination with Cimetidine

- unpredictable side effects in long-term treatment with centrally acting antihypertensives, beta blockers and anticoagulants when used in combination with benzodiazepines

Approval status:

- epilepsy in infants and all forms of status epilepticus

Sources:

- **Germany – SPC:**
  - **epilepsy (typical and atypical petit-mal epilepsy, primary or secondary generalized tonic-clonic seizures)**
    - oral
      - **infants:** initially 0.2 mg/d as 2 separate doses; maintenance with 0.5–1 mg/d as 3–4 separate doses
      - **young children:** 0.6 mg/d as 3 separate doses; maintenance with 1.5–3 mg/d as 3–4 separate doses
      - **school children:** initially 1 mg/d as 2 separate doses; maintenance with 3–6 mg/d as 3–4 separate doses
      - **note:** adjust individually to age and clinical response
- **USA – T:**
  - **seizure disorders:**
    - oral
      - **infants and children < 10 year or < 30 kg:** initially 0.01–0.03 mg/kg/d (max. 0.05 mg/kg/d) as 2–3 separate doses; increase by not more than 0.5 mg every third day until seizures are controlled or adverse effects seen
      - maintenance dose: 0.1–0.2 mg/kg/d as 3 separate doses, max. 0.2 mg/kg/d
      - **children ≥ 10 years and > 30 kg:** initially 1.5 mg/d as 3 separate doses; may be increased by 0.5–1 mg every third day until seizures are controlled or adverse effects seen.
      - maintenance dose: 0.05–0.2 mg/kg/d, max. 20 mg/d
- **United Kingdom – BNFC:**
  - **all forms of epilepsy**
    - oral
      - **children 1 month– 1 year:** initially 0.25 mg at night for 4 nights, increased over 2–4 weeks to the usual maintenance dose of 0.5–1 mg at night (may be given as 3 separate doses if necessary)
      - **children 1–5 years:** initially 0.25 mg at night for 4 nights, increased over 2–4 weeks to the usual maintenance dose of 1–3 mg at night (may be given as 3 separate doses if necessary)
      - **children 5–12 years:** initially 0.5 mg at night for 4 nights, increased over 2–4 weeks to the usual maintenance dose of 3–6 mg at night (may be given as 3 separate doses if necessary)
      - **children 12–18 years:** initially 1 mg at night for 4 nights, increased over 2–4 weeks to the usual maintenance dose of 4–8 mg at night (may be given as 3–4 separate doses if necessary)

Comments:

- efficacy and side effects vary widely between individual patients
- IV/rectal administration is also possible
- IV application as short or extended infusion. Fast injection or injection into small sclerotic veins increases the risk of thrombus formation and thrombophlebitis.

Clonidine

Dosage:
- ▸ initially and escalation regimen: 1.5–3 mcg/kg/d p.o. as 3 separate doses; if necessary, increase every 5–7 d
- ▸ maintenance dose:
  - sedation: 5–25 mcg/kg/d p.o., usually 37.5–150 mcg/d (max. 1.2 mg/d)
  - tic disorder: 3–10 mcg/kg/d p.o. (max. 300 mcg/d)
- ▸ gradual discontinuation: 75 % of dose for 2 d, 50 % of dose for 2 d, 25 % of dose for 2 d

Neuropaediatric indications:
- physical anxiety, especially after traumatic brain injury and chronic substance abuse (in overdosing or severe withdrawal symptoms)
- tic disorder

Mechanism of action:
- sympatholytic; stimulation of central presynaptic α_2-receptors with ensuing decreased presynaptic release of noradrenaline (norepinephrine) resulting in decreased sympathetic tone

Relevant contraindications:
- porphyria
- bradycardia < 50/min, AV block II/III, sick sinus syndrome

Relevant side effects and interactions:
- hypotension (esp. in IV)
- hypertensive crisis after sudden discontinuation
- drowsiness

Approval status:
- depends on the specific product (see SPC)

Sources:
- **Experts' recommendation**: abstinence phenomenon symptom: 20 mcg/kg/d as continuous IV infusion; may be increased
- **Germany – SPC:**
  - **hypertension**
    - oral
      - **children and adolescents < 18 years:** not recommended
- **USA – T:**
  - ADHD
    - oral
      - **children:** initially 0.05 mg/d; increase every 3–7 d by 0.05 mg/d to 3–5 mcg/kg/d as 3–4 separate doses. Some centers use doses as high as 8 mcg/kg/d or 0.5 mg/d
  - **analgesia**
    - epidural (continuous infusion)
      - **children:** initially 0.5 mcg/kg/h; adjust with caution, based on clinical effect; range: 0.5–2 mcg/kg/h, reserved for cancer patients with severe intractable pain
  - **neuropathic pain**
    - oral
      - **children:** initially 2 mcg/kg/dose every 4–6 h; increase incrementally over several days; range: 2–4 mcg/kg/dose every 4–6 h; may also be given as transdermal application (is approximately equivalent to the total oral daily dose)
- **United Kingdom – BNFC:** –

Comments:
- monitor blood pressure when concurrently using antihypertensive drugs

Clopidogrel

Dosage:
- ▸ 1 mg/kg/d (off-label)

Neuropaediatric indications:
- prevention of arterial thrombotic events after cerebral ischaemia in acetyl salicylic acid intolerance

Mechanism of action:
- Inhibition of the ADP-dependant pathway of platelet activation by irreversibly blocking the binding of ADP to the $P2Y_{12}$ receptor. This prevents fibrinogen binding to the glycoprotein IIb/IIIa receptor complex and thus inhibits platelet aggregation.

Relevant contraindications:
- severe renal or liver function disorders
- increased tendency for bleeding
- acute pathologic bleeding (gastrointestinal, cerebral)
- recent heart attack, unstable angina pectoris
- recent ischaemic stroke (less than 7 d ago)
- concurrent intake of coumarins

Relevant side effects and interactions:
- headache, vertigo
- flatulence, gastritis, gastrointestinal ulcers, nausea, vomiting
- increased tendency for bleeding

- hepatic function disorder
- rash, pruritus in hypersensitivity
- very rare: thrombotic-thrombocytopenic purpura
- concurrent intake of other anticoagulants (Phenprocoumon, Heparin, acetyl salicylic acid) increases risk of bleeding
- in combination with NSAIDs: increased risk of gastrointestinal bleedings

Approval status:
- not approved for paediatric treatment

Sources:
- **Germany – SPC:**
  - **prevention of atherothrombotic events**
    - oral
      - **children and adolescents < 18 years:** not recommended
- **USA – T:**
  - reduction of atherothrombotic events (in systemic-to-pulmonary artery shunt, intracardiac or intravascular stent, Kawasaki disease, or arterial graft)
    - **neonates and infants ≤ 24 months:** In PICOLO trial: 0.2 mg/kg/d as a SD, **note:** 79 % of patients received concomitant aspirin, patients < 2 kg and gestational age < 35 weeks)
    - **children > 2 years:** initially 1 mg/kg/d as a SD; titrate to response
- **United Kingdom – BNFC:** –

Comments:
- monitoring of antithrombotic therapy: ADP-induced platelet aggregation

Coenzyme Q10

(Ubiquinone)

Dosage:
- ▶ 400 mg/d p.o.

Neuropaediatric indications:
- usually, therapeutic option in ataxia (controversial)

Mechanism of action:
- Ubiquinone or Coenzyme Q_{10} is a 2,3-dimethoxy-5-methyl benzochinone with a side chain made up of 10 isoprenoid units. It is a natural component of eukaryotic organisms and has a central role in aerobic energy production via the mitochondrial electron transport chain. Coenzyme Q_{10} is the essential electron carrier involved in the oxidative phosphorylation of ADP to ATP and is therefore present in highest concentrations in tissues with high energy demands such as liver, lung, kidney and heart. Because of its variable red-ox state, it also functions as an important mitochondrial antioxidant.

Relevant contraindications:
- none

Relevant side effects and interactions:
- very rarely, increased efficacy of coumarins
- statins and some beta-blockers inhibit endogenous Coenzyme Q_{10}-synthesis by inhibiting mevalonic acid synthesis (cholesterol synthesis)

Approval status:
- not applicable

Sources:
- **Germany – SPC:** –
- **USA – T:** –
- **United Kingdom – BNFC:**
  - **mitochondrial disorders**
    - oral
      - **neonates:** initially 5 mg/dose once or twice daily with food; adjusted according to response up to 200 mg/d if required
      - **children 1 month-18 years:** initially 5 mg/dose once or twice daily with food, adjusted according to response up to 300 mg/d if required
      - note: not specified in SPC as indication of interest

Comments:
- plasma Q_{10} levels in healthy humans: 1 mcmol/l
- daily intake with food 3–10 mg
- physical and psychic exposure increase the demand for Coenzyme Q_{10}
- soluble in organic solvents (acetone, diethyl ether, chloroform) and fats; nearly insoluble in water
- food with high content of Coenzyme Q_{10}: sardines, pork, beef, olive oil, poultry, broccoli, sunflower oil, butter, cheese; whole-grain bread contains a lot of Coenzyme Q_9 that is metabolized to Coenzyme Q_{10} in the liver
- cooking can destroy Coenzyme Q_{10}
- various dosages have been published in common paediatric sources

Creatine monohydrate

Dosage:
- ▶ facio scapulo humeral muscular dystrophy:
  - initially 0.2 g/kg/d
  - maintenance with 0.1 g/kg/d
  - in some controlled studies limited efficacy; the value of frequently recommended intake breaks is questionable
- ▶ Duchenne/Becker muscular dystrophy:
  - 0.2 mg/kg/d, therapy trial over 4–6 weeks, then evaluate response and decide in each individual case whether or not to continue treatment in normal and mild muscle dystrophy, a 5–10 % increase of power and endurance can be achieved. Effect in very weak children is questionable.
- ▶ ensure sufficient fluid intake of at least 50 ml/kg

Neuropaediatric indications:
- facio scapulo humeral muscular dystrophy
- Duchenne/Becker muscular dystrophy

Mechanism of action:
- creatine phosphate provides the phosphoryl group that is required for re-phosphorylation of adenosine diphosphate (ADP), produced at contraction, to adenosine triphosphate (ATP)
- additionally, an increased expression of GLUT4 protein was observed

Relevant contraindications:
- none

Relevant side effects and interactions:
- odor intensive meteorism and diarrhea
- muscle cramps
- water retention in the muscle cells

Approval status:
- not applicable

Sources:
- Germany – SPC: –
- USA – T: –
- United Kingdom – BNFC: –
- Uptodate.com: –

Comments:
- the human body contains 120–150 g
- required daily intake: 2–4 g

Cyclophosphamide

Dosage:
- ▶ Opsoclonus Myoclonus Syndrome (OMS, Kinsbourne encephalitis): 2–8 mg/kg/d
- ▶ PACNS: 0.5–2 mg/kg/d
- ▶ induction of remission in Wegener's granulomatosis: 0.5–2 mg/kg/d
- ▶ myositis: IV, 0.7–1 mg/m^2 body area surface monthly

Neuropaediatric indications:
- Opsoclonus Myoclonus Syndrome (Kinsbourne encephalitis)
- threatening immune diseases (Wegener's granulomatosis, MS, SLE, PACNS, therapy-resistant severe myositis)

Mechanism of action:
- belongs to the group of nitrogen mustards with alkylating effect and is used to treat various types of cancer and immune diseases
- Prodrug, which is converted in the liver to the active metabolites. The most important one is 4-OH-cyclophosphamide/aldophosphamide which is mostly metabolized to carboxycyclophosphamide (by aldehyde dehydrogenase) while a minor proportion of aldophosphamide is degraded to acrolein and phosphoramide mustard. The latter is responsible for the irreversible crosslinking between and within DNA strands at guanidine-N7 positions leading especially in fast-dividing cells to double strand breaks and cell death.
- Important for the indications listed above is the immunosuppressant activity of Cyclophosphamide.

Relevant contraindications:
- severely impaired renal function
- urine passing disorders
- acute hemorrhagic cystitis
- acute infections
- severe bone marrow depression
- pregnancy
- careful use: electrolyte balance disorders, impaired hepatic or renal function

Relevant side effects and interactions:

- leukopenia (dose-dependant bone marrow depression)
- nausea, hair loss
- increased risk of malignant growth, especially leukemias and tumors of the bladder (primarily with high cumulated dosages)
- hemorrhagic cystitis (for prophylaxis, use protective comedication such as 2–5 mercaptoethane sulfonate sodium (MESNA) in parallel with Cyclophosphamide administration)
- infertility (cryopreservation of sperms/ova prior to first administration)
- no intake of alcohol, grapefruits or grapefruit juice
- increased effect of sulfonylurea on lowering blood sugar levels. Myelosuppressive effect with concurrent intake of allopurinol or hydrochlorothiazide
- previous or concurrent treatment with Phenobarbital, benzodiazepines, Phenytoin or Chloral hydrate: induction of microsomal liver enzymes
- decreased response to concurrent vaccination with influenza vaccines and to immunosuppressive drugs
- combination with depolarizing muscle relaxants: decrease of pseudocholinesterase concentration with consequences of long-persisting apnea attacks
- in combination with Chloramphenicol, prolonged half-life and delayed metabolism of Cyclophosphamide
- combination with Anthracyclines and Pentostatin: increased risk of cardiotoxic Cyclophosphamide effect
- combination with Indomethacin: risk of acute water intoxication

Approval status:

- various malignant and autoimmune diseases (see SPC)

Sources:

- **Germany – SPC:**
  - **severe and progredient forms of lupus nephritis, Wegener's granulomatosis**
    - IV
      - **adults:** initially 500–1000 mg/m² body surface
  - no published paediatric dosage for this indication
  - monitor white blood cell count and platelets
- **USA – T:**
  - **SLE**
    - IV
      - **children:** 500–750 mg/m² body surface every month, max. 1 g/m²
  - **nephrotic syndrome**
    - oral
      - **children:** 2–3 mg/kg daily for up to 12 weeks if corticosteroids are unsuccessful

- **vasculitis**
  - IV
    - **children:** 10 mg/kg every 2 weeks
- **United Kingdom – BNFC:**
  - **steroid-sensitive nephrotic syndrome**
    - oral
      - **children 3 months–18 years:** 2–3 mg/kg/d as a SD for 8 weeks
    - IV
      - **children 3 months–18 years:** 500 mg/m² body surface/dose once a month for 6 months
      - **note:** for all other indications consult local treatment protocol for details

D

Danaparoid sodium

Dosage:

▶ thrombosis prophylaxis: 20 U/kg/d as 2 separate doses SC (off-label)
▶ thromboembolism or dissection of brain-supplying arteries in Heparin intolerance II (HIT II): initially 30 U/kg, then 1.2–4 U/kg/h IV (off-label)

Neuropaediatric indications:

- parenteral anticoagulation in HIT II or status post HIT II

Mechanism of action:

- Heparinoid
- factor-X_a inhibition
- is categorized to LMWH by many, but is better tolerated by patients with Heparin intolerance

Relevant contraindications:

- hemorrhagic diathesis
- recent stroke or intracranial procedure
- other predisposition for bleeding
- bacterial endocarditis
- diabetic retinopathy
- advanced hepatic and renal insufficiency

Relevant side effects and interactions:
- bleeding
- thrombopenia
- allergic reactions

Approval status:
- no explicit paediatric approval

Sources:
- **Germany – SPC:**
  - **prophylaxis of deep vein thrombosis in HIT, treatment of thromboembolic disease in HIT**
    - injection
      - **children ≤ 17 years and < 55 kg:** expert knowledge is limited to data obtained with 36 children aged 2 weeks to 17 years.
    - dosing should be based on anti-factor Xa plasma levels of the patient

Clinical situation	Age	Dosage	Anti-factor Xa plasma level
Prophylaxis	≤ 2 years	8–144 U/kg/d	0.1–0.4 U/ml
	9–17 years	20–25 U/kg/d	
Treatment	≤ 2 years	No data	0.4–0.7 U/ml after IV-bolus
	9–17 years	Bolus IV 30 U/kg, 29–130 U/kg/d	0.4–0.8 U/ml in steady state U = Anti-factor Xa units

- **USA – T:** –
- **United Kingdom – BNFC:**
  - **thromboembolic disease in children with history of Heparin -induced thrombocytopenia**
    - IV
      - **neonates:** initially 30 U/kg by IV injection, then by continuous IV infusion with 1.2–2 U/kg/h adjusted according to coagulation activity
      - **children 1 month–16 years:** initially 30 U/kg (max. 1250 U if < 55 kg, 2500 U if ≥ 55 kg) by IV injection, then by continuous IV infusion with 1.2–2 U/kg/h adjusted according to coagulation activity
      - **children 16–18 years:** initially 2500 U (1250 U if < 55 kg, 3750 U if ≥ 90 kg) by IV injection, then by continuous IV infusion with 400 U/h for 2 h, then 300 U/h for 2 h, then 200 U/h for 5 d adjusted according to coagulation activity

Dantrolene

Dosage:
- ▶ initial dose and regimen of escalation:
  - spasticity: < 12 years, 0.5–1 mg/kg/d p.o. as a SD; increase every 7 d in steps of 0.5 mg/kg/d p.o. (then as 3–4 separate doses); > 12 years, 25 mg/d as a SD p.o.; increase every 7 d by 25 mg
  - malignant hyperthermia/severe rhabdomyolysis: 1–2.5 mg/kg IV bolus, repeat every 10 min up to the max. cumulative dose of 10 mg/kg
- ▶ maintenance dose: only spasticity: 8 mg/kg/d as 3–4 separate doses (max. 400 mg/d)

Neuropaediatric indications:
- spasticity (e.g. in cerebral palsy)
- malignant hyperthermia

Mechanism of action:
- prevents the release of Calcium from the sarcoplasmic reticulum presumably by inhibition of the ryanodine receptor

Relevant contraindications:
- hepatic diseases

Relevant side effects and interactions:
- drowsiness, fatigue, weakness, vomiting, diarrhea
- can cause hepatic damages (regular controls)

Approval status:
- spastic syndrome, children from 5 years on

Sources:
- **Germany – SPC:**
  - **spastic syndrome**
    - oral
      - **children (> 5 years, ≥ 25 kg body weight):** initially 1 mg/kg/d
      - week 1: 25 mg/d as a SD
      - week 2: 50 mg/d as 2 separate doses
      - week 3: 75 mg/d as 3 separate doses
      - **children ≥ 50 kg** (same dose as that used for adults)
      - max. 200 mg/d
      - if no response is seen after 6–8 weeks, consider stop of treatment
      - **children < 5 years:** not recommended

- USA – T:
  - **spasticity**
    - oral
      - **children:** initially 0.5 mg/kg/d as a SD for 7 d, increase to 1.5 mg/kg/d as 3 separate doses for 7 d, increase to 3 mg/kg/d as 3 separate doses for 7 d, and then increase to 6 mg/kg/d as 3 separate doses; max. 400 mg/d
      - **note:** titrate to desired effect; if no further benefit is observed at a higher dosage, decrease dose to previous lower dose
  - **malignant hyperthermia**
    - preoperative prophylaxis
    - note: no longer recommended as long as adequate perioperative patient management is provided and Dantrolene is promptly available if needed.
    - oral
      - **children:** 4–8 mg/kg/d as 3–4 separate doses for 1–2 d prior to surgery with the last dose administered approximately 3–4 h before scheduled surgery
    - IV
      - **children:** 2.5 mg/kg over 1 h, 1.25 h prior to surgery
    - crisis management: IV
      - **children:** 2.5 mg/kg; may be repeated as often as necessary until the hypermetabolic state normalized and all symptoms disappeared (typically 1–4 doses; if > 20 mg/kg is used without benefit, consider alternative diagnoses) (Malignant Hyperthermia Association of the U.S. (MHAUS))
    - post-crisis management: IV
      - **MHAUS for children recommendations:** continue therapy with 1 mg/kg/dose every 6 h for at least 24 h after control of symptoms
      - **European recommendations** for children: IV, continue therapy with 10 mg/kg/d for at least 36 h
      - **manufacturer's recommendations** for children: oral, 4–8 mg/kg/d as 4 separate doses for 1–3 d following crisis
- United Kingdom – BNFC: Dantrolene sodium is used
  - **malignant hyperthermia**
    - IV injection (rapid)
      - **children 1 month–18 years:** initially 2–3 mg/kg, then 1 mg/kg repeated as required (total max. dose: 10 mg/kg)
  - **chronic severe spasticity of voluntary muscle**
    - oral
      - **children 5–12 years:** initially 0.5 mg/kg/d as a SD; after 7 d increase to 1.5 mg/kg/d as 3 separate doses; every 7 d increase by further 0.5 mg/kg/dose until achieving satisfactory response, max. 2 mg/kg/dose 3–4 times daily, max. 400 mg/d
      - **children 12–18 years:** initially 25 mg/d as a SD; after 7 d increase to 75 mg/d as 3 separate doses; every 7 d, increase by further 0.5 mg/kg/dose until achieving satisfactory response, max. 2 mg/kg/dose 3–4 times daily, max. 400 mg/d

Comments:
- is typically used in the treatment of hospitalized patients (e. g. early rehabilitation after traumatic brain injury)
- slighter sedation than with Baclofen in effective spasmolytic doses

Dapsone

Dosage:
▶ 1–2 mg/kg/d for 1–2 weeks (off-label)

Neuropaediatric indications:
- relapsing episodes of Henoch Schonlein purpura (no influence on nephritis)

Mechanism of action:
- Dapsone is a sulfone that is thought to kill susceptible bacteria by a similar mode of action as that of sulfonamides, that is via inhibition of the bacterial dihydrofolic acid synthesis.
- immunomodulating and anti-inflammatory effect:
  - inhibits the chemotaxic response of neutrophils, the synthesis of IgG, IgA and of prostaglandins, the degranulation of mast cells and inhibits the lysosomal enzymes
  - inhibits via selective blocking of integrins the attachment of neutrophils to the endothelium and thus reduces diapedesis
  - decreases the release of the β-glucuronidase from macrophages

Relevant contraindications:
- Glucose-6-phosphate-dehydrogenase deficiency
- Hb < 10 g/dl
- hypersensitivity to sulfonamides
- severe hepatic diseases
- children < 5 years of age
- hereditary galactose intolerance, lactase deficiency, glucose-galactose malabsorption

Relevant side effects and interactions:
- dose-dependent hemolysis, agranulocytosis
- methemoglobinemia
- cyanosis
- headache, nausea, stomach trouble
- peripheral motoric neuropathy
- hypoalbuminemia

- exfoliative dermatitis, erythema multiforme
- Dapsone syndrome: fever, malaise, rash, jaundice, lymphadenopathy, mononucleosis, eosinophilia, anemia, methemoglobinemia
- probenecid inhibits elimination of Dapsone

Approval status:
- no explicit paediatric approval

Sources:
- **Germany – SPC:**
- **Leprosy**
  - oral
    - **children < 10 years:** doses have to be adjusted according to body weight
    - **children 10–14 years:** 50 mg/d as a SD
    - **children ≥ 15 years:** 100 mg/d as 2 separate doses
    - note: indication of interest not specified in SPC
- **USA – T:**
- **Prophylaxis against first episode of opportunistic disease caused by Toxoplasma gondii**
  - oral
    - **children ≥ 1 month:** 2 mg/kg or 15 mg/m² BSA (max. 25 mg/dose) once daily in combination with Pyrimethamine 1 mg/kg/d as a SD and Leucovorin 5 mg every 3 d
    - note: indication of interest not specified in SPC
- **United Kingdom – BNFC:** –

Desmopressin

Dosage:
- ▶ enuresis: 0.1–0.2 mg in the evening p.o.; in non-responders the dose can be doubled (= 0.2–0.4 mg)
- ▶ central diabetes insipidus: 5–10 mcg nasal spray (SPC)

Neuropaediatric indications:
- primary nocturnal enuresis
- central diabetes insipidus

Mechanism of action:
- synthetic V2-receptor-specific vasopressin analog
- binds to V2 receptor in the collecting duct system and increases water resorption
- due to the effect at the V1a receptor, endothelial cells secrete factor VIII and von Willebrand factor

Relevant contraindications:
- primary polydipsia
- gestosis
- hyponatremia
- diseases that require a treatment with diuretics
- SIADH (syndrome of inappropriate antidiuretic hormone secretion)
- raised intracranial pressure
- careful use: coronary heart diseases, disorders of the water and electrolyte balance, hypertension

Relevant side effects and interactions:
- frequent: weakness, flush phenomena, conjunctivitis, headache
- occasional: epistaxis, abdominal cramps, nausea, vomiting, decrease or increase in blood pressure, fatigue, red eyes
- rare: angina pectoris, thrombosis
- also possible: hypersensitivity reactions (pruritus, rash, fever, dyspnea, shock, bronchial spasm), hyponatremia, oedema with weight gain, seizures, unconsciousness, coma, raised intracranial pressure

Approval status:
- depends on the specific product (see SPC)

Sources:
- **Germany – SPC:**
  - **diabetes insipidus, polyuria and polydipsia**
    - oral
      - dosing has to be individually adjusted
      - **children:** 0.3 mg/d as 3 separate doses; adjust according to response; usual maintenance with 0.3–0.6 mg/d as 3 separate doses. Interrupt treatment and adjust dosing at signs of water retention/hyponatremia.
  - **primary nocturnal enuresis**
    - oral
      - **children ≥ 5 years:** initially 0.2 mg at bedtime. May be increased to 0.4 mg. Reduce fluid intake before and during bedtime.
      - usual treatment period: 3 months. Interrupt treatment at signs of water retention and/or hyponatremia (headache, vomiting/nausea, weight gain, severe cramps).
      - After 3 months, interrupt treatment for one week to check whether treatment needs to be continued.
- **USA – T:**
  - **diabetes insipidus**
    - oral
      - **children ≤ 12 years:** initially 0.1 mg/d as 2 separate doses, range: 0.1–0.8 mg/d

– **children > 12 years:** initially 0.1 mg/d as 2 separate doses; titrate to desired response, range: 0.1–1.2 mg/d as 2–3 separate doses
- intranasal
  - **children 3 months-12 years:** initially 5 mcg/d as 1–2 separate doses, range: 5–30 mcg/d; adjust morning and evening doses individually for an adequate diurnal rhythm of water turnover.
  - **children > 12 years:** initially 5–40 mcg/d as 1–3 separate doses, adjust morning and evening doses individually for an adequate diurnal rhythm of water turnover
- SC, IV
  - **children < 12 years:** initially 0.1–1 mcg as 1–2 separate doses (Cheetham T: Diabetes Insipidus in children: Pathophysiology, Diagnosis and Management. Paediatr Drugs 2002; 4: 785–796). Initiate at low dose and increase as necessary. Closely monitor serum sodium levels and urine output; fluid restriction is recommended.
  - **children ≥ 12 years:** 2–4 mcg/d as 2 separate doses, adjust morning and evening doses individually for an adequate diurnal rhythm of water turnover.
- **nocturnal enuresis**
  - oral
    - **children ≥ 6 years:** initially 200 mcg/d once before bedtime; titrate as needed to max. 0.6 mg; fluid intake should be limited to a minimum from 1 h before Desmopressin administration until the next morning or for at least 8 h after administration
- **United Kingdom – BNFC:**
  - **test for suspected diabetes insipidus (water deprivation test)**
    - intranasal
      - **neonates:** not recommended; use treatment trial
      - **children 1 month–2 years:** 5–10 mcg as a SD; not usually recommended
      - **children 2–12 years:** 10–20 mcg as a SD; not usually recommended
      - **children 12–18 years:** 20 mcg as a SD; not usually recommended
    - IM or SC injection
    - **neonates:** not recommended; use treatment trial
    - **children 1 month– 2 years:** 0.4 mcg as a SD; not usually recommended
    - **children 2–12 years:** 0.5–1 mcg as a SD; not usually recommended
    - **children 12–18 years:** 1–2 mcg as a SD; not usually recommended
  - **treatment of diabetes insipidus**
    - oral (as Desmopressin acetate)
      - **neonates:** initially 1–4 mcg/dose 2–3 times daily, adjusted according to response
      - **children 1 month–2 years:** initially 10 mcg/dose 2–3 times daily, adjusted according to response; range: 30–150 mcg/d
      - **children 2–12 years:** initially 50 mcg/dose 2–3 times daily, adjusted according to response; range: 100–800 mcg/d
      - **children 12–18 years:** initially 100 mcg/dose 2–3 times daily, adjusted according to response; range: 200–1200 mcg/d
    - sublingual (as Desmopressin base)
      - **children 2–18 years:** initially 60 mcg/dose 3 times daily, adjusted according to response; range: 40–240 mcg/dose 3 times daily
    - intranasal (as Desmopressin acetate)

– **neonates:** initially 0.1–0.5 mcg adjusted according to response; range: 1.25–10 mcg/d as 1–2 separate doses
- **children 1 month–2 years:** initially 2.5–5 mcg/dose 1–2 times daily, adjusted according to response
- **children 2–12 years:** initially 5–20 mcg/dose 1–2 times daily, adjusted according to response
- **children 12–18 years:** initially 10–20 mcg/dose 1–2 times daily, adjusted according to response
- IM, SC injection
  - **neonates:** initially 0.1 mcg/d as a SD, adjusted according to response
    - **note:** IM application only
  - **children 1 month–2 years:** initially 0.4 mcg/d as a SD, adjusted according to response
  - **children 12–18 years:** 1–4 mcg/d as a SD, adjusted according to response
- **primary nocturnal enuresis**
  - oral (as Desmopressin acetate)
    - **children 5–18 years:** 200 mcg at bedtime; increased to 240 mcg at bedtime only if lower dose not effective; reassess after 3 months by withdrawing treatment for at least 1 week
  - sublingual (as Desmopressin base)
    - **children 5–18 years:** 120 mcg at bedtime; increased to 240 mcg at bedtime only if lower dose not effective; reassess after 3 months by withdrawing treatment for at least 1 week

Dexamethasone

Dosage:

▶ tumor-associated cerebral oedema: 0.3 mg/kg/d
▶ pseudotumor cerebri: 1–2 mg/kg/d over 3–5 d; do not titrate, do not reduce gradually. Established maximum dose: 16–32 mg/d
▶ bacterial meningitis (children > 6 weeks): Dexamethasone 10–15 min prior to antibiotic therapy, 0.8 mg/kg/d as 2 separate doses for 2 d
▶ aseptic meningitis under chemotherapy: 0.4 mg/kg/dose every 6–8 h, according to symptoms
▶ opsoclonus Myoclonus Syndrome: 1–2 mg/kg/d, max.16–32 mg/d
▶ headache in radiation therapy: 8–24 mg per day
▶ radiation therapy-associated cerebral oedema: 40 mg bolus IV, then 12–24 mg/d as 3 separate doses IV/p.o. over 3 d

Neuropaediatric indications:

- emergency and perioperative management of tumor-associated cerebral oedema
- pseudotumor cerebri
- bacterial meningitis (> 6 weeks old)
- aseptic meningitis in chemotherapy
- immunomodulatory therapy in chorea minor
- opsoclonus Myoclonus Syndrome (OMS, Kinsbourne encephalitis)

- headache in radiation therapy
- radiation therapy-associated cerebral oedema
- chemotherapy of CNS tumors

Mechanism of action:

- synthetic long-acting glucocorticoid; acts about 30 times stronger than cortisone and does not possess any relevant mineralocorticoid effect

Relevant contraindications:

- acute systemic infection

Relevant side effects and interactions:

- frequent arterial hypertension and hyperglycemia
- irritability
- increased appetite and weight gain
- increased risk of infection
- gastrointestinal bleeding
- osteoporosis
- iatrogenic Cushing's syndrome

Approval status:

- depends on the specific product (see SPC)

Sources:

- Germany – SPC:
  - cerebral oedema
    - oral
      - **children:** 0.4 mg/kg/dose every 12 h for 2 d (as Dexamethasone dihydrogen phosphate), start prior to administration of antibiotics
- USA – T:
  - antiemetic (chemotherapy induced)
    - IV
      - **children:** initially 10 mg/m²/dose (max. 20 mg), then 20 mg/m²/d as 4 separate doses
  - anti-inflammatory
    - oral, IM, IV
      - **children:** 0.08–0.3 mg/kg body weight/d or 2.5–10 mg/m² BSA/d as separate doses every 6–12 h
  - bacterial meningitis
    - IV
      - **infants and children > 6 weeks:** 0.6 mg/kg/d as 4 separate doses for the first 2–4 d of antibiotic treatment; concomitant start of Dexamethasone use has not been shown to improve treatment outcome and is not recommended. For pneumococcal meningitis, available data has not shown clear benefits from Dexamethasone administration; risks and benefits should be considered prior to use.
  - cerebral oedema
    - oral, IV, IM
      - **children:** loading with 1–2 mg/kg/d as a SD; maintenance with 1–1.5 mg/kg/d (max. 16 mg/d) as separate doses every 4–6 h
- United Kingdom – BNFC:
  - inflammatory and allergic disorders
    - oral
      - **children 1 month–18 years:** 0.01–0.1 mg/kg/d as 1–2 separate doses, adjusted according to response; up to 0.3 mg/kg/d may be required in emergency situations
    - IM injection or slow IV injection or infusion
      - **children 1 month–12 years:** 0.083–0.333 mg/kg/d as 1–2 separate doses, max. 20 mg/d
      - **children 12–18 years:** initially 0.4–20 mg/d
  - life-threatening cerebral oedema
    - IV injection
      - **children < 35 kg:** initially 16.7 mg, followed by 3.3 mg every 3 h for 3 d, then 3.3 mg every 6 h for 1 d, then 1.7 mg every 6 h for 4 d, then decrease by 0.8 mg daily
      - **children ≥ 35 kg:** initially 20.8 mg, followed by 3.3 mg every 2 h for 3 d, then 3.3 mg every 4 h for 1 d, then 3.3 mg every 6 h for 4 d, then decrease by 1.7 mg daily
  - bacterial meningitis
    - slow IV injection
      - **children 3 months–18 years:** 0.15 mg/kg/dose (max. 10 mg) every 6 h for 4 d, starting before or with first antibacterial dose

Comments:

- good oral resorption
- vaccination with dead vaccines is possible. The immune reaction and thus the success of vaccination can be impaired when glucocorticoids are used in higher dosages.
- variable published dosage recommendations in common paediatric sources

3,4-Diaminopyridine

Dosage:

▶ no dosage recommendation for children/infants
▶ adult dose (off-label)
  - initial: 30 mg/d as 3 separate doses
  - increase in steps of 5 mg per SD
  - 80 mg/d maximum dose
  - 4-h dosing intervals

Neuropaediatric indications:

- presynaptic disruption of vesicle/transmitter release (e.g. Lambert Eaton (myasthenic) syndrome, LEMS)

Mechanism of action:

– reversible inhibition of voltage-gated (axoplasmic) potassium channels due to/based on interaction with the α-subunit of the channel protein
– leads to increased presynaptic release of acetylcholine (reason for treatment of LEMS)

Relevant contraindications:

– epilepsy

Relevant side effects and interactions:

– in the recommended dose range, no severe side effects are mentioned in the literature
– hypertonia, cardiac arrhythmia
– headache, fatigue, paresthesia, sleep disorder
– epileptic seizures
– states of confusion
– dystonia

Approval status:

– 3,4-Diaminopyridine-phosphate has been licensed as an orphan-drug for the treatment of LEMS in 2002 by the European Medicines Agency (EMA)

Sources:

– **Germany – SPC:** –
– **USA – T:** –
– **United Kingdom – BNFC:** –
– **Uptodate.com:** –

Diazepam (DZP)

Dosage:

▶ rectal (suppository, Diazepam-Rectiole): 0.5–0.7 mg/kg (< 15 kg: 5 mg; > 15 kg: 10 mg)
▶ IV: 0.25–0.5 mg/kg/dose
▶ generalized spasticity: loading dose, 0.25–0.5 mg/kg/d; maintenance dose, up to 1 mg/kg/d

Neuropaediatric indications:

– fever convulsion/cerebral seizure
– acute dystonic reaction
– chronic substance abuse (overdosing or severe withdrawal symptoms)
– status epilepticus
– generalized spasticity (e.g. in cerebral palsy)
– hereditary dysautonomia (Riley-Day syndrome)

Mechanism of action:

– benzodiazepine
– opens chloride channels and thus enhances the inhibitory function of GABAergic neurons, especially in the limbic system

Relevant contraindications:

– known hypersensitivity to benzodiazepines
– medication, drugs, alcohol addiction
– acute angle-closure glaucoma
– myasthenia gravis
– careful use: severe hepatic damage, ataxia, acute poisoning with alcohol, sopophorics or analgesics, neuroleptics, antidepressants, lithium, severe chronic respiratory insufficiency, sleep apnea syndrome, pregnancy

Relevant side effects and interactions:

– hypersensitivity reactions
– muscle weakness, dry mouth, gastrointestinal disorders
– temporary elevation of liver function parameters
– fatigue, weakness, vertigo, drowsiness
– headache, confusion, anterograde amnesia, depressive mood
– paradox reactions (e.g. acute agitation, temper tantrums)
– decreased libido
– decreased blood pressure, respiratory depression
– sedation (increased effect when used in combination with other medication, e.g. Phenobarbital)
– in high dosing and long-term treatment:
  – movement and gait problems
  – articulation disorders
  – vertigo
  – addiction, withdrawal syndrome (on sudden discontinuation after long-term treatment): sleeping disorder and increasing dreaming episodes, anxiety, tension, agitation, inner anxiety, shivering, sweating, increasing tendency for seizures, and/or symptomatic psychoses
  – impaired vision, double vision, nystagmus
– mutual effect enhancement with concurrent intake of centrally depressant drugs such as alcohol, barbiturates, opioids
– increased effect of muscle relaxants, analgesics and laughing gas
– reduced metabolic breakdown and thus increased effect and prolonged action of Diazepam certain when used in combination with Cimetidine or with proton pump inhibitors such as Omeprazole

- unpredictable side effects in long-term treatment with centrally acting antihypertensives, beta blockers and anticoagulants when used in combination with benzodiazepines

Approval status:
- depends on the specific product (see SPC)

Sources:
- Germany – SPC:
  - **status epilepticus**
    - IV, IM
      - **children ≤ 3 years, ≤ 15 kg:** 2–5 mg slow IV or 5–10 mg IM
      - **children > 3 years, > 15 kg:** 5–10 mg slow IV
      - **children > 5 years ≥ 22 kg:** 1 mg slow IV every 2–5 min up to max. 10 mg
      - **children:** max. 20 mg; may be repeated after 2–4 h
  - **muscle hypertonia**
    - **children:** adjust according to age and weight; range of 2–10 mg IM in the evening
    - treatment may be continued with oral dosage forms
- USA – T:
  - **status epilepticus**
    - IV
      - **neonates:** 0.1–0.3 mg/kg/dose injected over 3–5 min and repeated every 15–30 min, to max. total of 2 mg; **note:** not recommended as first-line agent; use only after various other antiepileptic drugs have failed; injection solution contains benzoic acid, sodium benzoate, and benzyl alcohol
      - **infants > 30 d and children:** 0.1–0.3 mg/kg/dose injected over 3–5 min, repeated every 5–10 min, max. 10 mg/dose
      - **manufacturer's recommendation: infants > 30 d and children < 5 years:** 0.2–0.5 mg slow IV every 2–5 min up to a max. dose of 5 mg; repeat in 2–4 h if needed
      - **children ≥ 5 years:** 1 mg slow IV every 2–5 min up to max. dose of 10 mg; repeat in 2–4 h if needed
      - **note:** not recommended as first-line agent
  - **convulsive disorders (acute treatment)**
    - rectal
      - **infants 1–< 6 months:** not recommended; product contains benzoic acid, sodium benzoate, benzyl alcohol, ethanol 10 %, and propylene glycol
      - **children 2–5 years:** 0.5 mg/kg
      - **children 6–11 years:** 0.3 mg/kg
      - **children ≥ 12 years:** 0.2 mg/kg
      - **note:** round dose to the nearest 2.5-mg increment, not exceeding 20 mg/dose; dose may be repeated in 4–12 h if needed; do not use more than 5 times per month or more than once every 5 d
    - **rectal:** undiluted 5 mg/ml; **parenteral:** 0.5 mg/kg/dose followed 10 min later by 0.25 mg/kg as SD if needed
  - **febrile seizure prophylaxis**
    - oral
      - **children:** 1 mg/kg/d as 3 separate doses; initiate therapy at first sign of fever and continue for 24 h after fever resolves
  - **sedation, muscle relaxation, anxiety**
    - oral
      - **children:** 0.12–0.8 mg/kg/d as 3–4 separate doses
    - IM, IV
      - **children:** 0.04–0.3 mg/kg/dose every 2–4 h to max. 0.6 mg/kg within an 8-h period if needed
- United Kingdom – BNFC:
  - **status epilepticus, febrile convulsions, convulsions caused by poisoning**
    - IV injection over 3–5 minutes
      - **neonates:** 0.3–0.4 mg/kg, repeated once after 10 minutes if necessary
      - **children 1 month–12 years:** 0.3–0.4 mg/kg (max. 10 mg), repeated once after 10 minutes if necessary
      - **children 12–18 years:** 10 mg, repeated once after 10 minutes if necessary
    - rectal (as rectal solution)
      - **neonates:** 1.25–2.5 mg, repeated once after 10 minutes if necessary
      - **children 1 month–2 years:** 5 mg, repeated once after 10 minutes if necessary
      - **children 1–12 years:** 5–10 mg, repeated once after 10 minutes if necessary
      - **children 12–18 years:** 10–20 mg, repeated once after 10 minutes if necessary
  - **muscle spasm in cerebral spasticity or in postoperative skeletal muscle spasm**
    - oral
      - **children 1–12 months:** initially 0.5 mg/kg/d as 2 separate doses
      - **children 1–5 years:** initially 5 mg/d as 2 separate doses
      - **children 5–12 years:** initially 10 mg/d as 2 separate doses
      - **children 12–18 years:** initially 20 mg/d as 2 separate doses, max. 40 mg/d

Comments:
- subtherapeutic blood level: < 0.2 mcg/ml
- half-life: 24–48 h
- suppository in status epilepticus:
  - advantage: standard preparation, usually fast onset of action
  - disadvantage: studies on efficacy and safety are dated and do not meet the evidence standards required today
  - in older children and adolescents socially not acceptable application
  - increased risk of accumulation after repeated administration due to the drug's long half-life in circulating blood and its lipophilic properties. The latter facilitates uptake and accumulation in fat tissue from where the drug can slowly diffuse back into the circulation (delayed drug clearance).

Diazoxide

Dosage:

▶ oral p.o. 15–20 mg/kg/d as 2–3 separate doses (SPC)

Neuropaediatric indications:

– hypoglycemia of different causes, especially persistent hypoglycemia due to increased insulin secretion

Mechanism of action:

– opens ATP-sensitive potassium channels in the pancreatic beta cell membrane leading to increased potassium influx into the cell and in turn to hyperpolarization of the cell membrane and closing of the voltage-dependent Ca^{2+} channels. As a result, the intracellular Ca^{2+} level decreases. Because the transmembrane transport of insulin depends on intracellular Ca^{2+} levels, lower Ca^{2+} levels result in decreased insulin secretion.

Relevant contraindications:

– heart attack or heart insufficiency
– careful use: coarctation of the aorta, AV shunt, cardiac diseases, hypotension, neonates with increased bilirubin level

Relevant side effects and interactions:

– allergic reactions
– fatigue, drowsiness, weakness, vertigo, headache
– limited development of lacrimal fluid, impaired vision
– pancreatitis, nausea, vomiting, epigastric problems, cramps, diarrhea
– hyperglycemia, glucosuria, hyperuricemia, prone to gout attacks, increased urea and creatinine levels
– hypotension
– aplastic anemia, leukopenia, agranulocytosis, thrombocytopenia
– increased blood pressure, decreasing effect of antihypertensive drugs
– decreased effect of oral antidiabetics
– water and sodium retention; may require administration of diuretics

Approval status:

– hypoglycemia of different causes in children and adults

Sources:

– **Germany – SPC:**
  – **leucine-sensitive hypoglycemia**
    – oral
      – **children:** 15–20 mg/kg/d as 2–3 separate doses

– **USA – T:**
  – **hyperinsulinemic hypoglycemia**
    – oral
      – **infants:** initially 10 mg/kg/d as 3 separate doses; usual range: 5–20 mg/kg/d as 3 separate doses
      – **children:** initially 3 mg/kg/d as 3 separate doses; usual range: 3–8 mg/kg/d as 2–3 separate doses
      – **note:** Some patients with refractory hypoglycemia may require higher doses.
– **United Kingdom – BNFC:**
  – **chronic intractable hypoglycemia**
    – oral, IV injection
      – **neonates:** initially 10 mg/kg/d as 2 separate doses to establish response; adjust dose according to response; usual maintenance with 1.5–3 mg/kg/dose 2–3 times daily; up to 12 mg/kg/d as 3 separate doses may be required in some cases, higher doses unlikely to be beneficial
      – **children:** initially 5.1 mg/kg/d as 3 separate doses to establish response; adjust dose according to response; usual maintenance with 1.5–3 mg/kg/dose 2–3 times daily; up to 15 mg/kg/d as 3 separate doses may be required in some cases, higher doses unlikely to be beneficial

Diclofenac

Dosage:

▶ acute migraine therapy: 1 mg/kg/dose p.o. (max. 50 mg)
▶ pain amplification syndrome: 2 mg/kg/d

Neuropaediatric indications:

– mild to moderate pain (e.g. migraine)

Mechanism of action:

– non-selective inhibitor of the cyclooxygenases (COX) I and II, resulting in inhibition of prostaglandin synthesis: analgetic, antiphlogistic, antipyretic and antirheumatic
– COX II > COX I

Relevant contraindications:

– hypersensitivity to NSAID
– active bleedings
– children < 15 years of age
– inflammatory bowel in the past
– pre-impaired kidney
– inducible porphyria
– after major surgery
– hematopoesis disorders
– gastrointestinal ulcers

- careful use: acute hepatic porphyria, bronchial asthma, hay fever, nasal polyps, chronic respiratory infections, cardiac insufficiency, hypertension, renal insufficiency, systemic lupus erythematodes and mixed collagenoses

Relevant side effects and interactions:
- gastrointestinal problems
- hematopoesis disorders
- photosensibility of the skin
- elevated transaminase
- vertigo, fatigue
- renal impairment

Approval status:
- depends on the specific product (see SPC)

Sources:
- Germany – SPC:
  - **inflammation and mild to moderate pain**
    - oral
      - **children ≥ 9 years and ≥ 35 kg:** 2 mg/kg/d as 3 separate doses
      - **note:** use low-dosed Diclofenac tablets (e.g. 25 mg)
- USA – T:
  - **acute treatment of mild to moderate pain**
    - oral
      - **children:** 2–3 mg/kg/d as 2–4 separate doses; max. 200 mg/d
- United Kingdom – BNFC:
  - **inflammation and mild to moderate pain**
    - oral, rectal
      - **children 6 months–18 years:** 0.3–1 mg/kg/dose (max. 50 mg) 3 times daily

Comments:
- duration of action: 4(–6) h, sustained release 8(–12) h
- if required, use gastric protection

Dimenhydrinate

Dosage:
- ▶ nausea and vomiting in vertigo:
  - 1–2 mg/kg (repeat every 6 h if necessary)
  - suppository:
    children 6–15 kg: 40 mg/d as a SD
    15–25 kg: 80–120 mg/d as 2–3 separate doses (à 40 mg each),
    25–40 kg: up to 160 mg/d as 4 separate doses (à 40 mg each),
    > 40 kg: up to 280 mg/d as 4 separate doses (à 70 mg each) (SPC)
- ▶ prophylaxis of motion sickness: 1–1.5 mg/kg; repeat after 6 h if necessary

Neuropaediatric indications:
- vertigo

Mechanism of action:
- antihistamine by blocking the H_1-receptors (antihistaminic agent of the first generation)
- also antimuscarinic effect
- readily crosses the blood-brain barrier, i.e. easy access to the CNS

Relevant contraindications:
- hypersensitivity to antihistamines
- acute asthma attack
- angle-closure glaucoma
- pheochromocytoma
- porphyria
- seizures
- last weeks of pregnancy
- concurrent administration of MAOIs
- careful use: pregnancy, impaired liver function, cardiac arrhythmias, chronic breathing problems, asthma, pyloric stenosis, long-term treatment, hypokalemia, hypomagnesemia, bradycardia, cardiac disorder (especially congenital long QT syndrome, coronary heart disease, cardiac conduction disorders (arrhythmias), combination with drugs that prolong the QT interval or lead to hypokalemia)

Relevant side effects and interactions:
- photosensitivity
- muscle weakness
- somnolence, drowsiness, vertigo, mood changes, temporary sleeping disorder
- especially in children: anxiety, agitation, insomnia, shivering

- impaired vision, elevated intraocular pressure
- nausea, pain, vomiting, constipation, diarrhea
- dry mouth, voiding disorders
- cholestatic jaundice
- tachycardia
- allergic skin reactions
- addiction (long-term treatment)
- mutually increased efficacy when used in combination with centrally depressant drugs (psychotropic drugs, hypnotic drugs, sedatives, analgesics, narcotics)
- increased anticholinergic effect of Dimenhydrinate when used together with other anticholinergic drugs
- concurrent intake of MAOIs: life-threatening bowel diseases, urinary retention, elevated intraocular pressure, decrease in blood pressure, respiratory impairment, imparement of brain function
- additive effects on prolongation of the QT interval when used in combination with other drugs that also prolong the QT interval
- torsade de pointes arrhythmias in combination with medication that leads to hypokalemia
- enhanced hypotension in combination with blood pressure decreasing medication
- masking of ototoxic effect with concurrent administration of aminoglycoside antibiotics
- can lead to false-positive results in allergy tests

Approval status:
- prophylaxis and symptomatic therapy of vomiting in children and adults

Sources:
- **Germany – SPC:**
  - **propylaxis and treatment of nausea and vomiting**
    - IM injection
      - **adolescents > 14 years:** 100–300 mg/d, max. 400 mg/d
      - **children 6–14 years:** 25–50 mg/dose 1–3 times daily, max. 150 mg/d
      - **children ≥ 6 kg:** 1.25 mg/kg/dose 1–3 times daily
    - IV injection
      - **adolescents > 14 years:** 62–186 mg/d, max. 400 mg/d
      - **children 6–14 years:** 25–50 mg/dose 1–3 times daily, max. 150 mg/d
      - **children ≥ 6 kg:** 1.25 mg/kg/dose 1–3 times daily
      - **CAUTION:** use very slow IV administration not exceeding 10 ml/2 min
- **USA – T:**
  - **treatment and prevention of nausea, vertigo, and vomiting associated with motion sickness**
    - oral
      - **children 2–5 years:** 12.5 mg–25 mg/dose every 6–8 h; max. 75 mg/d or 5 mg/kg/d or 150 mg/m² body surface/d as 4 separate doses; do not exceed 75 mg/d

- **children 6–12 years:** 25–50 mg/dose every 6–8 h; max.: 150 mg/d or 5 mg/kg/d or 150 mg/m²/d as 4 separate doses; do not exceed 150 mg/d
- **children ≥ 12 years:** 50–100 mg/dose every 4–6 h; do not exceed 400 mg/d
- IM
  - **children 2–5 years:** 1.25 mg/kg or 37.5 mg/m²/dose 4 times daily; max. 75 mg/d
  - **children 6–12 years:** 1.25 mg/kg or 37.5 mg/m²/dose 4 times daily; max. 150 mg/d
  - **children ≥ 12 years:** 50–100 mg/dose every 4 h (also as IV administration)
- **United Kingdom – BNFC:** –

Dipyridamole

Dosage:
▶ 2–5 mg/kg/d (off-label)

Neuropaediatric indications:
- secondary prevention of ischaemic strokes and transient ischaemic attacks

Mechanism of action:
- Inhibits platelet aggregation induced by collagen, ADP or platelet activating factor. In response to two different ways. (1) Inhibits adenosine uptake into and metabolism by erythrocytes, platelets and endothelial cells resulting in locally increased extracellular adenosine levels. Thus, less intracellular adenosine and less ATP are available for vasoconstriction.
- inhibition of phosphodiesterase 5; in thrombocytes an increase of cAMP arises that leads to a decrease of free Ca^{2+} in the cytosol of thrombocytes (reduced aggregation of the thrombocytes) and in the cytosol of smooth muscle cells (vasodilatation)

Relevant contraindications:
- hemorrhagic diathesis, gastrointestinal ulcers
- severe coronary heart diseases
- hereditary galactose-intolerance, deficiency of lactase, glucose-galactose malabsorption
- careful use:
  - analgesics intolerance/analgesics asthma
  - chronic and relapsing gastric or duodenal problems
  - genetically conditioned deficiency of glucose-6-phosphate dehydrogenase
  - pre-existing renal impairment
  - severe disorders of hepatic function
  - heart failure
  - concurrent administration of other anticoagulants, Valproic acid and acetyl salicylic acid (especially in infants and little children)

Relevant side effects and interactions:
- headache, vertigo, nausea, vomiting, diarrhea
- tinnitus, impaired vision or somnolence
- stomach pain, gastrointestinal micro bleeding
- disorders of the acid-base balance, sodium- and water retention
- hypoglycemia
- renal impairment
- decrease of uric acid elimination
- increased risk of bleeding in combination with other anticoagulants
- increased risk of gastrointestinal bleedings when used in combination with cortisone preparations, NSAIDs or alcohol
- enhanced efficacy of antihypertensive drugs and sulfonylurea
- dose adjustments when combined with adenosine intake
- enhanced efficacy of:
  - Digoxin, Triiodothyronine
  - Methotrexate, sulfonamides, Trimethoprim (Cotrimoxazole)
  - Valproic acid, barbiturates, Lithium
- decreased efficacy of:
  - cholinesterase inhibitors
  - spironolactone, canrenoate, loop diuretics, probenecid, sulfinpyrazone

Approval status:
- no explicit paediatric approval

Sources:
- Germany – SPC:
  - **prevention of ischaemic stroke**
    - oral
      - **children:** not recommended
- USA – T:
  - **maintain patency after surgical grafting procedures**
    - oral
      - **children:** 3–6 mg/kg/d as 3 separate doses
- United Kingdom – BNFC:
  - **Kawasaki syndrome (mucocutaneous lymph node syndrome)**
    - oral
      - **children 1 month–12 years:** 3 mg/kg/d as 3 separate doses
  - **prevention of thrombus formation after cardiac surgery**
    - oral
      - **children 1 month–12 years:** 5 mg/kg/d as 2 separate doses
      - **children 12–18 years:** 300–600 mg/d as 3 separate doses

Comments:
- monitoring of the antiplatelet therapy: ADP-induced platelet aggregation

Doxepin

Dosage:
▶ chronic substance abuse (overdosing or severe withdrawal symptoms): 10–100 mg/d

Neuropaediatric indications:
- chronic substance abuse (overdosing or severe withdrawal symptoms)

Mechanism of action:
- tricyclic antidepressive
- unselectively inhibits serotonin and noradrenaline reuptake at the presynaptic membrane thereby increasing their availability

Relevant contraindications:
- acute intoxication with hypnotic drugs, analgesics, psychotropic drugs, alcohol
- acute delirium
- untreated angle-closure glaucoma
- acute urinary retention
- paralytic ileus
- children < 12 years of age
- SC, i.a. or paravenous injection
- MAOI (discontinue 2 weeks prior to start of treatment)
- combination with QT-interval prolonging drugs
- careful use: severe liver damage, disorders of hematopoesis, organic brain syndrome (provocation of a drug-induced psychosis), increased predisposition for seizures, acute hypokalemia, bradycardia, clinically significant cardiac disorder, 12–18 years of age

Relevant side effects and interactions:
- especially anticholinergic side effects such as dry mouth, mydriasis, accommodation impairment, hypotension, tachycardia, gastrointestinal problems, voiding disorders, drug-induced psychosis
- cardiac arrhythmia
- change in blood count: leukopenia, agranulocytosis
- may increase the risk of breast cancer
- do not combine with drugs that prolong the QT interval or with medication that leads to hypokalemia

Approval status:

– depends on the specific product (see SPC)

Sources:
– **Germany – SPC:**
  – **sleeping disorders, agitation and anxiety due to depressive disorders or abstinence phenomenon symptom**
    – oral
      – **children < 12 years:** do not use in this patient group
      – **children > 12 years:** is not recommended. Only in exceptional cases: use significantly lower doses than in adults.
– **USA – T:**
  – **treatment of various forms of depression**
    – oral
      – **note:** not FDA approved for paediatric patients
      – **manufacturer's recommendation:** do not use in children < 12 years
      – some centers use the following doses:
      – **children:** 1–3 mg/kg/d as a SD or separate doses
      – **adolescents:** initially 25–50 mg/d as a SD or separate doses, gradually increase to 100 mg/d
– **United Kingdom – BNFC:**
  – **depressive illness, particularly where sedation is required**
    – oral
      – **children 12–18 years:** initially 75 mg/d as separate doses or as SD at bedtime, adjusted according to response; usual maintenance dose: 30–300 mg/d (> 100 mg/d as 3 separate doses)

Comments:
– during long-term treatment, the sedative effect often decreases
– the desired improvement in mood is usually attained after about 2–3 weeks of treatment
– closely monitor suicidal or severely depressive patients especially in the early stages of treatment
– before and during treatment, regularly monitor blood pressure, blood count, liver function, ECG and possibly EEG. If there are any abnormality, treatment should only continue if close monitoring is ensured

Doxycycline

Dosage:
▶ > 9 years: 2–4 mg/kg/d as 1–2 separate doses (max. 0.4 g/d); duration: 4 weeks

Neuropaediatric indications:
– neuroborreliosis (only in exceptional cases)

Mechanism of action:
– tetracycline
– inhibition of protein synthesis in susceptible bacteria. Doxycycline binds to the 30S subunit of the ribosome, preventing attachment of the charged aminoacyl-tRNA to the A site on the ribosome and thereby interrupting peptide chain elongation.

Relevant contraindications:
– hypersensitivity to tetracyclines
– severe hepatic dysfunction
– renal insufficiency
– < 8 years, use only in vital indications

Relevant side effects and interactions:
– pyrosis, abdominal or stomach tenderness, bloating, meteorism, diarrhea
– pseudomembranous colitis
– phototoxic reaction of light-exposed skin locations (erythema, skin oedema, development of blisters)
– exanthema, erythema, pruritus, urticaria, exfoliative dermatitis, fixed drug exanthema, erythema multiforme exsudativum (Stevens-Johnson syndrome), angiooedema, bronchial spasms, anaphylactic shock
– children < 8 years:
  – reversibly slowed-down bone growth
  – irreversible discolouration of the teeth and enamel damage
– increased intracranial pressure (headache, nausea, vomiting)
– leukopenia, thrombocytopenia, anemia, atypical lymphocytes, leukocytoses, toxic granulation of granulocytes
– hoarseness, difficulty swallowing, black hair tongue
– reduced Doxycycline absorption caused by antacids, milk, iron salts, Activated charcoal
– renal failure when used in combination with methoxyflurane
– enhanced efficacy of oral antidiabetics and oral anticoagulants
– accelerated break down of Doxycycline when used in combination with barbiturates, Carbamazepine, Phenytoin, Primidone

- increased Ciclosporin toxicity
- impaired efficacy of oral contraceptives
- increased digoxin plasma levels and Methotrexate toxicity

Approval status:
- depends on the specific product (SPC)

Sources:
- Germany – SPC:
  - lyme disease
    - oral
      - **children > 8 years or > 50 kg:** 200 mg/d for 2–3 weeks
- USA – T:
  - lyme disease
    - oral
      - **children ≥ 8 years and > 45 kg:** 200 mg/d as 2 separate doses for 14–21 d
- United Kingdom – BNFC:
  - lyme disease
    - oral
      - **children 12–18 years:** 200 mg/d for 10–14 d (for 28 d in lyme arthritis)
  - susceptible infections
    - oral
      - **children 12–18 years:** 200 mg/d on first day, then 100 mg/d; severe infections, 200 mg/d

E

Edrophonium chloride

Dosage:
▶ 0.1 mg/kg IV over 1 min (off-label)

Neuropaediatric indications:
- diagnostic agent in myasthenia gravis (Tensilon®test)

Mechanism of action:
- short-acting acetylcholinesterase inhibitor

Relevant contraindications:
- relative: bradycardiac arrhythmias, AV block
- absolute: bronchial asthma, mechanic obstruction of the gastrointestinal or the urogenital tract

Relevant side effects and interactions:
- only short duration of efficacy
- nausea, vomiting, diarrhea, sialorrhea and lacrimation
- increased bronchial secretion, bronchoconstriction, apnea
- Edrophonium combined with Atropine is not effective against depolarizing neuromuscular blocking agents.

Approval status:
- not applicable

Sources:
- Germany – SPC: –
- USA – T:
  - diagnosis of myasthenia gravis
    - IM, SC
      - **infants:** initial dose 0.5–1 mg
      - **children: ≤ 34 kg:** initially 2 mg
      - **children: > 34 kg:** initially 5 mg
    - IV
      - **infants:** initially 0.1 mg, followed by 0.4 mg (if no response); total dose = 0.5 mg
      - **children:** initially 0.04 mg/kg over 1 min, followed by 0.16 mg/kg given within 45 sec (if no response); max. dose = 10 mg in total
      - or manufacturer's recommendation:
        - **children ≤ 34 kg:** 1 mg; if no response after 45 sec, repeat injections in 1 mg increments every 30–45 sec to a total of 5 mg
        - **children > 34 kg:** 2 mg; if no response after 45 sec, repeat in 1 mg increments every 30–45 sec to a total of 10 mg
- United Kingdom – BNFC:
  - diagnostic test for myasthenia gravis
    - IV injection
      - **children 1 month–12 years:** 0.02 mg/kg, followed after 30 sec (if no adverse reaction has occurred) by 0.08 mg/kg
      - **children 12–18 years:** 2 mg, followed after 30 sec (if no adverse reaction has occurred) by 8 mg

Ephedrine

Dosage:

▶ 0.9–4 mg/kg/d as 3–4 separate doses; max. 60 mg/d p.o.

Neuropaediatric indications:

– disorders of cholinesterase (not all patients respond)

Mechanism of action:

– in contrast to adrenaline: central efficacy
– Ephedrine is a β-sympathomimetic, not selective to $β_1$- and $β_2$-adrenoreceptors
– in addition, indirectly α-sympathomimetic

Relevant contraindications:

– hypertension
– thyrotoxicosis
– pheochromocytoma
– angle-closure glaucoma
– voiding dysfunction with residual urine
– careful dosing in severe organic changes in heart and blood vessels and in cardiac arrhythmias

Relevant side effects and interactions:

– muscle tremor
– central agitation
– palpitations, ventricular arrhythmias
– difficulty voiding
– in overdosing: anxiety, voiding urge, central and myogenic tachycardia, increased blood pressure, extrasystoles, insomnia, optic and acoustic hallucination, seizures, hyperthermia, circulatory collapse, dyspnea
– cardiac arrhythmias in combination with Halothane
– combination with Guanethidine: direct α-sympathomimetic efficacy enhanced and Guanethidine efficacy antagonized

Approval status:

– not applicable

Sources:

– **Germany – SPC:** –
– **USA – T:**
  – **adjunctive agent in the treatment of shock: use the smallest effective dose for the shortest time**
  – IM, SC, IV

– **children < 12 years:** 3 mg/kg/d as 4–6 separate doses
– **children ≥ 12 years:** 25–50 mg (range: 10–50 mg); may repeat with a second dose of 50 mg; not to exceed 150 mg/24 h; IV: 10–25 mg; may repeat with a second dose in 5–10 min of 25 mg; not to exceed 150 mg/24 h
– **note:** indication of interest is not specified in SPC
– **United Kingdom – BNFC:** –

Eslicarbazepine

Dosage:

▶ maintenance dose: 800–1200 mg/d as 2 separate doses
▶ titration: first week 400 mg/d, increase according to target dose by 400 mg/d once weekly

Neuropaediatric indications:

– additional treatment of focal seizures with or without generalization

Mechanism of action:

– antiepileptic drug
– blocks sodium channels

Relevant contraindications:

– second- and third-degree atrioventricular block, known hypersensitivity to Eslicarbazepine or other ingredients of the preparation, carboxamide derivatives

Relevant side effects:

– vertigo, drowsiness
– headache, abnormal coordination, attention deficiency, tremor
– diplopia, blurred vision
– vertigo
– nausea, vomiting, diarrhea
– rash
– fatigue, gait disorders
– anemia
– hypersensitivity
– hypothyroidism
– increased/decreased appetite, hyponatremia, imbalance of electrolytes, cachexia, dehydration, obesity
– insomnia, apathy, depression, nervousness, agitation, ADHD/hyperactivity syndrome, confusion, mood changes, crying, psychomotor inhibition, stress, psychosis

- disturbed memory, disturbed sense of equilibrium, amnesia, sleep addiction, sedation, aphasia, dysesthesia, dystonia, lethargy, smell disorder, imbalance of the autnomous nervous system, cerebellar ataxia, cerebellar syndrome, generalized tonic-clonic seizures (grand mal seizures), peripheral neuropathy, nystagmus, speaking disorder, disorders in sleep pattern, dysarthria, hypoesthesia, loss of sense of taste (ageusia), burning body feeling
- impaired vision, oscillopsia, binocular eye movement disorder, okucar hyperemia, galvanic eye movement, ocular pain
- ear pain, defective hearing, tinnitus
- palpitations, bradycardia, sinus bradycardia
- hypertension, hypotension, orthostatic hypotension
- dysphonia, epistaxis
- dyspepsia, gastritis, stomach pain, dry mouth, abdominal/stomach malaise, flatulence, duodenitis, gingival hyperplasia, gingivitis, irritable bowel syndrome, tarry feces, painful swallowing, stomatitis, aching teeth
- hepatic diseases
- alopecia, dry, increased sweating, erythema, nail diseases, skin diseases
- muscle pain, back pain, neck pain
- nocturia
- irregular menstruation
- asthenia, malaise, shivering, peripheral oedema, peripheral cold sensation
- decreased blood pressure, weight loss, decreased diastolic blood pressure, increased blood pressure, decreased systolic blood pressure, decreased blood sodium, decreased hematocrit, decreased hemoglobin, increased heart rate, increased transaminase, increased triglycerides, decreased free tri-iodothyronine (T3), decreased free thyroxin (T4)
- joint injuries, intoxication, skin injuries
- thrombocytopenia, leukocytopenia
- pancreatitis

Interactions:
- interaction studies have only been performed in adults.
- Eslicarbazepine acetate is extensively converted to Eslicarbazepine, which is mainly eliminated by glucuronidation. *In vitro*, Eslicarbazepine is a weak inducer of CYP3A4 and UDP-glucuronyl transferases. *In vivo*, Eslicarbazepine increased the metabolic rate of drugs that are mainly eliminated via CYP3A4. Thus, the dose of those drugs may need to be increased when used concomitantly with Eslicarbazepine acetate. Eslicarbazepine *in vivo* may also increase the metabolic rate of drugs that are mainly eliminated by conjugation through the UDP-glucuronyl transferases. When initiating or discontinuing treatment with Zebinix or changing the dose, it may take 2 to 3 weeks to reach the new level of enzyme activity. This time delay must be taken into account when Zebinix is being used just prior to or in combination with other drugs that require dose adjustment when co-administered with Zebinix. Eslicarbazepine has inhibiting properties with respect to CYP2C19. Thus, interactions can arise when co-administering high doses of Eslicarbazepine acetate with drugs that are mainly metabolized via CYP2C19.

Interactions with other antiepileptic drugs
- *Carbamazepine:* In a study in healthy subjects, concomitant administration of Eslicarbazepine acetate 800 mg once daily and Carbamazepine 400 mg twice daily resulted in an average decrease of 32 % in exposure to the active metabolite Eslicarbazepine, most likely caused by an induction of glucuronidation. No change in exposure to Carbamazepine or its metabolite Carbamazepine-epoxide was noted. Based on individual response, the dose of Eslicarbazepine acetate may need to be increased if used concomitantly with Carbamazepine. Results from patient studies showed that concomitant treatment increased the risk of the following adverse reactions: diplopia (11.4 % of subjects with concomitant Carbamazepine, 2.4 % of subjects without concomitant Carbamazepine), abnormal coordination (6.7 % with concomitant Carbamazepine, 2.7 % without concomitant Carbamazepine), and dizziness (30.0 % with concomitant Carbamazepine, 11.5 % without concomitant Carbamazepine). The risk of increase of other specific adverse reactions caused by co-administration of Carbamazepine and Eslicarbazepine acetate cannot be excluded.
- *Phenytoin:* In a study in healthy subjects, concomitant administration of Eslicarbazepine acetate 1200 mg once daily and Phenytoin resulted in an average decrease of 31–33 % in exposure to the active metabolite, Eslicarbazepine, most likely caused by an induction of glucuronidation, and an average increase of 31–35 % in exposure to Phenytoin, most likely caused by an inhibition of CYP2C19. Based on individual response, the dose of Eslicarbazepine acetate may need to be increased and the dose of Phenytoin may need to be decreased.
- *Lamotrigine:* Glucuronidation is the major metabolic pathway for both Eslicarbazepine and Lamotrigine and therefore an interaction could be expected. A study in healthy subjects with Eslicarbazepine acetate 1200 mg once daily showed a minor average pharmacokinetic interaction (exposure of Lamotrigine decreased by 15 %) between Eslicarbazepine acetate and Lamotrigine and consequently no dose adjustments are required. However, due to inter-individual variability, the effect may be clinically relevant in some individuals.
- *Topiramate:* In a study in healthy subjects, concomitant administration of Eslicarbazepine acetate 1200 mg once daily and Topiramate showed no significant change in exposure to Eslicarbazepine but an 18 % decrease in exposure to Topiramate, most likely caused by a reduced bioavailability of Topiramate. No dose adjustment is required.

– *Valproic acid and Levetiracetam:* A population pharmacokinetics analysis of phase III studies in epileptic adult patients indicated that concomitant administration with Valproic acid or Levetiracetam did not affect the exposure to Eslicarbazepine but this has not been verified by conventional interaction studies.

Other drugs
– *oral contraceptives:* Administration of Eslicarbazepine acetate 1200 mg once daily to female subjects using a combined oral contraceptive showed an average decrease of 37 % and 42 % in systemic exposure to levonorgestrel and ethinylestradiol, respectively, most likely caused by an induction of CYP3A4. Therefore, women of childbearing potential must use adequate contraception during treatment with Zebinix, and up to the end of the current menstruation cycle after the treatment has been discontinued.
– *Simvastatin:* A study in healthy subjects showed an average decrease of 50 % in systemic exposure to Simvastatin when co-administered with Eslicarbazepine acetate 800 mg once daily, most likely caused by an induction of CYP3A4. An increase of the Simvastatin dose may be required when used concomitantly with Eslicarbazepine acetate.
– *Rosuvastatin:* There was an average decrease of 36–39 % in systemic exposure in healthy subjects when co-administered with Eslicarbazepine acetate 1200 mg once daily. The mechanism for this reduction is unknown, but could be due to interference of transporter activity for Rosuvastatin alone or in combination with induction of its metabolism. Since the relationship between exposure and drug activity is unclear, the monitoring of response to therapy (e. g., cholesterol levels) is recommended.
– *Warfarin:* Co-administration of Eslicarbazepine acetate 1200 mg once daily with Warfarin showed a small (23 %) but statistically significant decrease in exposure to S-Warfarin. There was no effect on the R-Warfarin pharmacokinetics or on coagulation. However, due to inter-individual variability in the interaction, special attention on monitoring of INR should be performed the first weeks after initiation or ending concomitant treatment of Warfarin and Eslicarbazepine acetate.
– *Digoxin:* A study in healthy subjects showed no effect of Eslicarbazepine acetate 1200 mg once daily on Digoxin pharmacokinetics, suggesting that Eslicarbazepine acetate has no effect on the transporter P-glycoprotein.
– *Monoamino Oxidase Inhibitors (MAOIs):* Based on the structural relationship of Eslicarbazepine acetate to tricyclic antidepressants, interaction between Eslicarbazepine acetate and MAOIs could be expected.

Approval status:
– adjunctive therapy in adults with partial-onset seizures with or without secondary generalization
– not approved for children and adolescents

Sources:
– **Germany – SPC:**
  – **adjunctive therapy in seizures:**
  – **children and adolescents < 18 years:** not recommended; safety and efficacy have not been established
– **USA – T:** –
– **United Kingdom – BNFC:** –
– **Uptodate.com:** –
  – **Drugdex®:** safety and efficacy have not been established in patients younger than 18 years

Comments:

no paediatric data is available

Etanercept

Dosage:
▶ 4–18 years: 0.4 mg/kg (max. 25 mg) 2 x/week in intervals of 3–4 d SC (positive effects in some cases are reported) (in myositis off-label)

Neuropaediatric indications:
– therapy-resistant severe myositis (positive effects in some cases are reported)

Mechanism of action:
– possesses the ligand binding domain of human TNF 2, which enables Etanercept to bind TNF-α and thus inhibits interaction of cytokines with membrane receptors
  – reduces the effect of naturally present TNF
  – is a TNF inhibitor, functioning as a decoy receptor that binds to TNF
  – is produced by monocytes, macrophages and activated T-cells and participates in many immunomediated inflammatory processes
  – activates the expression of adhesion molecules on the surface of endothelial cells that promote the influx of leukocytes into the interstitium
  – stimulates the release of metallomatrix proteases
  – under the influence of TNF-α, increased production of inflammatory-promoting cytokines such as interleukin-1, -6 and -8

Relevant contraindications:
– sepsis
– risk of sepsis
– active tuberculosis
– prematures and neonates
– < 3 years of age

- careful use: acute infections, < 3 years, inactive tuberculosis, HBV infections or suspected HBV infections, abnormal blood count, concurrent vaccination with live vaccines, varicella virus exposure, increased risk of infections, newly established CNS-demyelinating disease, heart failure, combination with anakinra or abatacept, Wegener's granulomatosis

Relevant side effects and interactions:

- local irritation at the injection site
- hypersensitivity reactions
- severe infections, deterioration of current infections
- interstitial lung disease, dyspnea, asthma
- hypertension
- thrombozytopenia, anemia, leukopenia, neutropenia, pancytopenia, aplastic anemia
- fever
- increased blood levels of hepatic enzymes
- pruritus, urticaria
- subacute cutaneous or discoid lupus erythematodes
- deep venous thrombosis, thrombophlebitis, lung embolism
- malignant diseases (especially breast cancer, bronchial cancer, lymphoma)
- membranous glomerulopathy, kidney stones, renal insufficiency
- heart failure, myocardial infarction
- syncope
- cerebral ischaemia
- pancreatitis, gastrointestinal bleeding
- especially in children and adolescents: headache, nausea, vomiting, abdominal pain, varicella infections with signs and symptoms of aseptic meningitis, appendicitis, gastroenteritis, depression/personality disorder, skin ulcers, esophagitis/gastritis, septic shock, diabetes type I, soft tissue infection, postoperative wound infection
- combination with sulfasalazine leads to decreased leukocytes
- combination with anakinra increases the risk of severe infections and neutropenia
- increased side effects when combined with abatacept

Approval status:

- active polyarticular juvenile idiopathic arthritis in children and adolescents (4–17 years) after insufficient response to or incompatibility with MTX-therapy

Sources:

- **Germany – SPC:**
- indication of interest is not specified in SPC
- **USA – T:**
- **Juvenile idiopathic arthritis**
  - SC
- **children 2–17 years:** 0.4 mg/kg/dose given twice weekly 72–96 h apart; max. dose: 25 mg; alternatively 0.8 mg/kg/dose once weekly; max. dose: 50 mg
- indication of interest is not specified in SPC
- **United Kingdom – BNFC:** –

Comments:

- approved indication: rheumatoid arthritis

Ethosuximide (ESM)

Dosage:

- ▶ initially 5–10 mg/kg/d; increase by 5 mg/kg/d every 4–7 d, maintenance with 20–40 mg/kg/d as 1–3 separate doses (SPC)
- ▶ absences: Monotherapy as a first choice: 15–30 mg/kg/d as 2–3 separate doses; target serum level: 40–100 mg/l
- ▶ juvenile myoclonic epilepsy: 15 mg/kg/d
- ▶ epilepsy in Angelman syndrome: 20 mg/kg/d as 2–3 separate doses

Neuropaediatric indications:

- absence epilepsy
- myoclonic seizures (juvenile myoclonic epilepsy)
- atypical benign partial epilepsy
- anticonvulsive therapy in Angelman syndrome

Mechanism of action:

- a T-type Ca^{2+} channel blocker that reduces Calcium influx into the thalamic neurons resulting in reduced neuronal excitability
- increases the GABAergic inhibitory synaptic transmission by inhibiting the intraictal Calcium influx into the cell

Relevant contraindications:

- porphyria
- known hypersensitivity
- careful dosing in patients with psychiatric diseases in anamnesis (e.g. anorexia)

Relevant side effects and interactions:

- nausea, vomiting, hiccup, fatigue, headache, vertigo, weight loss, appetite disorders
- exanthema up to Stevens-Johnson syndrome
- lupus erythematodes
- depression, movement disorder, psychoses

- rare: blood count changes (aplastic anemia, thrombocytopenia, leukopenia, pancytopenia, eosinophilia)
- enhanced efficacy of Phenytoin (increased plasma levels)
- Carbamazepine leads to decreased plasma levels of Ethosuximide
- Valproic acid leads to increased plasma levels of Ethosuximide

Approval status:

- childhood absence epilepsy (also called petit mal epilepsy; myoclonic-astatic, impulsive)

Sources:

- **Germany – SPC:**
  - **absences, myoclonic seizures, complex and atypical absences**
    - oral
      - **infants and children < 2 years:** initially 125 mg/d; increase gradually over a few days until seizures controlled.
      - **children 2–6 years:** initially 250 mg/d; increase gradually over a few days until seizures controlled.
      - **children ≥ 6 years:** initially 500 mg/d maintenance dose: Dosage may be gradually increased, for example every 5 to 7 days by 250 mg, until achieving optimal seizure control and reaching a dosage of 1000–1500 mg/d. Dosages up to 2000 mg/d could be necessary in some patients.
      - **children:** for most paediatric patients the optimal dose is 20 mg/kg/d as several separate doses; max. 1000 mg/d
- **USA – T:**
  - **management of absence (petit mal) epilepsy, of myoclonic seizures and akinetic epilepsy**
    - oral
      - **children < 6 years:** initially 15 mg/kg/d as 2 separate doses, max. 250 mg/dose, increase every 4–7 d; usual maintenance with 15–40 mg/kg/d as 2 separate doses; max. 1.5 g/d
      - **children> 6 years:** initially 500 mg/d as 2 separate doses: increase by 250 mg as needed every 4–7 d up to 1.5 g/d as 2 separate doses; usual maintenance with 20–40 mg/kg/d as 2 separate doses
- **United Kingdom – BNFC:**
  - **absence seizures, atypical absence, myoclonic seizures**
    - oral
      - **children 1 month–6 years:** initially 5 mg/kg/dose (max. 125 mg) twice daily; increase gradually over 2–3 weeks up to a maintenance dose of 10–20 mg/kg (max. 500 mg) twice daily; in isolated cases, total daily dose may be given as 3 separate doses
      - **children 6–8 years:** initially 500 mg/d as 2 separate doses; increased by 250 mg at intervals of 4–7 d to usual dose of 1000–1500 mg/d as 2 separate doses; occasionally, up to 2 g/d as 2 separate doses may be needed

Comments:

- the medication has an extremely unpleasant taste
- advise parents to immediately inform the physician if fever, ulcerations, haematomas or bleedings occur

F

Felbamate (FBM)

Dosage:
- ▶ 4–14 years: 7.5–45 mg/kg/d (max. 3600 mg/d) as 2–4 separate doses (SPC)
- ▶ > 14 years: 600–3600 mg/d (max. 3600 mg/d) as 2–4 separate doses (SPC)

Neuropaediatric indications:

- adjunctive therapy in therapy-resistant Lennox-Gastaut syndrome
- focal and secondary generalized seizures

Mechanism of action:

- has not been completely understood
- presumably inhibits the NMDA receptor by binding to its glycine-binding site
- also increases GABAergic signaling

Relevant contraindications:

- liver function disorder
- renal insufficiency
- neutropenia, thrombopenia
- hereditary galactose intolerance, lactase deficiency, glucose-galactose malabsorption

Relevant side effects and interactions:

- nausea, vomiting, loss of appetite, weight loss
- headache, sleeping disorder, blurred vision, disturbances of equilibrium
- dose-independent aplastic anemia (1 : 3000; lethal in approx. 30 %)
- acute hepatic failure (1 : 7000; lethal in approx. 60 %)
- combination with Carbamazepine may lead to increased plasma clearance of both Felbamate and Carbamazepine but decreased plasma clearance of Carbamazepine-10,11-epoxide. The resulting increased plasma Carbamazepine epoxide levels increase the risk of Carbamazepine side effects.
- inhibits Phenytoin – elimination; Phenytoin may decrease plasma Felbamate levels
- decreased plasma Valproic acid levels
- interactions of Clonazepam, Oxcarbazepine, and Vigabatrin with Felbamate can not be excluded
- interactions with medications that are metabolized by the cytochrome P-450 system

Approval status:
- add-on therapy for therapy-resistant Lennox-Gastaut syndrome in patients > 4 years of age

Sources:
- Germany – SPC:
  - adjunctive therapy for treatment of Lennox-Gastaut syndrome
    - oral
      - **children 4–14 years:**
      - **note:** in combination with Carbamazepine, Phenytoin, Phenobarbital or Valproic acid the frequency of adverse effects may rise.
        - initially 7.5–15 mg/kg/d as 2–3 separate doses. In the beginning, reduce concomitant antiepileptic drugs by 20–30 %. In intervals of at least 1 week titrate dose by 7.5–15 mg/kg up to max. 45 mg/kg/d (max. 3600 mg/d) as 3–4 separate doses (beware of accumulation of concomitant antiepileptic drugs). Possible accumulation of concomitant drugs should be assessed based on both steady state serum levels and clinical response.
- USA – T:
  - **Lennox-Gastaut syndrome**
    - oral
      - **children 2–14 years:** adjunctive therapy, initially 15 mg/kg/d as 3–4 separate doses; increase dose in 15-mg/kg increments at weekly intervals; max. 45 mg/kg/d or 3600 mg/d (whichever is less). At initiation of Felbamate, decrease dose of concomitant anticonvulsants (i.e., Carbamazepine, Phenytoin, Phenobarbital, Valproic acid) by 20 %; further dosage reductions of concurrent anticonvulsants may be needed.
  - **Severe epilepsy (partial seizures with and without secondary generalized seizures)**
    - **children > 14 years:** adjunctive therapy, initially 1200 mg/d as 3–4 separate doses; increase daily dose in 1200 mg-increments at weekly intervals; max. 3600 mg/d. At initiation of Felbamate, decrease dose of concomitant anticonvulsants (i.e., Carbamazepine, Phenytoin, Phenobarbital, Valproic acid) by 20 %; further dosage reductions of concurrent anticonvulsants may be needed.
    - **change to monotherapy:** initially 1200 mg/d as 3–4 separate doses; at week 2, increase daily dose by 1200 mg-increments at weekly intervals; max. 3600 mg/d. At initiation of Felbamate, decrease dose of concomitant anticonvulsants by ⅓ of their original dose, and when Felbamate dose is increased at week 2; continue to reduce any of the other anticonvulsants as clinically needed.
    - **monotherapy:** initially 1200 mg/d as 3–4 separate doses; titrate dosage upward to clinical response and monitor patients closely; increase daily dose in 600 mg-increments every 2 weeks to 2400 mg/d; max. dose: 3600 mg/d
- United Kingdom – BNFC: –

Comments:
- The indication of Felbamate therapy is very rigorous (stand-by medication) due to the risk of fulminant side effects.

Fentanyl

Dosage:
- ▶ 1–4 mcg/kg/dose (max. 200 mcg) IV
- ▶ analgosedation: 1–10 mcg/kg/h IV
  - transdermal patch: change dose patch every 3 d

Neuropaediatric indications:
- severe pain (also palliative)
- sedation in increased intracranial pressure

Mechanism of action:
- synthetic opioid
- pure agonist with high affinity to μ-receptors and lower affinity to κ-receptors
- 50 to 100-times more potent than Morphine

Relevant contraindications:
- therapy with MAOIs
- respiratory insufficiency or obstructive lung diseases
- careful use: bradyarrhythmia, head injuries, liver and renal impairment, children < 1 year of age, addiction to opioids, unconsciousness, hypotension in hypovolemia, obstructive or inflammatory bowel diseases, pheochromocytoma, increasing tendency for cerebral seizures, pancreatitis, myxoedema

Relevant side effects and interactions:
- respiratory depression, muscle rigidity, bradycardia, miosis, sweating, hypotensive response of the circulatory system
- sedation, vertigo, euphoria, anxiety, cognitive disorders
- headache, nausea, vomiting, constipation, dry mouth, voiding dysfunction
- tickle of throat in response to fast injections, pruritus, exanthema
- addiction, development of tolerance, withdrawal syndrome
- combination with MAOI: severe circulation and respiratory disorders (discontinue MAOI two weeks before beginning treatment with Fentanyl)
- interactions when using analgesic Fentanyl patches together with Furosemide, Glibenclamide, Omeprazole (by binding of 90 % plasma protein)
- because Fentanyl is metabolized via the cytochrome P 450 enzyme system, dose adjustment may be required in smokers and in combination with hypericum preparations or grapefruit juice
- do not use Fentanyl after administration of partial antagonists (Buprenorphine) because this could lead to intensified pain sensation

Approval status:

– depends on the specific product (see SPC)

Sources:

– **Germany – SPC:**
  – **management of severe chronic pain in patients receiving opioid therapy**
  – transdermal patch
    – In young children, the patch should preferably be applied to the upper back where it is not easily reached and possibly removed by the child. Fentanyl should be administered only to **opioid-tolerant paediatric patients (aged 2 to 16 years)** who already receive at least 30 mg of oral Morphine equivalents per day.
    – To convert paediatric patients from oral or parenteral opioids to transdermal patch, refer to the equianalgesic efficacy of drugs listed in Table 1 and use the recommended initial transdermal patch dose based upon the daily oral Morphine dose (see manufacturer's recommendation or SPC).
  – **Table 1:** Equianalgesic efficacy of drugs (mg)

active ingredient	Equianalgesic dose	
	parenteral (SC, IM, IV)	oral
Morphine	10	30–40
Hydromorphone	1.5	7.5
Oxycodone	10–15	20–30
Methadone	10	20
Pethidine	75	–
Codeine	–	200
Buprenorphine	0.4	0.8 (sublingual)
Ketobernidone	10	20–30

  – **Table 2:** Recommended initial dose of matrifen based on the daily oral dose of morphin

oral morphin-dose in 24 h (mg/kg) for paediatric patients	transdermal matrifen-dose (mcg/h) for paediatric patients
30–44	12
45–134	25

– The equivalent dose should not be used for changing from Fentanyl to other opioids due to overdosing. The first dose of transdermal patches will not develop its optimal analgesic effect within the first 24 h. Therefore, during the first 12 h after switching to Fentanyl, the patients should continue with the previous regular dose of analgesics. In the next 12 h, these analgesics should be given as the clinical need arises.
– For early detection of adverse events, which may include hypoventilation, patients should be monitored for at least 48 hours after initiation of Matrifen therapy or dose up-titration because it takes 12 to 24 h of

treatment for plasma Fentanyl to reach its peak levels. If the analgesic effect of Fentanyl is insufficient, supplementary Morphine or any other short-duration opioid should be administered. Depending on the additional analgesic needs and the pain status of the child, it may be decided to increase the dose. Dose adjustments should be done in 12.0 mcg/h steps.

– **USA – T:**
  – **analgesia**
  – **international evidence-based Group for Neonatal Pain**
    – slow IV bolus
      – **neonates:** 0.5–3 mcg/kg/dose or continuous IV infusion of 0.5–2 mcg/kg/h
  – **continuous sedation/analgesia**
    – slow IV bolus
      – **neonates and infants:** 1–4 mcg/kg/dose, may be repeated after 2–4 h
  – **continuous sedation/analgesia**
    – IV bolus
      – **neonates and infants:** initially 1–2 mcg/kg, then 0.5–1 mcg/kg/h; titrate upward;
      – mean required dose: **preterm neonates < 34 weeks of gestation:** 0.64 mcg/kg/h; **preterm neonates ≥ 34 weeks:** 0.75 mcg/kg/h
      – **older infants and children 1–12 years:** initially 1–2 mcg/kg, then 1 mcg/kg/h; titrate upward; usually 1–3 mcg/kg/h; some require 5 mcg/kg/h
  – **moderate to severe chronic pain**
    – transdermal patch
      – **children ≥ 2 years,** opioid-tolerant, receive at least 60 mg oral Morphine equivalents per day: initially 25 mcg/h patch system or higher, depending on conversion to Fentanyl equivalents and administration of equianalgesic dosage; use short-acting analgesics for first 24 h with supplementary PRN doses thereafter (for breakthrough pain); dose may be increased after 3 d, based on the daily dose of supplementary opioids required; use the ratio of 45 mg of oral Morphine equivalents per day to a 12.0-mcg/h increase in transdermal patch dosage; change patch every 72 h
      – **children > 12 years,** opioid-tolerant, receive at least 60 mg oral Morphine equivalents per day: initially 25 mcg/h patch system or higher; dose may be increased after 3 days based on the daily dose of supplementary PRN opioids required
  – **continuous sedation/analgesia during ECMO**
    – IV bolus:
      – **neonates and infants:** initially 5–10 mcg/kg slow IV bolus or over 10 min, then 1–5 mcg/kg/h; titrate upward; tolerance may develop; higher doses (up to 20 mcg/kg/h) may be needed by day 6 of ECMO
  – **breakthrough cancer pain: Transmucosal (Actiq®)**
    – **adolescents ≥ 16 years, opioid-tolerant:** titrate dose to provide adequate analgesia; initially 200 mcg; may repeat dose only once, 15 min after completion of first dose if needed. Do not exceed a max. of 2 doses for each episode of breakthrough cancer pain; patient has to wait for at least 4 h before treating another episode. Titrate dose up to next higher strength if several consecutive breakthrough episodes require treatment (> 1 Actiq® per episode); evaluate each new dose over several episodes of breakthrough cancer pain (generally 1–2 d) to determine proper dose of analgesia with acceptable side effects. Once dose has been determined, consumption should be limited to ≤ 4 units/d. Re-evaluate maintenance (around-the-clock) opioid dose if patient requires > 4 units/d. If signs of

excessive opioid effects occur before a dose is completed, the patch unit should be removed from the mouth immediately, and subsequently doses decreased.
- **United Kingdom – BNFC:**
  - **severe chronic pain**
    - transdermal
      - **children 2–16 years**, currently treated with strong opioid analgesic: initial dose based on previous 24 h opioid requirement (consult SPC)
      - **children 16–18 years**, not currently treated with strong opioid analgesic: one 12 or 25 mcg/h patch, replaced after 72 h; If patient currently treated with strong opioid analgesic, base initial dose on previous 24 h opioid requirement (consult SPC)

Comments:
- The strongly lipophilic properties make this drug difficult to control (uptake by and release from fat tissue). By now the use of related substances such as alfentanil, remifentanil, and sufentanil is given preference.
- subtherapeutic plasma levels: < 0.005 mcg/ml
- half-life in plasma: 1–3 h

Fluconazole

Dosage:
▶ 3–6 mg/kg/d in systemic infections; in infants < 2 weeks and children with very low birth weight, this dose should be given only every third day, in children aged 2–4 weeks only every other day (SPC)

Neuropaediatric indications:
- candidal meningoencephalitis

Mechanism of action:
- inhibits the fungal cytochrome P450 enzyme 14-α-demethylase (mammalian demethylase activity is much less sensitive to Fluconazole) and thus blocks conversion of lanosterol to ergosterol, an essential component of the fungal cytoplasmic membrane.
- susceptible fungi: Candida albicans, C. tropicalis, C. parapsilosis, C. guilliermondii, C. glabrata (in high dosages), Cryptococcus neoformans, dimorphic fungi (Histoplasma capsulatum, Blastomyces dermatitidis, Coccidioides immitis, Paracoccidioides brasiliensis), Penicillium species, dermatophytes
- resistant fungi: Candida krusei, Aspergillus species, Mucor species, Fusarium species, Scopulariopsis species, Pseudallescheria boydii, Scedosporium inflatum

Relevant contraindications:
- hypokalemia or hypomagnesemia
- prolonged QT or comedication that can lead to prolonged QT intervals (e.g. antiarrhythmics of class Ia or III)
- clinically relevant bradycardia
- cardiac arrhythmias
- pregnancy
- combination with cisapride, astemizole
- combination with terfenadine, if Fluconazole is repeatedly administered in dosages exceeding 400 mg/d
- careful use: AIDS and malignant diseases, severe liver function disorders, < 16 years of age, use of < 400 mg/d of Fluconazole in combination with Terfenadine

Relevant side effects and interactions:
- exanthema, alopecia, angiooedema, oedema of the face, pruritus
- headache, vertigo, peripheral nervous disorder
- nausea, vomiting, stomach pain, diarrhea, meteorism
- seizures
- taste disorder
- increased alkaline phosphatase, bilirubin, SGOT, SGTP up to severe liver function disorders with hepatitis and jaundice
- hypercholesterolemia, hypertriglyceridemia, hypokalemia
- leukocytopenia, neutropenia, agranulocytosis, thrombocytopenia
- change in kidney parameters
- enhanced efficacy and side effects of anticoagulants, benzodiazepines, oral sulfonylurea antidiabetics (Glibenclamide, Glipizide, Tolbutamide), Rifabutin, Tacrolimus, Sirolimus, Phenythoin, Ciclosporin, Theophylline, Terfenadine, Zidovudine
- decreased efficacy of Rifampicin
- increased serum Fluconazole levels caused by hydrochlorothiazide
- presumably no adverse effect on efficacy of oral contraceptives
- inhibition of glucocorticoid metabolism
- increased risk of myopathy or rhabdomyolysis in combination with HMG-CoA reductase inhibitors

Approval status:
- mycoses caused by yeast in adults and children

Sources:
- **Germany – SPC:**
  - **cryptococcal meningitis, candida infection**
    - IV
      - **term neonates (0–14 d):** 6–12 mg/kg/dose every 72 h; max. 12 mg/kg every 72 h
      - **term neonates (15–27 d):** 6–12 mg/kg/dose every 48 h; max. 12 mg/kg every 48 h
      - **infants and children 28 d–11 years:** 6–12 mg/kg/d
      - **children 12–17 years:** 3–12 mg/kg, depending on severity of illness

- **USA – T:**
  - **acute cryptococcal meningitis**
    - oral, IV
      - **neonates < 2 weeks:** initially 12 mg/kg on day 1, usually 6–12 mg/kg/dose every 72 h for 10–12 weeks after CSF culture becomes negative; relapse: 6 mg/kg/d
      - **neonates> 2 weeks, infants, children:** initially 12 mg/kg on day 1, usually 6–12 mg/kg/d for 10–12 weeks after CSF culture becomes negative; relapse: 6 mg/kg/d
- **United Kingdom – BNFC:**
  - **invasive candida infections and cryptococcal infections (including meningitis)**
    - oral, IV infusion
      - **neonates < 2 weeks:** 6–12 mg/kg/dose every 72 h; continue treatment according to response (at least 8 weeks for cryptococcal meningitis)
      - **neonates 2–4 weeks:** 6–12 mg/kg/dose every 48 h; continue treatment according to response (at least 8 weeks for cryptococcal meningitis)
      - **children 1 month–18 years:** 6–12 mg/kg/d (max. 800 mg); continue treatment according to response (at least 8 weeks for cryptococcal meningitis)
  - **prevention of relapse of cryptococcal meningitis in HIV-infected patients after completion of primary therapy**
    - oral, IV infusion
      - **children 1 month–18 years:** 6 mg/kg/d (max. 200 mg/d)

Comments:

- in reduced renal function the daily dose has to be reduced according to creatinine clearance

Flucytosine

Dosage:

- ▶ systemic candidiasis: Flucytosine 100–150 mg/kg/d as 4 separate doses IV + Amphotericin B conventional 0.5 mg/kg/d over 2–4 weeks; prematures and neonates, 50–100 mg/kg/d Flucytosine as 2 separate doses (SPC)
- ▶ cryptococcal meningitis: Flucytosine 100 mg/kg/d as 4 separate doses IV + Amphotericin B conventional 0.7–1 mg/kg/d over 6–10 weeks

Neuropaediatric indications:

- candidal and cryptococcal meningoencephalitis in combination with Amphotericin B

Mechanism of action:

- cytosine analog with two proposed modes of action that both lead to inhibition of fungal growth (impaired cell division)

- it is transported via a cytosine permease into the fungal cells where it is desaminated by cytosine deaminase to 5-fluoruracil (5-FU)
  - 5-FU is metabolized to 5-fluor-UMP via UMP pyrophosphorylase and then incorporated into the fungal RNA, resulting in impaired RNA synthesis
  - alternatively, 5-FU is metabolized to 5-fluor-dUMP, which is a potent inhibitor of thymidylate synthase, resulting in impaired DNA synthesis

Relevant contraindications:

- concurrent intake of Brivudine, Sorivudine and analogs (intake interval > 4 weeks)
- concurrent intake of dihydropyrimidine dehydrogenase inhibitors
- first trimester of pregnancy
- careful in second and third trimester of pregnancy

Relevant side effects and interactions:

- nausea, vomiting, diarrhea, gastric pain
- rash
- anemia, leukopenia, granulocytopenia, agranulocytosis, thrombocytopenia
- elevated liver enzymes
- hallucination, vertigo, headache, fatigue
- combination with Phenytoin can lead to Phenytoin intoxication
- nephrotoxic and cytostatic drugs impair renal elimination
- impaired two-step enzyme assay for measuring creatinine
- nucleoside analogues lead to strongly increased plasma levels of 5-fluorouracil
- in prematures and neonates the serum sodium concentration can lead to hypernatremia

Approval status:

- mycoses, especially systemic candidiasis and cryptococcal meningitis in adults and children

Sources:

- **Germany – SPC:**
  - **cryptococcal meningitis**
    - IV
      - **children with CNS infection:** 100 mg/kg/d, add 0.7–1.0 mg/kg/d Amphotericin B conventional for 6–10 weeks. Alternatively 0.7–1 mg/kg/d Amphotericin B conventional and add 100 mg/kg/d of Flucytosine over 2 weeks, followed by treatment with Fluconazole (400 mg/d) for at least 10 weeks.
- **USA – T:**
  - **candidal meningitis:**
    - oral (recommended: administer in combination with Amphotericin B)
      - **neonates:** initially 75–100 mg/kg/d for 3–20 d
      - **infants and children:** 50–150 mg/kg/d as 4 separate doses

- **United Kingdom – BNFC:**
  - **cryptococcal meningitis (adjunct to Amphotericin)**
    - oral, IV infusion
      - **neonates:** 100 mg/kg/d given as 2 separate doses
      - **children 1 month–18 years:** 100 mg/kg/d as 4 separate doses for 2 weeks

Comments:
- narrow therapeutic range

Flunarizine

Dosage:
▶ < 40 kg: 5 mg in the evening, > 40 kg: 10 mg in the evening (off-label)

Neuropaediatric indications:
- migraine prophylaxis, especially familial hemiplegic migraine

Mechanism of action:
- Calcium channel blocker
- inhibits Calcium influx into smooth muscle cells and erythrocytes in hypoxic conditions, resulting in vasodilatation and increased flexibility of erythrocytes

Relevant contraindications:
- known hypersensitivity to active ingredient or its class
- depression
- present or medical history of extrapyramidal symptoms

Relevant side effects and interactions:
- increased appetite and weight gain, nausea, drowsiness
- headache, depressions, anxiety, galactorrhea, dry mouth, muscle pain, bradykinesia, rigidity, akathisia, orofacial dyskinesia, tremor

Approval status:
- no precise approval for treatment of children

Sources:
- **Germany – SPC:**
- **children:** not recommended
- **USA – T:** –
- **United Kingdom – BNFC:** –
- **Uptodate.com:** no published paediatric dosage
- **migraine prophylaxis**
  - oral
  - **adults:** 5–10 mg once daily; incidence of adverse effects may be decreased by allowing 2 consecutive medication-free days each week. If no significant improvement is seen after 3 months of therapy, discontinue use.

Comments:
- reduced frequency of migraine is established after some weeks

Fluoxetine

Dosage:
▶ 0.5 mg/kg/d (max. 20 mg/d); increase to max. 2 mg/kg/d (max. 40 mg/d) as 2 separate doses p.o. (off-label)

Neuropaediatric indications:
- kinetic abnormalities (e.g. slow channel syndrome)
- depression
- obsessive-compulsive disorder

Mechanism of action:
- selective serotonin reuptake inhibitor (SSRI)
- main effect: inhibition of the reuptake of serotonin from the synaptic cleft
- further effects:
  - direct effects at 5-HT2C receptors
  - in high dosages: also inhibition of noradrenalin reuptake

Relevant contraindications:
- concurrent intake of non-selective MAOI; stop non-selective MAOI 14 d and reversible MAOI 1 d prior to medication start; if required, treatment with non-selective MAOI may be resumed at the earliest 5 weeks after last Fluoxetine dose
- careful use: history of seizures, < 18 years of age (lacking clinical experiences), obsession/hypomania, reduced liver or kidney function, acute heart diseases, diabetes, concurrent intake of oral anticoagulants or drugs that influence platelet function, history of bleeding, concurrent electroconvulsive therapy, intake of hypericum (serotonin syndrome), combination with other serotonergic substances or neuroleptics, pregnancy

Relevant side effects and interactions:
- photosensitivity
- hair loss, sweating, ecchymosis
- dermal or mucosal bleedings
- pruritus, rash, urticaria, vasculitis, angiooedema, toxic epidermal necrolysis (Lyell's syndrome)

- myalgia, arthralgias
- headache, nightmare, insomnia, vertigo, fatigue, euphoria
- twitching, ataxia, chills, myoclonus
- seizures, psychomotor anxiety
- blurred vision, mydriasis
- changed taste sensation
- diarrhea, nausea, vomiting, digestive disorder, difficulty swallowing, gastrointestinal bleeding
- galactorrhea
- hyponatremia
- orthostatic hypotension
- pharyngitis, dyspnea
- retention of urine, pollakiuria, delayed/lacking ejaculation, anorgasmia, priapism
- serotonin syndrome:
  - nausea, vomiting and diarrhea
  - restlessness, hallucination, loss of coordination
  - tachycardia, variation in blood pressure, elevated body temperature
  - increased muscle reflexes
- increased risk of serotonin syndrome when combined with MAOIs, drugs with serotonergic effect, lithium and tryptophan
- changes in Fluoxetine blood levels if combined with Phenytoin
- increased risk of coronary vasoconstriction and hypertension in combination with triptan drugs
- careful use: drugs with narrow therapeutic range that are metabolized by CYP2D6 (e.g. Flecainide, Encainide, Carbamazepine, tricyclic antidepressants)
- increased efficacy of oral anticoagulants
- prolonged seizures if combined with electroconvulsive treatment
- possibly higher incidence of side effects caused by hypericum

Approval status:

- depends on the specific product (see SPC)

Sources:

- **Germany – SPC:**
  - **major depression, obsessive-compulsive disorders**
    - oral
      - **children ≥ 8 years:** initially 10 mg/d; adjust to response and lowest effective dose for 1–2 weeks. May be increased to 20 mg/d. Limited data is available for doses > 20 mg and for duration of treatment > 9 weeks. If no satisfactory response after 9 weeks of treatment, interruption is indicated. In responding patients, treatment outcome should be evaluated after 6 months. Children with low body weight should receive lower doses of Fluoxetine.

- **USA – T:**
  - **depressions**
    - oral
      - **manufacturer's recommendation: children and adolescents 8–18 years:** initially 10–20 mg/d; in patients started at 10 mg/d, dose may be increased to 20 mg/d after 1 week. **children with lower weight:** initially 10 mg/d; usual maintenance with 10 mg/d; may be increased to 20 mg/d after several weeks, if required.
      - **note: some experts recommend lower doses: children ≤ 11 years,** initially 5 mg/d; **children ≥ 12 years,** initially 10 mg/d; clinically, doses have been titrated up to 40 mg/d in paediatric patients
  - **obsessive-compulsive disorders**
    - oral
      - **children 7–18 years: lower-weight children:** initially 10 mg/d; if needed, dose may be increased after several weeks; usual range 20–30 mg/d; minimal experience with doses > 20 mg/d; no experience with doses > 60 mg/d
      - **higher-weight children:** initially 10 mg/d; dose may be increased to 20 mg/d after 2 weeks, and increased again after several further weeks, if needed; usual range: 20–60 mg/d
  - **elective mutism**
    - oral
      - **study (n = 6, 6–12 years):** initially 0.2 mg/kg/d for 1 week, then 0.4 mg/kg/d for 1 week, then 0.6 mg/kg/d for 10 weeks
- **United Kingdom – BNFC:**
  - **major depression**
    - oral
      - **children 8–18 years:** 10 mg/d as a SD, increased after 1–2 weeks if necessary, max. 20 mg/d as a SD; CAUTION: long duration of action; keep in mind the long half-life of Fluoxetine when adjusting dosage (or in overdosage)

Comments:

- relatively long half-life of 4–6 d; active metabolite (norfluoxetine), 4–16 d

Flupirtine

Dosage:

- ▶ acute treatment of tension-type headaches: 2–3 mg/kg/dose
- ▶ tension-type headache: 6–9 mg/kg/d as 3 separate doses (possibly for 1–4 weeks, especially in muscle tensions)
- ▶ therapeutic efficacy level in the blood: 0.5–1.5 mcg/ml
- ▶ suppository: from 6 years on, 75 mg/dose 3–4 times a day (SPC)

Neuropaediatric indications:

- strong to severe acute or chronic pain

- acute therapy and prophylaxis of tension-type headaches

Mechanism of action:
- centrally effective muscle relaxant and non-opioid analgesic

Relevant contraindications:
- liver diseases
- reduced renal function
- hepatic encephalopathy
- cholestasis
- myasthenia gravis

Relevant side effects and interactions:
- signs of fatigue, vertigo
- increased liver enzymes, hepatitis
- no combination with Paracetamol and Carbamazepine

Approval status:
- depends on the specific product (see SPC)

Sources:
- Germany – SPC: – not longer approved in this indication for paediatric patients (07/2013)
- USA – T: –
- United Kingdom – BNFC: –

Comments:
- control liver function parameters; this drug is suspected to cause liver damage
- is also used experimentally in the treatment of neuronal ceroid lipofuscinoses (NCL)

Folinic acid

Dosage:
▶ 3 mg/kg/d IV as 3 separate doses (maintenance therapy p.o.)

Neuropaediatric indications:
- cryptogenic therapy-resistant neonatal seizures

Mechanism of action:
- 5-formyl derivative of tetrahydrofolic acid (THF)

Relevant contraindications:
- megaloblastic anemia caused by Vitamin B_{12} deficiency (CAUTION: irreversible neurological disorder)

Relevant side effects and interactions:
- rare and only in very high dosages
- CNS disorders (sleeping problems, agitation, depression)
- gastrointestinal disorders
- decreased efficacy of folic acid antagonists (see below) and anticonvulsants
- enhanced efficacy of 5-fluoruracil (see below)

Approval status:
- depends on the specific product (see SPC)

Sources:
- Germany – SPC: –
- USA – T: –
- United Kingdom – BNFC: –
- Uptodate.com:
- Treatment of weak Folinic acid antagonist overdosage (e.g., Pyrimethamine, Trimethoprim)
  – oral
    - **children:** 5–15 mg/d for 3 d or until blood counts are normal, or 5 mg every 3rd day; doses of 6 mg/d are needed for patients with platelet counts < 100 000/mm^3

Comments:
- synergistic effect with 5-fluoruracil in chemotherapy: Folinic acid binds to thymidilate synthase resulting in a decrease of the intracellular thymidilate concentration and thus enhanced cytostatic effect of 5-fluoruracil.
- "leucovorin-rescue":
  – antidote in therapy with Methotrexate
  – Methotrexate acts as a folic acid antagonist and competitively and reversibly inhibits dihydrofolate reductase
  – in high-dose Methotrexate administrations, the Methotrexate effect should be continuously antagonized to reduce severe intoxication of the bone marrow and mucous membranes (mucositis).

Foscarnet

Dosage:
▶ 180 mg/kg/d IV as 3 separate doses; 14–21 d (off-label)

Neuropaediatric indications:
- CMV encephalitis
- HSV encephalitis (second line)

Mechanism of action:

- mimics the structure of pyrophosphate
- inhibits selectively the pyrophosphate binding site on viral DNA polymerases at concentrations that are too low for affecting human DNA polymerases.
- Foscarnet is not activated by thymidine kinases, making it useful in Aciclovir- or Ganciclovir-resistant infections

Relevant contraindications:

- patients receiving pentamidine IV
- careful use: dialysis-dependent patients, renal insufficiency, < 18 years of age

Relevant side effects and interactions:

- nausea, vomiting, diarrhea, anorexia, abdominal pain, constipation, indigestions
- shivering, fever, exanthema
- fatigue, headache, vertigo, seizures, tremor, hypoesthesia, ataxia, neuropathy
- asthenia
- elevated serum creatinine, renal impairment, pain in the kidneys
- hypocalcemia, hypokalemia, hyponatremia, hypomagnesemia, hypophosphatemia, hyperphosphatemia
- ECG changes, palpitations, hypertension, hypotension
- anemia, granulocytopenia, leukopenia, thrombopenia
- temporary elevation of liver enzymes in the serum (AST, ALT, gamma-GT, LDH, alkaline phosphatase)
- anxiety, depression, confusion

Approval status:

- not approved for children (< 18 years of age)

Sources:

- **Germany – SPC:**
  - **life-threatening infections with CMV**
    - IV
      - **note:** use only in immunocompromised patients (until efficacy and safety are established)
      - **adolescents:** initially 60 mg/kg/dose Foscarnet sodium hexahydrate over 1 h 3 times daily or 90 mg/kg/dose over 2 h twice daily
      - maintenance for prophylaxis of relapse: 90–120 mg/kg/d Foscarnet sodium hexahydrate over 2 h for 7 d. Start therapy with 90 mg/kg and titrate up to 120 mg/kg. Patients not responding to the maintenance regimen may again be treated with the initial dose regimen. After stabilization of these patients, switch to the maintenance regimen.
- **USA – T:**
  - **Aciclovir -resistant herpes simplex virus infection**
    - IV

- **children:** 40 mg/kg/dose every 8–12 h for up to 3 weeks or until lesions heal: repeated treatment may lead to the development of resistance
- **United Kingdom – BNFC:**
  - **CMV disease**
    - IV infusion
      - **children 1 month–18 years:** initially 180 mg/kg/d as 3 separate doses for 2–3 weeks, then maintenance with 60 mg/kg/d, increase to 90–120 mg/kg/d if tolerated; if disease progresses on maintenance dose, repeat initial dose regimen
  - **mucocutaneous herpes simplex infection**
    - IV infusion
      - **children 1 month–18 years:** 120 mg/kg/d as 3 separate doses for 2–3 weeks or until lesions heal

Furosemide

Dosage:

▶ diuresis: 0.5–2 mg/kg/dose p.o. (max. 40 mg/d); adults and adolescents > 15 years, 20–40 mg IV (repeated administration of this dose if required); infants and children under the age of 15: max. 0.5–1 mg/kg/d IV (SPC)

Neuropaediatric indications:

- forced diuresis (e.g. in intoxications)
- pseudotumor cerebri: add-on to Acetazolamide

Mechanism of action:

- loop diuretic
- inhibits the sodium-potassium-chloride cotransporter and thus the reuptake of sodium, potassium and chloride from the tubulus lumen in the ascending part of the nephrotic loop (Henle's loop)

Relevant contraindications:

- severe liver function disorders
- severe hypokalemia
- hyponatremia
- hypovolemia
- renal insufficiency with enuresis (because Furosemide would be ineffective)
- careful use: diabetes mellitus, gout, disorders of cerebral blood circulation, coronary insufficiency, hypoproteinemia, urinary obstruction

Relevant side effects and interactions:

- apathy, drowsiness, confusion, excessive thirst, loss of appetite
- orthostatic hypotension, cardiac arrhythmias
- muscle weakness, paresthesia, pareses, flatulence

- exanthema, dermatitis, dermal photosensibility
- hypomagnesemia (cramps, cardiac arrhythmias)
- in long term use:
  - muscle tension, pressure in the head, vertigo, weakness, hypotension
  - impaired vision, hearing disorder, dry mouth, gastrointestinal disorders, pancreatitis
  - hyperuricemia, hypercholesterolemia, hypertriglyceridemia, deterioration of a metabolic alkalosis, vasculitis, anemia, leukopenia, thrombocytopenia, agranulocytosis, hyperuricemia, increase of serum creatinine levels
  - salt loss (sodium, potassium and Calcium)

Approval status:
- depends on the specific product (see SPC)

Sources:
- **Germany – SPC:**
- **management of oedema associated with heart failure and hepatic or renal disease**
  - IV
    - **children:** usual dose, 1(-2) mg/kg/d, max. 40 mg/d
    - **note:** indication of interest is not specified in SPC
- **USA – T:**
- **management of oedema associated with heart failure and hepatic or renal disease**
  - oral
    - **infants and children:** 2 mg/kg/d as a SD; if ineffective, may be increased in increments of 1–2 mg/kg/dose every 6–8 h; do not exceed 6 mg/kg/dose. In most cases, it is not necessary to exceed individual doses of 4 mg/kg or a dosing frequency of once or twice daily.
  - IM, IV
    - **infants and children:** 1–2 mg/kg/dose every 6–12 h
  - continuous infusion
    - **infants and children:** 0.05 mg/kg/h; titrate dosage to clinical effect
    - **note:** indication of interest is not specified in SPC
- **United Kingdom – BNFC:**
  - oliguria
    - oral
      - **children 12–18 years:** initially 250 mg/d; if necessary, increase dose in steps of 250 mg given every 4–6 h; max. single dose 2 g (rarely used)
    - IV infusion
      - **children 1 month–12 years:** 2–5 mg/kg/dose up to 4 times daily, max. 1000 mg/d
      - **children 12–18 years:** initially 250 mg over 1 h (rate not exceeding 4 mg/min); increase to 500 mg over 2 h if not achieving satisfactory urine output, then give a further 1 g over 4 h if no satisfactory response within subsequent hour; if still no response, dialysis is probably required; effective dose (up to 1 g) can be repeated every 24 h

G

Gabapentin (GBP)

Dosage:
- epilepsy: 10–25(–50) mg/kg/d p.o. as 2–3 separate doses (SPC/off-label)
- essential tremor: 10(–50) mg/kg/d (off-label)
- myotonic dystrophy: day 1, 10 mg/kg/d as a SD; day 2, 20 mg/kg/d as 2 separate doses; day 3, 30 mg/kg/d as 3 separate doses (off-label)
- neurogenic pain: within 3 and 7 d titrate to: 15–30 mg/kg/dose 3 times daily p.o.

Neuropaediatric indications:
- neurogenic pain and dysesthesia (peripheral neuropathic pain)
- CRPS (complex regional pain syndrome)
- adjunctive therapy of focal epilepsy
- essential tremor
- myotonic dystrophy

Mechanism of action:
- GABA analogue, binds to sites associated with α_2-δ-subunits of voltage-dependent Calcium channels leading to a decreased release of monoamine neurotransmitters

Relevant contraindications:
- acute pancreatitis
- galactosemia
- dose adjustments in renal insufficiency
- relative contraindication: < 12 years of age
- primary generalized epilepsy (e.g. absences)
- careful use in pregnancy
- tablets: hypersensitivity to peanuts or soy beans

Relevant side effects and interactions:
- viral infections, pneumonia, urinary tract infections, otitis media
- leukopenia
- fatigue, vertigo, headache
- nausea, vomiting, weight gain, loss of appetite
- nervousness, insomnia
- ataxia, nystagmus, paresthesia, seizures, hyperkinesia, dysarthria, tremor, limited reflexes
- impaired vision

- pruritus
- hypersensitivity reactions
- resorption of Gabapentin is influenced by Calcium- or Magnesium-containing antacids
- Morphine and alcohol can increase the efficacy and side effects of Gabapentin
- Gabapentin can influence urin test results for proteins (higher rate of false-positive results)

Approval status:

- monotherapy or adjunctive therapy: > 12 years of age with focal and secondary generalized seizures
- anticonvulsive add-on therapy in children > 6 years with focal and generalized secondary seizures
- not approved for pain in children

Sources:

- Germany – SPC:
  - epilepsy
    - oral
      - **children 6–12 years:** initially 10–15 mg/kg/d; increase over 3 d to 25–35 mg/kg/d as 3 separate doses, max. 50 mg/kg/d. Intervals between the doses should not exceed 12 h.
      - administer daily doses as 2–3 separate doses
      - Concomitant antiepileptic drugs have no influence on plasma Gabapentin levels.
      - **children > 12 years:** day 1, 300 mg/d; day 2, 600 mg/d as 2 separate doses; day 3, 900 mg/d as 3 separate doses; titrate to response every 2–3 d in 300 mg/d increments up to max. 1800 mg/d in week 1, max. 2400 mg/d in week 2 and max. 3600 mg/d in week 3. In clinical long-term studies, up to 4800 mg/d were well tolerated. Intervals between the doses should not exceed 12 h. Administer daily doses as 2–3 separate doses.
      - **note:** also used as adjunctive therapy in children > 6 years and as monotherapy for children > 12 years
- USA – T:
  - epilepsy
    - oral
      - **children 3–12 years:** initially 10–15 mg/kg/d as 3 separate doses; titrate dose upward over 3 d
      - **usual dose:**
      - **children 3–4 years:** 40 mg/kg/d as 3 separate doses
      - **children ≥ 5–12 years:** 25–35 mg/kg/d as 3 separate doses; 50 mg/kg/d well tolerated in one long-term study
      - **children > 12 years:** initially 900 mg/d as 3 separate doses; titrate dose upward if needed; usual dose, 900–1800 mg/d divided in 3 doses; doses up to 2400 mg/d as 3 separate doses were well tolerated long-term; max. 3600 mg/d
      - **note:** do not exceed 12 h between doses with 3 times/d dosing

- **neuropathic pain**
  - oral
    - **children:** limited information is available; some centers use initially 5 mg/kg/dose at bedtime; day 2, increase to 10 mg/kg/d as 2 separate doses; day 3, increase to 15 mg/kg/d as 3 separate doses; titrate to response; usual dosage range, 8–35 mg/kg/d as 3 separate doses
- United Kingdom – BNFC:
  - **adjunctive treatment of focal seizures with or without secondary generalization**
    - oral
      - **children 2–6 years:** day 1, 10 mg/kg/d as a SD; day 2, 20 mg/kg/d as 2 separate doses; day 3, 30 mg/kg/d as 3 separate doses; depending on response, increase to the usual dose of 30–70 mg/kg/d as 3 separate doses
      - **children 6–12 years:** day 1, 10 mg/kg/d (max. 300 mg) as a SD; day 2, 10 mg/kg/dose (max. 300 mg) twice daily; day 3, 10 mg/kg/dose (max. 300 mg) 3 times daily; usual dose, 25–35 mg/kg/d as 3 separate doses; max. 70 mg/kg/d as 3 separate doses
      - **children 12–18 years:** day 1, 300 mg/d as a SD; day 2, 600 mg/d as 2 separate doses; day 3, 900 mg/d as 3 separate doses or day 1, 900 mg/d as 3 separate doses; then increased according to response in steps of 300 mg (as 3 separate doses) every 2–3 d; usual dose, 0.9–3.6 g/d as 3 separate doses
  - **monotherapy for focal seizures with or without secondary generalization**
    - oral
      - **children 12–18 years:** day 1, 300 mg/d as a SD; day 2, 600 mg/d as 2 separate doses; day 3, 900 mg/d as 3 separate doses or day 1, 900 mg/d as 3 separate doses; then increased according to response in steps of 300 mg (as 3 separate doses) every 2–3 d; usual dose, 0.9–3.6 g/d as 3 separate doses

Comments:

- usually well tolerated even in high dosages
- efficacy is discussed controversially

Ganciclovir

Dosage:

- ▶ 10–15 mg/kg/d as 3 separate doses IV (short infusion over 1 h) for 2–3 weeks (infants < 3 months, 10 mg/kg/d) (off-label)
- ▶ maintenance therapy: 5 mg/kg/d IV (over 1 h) (off-label)

Neuropaediatric indications:

- CMV infections/CMV encephalitis

Mechanism of action:

- a synthetic guanine analogue that selectively inhibits replication of herpes viruses and is especially active against CMV.
- Ganciclovir is first phosphorylated to Ganciclovir monophosphate by virus-encoded enzymes and then further phosphorylated to the di- and triphosphate by cellular

enzymes. The triphosphate of Ganciclovir competitively inhibits incorporation of deoxyguanosine triphosphate (dGTP) via DNA polymerase into DNA. Because Ganciclovir triphosphate inhibits the viral DNA polymerase far more effectively than the host-cell DNA polymerase, the result is a preferential cessation of chain elongation in the viral DNA.

Relevant contraindications:

- hypersensitivity to Aciclovir, Ganciclovir and Valganciclovir
- severe neutropenia
- severe thrombocytopenia
- Hb < 8 g/dl
- careful use: patients with cytopenia, < 18 years, patients with radiation therapy

Relevant side effects and interactions:

- neutropenia: cell count under 1000 neutrophils/µl (up to 50 %)
- thrombocytopenia: < 50 000 thrombocytes/µl (approximately 20 %)
- anemia, eosinophilia, pancytopenia
- dyspnea
- sepsis
- urinary tract infection
- oral candidiasis
- increase of transaminases and alkaline phosphatase
- increase of urea and plasma creatinine concentration
- vertigo, headache, hallucination, loss of appetite, anorexia, depression, insomnia
- seizures
- hypoesthesia, paresthesia, peripheral neuropathy
- nausea, vomiting, diarrhea, abdominal pain, obstipation, flatulence, dysphagia, dyspepsia
- exanthema, dermatitis, pruritus
- oedema of the macula, retinal detachment
- myalgia, arthralgia, muscle cramps

Approval status:

- not approved for use in children

Sources:

- **Germany – SPC:**
  - **CMV infections**
    - IV
      - **children:** efficacy and safety have not been established, thus the use in this patient group is not recommended
- **USA – T:**
  - **congenital CMV infection**
    - slow IV
      - **neonates and infants:** 12 mg/kg/d as 2 separate doses for 6 weeks
  - **other CMV infections**
    - slow IV
      - **children:** initially 10 mg/kg/d as 2 separate doses for 14–21 d or 7.5 mg/kg/d as 3 separate doses; maintenance therapy: 5 mg/kg/d as a SD for 7 d or 6 mg/kg/d for 5 d/week
- **United Kingdom – BNFC:**
  - **congenital cytomegalovirus infection of the CNS**
    - IV infusion
      - **neonates:** 12 mg/kg/d as 2 separate doses for 6 weeks
  - **life-threatening or sight-threatening cytomegalovirus infections in immunocompromised patients**
    - IV infusion
      - **children 1 month–18 years:** initially 10 mg/kg/d as 2 separate doses for 14–21 d for treatment or for 7–14 d for prophylaxis; maintenance (for patients at risk of retinitis relapse), 6 mg/kg/d on 5 d per week or 5 mg/kg/d until adequate recovery of immunity; if retinitis progresses, the initial treatment regimen may be repeated

Comments:

- distinctly more side effects than Aciclovir, because Ganciclovir tends to be more readily phosphorylated even in non-infected cells than Aciclovir

Gentamicin

Dosage:

▶ 4–5 mg/kg/d as 2 separate doses or 4.5–7.5 mg/kg/d as a SD

Neuropaediatric indications:

- meningitis in the first six weeks of life
- shunt infections

Mechanism of action:

- aminoglycoside antibiotic
- inhibits bacterial protein synthesis by binding to the 30S ribosomal subunit leading to inaccurate mRNA translation and in turn to early termination of peptide chain elongation or to formation of aberrant proteins
- is mainly effective in Gram-negative bacteria (Escherichia coli, Enterobacter, Klebsiella, Proteus, Pseudomonas aeruginosa, Citrobacter, Serratia, Yersinia enterocolitica), and Gram-positive staphylococci
- ineffective in anaerobic bacteria (uptake into bacterial cells is oxygen dependant)

Relevant contraindications:

- preexisting impairement of vestibular or cochlear organs
- terminal renal failure
- pregnancy
- careful use: in impaired renal function and in prematures and neonates

Relevant side effects and interactions:

- myalgia, paresthesia
- neuromuscular block, ocular muscle palsy, scotoma
- respiratory depression
- impairement of vestibular or cochlear organ (especially when used in neonates)
- mild temporary increase of SGOT, SGPT and AP
- renal damages
- granulocytopenia, thrombocytopenia, leukopenia, anemia, eosinophilia
- exanthema, pruritus, urticaria
- enhanced oto- or nephrotoxicity in combination with cephalosporins, Amphotericin B, Colistin, Ciclosporin, Cisplatin, loop diuretics, methoxyflurane
- enhances the neuromuscular block via halothane and curare-like muscle relaxants

Approval status:

- depends on the specific product (see SPC)

Sources:

- **Germany – SPC:**
  - **treatment of severe infections caused by Gentamicin sensitive bacteria (e.g. meningitis)**
    - IM, slow IV injection, short IV infusion
      - **children:** initial: 1.5–2.0 mg/kg, usual: 3–6 mg/kg/d as 1–2 separate doses (patients with normal renal function)
      - **neonates:** 4–7 mg/kg/d as a SD
      - **infants ≥ 1 month:** 4.5–7.5 mg/kg/d as 1–2 separate doses
      - patients with reduced renal function should receive reduced doses (adjust according to response)
- **USA – T:** indication of interest is not specified in SPC
- **United Kingdom – BNFC:**
  - **meningitis and other CNS infections**
    - IM, slow IV injection over at least 3 minutes
      - **children 1 month–12 years:** 7.5 mg/kg/d as 3 separate doses
      - **children 12–18 years:** 6 mg/kg/d given as 3 separate doses
  - **bacterial ventriculitis and CNS infection (supplement to systemic therapy)**
    - Intrathecal or intraventricular injection
      - **neonates:** seek specialist's advice
      - **children 1 month–18 years:** 1 mg/d, increase to 5 mg/d if necessary

Comments:

- poor tissue penetration
- ineffective in acidic conditions
- control serum levels (bottom level < 2 mg/l, peak level 5–10 mg/l)

Glatiramer acetate

Dosage:

▶ 20 mg/d as a SD SC (off-label)

Neuropaediatric indications:

- immunomodulatory therapy in MS

Mechanism of action:

- a random polymer of glutamic acid, alanine, tyrosine and lysine
- mechanism of action is not completely understood
- presumably Glatiramer acetate modifies the immune processes and influences especially T cells (reduction of proinflammatory Th1 and increase of regulatory Th2 cells)

Relevant contraindications:

- hypersensitivity to Glatiramer acetate or Mannitol
- careful use: current heart disease, < 18 years of age, impaired renal function

Relevant side effects and interactions:

- distinctly fewer side effects than Interferon beta
- reactions at the injection site (flush, induration, small haematoma)
- flu-like symptoms (fever, headache, weakness, shivering, myalgia, arthralgias)
- diarrhea, nausea, constipation
- increased muscle tone, back pain
- tachycardia, dyspnea, pectoral pain
- depression, anxiety
- exanthema, sweating
- with concurrent intake of cortisone medication, reactions at the injection site occur more often
- interactions between glatiramer and other medication has not been investigated

Approval status:

- not approved for patients < 18 years of age

Sources:
- Germany – SPC:
  - **multiple sclerosis**
  - SC
    - There have not been any prospective, randomized, controlled clinical trials regarding pharmacokinetics in children and adolescents. Based on the limited data available, a dose of 20 mg/d for children aged 12–18 years appears to be safe and comparable to the safety profile in adults.
    - **children < 12 years:** do not use in this age group
- USA – T: –
- United Kingdom – BNFC: –
- **Uptodate.com:** no published paediatric dosage
- **multiple sclerosis**
- **adults:** 20 mg/d SC

Glucagon

Dosage:
▶ 5–10 mcg/kg/h continuous IV infusion

Neuropaediatric indications:
- severe hypoglycemic reactions in patients with insulin-dependent diabetes

Mechanism of action:
- This single-chain polypeptide hormone occurs naturally in pancreatic alpha cells and has a significant physiological role in the regulation of glucose and ketone body metabolism. Glucagon for clinical use is now usually produced by recombinant techniques.
- Binds to its specific, G-protein coupled receptor in the plasma membrane of the target cell, setting off a complex signaling pathway, which involves adenylate cyclase activation and increased rate of cAMP formation.
- cAMP leads to
  - glycogenolysis via activation (phosphorylation) of glycogen phosphorylase
  - gluconeogenesis, the new synthesis of glucose from amino acids, via stimulation of protein catabolism (which is accompanied by a rise in serum urea levels)
  - activation of lipases: increase of fatty acids' levels in the blood

Relevant contraindications:
- pheochromocytoma
- careful use: glucagonoma and insulinoma

Relevant side effects and interactions:
- nausea, vomiting, stomach pain
- subsequent hypoglycemia, diabetic coma
- brady-/tachycardia, hypo-/hypertension
- antagonistic effect to insulin
- indometacin causes decreased efficacy
- can enhance the anticoagulant effect of Warfarin

Approval status:
- severe hypoglycemic reactions in diabetic patients under insulin therapy in children and adults

Sources:
- Germany – SPC:
  - **hypoglycemia associated with diabetes**
    - SC, IM injection
      - **children > 25 kg or older than 6–8 years:** 1 mg
      - **children < 25 kg or younger than 6–8 years:** 0.5 mg
      - patients usually respond within 10 min to injection. If so, the patient should receive glucose IV. If patient does not respond, administer oral carbohydrates to recover glycogen and to prevent hypoglycemia.
- USA – T:
  - **hypoglycemia**
    - IM, IV, SC
      - **neonates:** 0.02–0.2 mg/kg/dose (max. dose 1 mg); may be repeated after 20 min if needed; **note:** doses vary widely between manufacturer's labeling and published case reports.
      - **infants, children ≤ 20 kg:** 0.02–0.03 mg/kg or 0.5 mg
      - **children > 20 kg:** 1 mg
- United Kingdom – BNFC:
  - **hypoglycemia associated with diabetes**
    - SC, IM, IV injection
      - **neonates:** 0.02 mg/kg
      - **children 1 month–2 years:** 0.5 mg
      - **children 2–18 years:** < 25 kg: 0.5 mg; > 25 kg: 1 mg

Comments:
- variable published dosage recommendations in common paediatric sources

Glycopyrronium bromide

Dosage:

▶ 120–400 mcg/kg/d as 3–4 separate doses, max. 3–6 mg/d (off-label)

Neuropaediatric indications:

- sialorrhea

Mechanism of action:

- anticholinergic agent with quaternary ammonium structure
- competitive antagonist at muscarinergic acetylcholine receptors

Relevant contraindications:

- angle closure glaucoma
- voiding dysfunction with residual urine
- mechanic stenosis in the gastrointestinal tract, megacolon
- tachyarrhythmia
- acute pulmonary oedema
- severe cerebral sclerosis
- careful use: liver and kidney diseases, hyperthyroidism, hiatus hernia with reflux-esophagitis

Relevant side effects and interactions:

- decreased perspiration
- flush
- anxiety, hallucination
- accommodation impairment of the eye, may provoke glaucoma attacks
- dry mouth
- tachycardia
- micturition disorder
- enhanced anticholinergic effect by Amantadine, Chinidin, tri- and tetracyclic antidepressants, neuroleptics
- mutual decrease in efficacy of Glycopyrronium bromide and dopamine antagonists (e.g. Metoclopramide)

Approval status:

- approved for preoperative anesthetic procedure in children and adults

Sources:

- **Germany – SPC:**
  - **premedication at induction**
    - SC, IV (only if monitored closely)
      - **children:** 4–8 mcg/kg, max. 200 mcg

- USA – T: –
- **United Kingdom – BNFC:**
  - **premedication at induction**
    - IV, IM injection
      - **neonates:** 5 mcg/kg
      - **children 1 month–12 years:** 4–8 mcg/kg (max. 200 mcg)
      - **children 12–18 years:** 200–400 mcg or 4–5 mcg/kg (max. 400 mcg)
  - **control of upper airways secretion and hypersalivation**
    - oral
      - **children 1 month–18 years:** 40–100 mcg/kg/dose (max. 2 mg) 3–4 times daily, adjusted according to response
    - SC, IV, IM injection
      - **children 1 month–12 years:** 4–10 mcg/kg (max. 200 mcg) 4 times daily if required
      - **children 12–18 years:** 200 mcg/dose every 4 h if required
    - SC infusion
      - **children 1 month–12 years:** 12–40 mcg/kg/d (max. 1.2 mg)
      - **children 12–18 years:** 600–1200 mcg/d

Comments:

- variable published dosage recommendations in common paediatric sources

H

Haloperidol

Dosage:

▶ tic disorder: 0.25–0.5 mg/d as 2 separate doses (initial dose)
▶ chronic substance abuse (in overdosing or severe withdrawal symptoms): 1–10 mg/d
▶ all other: IV or p.o.
  - initially 0.02–0.05 mg/kg/d as 2 separate doses (max. 0.5 mg/dose)
  - increase up to 0.08–0.2 mg/kg/d
  - rarely up to 4 mg/kg/d as 2 separate doses (max. 100 mg/dose)

Neuropaediatric indications:

- severe chorea
- benign hereditary chorea (cautious indication definition)
- tic disorder
- emergency therapy in high aggressiveness
- chronic substance abuse (in overdosing or severe withdrawal symptoms)

Mechanism of action:
- antagonist of central nervous dopamine receptors

Relevant contraindications:
- severe liver or renal impairment
- voiding dysfunction, glaucoma
- acute intoxication with centrally depressant drugs
- known neuroleptic malignant syndrome
- hypokalemia, bradycardia, congenital long-QT syndrome, other cardiac disorders
- brain disorders, history of seizures

Relevant side effects and interactions:
- extrapyramidal disorders
- early dyskinesia (reversible)
- tardive dyskinesia (partially only incompletely reversible): involuntary swallowing and pharynx movements, speech disorder, dystonic movements
- fatigue, akathisia, tasikinesia
- hypotension (especially in current volume deficiency), orthostatic dysregulation, cardiac conduction disorders (AV block, bundle branch block)
- speech disorder
- neuroleptic malignant syndrome (very rare)
- paradox hypotension and tachycardia after administration of adrenaline
- antiarrhythmics of class IA or III, macrolide antibiotics, antihistamines, Cimetidine, Fluoxetine, amphetamine, dopamine

Approval status:
- depends on the specific product (see SPC)

Sources:
- **Germany – SPC:**
  - **dyskinetic syndrome and tic disorders (e.g. Huntington`s chorea, Tourette syndrome)**
    - oral
      - **children ≥ 3 years:** initially 0.025–0.05 mg/kg, may be increased to max. 0.2 mg/kg in appropriate application form
      - **note:** Use in children < 3 years is not recommended.
- **USA – T:**
  - oral
    - **children 3–12 years, 15–40 kg:**
      - initially 0.25–0.5 mg/d as 2–3 separate doses; increase by 0.25–0.5 mg every 5–7 d; max. 0.15 mg/kg/d
      - usual maintenance:
        - agitation or hyperkinesia: 0.01–0.03 mg/kg/d once daily
        - Tourette syndrome or nonpsychotic behaviour disorders: 0.05–0.075 mg/kg/d as 2–3 separate doses
        - psychotic disorders: 0.05–0.15 mg/kg/d as 2–3 separate doses
      - **note:** Maximum effective dosage has not been established; doses > 6 mg/d have not been shown to further enhance behaviour improvement. Preliminary findings of a double-blind, placebo controlled study reported the mean optimal dose in 12 schizophrenic children aged 5–12 years to be 2 mg/d (range 0.5–3.5 mg/d or 0.02–0.12 mg/kg/d) as 3 separate doses.
  - IM (as lactate)
    - **children 6–12 years:** 1–3 mg/dose every 4–8 h to max. 0.15 mg/kg/d, switch to oral therapy as soon as possible
    - **note:** Gradually decrease to the lowest effective maintenance dosage once satisfactory therapy response is obtained
- **United Kingdom – BNFC:**
  - **excitement and violent or dangerously impulsive behaviour, schizophrenia and other psychoses, manic episode, short-term adjunctive management of psychomotor agitation**
    - oral
      - **children 12–18 years:** initially 0.5–3 mg/dose 2–3 times daily or 3–5 mg/dose 2–3 times daily in severely affected or resistant disease; in resistant schizophrenia, up to 30 mg/d may be needed; adjust according to response to lowest effective maintenance dose (as low as 5–10 mg/d)
  - **motor tics (including Tourette syndrome)**
    - oral
      - **children 5–12 years:** 0.025–0.05 mg/kg/d as 2 separate doses; adjust according to response up to 10 mg/d
      - **children 12–18 years:** 4.5 mg/d as 3 separate doses; adjust according to response up to 10 mg/d

Heparin

low molecular weight Heparin = LMWH; unfractionated Heparin = UFH

Dosage:

▶ common dosing of LMWH:

	Target level [Anti-FXa U*/ml]	Enoxaparin (Clexane®)	Dalteparin (Fragmin®)
Prophylaxis	0.2–0.4	< 2 months: 1.5 mg*/kg/d > 2 months: 1.0 mg/kg/d	50–100 U*/kg/d (as 1 separate dose)
Therapy	0.4–0.8–(1.0)	< 2 months: 3 mg/kg/d > 2 months: 2 mg/kg/d	120–200 U/kg/d (as 1–2 separate doses)

* U = Anti-FXa international units (Enocoparin: 1 mg = 100 U)

▶ sinus vein thrombosis (SVT) with concurrent bleeding:
  - acute: 100–200 U/kg/d UFH IV (target PTT not or just slightly prolonged)

– long-term therapy: if there is no or stable bleeding, consider changing to LMWH in prophylactic dose for 6–12 months depending on aetiology and current risk factors
▶ SVT without concurrent bleeding:
– acute: 200–400 (–600) U/kg/d UFH IV (target PTT 50–60s)
– subacute: as soon as the condition is under control, change to LMWH (target Anti-FXa: 0.6–0.8 U/ml): < 1 year: 2 × 1.5 mg/kg enoxaparin/d SC; > 1 year: 2 × 1 mg/kg enoxaparin/d SC or other appropriately weight adapted LMWH
– maintenance therapy: after 4 weeks, change to LMWH in prophylactic dose (target Anti-FXa: 0.2–0.6 U/ml): < 1 year: 1 × 1 mg/kg enoxaparin/d SC; > 1 year: 2 × 0.75 mg/kg enoxaparin/d SC or other weight adapted LMWH, depending on aetiology or predicted future risk factors for 6–12 months
▶ dissection of brain supplying arteries without SAH: acute and subacute, target PTT 2–3 times increased

Neuropaediatric indications:

– thromembolism-therapy and -prophylaxis
– venous thrombosis-therapy and -prophylaxis

Mechanism of action:

– LMWH and UFH bind to antithrombin III and accelerate about 1000-fold the inactivation of activated coagulation factors
– LMWH inactivates the prothrombinase complex (activated factor X, activated factor V, Calcium ions and phospholipids)
– UFH inactivates the prothrombinase complex and additionally, activated factor II (= thrombin). Thus, UFH is a faster-acting anticoagulant than LMWH.
– further inactivation of factors IX, XI, XII and kallikrein

Relevant contraindications:

– significant liver or kidney diseases (mostly UFH; dose adjustments)
– epidural anesthesia, pancreas diseases, deficiency of coagulation factors (exception: disseminated intravascular coagulation in the hypercoagulation phase)
– present or possibility of future inner bleedings
– puncture at arteries and parenchymatous organs, intramuscular injections (< 7 d)
– upcoming or recent surgical procedures

Relevant side effects and interactions:

– bleeding
– osteoporosis and spontaneous fractures after long-term treatment (less frequent with LMWH)

– allergic reactions
– HIT

Approval status:

– depends on the specific product (see SPC)
– LMWHs are not approved for the treatment of children, but are the standard of antithrombotic therapy; there is sufficient experience even with prematures.

Sources:

– **Germany – SPC: UFH**
  – **treatment of venous and arterial thromboembolic disorders**
    – continuous IV infusion for existing clots
      – **children:** initially 50 U/kg, followed by 20 U/kg/h
    – if continuous infusion is not possible, SC administration may be considered: 10 000–12 500 U/12 h (monitor carefully)
    – Monitoring and dosing adjustments according to activated partial thromboplastin time (aPTT), which should be 1.5–2.5-fold elevated compared to normal aPTT. Measure aPTT at 1–2 h, 6 h, and 12 h after start of therapy.
– **USA – T: enoxaparin**
  – **prophylaxis of thromboembolic disorders**
    – SC
      – **infants < 2 months:** initially 1.5 mg/kg/d as 2 separate doses
      – **infants > 2 months:** initially 1 mg/kg/d as 2 separate doses
  – **therapy of thromboembolic disorders**
    – SC
      – **infants < 2 months:** initially 3 mg/kg/d as 2 separate doses
      – **infants > 2 months:** initially 2 mg/kg/d as 2 separate doses
    – Maintenance therapy

Anti-factor Xa	Dosage titration	Control of Anti-factor Xa
< 0.35 U/ml	Increase dose by 25 %	4 h after next dose
0.35–0.49 U/ml	Increase dose by 10 %	4 h after next dose
0.5–1 U/ml	Keep same dosage	Next day, then 1 week later, then monthly (4 h after dose)
1.1–1.5 U/ml	Decrease dose by 20 %	Before next dose
1.6–2 U/ml	Hold dose for 3 h and then decrease dose by 30 %	Before next dose, then 4 h after next dose
> 2 U/ml	Hold all doses until anti-factor Xa = 0.5 U/ml, then decrease dose by 40 %	Before next dose and every 12 h until anti-factor Xa < 0.5 U/ml

- **United Kingdom – BNFC: dalteparin sodium**
  - treatment of thrombotic episodes
    - SC injection
      - **neonates:** 200 U/kg/d as 2 separate doses
      - **children 1 month–12 years:** 200 U/kg/d as 2 separate doses
      - **children 12–18 years:** 200 U/kg/d (max. 18 000 U) as a SD, if increased risk of bleeding reduced to 200 U/kg/d as 2 separate doses
  - prophylaxis of thrombotic episodes
    - SC injection
      - **neonates:** 100 U/kg/d as a SD
      - **children 1 month–12 years:** 100 U/kg/d as a SD
      - **children 12–18 years:** 2500–5000 U/d as a SD
- **United Kingdom – BNFC: enoxaparin sodium**
  - treatment of thrombotic episodes
    - SC injection
      - **neonates:** 3–4 mg/kg/d as 2 separate doses
      - **children 1–2 months:** 3 mg/kg/d as 2 separate doses
      - **children 2 months–18 years:** 2 mg/kg/d as 2 separate doses
  - prophylaxis of thrombotic episodes
    - SC injection
      - **neonates:** 1.5 mg/kg/d as 2 separate doses
      - **children 1–2 months:** 1.5 mg/kg/d as 2 separate doses
      - **children 2 months–18 years:** 1 mg/kg/d as 2 separate doses, max. 40 mg/d
- **United Kingdom – BNFC: UFH**
  - treatment of thrombotic episodes
    - IV
      - **neonates:** initially 75 U/kg (50 U/kg, if under 35 weeks postmenstrual age) by IV injection, then by continuous IV infusion 25 U/kg/h, adjusted according to aPTT
      - **children 1 month–1 year:** initially 75 U/kg by IV injection, then by continuous IV infusion 25 U/kg/h, adjusted according to aPTT
      - **children 1–18 years:** initially 75 U/kg by IV injection, then by continuous IV infusion 20 U/kg/h, adjusted according to aPTT
    - SC injection
      - **children 1 month–18 years:** 250 U/kg/dose twice daily, adjusted according to aPTT
  - prophylaxis of thrombotic episodes
    - SC injection
      - **children 1 month–18 years:** 100 U/kg/dose (max. 5000 U) twice daily, adjusted according to aPTT

Comments:

- advantage of LMWH: extended efficacy; in SC thrombosis prophylaxis, control of coagulation is rarely necessary
- monitoring:
  - UFH: target a 1.5 times increased aPTT (PTT ~ 50 sec)
  - LMWH:
    - children up to 3 years: first control, 2–3 h after the second or third SC administration then according to dose changes (approximately 20–30 U/kg/dose) control up to stable level
    - children > 3 years: first control 4 h after second or third SC administration then according to dose changes (approximately 20–30 U/kg/dose)
    - stable levels: 1(–2) x/week in the first 4 weeks then 1 x/month

Hydroxocobalamin

(Vitamin B$_{12}$, Cyanocobalamin)

> **Dosage:**
> ▶ 100 mcg/kg/dose (max. 1 mg) IM for 15 d, then weekly or monthly for prophylaxis (off-label)

Neuropaediatric indications:
- Vitamin B$_{12}$ deficiency (subacute combined degeneration of spinal cord)

Mechanism of action:
- Vitamin B$_{12}$ or coenzyme B$_{12}$ participates in 2 reactions in the human body:
  - N-methyltetrahydrofolate-homocysteine S-methyltransferase (= methionine synthase): re-methylation of homocysteine to methionine. In Vitamin B$_{12}$ deficiency, N-methyltetrahydrofolate accumulates, thus decreasing the availability of tetrahydrofolate for the synthesis of Thymidine, Adenine and Guanine.
  - methylmalonyl-CoA mutase: catalyzes the break down of methylmalonyl-CoA to succinyl-CoA (part of citric acid cycle). In Vitamin B$_{12}$ deficiency, methylmalonyl-CoA levels increase in blood and urine leading to methylmalonic acidemia.

Relevant contraindications:
- none

Relevant side effects and interactions:
- dermal reactions, iron deficiency, folic acid deficiency, hypokalemia

Approval status:
- depends on the specific product (see SPC)

Sources:
- **Germany – SPC:**
  - **Vitamin B$_{12}$ deficiency**
  - oral
    - sustained treatment of pernicious anemia: 300 mcg/d. May be increased to 600 mcg/d.

- IV
  - 1 mg/week as long as signs and symptoms persist. If a lifelong treatment is indicated (e.g. approved Vitamin B_{12} resorption disorder): 1 mg/month
  - **note:** no special paediatric dosing is specified in SPC
- **USA – T:**
  - **Schilling test (diagnostic for Vitamin B_{12} deficiency)**
    - IM
      - **children:** 1 mg once
  - **congenital transcobalamin deficiency**
    - IM
      - **neonates:** 1 mg/dose twice weekly
  - **Vitamin B_{12} deficiency or pernicious anemia**
    - IM
      - **children:** initially 100 mcg/d for 10–15 d (total dose: 1–5 mg); maintenance with 60 mcg/month or 30–50 mcg/d for at least 2 weeks (total dose: 1–5 mg), followed by 100 mcg/month
  - **cobalamin C disease**
    - IM
      - **neonates:** 1 mg/dose once daily was used in a single full-term neonate in conjunction with carnitine and Folinic acid
- **United Kingdom – BNFC:**
  - **prophylaxis of macrocytic anemias associated with Vitamin B_{12} deficiency**
    - IM
      - **children 1 month–18 years:** 1 mg every 2–3 months
  - **congenital transcobalamin II deficiency**
    - IM
      - **neonates:** 1 mg/dose 3 times a week; reduce after 1 year to 1 mg/dose once weekly or as appropriate
      - **children 1 month–18 years:** 1 mg/dose 3 times a week; reduce after 1 year to 1 mg/dose once weekly or as appropriate

Comments:
- daily demand approximately 1 mcg

Ibuprofen

Dosage:
▶ acute therapy of tension-type headache: 10–15 mg/kg/dose p.o./supp.
▶ acute therapy of migraine: 10–15 mg/kg/dose p.o./supp.
▶ pain amplification syndrome: 20 mg/kg/d
▶ fever in fever convulsion: 2.5–10 mg/kg/dose (max. 600 mg/dose) every 6–8 h

Neuropaediatric indications:
- mild to moderate pain (tension-type headache, migraine)
- fever, fever convulsion

Mechanism of action:
- non-selective inhibitor of the cyclooxygenases I and II, development of prostaglandins is inhibited: analgesic, antiphlogistic, antipyretic
- reversible inhibition of platelet aggregation

Relevant contraindications:
- disorders of hematopoesis
- gastrointestinal ulcers
- acute hepatic porphyria
- bronchial asthma, hay fever, nasal polyps, chronic respiratory infections
- cardiac or hepatic insufficiency, hypertension
- renal insufficiency (possible deterioration of renal function by inhibition of prostaglandin synthesis; also nephrotoxic)
- systemic lupus erythematodes and various connective tissue diseases
- special caution in chronic inflammatory bowel diseases (Crohn's disease, ulcerative colitis) (Ibuprofen can cause relapses)

Relevant side effects and interactions
- pyrosis, nausea, diarrhea (these gastrointestinal side effects can be reduced by concurrent intake of food)
- if addicted to or long-term use: gastrointestinal bleedings, stomach ulcer, gastritis, anemia
- rash, pruritus
- headache, fatigue, vertigo, impaired vision, hearing disorder (rare)
- sodium and water retention (oedema)

- renal impairment, rare (e.g. nephrotic syndrome, in some cases acute renal failure. Ibuprofen can also lead to interstitial nephritis in some patients, long-term use may lead to papillary necrosis)
- hematopoetic disorder
- hypersensitive reactions (e.g. dermal reactions, bronchial spasms, decreasing blood pressure up to shock. In some patients Ibuprofen, Diclofenac, naproxen, tolmetin can cause aseptic meningitis with headache, nausea, vomiting, fever, neck stiffness or disorientation)
- mild anticoagulative effect
- anticoagulants and thrombolytics increase the bleeding risk
- Lithium: Ibuprofen increases the plasma concentration of Lithium due to decreased renal elimination (risk of Lithium-intoxication)
- Acetylsalicylic acid: concurrent intake of Ibuprofen can nearly eliminate the anticoagulative effect of Acetylsalicylic acid.

Approval status:
- depends on the specific product (see SPC)

Sources:
- Germany – SPC:
  - **mild to moderate pain, fever**
  - oral

body weight, age	max. daily dose for children
20–29 kg, 6–9 years:	600 mg
30–39 kg, 10–12 years:	800 mg
≥ 40 kg, ≥ 12 years:	1200 mg

- USA – T:
  - **note:** to reduce the risk of adverse cardiovascular and GI effects, use the lowest effective dose for the shortest period of time
  - **analgesic**
    - oral
      - **infants and children:** 4–10 mg/kg/dose every 6–8 h, max. 40 mg/kg/d
  - **antipyretic**
    - oral
      - **infants and children 6 months–12 years:** < 102.5°F (< 39°C): 5 mg/kg/dose, ≥ 102.5°F (≥ 39°C): 10 mg/kg/dose every 6–8 h, max. 40 mg/kg/d
  - **OTC paediatric labeling (analgesic, antipyretic)**
    - oral
      - **children 6 months–11 years:** 7.5 mg/kg/dose every 6–8 h, max. 30 mg/kg
      - manufacturer's recommendation: **note:** use of weight to select dose is preferred; if weight is not available, then use age; doses may be repeated every 6–8 h; max. 4 doses/d; treatment for > 10 d is not recommended unless directed by healthcare provider; treatment of sore throat for > 2 d or use in children < 3 years of age with sore throat is not recommended unless directed by healthcare provider

Bodyweight in kg	age	dosage in mg
5.4–7.7	6–11 months	50
8.2–10.4	12–23 months	75
10.9–15.9	2–3 years	100
15.9–21.3	4–5 years	150
21.8–26.8	6–8 years	200
27.2–32.2	9–10 years	250
32.7–43.1	11 years	300

- United Kingdom – BNFC:
  - **mild to moderate pain, pain and inflammation of soft-tissue injuries, pyrexia with discomfort**
    - oral
      - **children 1–3 months:** 5 mg/kg/dose, 3–4 times daily
      - **children 3–6 months:** 50 mg/dose, 3 times daily, max. 30 mg/kg/d as 3–4 separate doses
      - **children 6 months–1 year:** 50 mg/dose, 3–4 times daily, max. 30 mg/kg/d as 3–4 separate doses
      - **children 1–4 years:** 100 mg/dose, 3 times daily, max. 30 mg/kg/d as 3–4 separate doses
      - **children 4–7 years:** 150 mg/dose, 3 times daily, max. 30 mg/kg/d as 3–4 separate doses
      - **children 7–10 years:** 200 mg/dose, 3 times daily, max. 30 mg/kg/d (max. 2.4 mg) as 3–4 separate doses
      - **children 10–12 years:** 300 mg/dose 3 times daily, max. 30 mg/kg/d (max. 2.4 mg) as 3–4 separate doses
      - **children 12–18 years:** initially 300–400 mg/dose, 3–4 times daily; increase if necessary to max. 600 mg/dose, 4 times daily; maintenance dose of 200–400 mg/dose, 3 times daily, may be adequate

Comments:
- duration of action: 4(–6) h; sustained release tablets 8(–12) h
- consider prophylactic gastric protection
- advantages in comparison to Acetylsalicylic acid and Paracetamol
  - risk of side effects "low", good therapeutic range
  - no association with Reye's syndrome
  - influence on coagulation is low
  - good gastric solubility of Ibuprofen lysinate (salt of Ibuprofen and lysine) facilitates fast resorption and fast onset of action, bucco-lingual administration

Idebenone

Dosage:
- ▶ 15–45 mg/kg/d

Neuropaediatric indications:
- therapeutic option in ataxia

Mechanism of action:
- synthetically produced analogue of Coenzyme Q_{10}
- Coenzyme Q_{10}:
  - essential electron and proton carrier between complex I and complex II of the respiratory chain
  - organs with highest energy requirements such as liver, lung, kidney and heart have the highest concentration of Coenzyme Q_{10}
  - additionally, important mitochondrial antioxidant
- efficacy in the treatment of Friedreich's ataxia has not been sufficiently proven; effects are reported for cardiomyopathies

Relevant contraindications:
- none

Relevant side effects and interactions:
- no side effects have been reported

Approval status:
- in Europe: orphan drug status in Friedreich's ataxia, Leber's optic neuropathy, Duchenne/Becker muscular dystrophy

Sources:
- Germany – SPC: –
- USA – T: –
- United Kingdom – BNFC: –
- Uptodate.com: –

Comments:
- ongoing clinical studies in Friedreich's ataxia, Leber's optic neuropathy, Duchenne/Becker muscular dystrophy, debatable efficacy

Imipenem

Dosage
- ▶ < 3 months: 50 mg/kg/d as 2–3 separate doses
- ▶ > 3 months: 60 mg/kg/d as 4 separate doses (max. 2 g/d) (SPC)

Neuropaediatric indications
- neuroborreliosis in cephalosporin allergy
- bacterial meningitis

Mechanism of action
- carbapenem (β-lactam antibiotics)
- bacteriostatic, because the opening and binding of the β-lactam-ring inhibits cross-linking of the peptidoglycans preventing assembly of new membranes
- broad spectrum efficacy in the Gram-positive, Gram-negative, aerobic and anaerobic area
- only moderate efficacy in pseudomonads
- resistant are Clostridium difficile, Enterococcus faecium, legionella, mycoplasmae, MRSA, Stenotrophomonas maltophilia

Relevant contraindications:
- hypersensitivity to β-lactam antibiotics such as penicillin or cephalosporins (cross allergy possible)

Relevant side effects and interactions:
- exanthema
- eosinophilia, leukopenia, thrombocytopenia, thrombocytosis, rarely agranulocytosis
- elevated levels of transaminase, alkaline phosphatase and creatinine possible
- gastrointestinal disorders
- vertigo, seizures
- phlebitis
- brown colouration of the tongue
- combination with Ganciclovir and Valganciclovir (rarely Theophylline): seizures possible
- lowers the serum concentration of Valproic acid
- probenecid can increase the serum level of Imipenem

Approval status:
- severe infections in children and adults

Sources:
- Germany – SPC:
  - treatment of severe or life threatening infections caused by Imipenem -sensitive bacteria
    - IV
      - **children < 1 year:** not recommended
      - **children > 1 year:** 60 mg Imipenem + 60 mg Cilastatin/kg/d as 4 separate doses up to 100 mg Imipenem + 100 mg Cilastatin/kg/d as 4 separate doses
      - **adolescents:** 2 g Imipenem + 2 g Cilastatin/d as 4 separate doses or 3 g Imipenem+ 3 g Cilastatin/d as 3 separate doses or 4 g Imipenem + 4 g Cilastatin/d as 4 separate doses
- USA – T:
- **note:** Dosage recommendations are based on Imipenem component; however, not the preferred Carbapenem for preterm infants due to Cilastatin accumulation and possible adverse effects.
  - non-CNS infection caused by multidrug-resistant Gram-negative bacteria
    - IV
      - **neonates < 7 d:** 25 mg/kg/dose every 12 h
      - **neonates ≥ 7 d and < 1200 g:** 25 mg/kg/dose every 12 h
      - **neonates ≥ 7 d and ≥ 1200 g:** 25 mg/kg/dose every 8 h
    - IV, IM
      - **infants 1–3 months:** 100 mg/kg/d as 4 separate doses
      - **infants ≥ 3 months and children:** 60–100 mg/kg/d as 4 separate doses; max. 4 g/d
- United Kingdom – BNFC: –

Comments:
- in renal impairment: dose reduction
- variable published dosage recommendations in common paediatric sources

Infliximab

Dosage:
- initially 3 mg/kg IV, then in week 2 and 6 the same dose, then every 8 weeks (off-label)

Neuropaediatric indications:
- in relapsing dermatomyositis with calcinosis (positive effect in some cases)

Mechanism of action:
- chimeric monoclonal antibodies against TNF-α
- Infliximab neutralizes the biological activity of TNF-α by binding with high affinity to the soluble and transmembrane forms of TNF-α
  - TNF-α is produced by monocytes, macrophages and activated T-cells and participates in many immune-mediated inflammatory processes
  - activates the expression of adhesion molecules on the surface of endothelial cells that promote the influx of leukocytes into the interstitium
  - stimulates the release of metallomatrix proteases
  - under the influence of TNF-α: increased production of inflammatory-promoting cytokines like interleukin-1, -6 and -8

Relevant contraindications:
- tuberculosis or other severe infections
- hypersensitivity to murine proteins
- heart failure (NYHA III and IV)
- pregnancy
- careful use: Crohn's disease with fistulas, other infections, previous or present demyelinating diseases, past malignant diseases, psoriasis, heart failure (NYHA I and II), liver and kidney diseases, < 18 years

Relevant side effects and interactions:
- headache, vertigo, drowsiness, fatigue
- nausea, diarrhea, abdominal pain, dyspepsia, gastroesophageal reflux, cheilitis, diverticulitis
- rash, pruritus, urticaria, increased sweat secretion, seborrhea, fever
- increased viral and bacterial infections
- dyspnea, asthma, oedema of the lung
- elevated liver transaminases, liver function disorders
- depression, confusion, agitation, insomnia, amnesia, apathy, nervousness
- wound healing disorders
- thrombocytopenia, anemia, leukopenia, lymphadenopathy, lymphocytosis, lymphopenia, neutropenia
- deterioration of demyelinating diseases
- lupus-like syndrome
- hypersensitivity reactions
- syncope
- bradycardia, awareness of heart beat, cyanosis, arrhythmia, deterioration of a heart failure, hypertension, hypotension
- ecchymosis, petechia
- thrombophlebitis, peripheral ischaemia, epistaxis, bronchial spasm
- oedema of the lung
- myalgia, arthralgias
- severe side effects especially in paediatric patients: hepatosplenic T-cell lymphoma (increased risk in Crohn's disease and concurrent administration of Azathioprine or 6 mercaptopurine)

Approval status:

– approved in children with Crohn's disease between the age of 6 and 17 years

Sources:

– **Germany – SPC:**
  – **severe active Crohn's disease**
    – IV
    – no additional information to USA – T or United Kingdom – BNFC
    – indication of interest is not specified in SPC
– **USA – T:**
  – **Crohn's disease**
    – IV infusion
      – **note:** premedication with antihistamines (H_1-antagonist and/or H_2-antagonist), Acetaminophen and/or corticosteroids may be considered to prevent and/or manage infusion-related reaction
      – **children:** initially 5 mg/kg/dose; repeat 5 mg/kg/dose at 2 and 6 weeks after the first infusion; maintenance with 5 mg/kg/dose every 8 weeks. If the response is incomplete, may has to be increased up to 10 mg/kg
– **United Kingdom – BNFC:**
  – **severe active Crohn's disease**
    – IV infusion
      – **children 6–18 years:** initially 5 mg/kg, then 5 mg/kg 2 weeks and 6 weeks after initial dose, then 5 mg/kg every 8 weeks; interval between maintenance doses adjusted according to response; discontinue if no response within 10 weeks of initial dose
  – **fistulating Crohn's disease**
    – IV infusion
      – **children 6–18 years:** initially 5 mg/kg, then 5 mg/kg 2 weeks and 6 weeks after initial dose. If the patient's condition has responded to treatment, consult literature for guidance on further doses.

Comments:

– is used for rheumatic diseases and in Crohn's disease
– variable published dosage recommendations in common paediatric sources

Interactions of anticonvulsive drugs

		First AED																	
		CBZ	CLB	FBM	GBP	LCM	LTG	LEV	OXC	PB	PHT	PGB	PRM	RFN	STP	TGB	TPM	VPA	VGB	ZNS
ADDED AED	CBZ	AI	CLB↓↓ DMCLB↑↑	FBM↓↓	⇌	⇌	LTG↓↓	⇌	H-OXC↓	⇌	PHT↑↓	⇌	PRM↓ PB↑	RFN↓	STP↓↓	TGB↓↓	TPM↓↓	VPA↓↓	⇌	ZNS↓↓
	CLB	?	–	?	NU	NU	?	⇌	⇌	?	PHT↑	NU	PRM↑	?	?	?	?	VPA↑	NU	?
	FBM	CBZ↓ CBZ-E↑	CLB↓↓ DMCLB↑↑	–	NU	NU	⇌	NU	⇌	PB↑↑	PHT↑↑	NU	?	?	?	?	?	VPA↑↑	⇌	?
	GBP	⇌	NU	FBM↑	–	NU	NU	⇌	NU	⇌	⇌	?	NU	NU	NU	NU	⇌	⇌	NU	NU
	LCM	⇌	NU	NU	NU	–	⇌	⇌	⇌	NU	⇌	NU	NU	NU	NU	NU	⇌	⇌	NU	NU
	LTG	⇌	⇌	NU	NU	⇌	–	⇌	NU	⇌	⇌	⇌	⇌	⇌	?	NU	⇌	VPA↓	NU	⇌
	LEV	⇌	⇌	NU	⇌	⇌	⇌	–	NU	⇌	⇌	⇌	⇌	NU	NU	NU	NU	⇌	NU	NU
	OXC	CBZ↓	⇌	?	?	⇌	LTG↓	NU	–	PB↑	PHT↑	NU	?	?	?	?	TPM↓	⇌	NU	?
	PB	CBZ↓↓	CLB↓↓ DMCLB↑↑	FBM↓↓	⇌	NU	LTG↓↓	⇌	H-OXC↓	AI	PHT↑↓	⇌	1)	RFN↓↓	STP↓↓	TGB↓↓	TPM↓↓	VPA↓↓	⇌	ZNS↓↓
	PHT	CBZ↓↓	CLB↓↓ DMCLB↑↑	FBM↓↓	⇌	⇌	LTG↓↓	⇌	H-OXC↓	PB↑	AI	⇌	PRM↓ PB↑	RFN↓↓	STP↓↓	TGB↓↓	TPM↓↓	VPA↓↓	⇌	ZNS↓↓
	PGB	⇌	NU	NU	?	NU	⇌	⇌	NU	⇌	⇌	–	NU	NU	NU	⇌	⇌	⇌	NU	NU
	PRM	CBZ↓↓	CLB↓↓ DMCLB↑↑	FBM↓↓	⇌	NU	LTG↓↓	⇌	?	1)	PHT↑↓	NU	–	RFN↓↓	STP↓↓	TGB↓↓	TPM↓↓	VPA↓↓	⇌	ZNS↓↓
	RFN	CBZ↓	?	?	NU	NU	LTG↓	NU	?	PB↑	PHT↑	NU	?	–	?	?	?	⇌	NU	?
	STP	CBZ↑↑	CLB↑↑ DMCLB↑↑	?	NU	NU	?	NU	?	PB↑↑	PHT↑↑	NU	PRM↑↑	?	–	?	?	VPA↑↑	NU	?
	TGB	⇌	NU	NU	NU	NU	NU	NU	NU	⇌	⇌	⇌	?	?	?	–	NU	⇌	NU	?
	TPM	⇌	?	?	NU	⇌	⇌	⇌	NU	?	PHT↑	⇌	?	?	?	?	–	VPA↓	NU	?
	VPA	CBZ-E↑↑	?	FBM↑	⇌	⇌	LTG↑↑	⇌	⇌	PB↑↑	PHT↓*	⇌	PB↑↑	RFN↑	?	⇌	TPM↓	–	⇌	ZNS↓↓
	VGB	⇌	NU	⇌	NU	NU	NU	NU	NU	⇌	PHT↓	NU	⇌	RFN↓	NU	NU	NU	⇌	–	NU
	ZNS	CBZ↑↓	?	?	NU	NU	⇌	NU	?	⇌	PHT↑	NU	⇌	?	?	NU	NU	⇌	NU	–

– CBZ = Carbamazepine; CBZ-E = Carbamazepine-10,11-Epoxid (active metabolite of CBZ); CLB = Clobazam; NDCLB = N-Desmethyclobazam (active metabolite of CLB); FBM = Felbamat; GBP = Gabapentin; H-OXC = 10-Hydroxy-Oxcarbazepin (active metabolite of OXC); LCM = Lacosamide; LEV = Levetiracetam; LTG = Lamotrigine; OXC = Oxcarbazepine; PB = Phenobarbital; PHT = Phenytoin; PGB = Pregabalin; PRM = Primidone; RFN = Rufinamide; STP = Stiripentol; TGB = Tiagabine; TPM = Topiramate; VPA = Valproic acid; VGB = Vigabatrin; ZNS = Zonisamide; AI = Autoinduction; NU = not investigated; 1) = not generally co-prescribed; ⇌ = no changes; ↓ = usually only small (or inconsistent) decrease of plasma levels; ↓↓ = usually clinically significant reduction of plasma levels; ↑ = usually small (or inconsistent) increase of plasma levels; ↑↑ usually clinically significant increase of plasma levels; * = free/other (pharmacologically aktive) possible increase of plasma levels. (Quelle: Patsalos PN (2010), Drug to Drug Interactions of Antiepileptic Drugs (adivided doses): I. Interactions between divided dosess. In: Panayiotopoulos CP et al. (ed.) Atlas of epilepsies. London: Springer, pp. 1459–1463.)

Interferon beta-1a

Dosage:
▶ consider using a lower initial dose in children younger than 10 years or < 30 kg
▶ preparation Avonex®: 30 mcg 1×/week
▶ preparation Rebif®: 22–44 mcg 3×/week

Neuropaediatric indications:
– immunomodulatory therapy in multiple sclerosis

Mechanism of action:
– from mammalian cell cultures (Chinese hamster ovarian cells)
– molecular structure is identical to human Interferon-beta
– physiologically produced by fibroblasts in the body
– stimulates monocytes in vivo; cytotoxic cell activity
– T-cell-activity is inhibited
– precise mechanism of action in MS is unknown. Presumably Interferon beta-1a acts by downregulating myelin-damaging autoimmune reactions of the body.

Relevant contraindications:
– acute severe depression
– hypersensitivity to natural or recombinant interferon or human albumin
– current pregnancy
– careful use: children younger than 12 y (Avonex®) and children younger than 16 y (Rebif®), other affective disorders, previous seizures, heart diseases, severe hepatic and renal impairment, myelosuppression, co-administration of other medication with a narrow therapeutic range and metabolization by the cytochrom-P450 system

Relevant side effects and interactions:
– local skin reaction at the injection site (exanthema, pruritus, swelling)
– flu-like symptoms (fever, sweating, shivering, weakness, fatigue, myalgia, arthralgias, headache), mostly in the first hours after injection; usually less frequent with increasing duration of treatment
– CNS disorders (e.g. tremor, depressions, confusion, anxiety, drowsiness, somnolence, coma, cerebral seizures)
– hair loss
– loss of appetite, nausea, vomiting, stomach pain, diarrhea
– elevation of transaminases
– arrhythmia, tachycardia, palpitations
– granulocytopenia, thrombopenia, anemia
– development of antibodies

– interaction with other drugs has not been investigated

Approval status:
– not approved for children younger than 12 years (Avonex®) and under 16 years of age (Rebif®)

Sources:
– **Germany – SPC:**
  – **multiple sclerosis (progressive and relapsing)**
    – **children:** efficacy and safety have not been established in patients < 18 years. A dosing recommendation cannot be given.
– **USA – T:** –
– **United Kingdom – BNFC:** –
– **Uptodate.com:** no published paediatric dosage
– **Multiple sclerosis**
  – IM (Avonex®):
    – **adults:** U.S. labeling: 30 mcg once weekly
    – **adults:** Canadian labeling: 30 mcg once weekly; consider increasing to 60 mcg once weekly in progressive relapsing MS or secondary progressive MS with recurrent neurologic dysfunction

Interferon beta-1b

Dosage:
▶ consider using a lower dose in children younger than 10 years or < 30 kg
▶ betaferon: 250 mcg (8 Mio U) every other day

Neuropaediatric indications:
– immunomodulatory therapy in multiple sclerosis

Mechanism of action:
– produced by synthesis in E. coli
– compared to human Interferon beta, modified sequence: point mutation resulting in different protein and glycosylation patterns
– produced physiologically by fibroblasts in the body
– stimulates monocytes in vivo
– T-cell-activity is inhibited
– precise mechanism of action in MS is unknown; presumably Interferon beta-1b acts by down regulating myelin-damaging autoimmune reactions of the body

Relevant contraindications:
– acute severe depression
– hypersensitivity to natural or recombinant interferon or human albumin

470

- pregnancy
- decompensated liver insufficiency
- medication-resistant epilepsy
- careful use: < 12 years, other affective disorders, previous seizures, heart diseases, severe hepatic and renal impairment, myelosuppression, co-administration of other medication with a narrow therapeutic range and metabolization by the cytochrom-P450 system, co-administration of medication with influence on hematopoesis

Relevant side effects and interactions:

- local skin reaction at the injection site (exanthema, pruritus, swelling)
- flu-like symptoms (fever, sweating, shivering, weakness, fatigue, myalgia, arthralgias, headache), mostly in the first hours after injection; usually less frequent with increasing duration of treatment
- CNS disorders (e.g. tremor, depression, confusion, anxiety, drowsiness, somnolence, coma, cerebral seizures)
- hair loss
- loss of appetite, nausea, vomiting, stomach pain, diarrhea
- elevation of transaminases
- arrhythmia, tachycardia, palpitations
- granulocytopenia, thrombopenia, anemia
- development of antibodies
- interaction with other drugs has not been investigated

Approval status:

- not approved for children younger than 12 years

Sources:

- **Germany – SPC:**
  - **treatment of progressive relapsing or secondary progressive multiple sclerosis**
    - SC
      - **children and adolescents:** There have not been any clinical or pharmacokinetic studies. Limited data indicates that safety is comparable to use in adults when using 8 Mio U every other day in children aged 12 to 16.
      - **children < 12 years:** no data is available, therefore use is not recommended
- **USA – T:** –
- **United Kingdom – BNFC:** –
- **Uptodate.com:** not recommended in children aged < 18 years

Intravenous immunoglobulins (IVIG)

Dosage:

- Guillain-Barré syndrome: 0.4 g/kg/d for 5 consecutive days; in progression or secondary deterioration after 4–6 weeks (primarily SIDP or CIDP), 1 g/kg/d for 2 d; for subsequent episodes of deterioration, repeat every 4 weeks and titrate down to lowest effective dose
- opsoclonus myoclonus syndrome (OMS, Kinsbourne encephalitis): 0.4 g/kg/d for 4 d or 1 g/kg/d for 2 d or 2 g/kg as a SD
- MS-relapse therapy/ADEM: 2 g/kg/month over 2–5 d
- Kawasaki syndrome: 2 g/kg/dose
- myositis: 2 g/kg/dose; initially 5 times every 2 weeks, then in intervals of 4 weeks
- myasthenic crisis: 2 g/kg over 2–5 d

Neuropaediatric indications:

- Guillain-Barré syndrome, chronic inflammatory demyelinating polyneuropathy (CIDP)
- MS relapse therapy if Interferon beta and Glatiramer acetate are contraindicated
- ADEM
- Kawasaki syndrome
- myasthenic crisis
- opsoclonus myoclonus syndrome (OMS, Kinsbourne encephalitis)
- severe myositis after non-response to corticosteroids and MTX
- therapy-resistant epileptic encephalopathies

Mechanism of action:

- Human normal immunoglobulin contains the IgG antibodies present in the normal population. It is usually prepared from pooled plasma from not fewer than 1000 donations.
- The mechanism of action in indications other than replacement therapy is not fully elucidated, but includes immunomodulatory effects. These effects can vary depending on the disease treated:
  - via Fc-receptor block of Fc-receptors at macrophages and effector cells
  - anti-inflammatory effect: decrease of immune-complex mediated inflammatory reactions, the release of inflammatory mediators, or via induction of anti-inflammatory cytokines
  - decreased production of auto-antibodies via inhibition of B-cell activity (anti-idiotypic effect)
  - activation of regulatory T-cells
  - influence of cell growth via regulation of apoptosis and inhibition of lymphocyte proliferation

- solubilization of immune complexes
- inhibition of myotoxic cytokines, such as TNF-a and IL-1
- interference with Fc-receptor-mediated phagocytosis via blocking Fc-receptors of endomysial macrophages
- inhibition of the development of immune-complex residues, which can damage membranolytically the endomysial capillaries

Relevant contraindications:

- absolute: known hypersensitivity to immunoglobulins, selective IgA deficiency, known Anti-IgA antibody
- relative: thrombosis, hyperviscosity, renal diseases, nephrotoxic add-on medication, hypovolemia

Relevant side effects and interactions:

- severe side effects in 1–2.5 % of treated patients, in 10–50 % of the patients mild adverse reactions
- redness of face, feeling of tightness in breast, back pain, nausea, shivering, fever, sweating, headache and decreasing blood pressure
- anaphylaxis, acute renal failure, hemolysis, aseptic meningitis, thromboembolics, proteinuria
- possible transmission of infections
- the efficacy of some vaccines is partially decreased (especially in attenuated life vaccination against measles, rubella or mumps); these vaccines should be administered at least 3 months after last infusion of immunoglobulins
- interpretation of serologic results obtained directly after IVIG administration can be difficult (especially with regard to infections, Coombs test, ANA titer or rheumatic factors)

Approval status:

- depends on the specific product (see SPC)

Sources:

- **Germany – SPC:**
  - **Kawasaki syndrome**
    - IV
      - **children:** 1.6–2 g/kg as separate doses over 2 to 5 d or as a SD 2 g/kg. Patient should receive aspirin treatment as well.
  - **Guillain-Barré syndrome**
    - IV
      - **children:** 0.4 g/kg/d for 5 d
  - **chronic inflammatory demyelinating polyneuropathy**
    - IV
      - **children:** only limited data available

- **USA – T:**
  - **Kawasaki syndrome**
    - IV
      - **children:** 2 g/kg/d as a SD over 10–12 h; must be used in combination with aspirin; if signs and symptoms persist ≥ 36 h after completion of infusion, retreatment with a second 2 g/kg infusion should be considered
  - **Guillain-Barré syndrome**
    - IV
      - **children:** 0.4 g/kg/d for 5 d or 1 g/kg/d for 2 d or 2 g/kg as a SD
  - **refractory dermatomyositis, refractory polymyositis**
    - IV
      - **children:** 2 g/kg/month over 2–5 d
  - **chronic inflammatory demyelinating polyneuropathy**
    - IV
      - **children:** 0.4 g/kg/d for 5 d once every month or 1 g/kg/d for 2 d once every month
- **United Kingdom – BNFC:**
  - **Kawasaki syndrome**
    - IV infusion
      - **children:** 2 g/kg as a SD should be given with concomitant aspirin within 10 d of onset of symptoms

Comments:

- especially careful use: patients receiving human immunoglobulin for the first time, change of preparation, and after long discontinuation of treatment with IVIG
- monitor each patient during and after administration:
  - vital signs
  - pay attention to early signs of anaphylactic shock (keep adrenaline and glucocorticoids on standby as circumstances may require shock treatment)
  - balance of urine elimination and serum creatinine concentration
  - hypersensitivity reactions may occur even after infusion is completed
- GBS:
  - in efficacy comparable to plasmapheresis. Low rate of complications (evidence class I studies)
  - 20–25 % do not respond
  - can be repeated after 2–3 weeks of initial non-response (evidence class IV)
  - efficacy of combined treatment with plasmapheresis and IVIG is not superior to that of treatment with single components (evidence class I)

Itraconazole

Dosage:
- ▶ 4–8(–12) mg/kg/d p.o. as 2 separate doses

Neuropaediatric indications:
- aspergillus meningoencephalitis

Mechanism of action:
- inhibits the 14-alpha-demethylase of the cytochrom-P450 system in fungal cells (human demethylase is far less inhibited)
- Thus, lanosterol can not be converted to ergosterol resulting in dysfunction of the fungal cell wall.
- broad spectrum efficacy: effective against yeasts, dimorphic fungi such as Candida, Aspergillus, Cryptococcus neoformans and others
- limited efficacy to Fusarium and Zygomycetes, some Candida forms, such as Candida glabrata or krusei, which are resistant to Fluconazole have been shown to be sensitive to Itraconazole

Relevant contraindications:
- concurrent intake of medication metabolized via CYP450–3A4
- concurrent administration of HMG-CoA-reductase inhibitors and ergolines
- hypokalemia or hypomagnesemia
- QT-prolonging or concurrent intake of medication that can lead to a QT-prolonging (e.g. antiarrhythmics of class Ia or III)
- combination with Cisapride, Astemizole
- combination with Terfenadine
- careful use: AIDS and malignant diseases, severe liver function disorders, < 16 years of age, cardiac arrhythmias, coronary heart diseases, pulmonary function disorder, renal diseases or other diseases that can lead to oedema or immunosuppression

Relevant side effects and interactions:
- exanthema, alopecia, angiooedema, oedema of the face, pruritus
- headache, vertigo, peripheral nerve impairment, unconsciousness
- nausea, vomiting, stomach pain, diarrhea, meteorism
- seizures
- gustatory sense disorder
- increase of alkaline phosphatase, bilirubin, SGOT, SGTP up to liver function disorders with hepatitis and jaundice
- hypercholesterolemia, hypertriglyceridemia, hypokalemia
- hypertension, tendency of oedema
- leukocytopenia, neutropenia, agranulocytosis, thrombocytopenia
- changes of renal function parameters
- enhanced efficacy and side effects of anticoagulants, benzodiazepines, oral antidiabetics of sulfonylurea type (Glibenclamide, Glipizide, Tolbutamide), Rifabutin, Tacrolimus, Sirolimus, Phenythoin, Cyclosporine, Theophylline, Terfenadine, Zidovudine
- reduced efficacy of Rifampicin
- presumably no unfavourable effect on the efficacy of oral contraceptives
- inhibition of glucocorticoid metabolization
- increased risk of myopathy or rhabdomyolysis in combination with HMG-CoA reductase inhibitors

Approval status:
- depends on the specific product (see SPC)

Sources:
- **Germany – SPC:**
- **Systemic fungal infections**
  - oral
    - **children and adolescents:** only limited data available, therefore the use is not recommended.
- **USA – T:**
  - **treatment of susceptible systemic fungal infections**
    - oral
      - **children:** Efficacy of Itraconazole has not been established; a limited number of children have been treated with Itraconazole using doses of 3–5 mg/kg/d once daily; doses as high as 5–10 mg/kg/d as 1–2 separate doses have been used in 32 patients with chronic granulomatous disease for prophylaxis against Aspergillus infection; doses of 6–8 mg/kg/d have been used in the treatment of disseminated histoplasmosis.
- **United Kingdom – BNFC:**
  - **systemic aspergillosis, candidiasis and cryptococcosis including cryptococcal meningitis where other antifungal drugs are inappropriate or ineffective**
    - oral
      - **children 1 month–18 years:** 5 mg/kg/d (max. 200 mg) as a SD; increase in invasive or disseminated disease and in cryptococcal meningitis to 5 mg/kg/dose (max. 200 mg) twice daily
    - IV infusion
      - **children 1 month–18 years:** 2.5 mg/kg/dose (max. 200 mg) every 12 h for 2 d, then 2.5 mg/kg/dose (max. 200 mg) once daily for max. 12 d

Comments:
- insufficient resorption after oral intake
- variable published dosage recommendations in common paediatric sources

K

Ketamine

Dosage
▶ anesthesia:
  – initially 2–4 mg/kg IV, or nasal administration of 3 mg/kg in 0.1 ml sodium chloride 0.9 %
  – repeat doses every 5–15 min: 1–2 mg/kg IV or 5–10 mg/kg IM
▶ analgesic (e.g. lumbar puncture): in combination with Midazolam, e.g. 0.2–0.3 mg/kg; monitor patient closely

Neuropaediatric indications
– anesthesia in emergency medicine
– alternative therapeutic to anesthesia in therapy-resistant non-convulsive status epilepticus
– analgesia (e.g. lumbar puncture, interventional neuropaediatrics)

Mechanism of action
– N-methyl-D-aspartate (NMDA) receptor antagonist at the phencyclidine-binding location
– influences the cholinergic system by inhibition of the NMDA-receptor-dependent acetylcholine release
– weak agonist at opioid receptors
– affinity to GABA receptors
– inhibits peripheral re-uptake of catecholamines (noradrenaline and dopamine) at the synaptic endplate with enhanced of endogenous and exogenous catecholamine effect

Relevant contraindications
– increased intracranial pressure, traumatic brain injury
– coronary heart diseases
– pulmonary diseases
– hyperthyroidism
– increased intraocular pressure, perforated eye injuries

Relevant side effects and interactions:
– increased intracranial pressure
– respiratory depression
– psychotropic effect, nightmare, hallucination
– decreased seizure threshold
– increased blood pressure and pulse
– increased bronchial and salivary secretion
– hydronephrosis in frequent use
– intoxication:
  – apnea, especially in too fast IV injection
  – variation in blood pressure, cardiac arrhythmias
  – in individual hypersensitivity: day dreams, hallucination with confusion and increased muscle tone
– extended duration of action and decreased side effects if combined with benzodiazepines (can partially prevent nightmares and hallucination in the wake-up phase) or neuroleptics
– extended duration of action of non-depolarizing muscle relaxants
– decreased seizure-threshold with concurrent intake of Aminophylline
– concurrent intake of thyroid gland hormones and sympathomimetics can increase blood pressure and pulse
– enhanced efficacy of Halothane
– cardiac arrhythmias if combined with Halothane or Epinephrine
– do not combine with barbiturates (precipitations)

Approval status:
– depends on the specific product (see SPC)

Sources:
– **Germany – SPC:**
  – **anesthesia in emergency**
    – IV 0.25–0.5 mg/kg
    – IM 0.5–1.0 mg/kg
    – no published paediatric dosage
– **USA – T:**
  – **anesthesia**
    – oral
      – **children:** 6–10 mg/kg for 1 dose (mixed in cola or other beverage) given 30 min before the procedure
    – IM
      – **children:** 3–7 mg/kg
    – IV
      – **children:** range of 0.5–2 mg/kg, (0.5–1 mg/kg for sedation for minor procedures); usual induction dose is 1–2 mg/kg; for maintenance use supplemental doses of ⅓ to ½ of initial dose
      – **neonates:** Some neonatal experts do not recommend the use of Ketamine in neonates; an increase in neuronal apoptosis has been observed in neonatal animal studies
      – limited data available; dose not established; titrate dose to effect

- procedural sedation/analgesia: full-term neonates receive 0.2–1 mg/kg/dose; may be repeated with 0.5 mg/kg/dose as needed; the use is most frequently reported in cardiac catheterization and ROP corrective procedures
- **United Kingdom – BNFC:**
  - **sedation prior to invasive or painful procedures**
    - IV injection
      - **children 1 month–18 years:** 1–2 mg/kg/dose as a SD
  - **induction and maintenance of anesthesia (short procedures)**
    - IV injection over at least 60 sec
      - **neonates:** 1–2 mg/kg produces 5–10 minutes of surgical anesthesia; adjust according to response
      - **children 1 month–12 years:** 1–2 mg/kg produces 5–10 minutes of surgical anesthesia; adjust according to response
      - **children 12–18 years:** 1–4.5 mg/kg adjusted according to response (2 mg/kg usually produces 5–10 minutes of surgical anesthesia)
    - IM injection
      - **neonates:** 4 mg/kg usually produces 15 minutes of surgical anesthesia; adjust according to response
      - **children 1 month–18 years:** 4–13 mg/kg (4 mg/kg sufficient for some diagnostic procedures); adjust according to response; 10 mg/kg usually produces 12–25 minutes of surgical anesthesia
  - **induction and maintenance of anesthesia (longer procedures)**
    - IV
      - **neonates:** initially 0.5–2 mg/kg by IV injection, followed by a continuous IV infusion of 8 mcg/kg/minute adjusted according to response; up to 30 mcg/kg/minute may be used to produce deep anesthesia
      - **children 1 month–18 years:** initially 0.5–2 mg/kg by IV injection followed by a continuous IV infusion of 10–45 mcg/kg/minute adjusted according to response

Comments:
- can also be taken orally (!!!) in fruit juice

L

Lacosamide

Dosage:
- maintenance dose: 200–400 mg for patients aged 16 years or older
- titration schedule: first week 2 × 50 mg/d, increase according to desired target dose by 50–100 mg/week
- IV solution: dosing as specified above; bioequivalent with oral administration; infusion over 15–60 min

Neuropaediatric indications:
- adjunctive therapy in the treatment of partial-onset seizures with or without secondary generalization in adult and adolescent (16–18 years) patients with epilepsy

Mechanism of action:
- The precise mechanism by which Lacosamide exerts its antiepileptic effect in humans remains to be fully elucidated. In vitro electrophysiological studies have shown that Lacosamide selectively enhances slow inactivation of voltage-gated sodium channels, resulting in stabilization of hyperexcitable neuronal membranes.

Relevant contraindications:
- hypersensitivity to the active substance or to any of the excipients, known second or third degree atrioventricular (AV) block

Relevant side effects:
- vertigo, headache
- diplopia
- nausea
- depression, confusions
- disturbances of equilibrium, coordination disorders, disturbances of memory, cognitive disorder, somnolence, tremor, nystagmus, hypoesthesia, dysarthria, attention deficiency disorder
- blurred vision
- vertigo, tinnitus
- vomiting, constipation, flatulence, dyspepsia, dry mouth
- pruritus, rash
- muscle spasms
- walking disorder, asthenia, fatigue, irritability
- falling, skin wounds
- atrioventricular block, bradycardia

Interactions:
- Lacosamide should be used with caution in patients treated with drugs known to be associated with EEG-PR prolongation (e. g. Carbamazepine, Lamotrigine, Pregabalin) and in patients treated with class I antiarrhythmic drugs. However, subgroup analysis did not identify an increased magnitude of PR prolongation in patients with concomitant administration of Carbamazepine or Lamotrigine in clinical trials.
- *in vitro* data: Data generally suggest that Lacosamide has a low interaction potential. In vitro studies indicate that the enzymes CYP1A2, 2B6, and 2C9 are not induced and that CYP1A1, 1A2, 2A6, 2B6, 2C8, 2C9, 2D6, and 2E1 are not inhibited by Lacosamide at plasma concentrations observed in clinical trials. An in vitro study indicated that Lacosamide is not transported by P-glycoprotein in the intestine. In vitro data show

that CYP2C9, CYP2C19 and CYP3A4 are capable of catalyzing the formation of the o-desmethyl metabolite.

– *in vivo* data: Lacosamide does not inhibit or induce CYP2C19 and 3A4 to a clinically relevant extent. Lacosamide did not affect the AUC of Midazolam (metabolized by CYP3A4; Lacosamide dose: 200 mg b.i.d.) but C_{max} of Midazolam was slightly increased (30 %). Lacosamide did not affect the pharmacokinetics of omeprazole (metabolized by CYP2C19 and 3A4; Lacosamide dose: 300 mg b.i.d.). The CYP2C19 inhibitor omeprazole (40 mg q.d.) did not give rise to a clinically significant change in Lacosamide exposure. Thus moderate inhibitors of CYP2C19 are unlikely to affect systemic Lacosamide exposure to a clinically relevant extent. Caution is recommended in concomitant treatment with strong inhibitors of CYP2C9 (e.g. Fluconazole) and CYP3A4 (e.g. Itraconazole, Ketoconazole, Ritonavir, Clarithromycin), which may lead to increased systemic exposure of Lacosamide. Such interactions have not been established in vivo but are possible based on in vitro data. Strong enzyme inducers such as rifampicin or St John´s wort (Hypericum perforatum) may moderately reduce the systemic exposure of Lacosamide. Therefore, starting or ending treatment with these enzyme inducers should be done with caution.

– *antiepileptic drugs:* In interaction trials Lacosamide did not significantly affect the plasma concentrations of Carbamazepine and Valproic acid. Lacosamide plasma concentrations were not affected by Carbamazepine and by Valproic acid. A population pharmakokinetic analysis estimated that concomitant treatment with other antiepileptic drugs known to be enzyme inducers (Carbamazepine, Phenytoin, Phenobarbital, in various doses) decreased the overall systemic exposure of Lacosamide by 25 %.

– *oral contraceptives:* In an interaction trial there was no clinically relevant interaction between Lacosamide and the oral contraceptives ethinyl estradiol and levonorgestrel. Progesterone concentrations were not affected when the drugs were co-administered.

– *others:* Interaction trials showed that Lacosamide had no effect on the pharmacokinetics of digoxin. There was no clinically relevant interaction between Lacosamide and metformin.

– No data on the interaction of Lacosamide with alcohol are available.

– Lacosamide has a low protein binding of less than 15 %. Therefore, clinically relevant interactions with other drugs through competition for protein binding sites are considered unlikely.

Approval status:

adjunctive therapy in the treatment of partial-onset seizures with or without secondary generalization in adult and adolescent (16–18 years) patients with epilepsy

Sources:

– Germany – SPC:
  – **adjunctive treatment of focal seizures with or without secondary generalization**
    – oral
      – **children < 16 years:** not recommended due to lack of data regarding efficacy and safety
      – **children ≥ 16 years:** initially 100 mg/d as 2 separate doses, increase after 1 week to 200 mg/d as 2 separate doses. According to response the maintenance dose can be titrated by 50-mg increments twice daily up to max. 400 mg/d as 2 separate doses. If it is indicated to interrupt therapy then reduce slowly (e.g. reduce by 200 mg/week).
– USA – T: –
– United Kingdom – BNFC:
  – **adjunctive treatment of focal seizures with or without secondary generalization**
    – IV infusion over 15–60 minutes (for up to 5 d) or oral
      – **children 16–18 years:** initially 50 mg/dose twice daily; increase in steps of 50 mg/dose twice daily every week; max. 200 mg/dose twice daily

Comments:

until now no paediatric data

Lamotrigine (LTG)

Dosage:

▶ monotherapy: 1–15 mg/kg/d as 2 separate doses (target plasma level: 2–12 mg/l)
  – adjunctive therapy (with Valproic acid): 1–5 mg/kg/d as 2 separate doses
▶ juvenile myoclonic epilepsy: 3 mg/kg/d p.o.
▶ West syndrome: 1–10 mg/kg/d p.o. as 2(–4) separate doses

Neuropaediatric indications:

– focal, generalized and absence epilepsy

Mechanism of action:

– blocks sodium and voltage dependant Calcium channels of neurons and thus, prevents the release of excitatory neurotransmitters aspartate and glutamate

Relevant contraindications:

– hypersensitivity to Carbamazepine or Phenytoin (cross reactions possible)
– < 18 years in manic-depressive diseases
– careful use: liver and renal impairment, prevention of manic episodes of bipolar patients, pregnancy

Relevant side effects and interactions:

- too fast titration: skin and mucosa reactions such as exanthema, exfoliative dermatitis, Stevens-Johnson syndrome
- rare: double vision, vertigo, headache, nausea, ataxia, tremor, Lyell's syndrome, agranulocytosis, leukopenia, thrombocytopenia, sleeping disorder, behavioural disorder
- in 3 % of the patients seizures may increase
- oral contraceptives and pregnancy reduce the plasma level of Lamotrigine up to 50 %
- Valproic acid decelerates the break down of Lamotrigine
- Carbamazepine, Phenytoin, Primidone, Phenobarbital, Rifampicin and Ethinyl estradiol/Levonorgestrel combinations (possibly also other oral contraceptives and HRT therapies) accelerate the break down of Lamotrigine

Approval status:

- monotherapy or adjunctive therapy in generalized, focal and secondary generalized seizures and "mixed" epilepsy-types in patients aged > 12 years
- anticonvulsive add-on medication for children between the age of 2 and 11 years.

Sources:

- **Germany – SPC:**
  - epilepsy
    - oral
- No additional information to USA – T or United Kingdom – BNFC
- **USA – T:**
  - children 2–12 years
  - note: only whole tablets should be used for dosing; children 2–6 years will likely require maintenance doses at higher end of recommended range; patients weighing < 30 kg may need as much as a 50 % increase in maintenance dose, compared with patients weighing > 30 kg; titrate dose to clinical effect.

Treatment schedule	Week 1 and 2	Week 3 and 4	Maintenance dose
Patients receiving antiepileptic drugs other than Carbamazepine, Phenytoin, Phenobarbital, Primidone, or Valproic acid	0.3 mg/kg/d as 1–2 separate doses; round dose down to the nearest whole tablet	0.6 mg/kg/d as 2 separate doses; round dose down to the nearest whole tablet	4.5–7.5 mg/kg/d as 2 separate doses; max. 300 mg/d. Titrate dose to effect; after week 4, increase dose every 1–2 weeks by a calculated increment; calculate increment as 0.6 mg/kg/d rounded down to the nearest whole tablet; add this amount to the previously administered daily dose
Patients receiving divided dose regimens containing Valproic acid	0.15 mg/kg/d as 1–2 separate doses; round dose down to the nearest whole tablet; 2 mg every other day for patients (> 6,7 and < 14 kg)	0.3 mg/kg/d as 1–2 separate doses; round dose down to the nearest whole tablet	1–5 mg/kg/d as 1–2 separate doses, max. 200 mg/d. In children adding Lamotrigine to Valproic acid alone: 1–3 mg/kg/d. Titrate dose to effect; after week 4, increase dose every 1–2 weeks by a calculated increment; calculate increment as 0.3 mg/kg/d rounded down to the nearest whole tablet; add this amount to the previously administered daily dose.
Patients receiving enzyme-inducing divided dose regimens without Valproic acid	0.6 mg/kg/d as 2 separate doses; round dose down to the nearest whole tablet	1.2 mg/kg/d as 2 separate doses; round dose down to the nearest whole tablet	5–15 mg/kg/d as 2 separate doses; max. 400 mg/d. Titrate dose to effect; after week 4, increase dose every 1–2 weeks by a calculated increment; calculate increment as 1.2 mg/kg/d rounded down to the nearest whole tablet; add this amount to the previously administered daily dose

- children > 12 years (immediate release formulation):

Treatment schedule	Week 1 and 2	Week 3 and 4	Maintenance dose
Patients receiving antiepileptic drugs other than Carbamazepine, Phenytoin, Phenobarbital, Primidone, or Valproic acid	25 mg/d	50 mg/d	225–375 mg/d as 2 separate doses; titrate dose to effect; after week 4, increase dose every 1–2 weeks by 50 mg/d

Treatment schedule	Week 1 and 2	Week 3 and 4	Maintenance dose
Patients receiving anti-epileptic drug regimens containing Valproic acid	25 mg every other day	25 mg/d	100–400 mg/d as 1–2 separate doses (patients receiving Valproic acid and other drugs that induce glucuronidation); usual maintenance in patients adding Lamotrigine to Valproic acid alone: 100–200 mg/d. Titrate dose to effect; after week 4, increase dose every 1–2 weeks by 25–50 mg/d
Patients receiving anti-epileptic drug regimens without Valproic acid	50 mg/d	100 mg/d as 2 separate doses	300–500 mg/d as 2 separate doses. Titrate dose to effect; after week 4, increase dose every 1–2 weeks by 100 mg/d; doses as high as 700 mg/d as 2 separate doses have been used

- United Kingdom – BNFC:
  - monotherapy and adjunctive treatment of focal seizures and primary and secondary generalized tonic-clonic seizures; seizures associated with Lennox-Gastaut syndrome
    - oral
      - children 2–12 years:

Treatment schedule	Week 1 and 2	Week 3 and 4	Maintenance dose
Adjunctive therapy of seizures with Valproic acid	0.15 mg/kg/d as a SD; those weighing under 13 kg may receive 2 mg on alternate days	0.3 mg/kg/d as a SD	After week 4 increase by max. of 0.3 mg/kg every 7–14 d 1–5 mg/kg/d as 1–2 separate doses (max. SD 100 mg)
Adjunctive therapy of seizures (with enzyme inducing drugs) without Valproic acid	0.6 mg/kg/d as 2 separate doses	1.2 mg/kg/d as 2 separate doses	Increase by max. 1.2 mg/kg every 7–14 d; usual maintenance 2.5–7.5 mg/kg/dose (max. SD 200 mg) two times daily

Treatment schedule	Week 1 and 2	Week 3 and 4	Maintenance dose
Adjunctive therapy of seizures (without enzyme inducing drugs) without Valproic acid	0.3 mg/kg/d as 1–2 separate doses	0.6 mg/kg/d as 1–2 separate doses	Increase by max. 0.6 mg/kg every 7–14 d; usual maintenance 1–10 mg/kg/d as 1–2 separate doses; max. 200 mg/d

  - children 12–18 years:

Treatment schedule	Week 1 and 2	Week 3 and 4	Maintenance dose
Adjunctive therapy of seizures with Valproic acid	25 mg on alternate days	25 mg/d as a SD	Increase by max. 50 mg every 7–14 d; usual maintenance 100–200 mg/d as 1–2 separate doses
Adjunctive therapy of seizures (with enzyme inducing drugs) without Valproic acid	50 mg/d as a SD	100 mg/d as 2 separate doses	Increased by max. 100 mg every 7–14 d; usual maintenance 200–400 mg/d as 2 separate doses (up to 700 mg/d has been required)
Adjunctive therapy of seizures (without enzyme inducing drugs) without Valproic acid	25 mg/d as a SD	50 mg/d as a SD	Increase by max. 100 mg every 7–14 d; usual maintenance 100–200 mg/d as 1–2 separate doses
Monotherapy	25 mg/d as a SD	50 mg/d as a SD	Increase by max. 100 mg every 7–14 d; usual maintenance 100–200 mg/d as 1–2 separate doses (up to 500 mg/d has been required)

- monotherapy of typical absence seizures
  - oral
    - children 2–12 years:

Treatment schedule	Week 1 and 2	Week 3 and 4	Maintenance dose
	0.3 mg/kg/d as 1–2 separate doses	0.6 mg/kg/d as 1–2 separate doses	Increase by max. 0.6 mg/kg every 7–14 d; usual maintenance 1–10 mg/kg/d as 1–2 separate doses (up to 15 mg/kg/d has been required)

Comments:
- initial de-sensitization dose reduces the development of skin problems (gradual titration!).
- inform parents: if skin problems occur, prompt stop of the medication and immediate consultation of a physician is necessary
- efficacy enhancement when combined with Valproic acid

Lepirudin

Dosage:
- ▶ thromboembolism or dissection of arteries supplying the brain at HIT II: initially 0.4 mg/kg, then 0.15 mg/kg/h IV (off-label)
- ▶ dosing according to PTT

Neuropaediatric indications:
- parenteral anticoagulation at HIT II or status post HIT II

Mechanism of action:
- Hirudin is a product of the pancreas of the European leech (Hirudo medicinalis) and consists of various isoforms
- Lepirudin is a recombinant hirudin produced in yeast cells
- binds non-covalently and without co-factors to thrombin and inhibits its prothrombotic activity
- binding to free and to already fibrin-connected thrombin can prevent the activity of thrombocytes and coagulation factors and the generation of free fibrin monomers from fibrinogen, and thus can prevent the coagulation promoting activity of already existing clots.

Relevant contraindications
- known hypersensitivity to hirudin
- hemorrhagic diathesis
- recent stroke or intracranial procedures
- increased tendency to bleed
- bacterial endocarditis
- advanced renal insufficiency

Relevant side effects and interactions:
- bleeding complications
- allergic reactions
- fever
- concurrent intake of thrombolytics like alteplase or streptokinase can enhance the anticoagulant effect of Lepirudin

Approval status:
- not approved for children

Sources:
- **Germany – SPC:**
  - **anticoagulation**
    - IV
      - **children:** Efficacy and safety have not been established.
- **USA – T:** –
- **United Kingdom – BNFC:** –
- **Uptodate.com:** no published paediatric dosage

Levetiracetam (LEV)

Dosage:
- ▶ usually 20–40(–50) mg/kg/d as 2 separate doses (SPC/off-label)
- ▶ juvenile myoclonic epilepsy: 30 mg/kg/d as 2 separate doses
- ▶ West syndrome: 20–60 mg/kg/d p.o./IV as 2(–4) separate doses

Neuropaediatric indications
- focal, generalized and absence epilepsy
- neonatal seizures (small number of cases or case reports)

Mechanism of action
- mechanism of action is unknown and does not match the other antiepileptics
- probable effect on the synaptic vesicle protein 2A (SV2A) and thus blocking transmitter release

Relevant contraindications:
- CAUTION in behavioural disorders, aggressive behaviour, depression, suicidal tendencies
- hypersensitivity to Levetiracetam
- pregnancy
- use carefully in patients with impaired renal and/or liver function

Relevant side effects and interactions:
- frequent: drowsiness, weakness, vertigo
- rare: headache, anorexia, diarrhea, dyspepsia, abdominal pain, ataxia, depression, emotional lability, aggression, suicidal tendency, increased irritability, insomnia,

tremor, exanthema, eczema, pruritus, diplopia, increased coughing, vomiting, agitation, myalgia, thrombocytopenia
– no interaction with other drugs

Approval status:

– monotherapy: > 16 years of age in focal seizures with or without generalization
– anticonvulsive adjunctive therapy: > 1 month of age (since 1/2010) in focal seizures with or without generalization; > 12 years in primary generalized tonic-clonic and myoclonic seizures in myoclonic epilepsy

Sources:

– **Germany – SPC:**
  – **adjunctive therapy of partial seizures with or without secondary generalization**
    – IV
      – **children 4–17 years, < 50 kg:** initially 20 mg/kg/d as 2 separate doses. According to response, titrate dose to 60 mg/kg/d as 2 separate doses. Dosing adjustments should not exceed 20 mg/kg as 2 separate doses every 2 weeks. Use lowest effective dose. Dosing of children weighing > 50 kg is equal to adults' dosing.
– **USA – T:**
  – **epilepsy**
    – oral
      – **infants, children 6 months–4 years:** (dose not established, limited data available) initially 10–20 mg/kg/d as 2 separate doses; may be increased once every week by 10 mg/kg/d (max. reported dose: 62 mg/kg/d). Dosing based on retrospective reports (n = 122, n = 81) with mean effective doses of 23 mg/kg/d and 41 mg/kg/d, respectively
  – **myoclonic seizures**
    – oral
      – **children ≥ 12 years,** immediate release: initially 1000 mg/d as 2 separate doses; increase dosage every 2 weeks by 500 mg/dose, given twice daily, to the recommended dose of 3000 mg/d as 2 separate doses. Efficacy of doses other than 3000 mg/d has not been established.
    – IV
      – **children ≥ 16 years:** initially 1000 mg/d as 2 separate doses; increase dosage every 2 weeks by 500 mg/dose, given twice daily, to the recommended dose of 3000 mg/d as 2 separate doses. Efficacy of doses other than 3000 mg/d has not been studied.
      – **note:** when switching from oral to IV formulation, the total daily dose should remain the same
  – **partial onset seizures**
    – oral
      – **children 4–< 16 years,** immediate release: initially 20 mg/kg/d as 2 separate doses; may be increased every 2 weeks by 10 mg/kg/SD given twice daily, if tolerated, to a maximum of 60 mg/kg/d; mean required dose: 52 mg/kg/d
      – **children ≥ 16 years,**
      – immediate release: initially 1000 mg/d as 2 separate doses; may be increased every 2 weeks by 500 mg/dose given twice daily, if tolerated, to a maximum of 3000 mg/d as 2 separate doses; doses > 3000 mg/d have been used in trials; however, there is no evidence of increased benefit.

– extended release: initially 1000 mg/d as a SD, may increase every 2 weeks by 1000 mg/d to max. 3000 mg/d as a SD
    – IV
      – **children ≥ 16 years:** initially 1000 mg/d as 2 separate doses; may be increased every 2 weeks by 500 mg/dose given twice daily, if tolerated, to a maximum of 3000 mg/d as 2 separate doses; oral doses of > 3000 mg/d have been used in trials; however, there is no evidence of increased benefit.
      – **note:** when switching from oral to IV formulation, the total daily dose should remain the same
  – **primary generalized tonic-clonic seizures**
    – oral
      – **children 6–< 16 years,** immediate release: initially 20 mg/kg/d as 2 separate doses; increase dosage every 2 weeks by 10 mg/kg/dose twice daily, to the recommended dose of 60 mg/kg/d as 2 separate doses. Efficacy of doses other than 60 mg/kg/d has not been established.
      – **children ≥ 16 years,** immediate release: initially 1000 mg/d as 2 separate doses; increase dosage every 2 weeks by 500 mg/dose given twice daily, to the recommended dose of 3000 mg/d as 2 separate doses. Efficacy of doses other than 60 mg/kg/d has not been established.
    – IV use for children < 16 years is not recommended
– **United Kingdom – BNFC:**
  – **monotherapy of focal seizures with or without secondary generalization**
    – oral, IV infusion
      – **children 16–18 years:** initially 250 mg/d as a SD increased after 1 week to 500 mg/d as 2 separate doses, thereafter, increased according to response in steps of 250 mg/dose twice daily every 2 weeks; max. 3000 mg/d as 2 separate doses
  – **adjunctive therapy of focal seizures with or without secondary generalization**
    – IV infusion
      – **children 4–18 years (children 12–18 years in myoclonic seizures and tonic-clonic seizures), < 50 kg:** initially 10 mg/kg/d as a SD, increased gradually by max. 10 mg/kg twice daily every 2 weeks; max. 60 mg/kg/d as 2 separate doses
      – **children 12–18 years (children 12–18 years in myoclonic seizures and tonic-clonic seizures), > 50 kg:** initially 500 mg/d as 2 separate doses, increased gradually by 500 mg twice daily every 2 weeks; max. 3000 mg/d
  – **adjunctive therapy of focal seizures with or without secondary generalization**
    – oral
      – **children 1–6 months:** initially 7 mg/kg/d as a SD, increased gradually by max. 7 mg/kg twice daily every 2 weeks; max. 42 mg/kg/d as 2 separate doses
      – **children 6 months–18 years, < 50 kg:** initially 10 mg/kg/d as a SD, increased gradually by max. 10 mg/kg twice daily every 2 weeks; max. 60 mg/kg/d as 2 separate doses
      – **children 12–18 years, > 50 kg:** initially 500 mg/d as 2 separate doses, increased gradually by 500 mg twice daily every 2 weeks; max. 3000 mg/d as 2 separate doses

Comments:

– therapeutic serum level between 21 and 64 mg/ml
– mainly good tolerance
– is not metabolized in the liver and thus combination with all other antiepileptics is possible without any interactions

- treatment of status:
  - limited experiences so far
  - exact duration to onset of action is unclear, presumably < 30 min

Levodopa

(L-Dopa)

Dosage:

- ▶ primary generalized dystonia or L-dopa-responsive dystonia or hereditary degenerative or secondary dystonia (e.g. dyskinetic cerebral palsy): p.o.: 1 mg/kg/d as 4 separate doses (0.25 mg/kg/dose), increase by 1 mg/kg/week; no response to 10 mg/kg/d after four months indicates a non-dopamine-responsive dystonia
- ▶ restless legs syndrome: 100/25 mg/dose (L-dopa/carbidopa or L-dopa/benserazide) 1 h prior to bedtime, dose reduction or dose doubling is possible according to age/symptoms

Neuropaediatric indications:

- dopa-responsive diseases: L-dopa-responsive dystonia, disorder of tetrahydrobiopterin synthesis
- primary generalized dystonia
- hereditary degenerative or secondary dystonia (e.g. cerebral palsy)
- restless legs syndrome

Mechanism of action:

- L-3,4-dihydroxyphenylalanine
- prodrug; passes the blood-brain barrier, uptake in dopaminergic nerves, decarboxylation to dopamine and agonistic effect at the dopamine receptors
- concurrent intake of decarboxylase inhibitors (carbidopa, benserazide) is said to prevent the early breakdown to dopamine before entering the cerebrospinal compartment

Relevant contraindications:

- angle-closure glaucoma
- concurrent intake of MAOIs
- severe cardiovascular diseases, severe liver and renal diseases
- severe psychiatric diseases

Relevant side effects and interactions:

- depressions, euphoria, confusion, hallucination and nightmares
- nausea, loss of appetite
- movement disorder
- rare: changes in blood cell count, disorder in blood pressure regulation
- do not combine with MAOIs
- reserpine and other antidepressive drugs decrease the effect

Approval status:

- depends on the specific product (see SPC)

Sources:

- **Germany – SPC:**
  - **Parkinson's disease**
    - oral
      - **children:** Safety has not been established in patients < 18 years. The use is not recommended in children.
- **USA – T:** –
- **United Kingdom – BNFC:**
  - **dopamine-sensitive dystonias (including Segawa syndrome and dystonias related to cerebral palsy)**
    - oral (as L-dopa)
      - **children 3 months–18 years:** initially 0.25 mg/kg/dose 2–3 times daily of a preparation containing 1 : 4 carbidopa: L-dopa; increase according to response every 2–3 d to max. 3 mg/kg/d as 3 separate doses
  - **treatment of defects in tetrahydrobiopterin synthesis and dihydrobiopterin reductase deficiency**
    - oral (as L-dopa)
      - **neonates:** initially 1–2 mg/kg/d as 4 separate doses of a preparation containing 1 : 4 carbidopa: L-dopa; increase according to response every 4–5 d to maintenance dose of 10–12 mg/kg/d as 4 separate doses; at higher doses consider a preparation containing 1 : 10 carbidopa: L-dopa; review regularly (every 3–6 months)
      - **children 1 month–18 years:** initially 1–2 mg/kg/d as 4 separate doses of a preparation containing 1 : 4 carbidopa: L-dopa; increase according to response every 4–5 d to maintenance dose of 10–12 mg/kg/d as 4 separate doses; at higher doses consider a preparation containing 1 : 10 carbidopa: L-dopa; review regularly (every 3–6 months in early childhood)

Comments:

- combination preparation with carboxylase inhibitors
- protein rich meals impair the uptake

Lidocaine

Dosage:

- ▶ failure to control neonatal seizures:
  - loading dose: 2 mg/kg in 10 min IV
  - dosage schedule: continuous administration with gradually decreased dosing: 6 mg/kg/h over 6 h; 4 mg/kg/h over 12 h; 2 mg/kg/h over 12 h while monitoring serum levels
- ▶ superficial anesthesia with EMLA® patch: about 30 min before drug infusion
- ▶ infiltration anesthesia with Lidocaine 1 %:
  - with Lidocaine 1 % solution 25(–27,–30) G-needles
  - without adrenaline max. 0.4 ml/kg, with adrenaline max. 0.7 ml/kg
  - aspirate to exclude intravascular injection

Neuropaediatric indications:

- failure to control neonatal seizures
- analgesia (e.g. lumbar puncture)

Mechanism of action:

- blocks voltage dependant sodium channels in nerve cell membranes and thus inhibits the fast Na^+ influx during the depolarization phase. As a result, this phase is prolonged and development of the action potential is inhibited

Relevant contraindications:

- AV block II. and III. degree
- acute decompensated heart failure
- careful use: sick sinus syndrome, AV block 1st degree, bradycardia (< 50/min), non-rhythmogenic hypotension (< 90 mmHg systolic), severe liver function disorders, decreased hepatic blood flow, renal insufficiency, pregnancy

Relevant side effects and interactions:

- pain in legs and back
- increased blood pressure
- vertigo, tinnitus, impaired vision
- loss of orientation, tremor, prickling, cramps, absence
- breathing disorder, decrease in blood pressure, enhancement of cardiac arrhythmia
- allergic reactions with urticaria, oedema, bronchial spasms
- paresis, paresthesia, incontinence
- temperature increase
- changes in taste or numb tongue

- additive inhibitory effect to the AV conduction, intraventricular nerve conduction and the power of contraction with other antiarrhythmics, beta receptor blockers, Calcium antagonists
- Cimetidine decreases the Lidocaine clearance
- accelerated breakdown of Lidocaine by CYP 450 enzyme inductors

Approval status:

- depends on the specific product (see SPC)

Sources:

- **Germany – SPC:**
  - **local and regional nerve block due to pain therapy**
    - **children > 15 years:** various concentrations of Lidocaine hydrochloride injection solutions are used:

surface anesthesia	up to 300 mg	independent of dosage form
Infiltration	up to 300 mg	0.5–2 %
Infiltration in dentistry	up to 300 mg	2 %
Peripheral nerve block	up to 300 mg	1–2 %
Stellate block	up to 100 mg	1 %
Truncus sympathicus block	up to 300 mg	1 %
Paravertebral anesthesia	up to 300 mg	1 %
Peridural anesthesia	up to 300 mg	0.5–2 %
Field block	up to 500 mg	0.5–2 %
IV regional anesthesia	up to 300 mg	0.5 %
Urticaria, intracutaneous per wheal	up to 4 mg	0.5–1 %

  - **Lumbar region**
    - **5-years:** 0.5 ml per segment
    - **10-years:** 0.9 ml per segment
    - **15-years:** 1.3 ml per segment
  - calculate dosing individually for children and therefore adjust according age and weight. For children, preferably use solutions with a low drug concentration.
- **USA – T:**
  - **antiarrhythmic**
    - IV, i.o.
      - **note:** use for patients with pulseless VT or VF if amiodarone is not available; give after defibrillation attempts, CPR, and epinephrine:
      - **neonates:** loading dose of 1 mg/kg/dose; follow with continuous IV infusion or repeated bolus injections

- **infants, children:** loading dose: 1 mg/kg/dose (max. 100 mg/dose); follow with continuous IV infusion; consider administering second bolus of 0.5–1 mg/kg/dose if delay between bolus and start of infusion is > 15 min;
  - **note:** Patients with reduced hepatic function or decreased hepatic blood flow should receive ½ the usual loading dose.
- continuous IV infusion
  - **neonates:** 20–50 mcg/kg/min; use lower dose for neonates with shock, hepatic disease, cardiac arrest or CHF
  - **infants, children:** 20–50 mcg/kg/min. The manufacturer recommends a max. of 20 mcg/kg/min in patients with shock, hepatic disease, cardiac arrest or CHF.
- endotracheal
  - **children:** 2–3 mg/kg/dose, flush with 5 ml of saline and follow with 5 assisted manual ventilations
- anesthesia
  - **local injection:** in children the dose varies with procedure, degree of anesthesia needed, blood supply of tissues, duration of anesthesia required, and physical condition of patient; max. 4.5 mg/kg, do not exceed 300 mg.
  - **topical:** see manufacturer's recommendations for the respective formulation to be used
- United Kingdom – BNFC:
  - neonatal seizures
    - IV infusion
      - neonates: initially 2 mg/kg over 10 minutes, followed by 6 mg/kg/h for 6 h; reduce dose over the following 24 h (4 mg/kg/h for 12 h, then 2 mg/kg/h for 12 h)
  - anesthesia
    - infiltration anesthesia
      - **neonates:** according to nature of procedure, up to 3 mg/kg (0.3 ml/kg of 1 % solution), repeated not more often than every 4 h
      - **children 1 month–12 years:** according to nature of procedure, up to 3 mg/kg (0.3 ml/kg of a 1 % solution), repeated not more than every 4 h
      - **children 12–18 years:** according to weight of child and nature of procedure, max. 200 mg, repeated not more than every 4 h
  - **preparation EMLA®:** anesthesia before minor skin procedures including venipuncture
    - **neonates:** apply max. 1 g under occlusive dressing for max. 1 h before procedure; max. 1 dose in 24 h
    - **children 1–3 months or < 5 kg:** apply max. 1 g under occlusive dressing for max. 1 h before procedure; max. 1 dose in 24 h
    - **children 3 months–1 year or > 5 kg:** apply max. 2 g under occlusive dressing for max. 4 h before procedure; max. 2 doses in 24 h
    - **children 1–18 years:** apply thick layer under occlusive dressing 1–5 h before procedure (2–5 h before procedures on large areas, e.g. split skin grafting); max. 2 doses in 24 h for children 2–12 years
  - **Xylocain® pumpspray:** endotracheal intubation
    - **children up to 18 years:** up to 3 mg/kg

Lorazepam (LZP)

Dosage:
- fever convulsion: 0.05–0.1 mg/kg/dose buccal, IV
- acute dystonic reaction: 0.1 mg/kg (in 2 mg portions, max. 4 mg/dose)
- anxiolytic agent for procedures: 0.05–0.2 mg/kg/dose
- acute treatment of singular cerebral seizure after stroke: 0.1 mg/kg buccal, IV
- epilepsy in Angelman syndrome: 0.05 mg/kg/d
- status epilepticus (initially up to max. 4 mg/dose):
  - initially, buccal or IV: 0.05–0.1 mg/kg (over 30–60 sec)
  - after 5–20 min: 0.05–0.1 mg/kg (over 30–60 sec)
- generalized spasticity: initially 0.05 mg/kg/d; for long term treatment, up to 0.15–0.3 mg/kg/d as 3 separate doses

Neuropaediatric indications:
- emergency medication for singular cerebral seizure and status epilepticus
- fever convulsion
- anxiolytic agent for procedures
- acute dystonic reaction
- anticonvulsive treatment of epilepsy in Angelman syndrome
- status epilepticus (if IV route is already established)
- generalized spasticity (e.g. in cerebral palsy short-term)

Mechanism of action:
- benzodiazepine
- opens chloride channels and thus enhances GABAergic neuronal inhibition especially in the limbic system

Relevant contraindications:
- known hypersensitivity to benzodiazepines
- addiction (medication, drugs, alcohol)
- acute angle-closure glaucoma
- myasthenia gravis
- careful use: severe liver damage, ataxia, acute poisoning with alcohol, analgesics or sopophorics, neuroleptics, antidepressants, lithium, severe chronic respiratory insufficiency, sleep apnea syndrome, pregnancy

Relevant side effects and interactions:
- hypersensitivity reactions
- muscle weakness, dry mouth, gastrointestinal disorders
- temporary elevation of liver function parameters

- fatigue, drowsiness, weakness, vertigo, drowsiness
- headache, confusion, anterograde amnesia, depressive mood
- paradox reactions (e.g. acute agitation, anger)
- libido reduction
- decrease in blood pressure, respiratory depression
- sedation (increased risk when combined with other medication, e.g. Phenobarbital)
- high dosing and long-term treatment:
  - unstable walking
  - articulation disorders
  - vertigo
  - addiction, withdrawal syndrome (abrupt stop after long-term treatment): sleeping disorder and increased dreaming, anxiety, tonicity, agitation, shivering, sweating, increased tendency of seizures or symptomatic psychosis
  - impaired vision, double vision, nystagmus
- mutually enhanced effect with concurrent intake of centrally depressant drugs and alcohol
- increased effect of muscle relaxants, analgesics and laughing gas
- increased and prolonged effect of certain benzodiazepines due to delayed breakdown when combined with Cimetidine
- unpredictable side effects in long-term treatment with centrally depressant anti-hypertensives, beta blockers and anticoagulants when combined with benzodiazepines

Approval status:

- depends on the specific product (see SPC)

Sources:

- **Germany – SPC:**
  - **status epilepticus**
    - IV, IM
      - **children and adolescents:** initially 0.05 mg/kg; if seizures do not disappear within 10–15 min, give another dose of 0.05 mg/kg
      - **children < 18 years** should not be treated with preparation Tavor® inject except for status epilepticus.
    - **benzyl alcohol can cause toxic and anaphylactic reactions in infants and children < 3 years of age.**
      - **CAUTION:** children may hyperreact to benzyl alcohol. Central nervous symptoms (i.e. seizures, intraventricular haemorrhage), non-receptiveness, tachypnea, tachycardia and sweating were related to toxicity of propylene glycol. Although normal range dosages contain very small amounts of this substance, newborns, infants and those with low birth weight who received higher doses of Lorazepam, may still be susceptible to the toxic effects.

- **USA – T:**
  - **sedation prior to procedure**
    - oral, .IM, IV
      - **infants and children:** 0.05 mg/kg, range: 0.02–0.09 mg/kg; use lower doses for IV (0.01–0.03 mg/kg), repeat every 20 min, titrate to response
  - **status epilepticus**
    - IV
      - **neonates:** 0.05 mg/kg slow IV over 2–5 min; may be repeated in 10–15 min (CAUTION: benzyl alcohol)
      - **infants and children:** 0.05–0.1 mg/kg (max. 4 mg/dose) slow IV over 2–5 min (max. 2 mg/min); may be repeated every 10–15 min if needed
      - **adolescents:** 0.07 mg/kg (max. 4 mg/dose) slow IV over 2–5 min (max. 2 mg/min), may be repeated every 10–15 min if needed; usual total max. dose: 8 mg
      - **note:** Dilute injection prior to IV use with equal volume of compatible diluent (DSW, NS, SWI); do not inject intraarterially, arteriospasm and gangrene may occur. Injection contains 2 % benzyl alcohol, polyethylene glycol, and propylene glycol, which may be toxic to newborns in high doses; benzyl alcohol may cause allergic reactions in susceptible individuals; large amounts of benzyl alcohol ($\geq$ 99 mcg/kg/d) have been associated with a potentially fatal toxicity ("gasping syndrome") in neonates; the "gasping syndrome" consists of metabolic acidosis, respiratory distress, gasping respirations, CNS dysfunction (including convulsions, intracranial haemorrhage), hypotension and cardiovascular collapse; use Lorazepam products containing benzyl alcohol with special caution in neonates; in vitro and animal studies have shown that benzoate, a metabolite of benzyl alcohol, displaces bilirubin bound to protein.
- **United Kingdom – BNFC:**
  - **status epilepticus, febrile convulsions, convulsions caused by poisoning**
    - slow IV injection
      - **neonates:** 0.1 mg/kg as a SD, repeated once after 10 minutes if necessary
      - **children 1 month–12 years:** 0.1 mg/kg (max. 4 mg) as a SD, repeated once after 10 minutes if necessary
      - **children 12–18 years:** 4 mg as a SD, repeated once after 10 minutes if necessary
  - **premedication**
    - oral
      - **children 1 month–12 years:** 0.05–0.1 mg/kg as separate doses (max. 4 mg) at least 1 h before procedure
      - **children 12–18 years:** 1–4 mg at least 1 h before procedure
      - **note:** same dose may be given the night before procedure in addition to, or instead of, the dose just before procedure
    - IV injection
      - **children 1 month–18 years:** 0.05–0.1 mg/kg (max. 4 mg), 30–45 minutes before procedure

IM and IV comments:

- Appropriate benzodiazepine, whose peak and duration of anticonvulsive effect is considered superior. Buccal administration is a perfect alternative if the rectal

application is socially and situationally inadequate. The fast buccal resorption is controversially discussed.
- Lorazepam tends to be more effective, has fewer relapsing rates, and is less depressive on breathing than Diazepam. The duration of effect (against seizures) is higher (12–24 h) than for Diazepam (< 1 h).
- buccal administration in status epilepticus:
  - advantage: simple application in daily routine
  - disadvantage: fast onset of action is not unequivocally proven; unreliable resorption by the stomach mucosa

M

Magnesium

Dosage:
▶ 400 (200–600) mg/d of elemental Magnesium

Neuropaediatric indications:
- migraine prophylaxis (preferably (only empirical) Magnesium aspartate)

Mechanism of action:
- Mg^{2+} is a physiological Ca^{2+}-antagonist and thus presumably has a vasodilative effect

Relevant contraindications:
- distinct bradycardia
- myasthenia gravis
- AV block
- severe renal impairment
- phenylketonuria
- hypophosphatemia
- dehydration
- Calcium Magnesium Ammonium phosphate stone diathesis

Relevant side effects and interactions:
- high dosages: pasty feces, diarrhea
- for long-term intake of high dosages and in renal impairment: hypermagnesemia up to Magnesium intoxication (CNS disorder, muscle weakness, respiratory depression, lacking reflexes, fatigue, paresis, coma and cardiac arrhythmias

- 1–2 h between oral intake of Magnesium-containing compounds and:
  - iron
  - tetracyclines
  - sodium fluoride

Approval status:
- depends on the specific product (see SPC)

Sources:
- Germany – SPC: –
- USA – T: –
- United Kingdom – BNFC: –

Mannitol

Dosage:
▶ Mannitol 20 %: 1,25 ml/kg/dose every 4–8 h (0.25 g/kg/dose every 4–8 h)
▶ CAUTION: rebound effect (however, insufficient evidence)
▶ CAUTION: control serum osmolality, target: < 320 mosm/l
▶ radiotherapy-associated cerebral oedema: 3–6 × 125 ml/d (3–6 × 25 g/d) over 3–5 d

Neuropaediatric indications
- emergency treatment of known or suspected cerebral oedema, especially after head trauma (tumor oedema only in connection with massive swelling)

Mechanism of action:
- osmotic diuretic
- Is freely filtered at the glomeruli of the kidney, but only poorly reabsorbed by the renal tubule, leading to increased osmotic pressure of the blood plasma. As a result, water is shifted from tissues into the interstitial space and blood plasma thus reducing cerebral oedema and intracranial pressure.

Relevant contraindications:
- cardiac failure, pulmonary oedema
- hypernatremia, hypovolemia

Relevant side effects and interactions:
- hypovolemia caused by obligatory water diuresis
- changes of blood osmolarity

Approval status:
- depends on the specific product (see SPC)

Sources:

- **Germany – SPC:**
  - **reduction of increased intracranial, intraocular pressure**
    - IV
    - the SPC does not specify any paediatric dosage
      - initial dose: 1.5–2 g/kg infused over 30–60 min. To achieve an adequate effect, administer dose 1–1.5 h prior to procedure.
    - **diuresis in case of intoxication**
      - initially 25 g; adjust according to diuresis (at least 100 ml/h; ensure a positive fluid balance of 1–2 L).
      - **CAUTION:** children with reduced renal function should receive a test dose of 0,2 g/kg over 3–5 min. Usual dose is 0.5–1.5 g/kg. May be repeated once or twice in intervals of 4–8 h. For treatment of increased intracranial/intraocular pressure in children, infuse over 30–60 min.
- **USA – T:**
  - **reduction of increased intracranial pressure associated with cerebral oedema**
    - IV:
      - neonates, acute renal failure: 0.5–1 g/kg/dose; some experts recommend against routine use due to the risk of IVH in low birthweight neonates (solution is hypertonic) or the precipitation of CHF if a lack of response occurs (Andreoli SP, "Acure Renal Failure in the Newborn", Semin Perinatol, 2004, 28(2): 112–23)
      - **children:** test dose (to assess adequate renal function), 0,2 g/kg (max. 12.5 g) over 3–5 min to produce a urine flow of at least 1 ml/kg/h for 1–3 h; initial dose, 0.5–1 g/kg; maintenance with 0.25–0.5 g/kg/dose every 4–6 h
- **United Kingdom – BNFC:**
  - **cerebral oedema, raised intraocular pressure**
    - IV infusion over 30–60 minutes
      - **children 1 month–12 years:** 0,25–1,5 g/kg/dose, repeated 1–2 times after 4–8 h if necessary
      - **children 12–18 years:** 0,25–2 g/kg/dose, repeated 1–2 times after 4–8 h if necessary

Comments:

- note: only effective for some hours (max. few days), then rebound/deterioration is possible
- at first administration: temporary hypertensive hyponatremia
- limitations of long-term or frequent administration due to the development of hypernatremia
- Uptake of Mannitol by the bowel linings is very poor. Therefore, parenteral administration is necessary.

Melatonin

Dosage:

▶ sleeping disorder e.g. in syndromes/neurodegenerative diseases: small children 3–5 mg; school-aged children 6–10 mg; adolescents slightly less, e.g. 6 mg
▶ circadian sleeping disorder in cerebral palsy: 5–15 mg
▶ psychologically conditioned sleeping disorder: 3(–6) mg in the evening

Neuropaediatric indications:

- sleeping induction for EEG
- circadian rhythm disorders in particular for children with neurological disorders (e.g. impaired vision, cerebral palsy)
- psychologically conditioned sleeping disorder

Mechanism of action:

- Biosynthesis of the circadian neurohormone Melatonin by the pineal gland is inhibited by light to the retina while rapidly increasing during periods of darkness. At night (in darkness) Melatonin is increasingly secreted and promotes sleepiness (reduces early sleeping phases and prolongs REM-phases).

Relevant contraindications: –

Side effects and interactions (in theory):

- fatigue, vertigo, headache, irregular circadian rhythm, ataxia, nightmares
- nausea, vomiting, abdominal cramps
- decreased tendency of seizures
- psychoses, hallucination, dysphoria
- hypotension, cardiac arrhythmias
- increased serum glucose levels
- gynecomastia
- coagulation disorder, leukocytosis, increased risk of leukemia
- inhibition of the natural Melatonin production by alpha-blocker, beta-blocker, Caffeine, NSAID, SSRI

Approval status:

- not applicable

Sources:
- **Germany – SPC:**
  - **Insomnia**
    - oral
      - **children < 18 years:** because and safety have not been established, the use in this age group is not recommended (medico-legal argumentation)
- **USA – T:** –
- **United Kingdom – BNFC:**
  - **sleep onset insomnia and delayed sleep phase syndrome**
    - oral
      - **children 1 month–18 years:** initially 2–3 mg/d before bedtime, increased if necessary after 1–2 weeks to 4–6 mg/d before bedtime; max. 10 mg/d

Metamizole

Dosage:
- ▶ fever in fever convulsion: 10 mg/kg/dose every 4–6 h p.o./IV
- ▶ acute therapy of migraine and tension-type headache: 10–20 mg/kg/dose p.o./IV
- ▶ other pain and colic: 15 mg/kg (max. 75 mg/kg/d)
- ▶ headache in radiotherapy: 2000–4000 mg/d as 4 separate doses
- ▶ avoid multiple high doses in patients with impaired renal or liver function

Neuropaediatric indications:
- colic-like pain
- acute severe pain (migraine, headache in radiotherapy)
- high fever
- fever convulsion

Mechanism of action:
- reversible inhibition of cyclooxygenase I and II and thus reduced synthesis of prostaglandins
- strongly analgesic and antipyretic, mildly antiphlogistic
- spasmolytic
- highest analgesic and antipyretic effect of all NSAID
- presumably a further analgesic effect by functioning as a cannabis receptor ligand in the CNS

Relevant contraindications:
- disorders of the bone marrow function/diseases of the hematopoetic system
- genetically conditioned glucose-6-phosphate-dehydrogenase deficiency (risk of hemolysis)
- acute hepatic porphyria
- injection solution: known hypotension and instable circulation
- careful use: analgesics asthma syndrome, bronchial asthma, chronic urticaria, high fever (hypotensive reaction possible)
- hypotension and instable circulation

Relevant side effects and interactions:
- exanthema, pruritus, burning of the skin, flush, urticaria, tumescences
- gastrointestinal disorder
- hypotensive reaction up to severe decrease in blood pressure after administration, cardiac arrhythmia
- severe angiooedema
- dyspnea, severe bronchial spasms
- leukopenia
- renal impairment
- agranulocytosis:
  - risk increases, if administered for > 1 week; may occur even after multiple administrations without any apparent complications
  - symptoms: sore throat, high fever, shivering, swallowing problems, inflammation in the mouth, nose, pharynx, genital or anal region
  - strongly accelerated decrease in blood pressure
  - no or mild swelling of lymph nodes or spleen
  - granulocytes considerably diminished/lacking
  - mostly normal hemoglobin, erythrocytes and thrombocytes
  - therapy: immediate stop
- Interactions: Captopril, Methotrexate, Lithium, Triamterene, oral anticoagulants, changed efficacy of antihypertensive drugs and diuretics
- severe hypothermia is possible if combined with Chlorpromazine

Approval status:
- depends on the specific product (see SPC)

Sources:
- **Germany – SPC:**
  - **acute/chronic pain**
    - oral

Age, body weight	Single dose	Maximum daily dose
3–11 months, 5–8 kg	50–100 mg	300 mg
1–3 years, 9–15 kg	75–250 mg	750 mg
4–6 years, 16–23 kg	125–375 mg	1125 mg

Age, body weight	Single dose	Maximum daily dose
7–9 years, 24–30 kg	200–500 mg	1500 mg
10–12 years 31–45 kg	250–750 mg	2250 mg
13–14 years, 46–53 kg	375–875 mg	2625 mg
≥ 15 years, (> 53 kg)	500–1000 mg	3000 mg

- **USA – T:** –
- **United Kingdom – BNFC:** –

Comments:

- slow IV infusion to check possible hypotension (may occur with a delay of > 30 min)
- duration of effect: 4(–6) h

Methotrexate (MTX)

Dosage:

▶ Henoch Schonlein purpura (for severe relapsing episodes used as a steroid saving medication when administration of high steroid dosages): 10–20 mg/m² BSA
▶ retention of remission in Wegener's granulomatosis: 10–20 mg/m² BSA
▶ myositis: p.o./SC, 15 mg/m² BSA
▶ chemotherapeutic regime only under specialist's advise

Neuropaediatric indications:

- Henoch Schonlein purpura
- Wegener's granulomatosis
- medulloblastoma, ependymoma
- chemotherapy of CNS tumors
- mild/moderate myositis in insufficient response to corticosteroids or in severe cases of myositis as add-on therapy

Mechanism of action:

- analog of folic acid
- competitive inhibitor of dihydrofolate reductase

Relevant contraindications:

- pregnancy
- severe infections
- ascites
- pleural effusion
- concurrent UV radiotherapy
- renal impairment (creatinine clearance < 60 ml/min)
- liver damage
- diseases of the blood forming system
- increased alcohol consumption
- immunodeficiency
- gastrointestinal ulcers
- careful use: impaired pulmonary function, insulin-dependent diabetes mellitus, inactive chronic infections, conditions that lead to dehydration, intake of other liver-damaging drugs, children (limited experiences), folic acid deficiency or concurrent administration of drugs that lead to folate deficiency, vaccination with live vaccines

Relevant side effects and interactions:

- loss of appetite, nausea, vomiting, diarrhea, gastrointestinal bleeding
- stomatitis
- anemia, leukopenia, thrombopenia
- defective spermatogenesis and oogenesis
- hair loss, pruritus
- pneumonitis, alveolitis
- especially in long-term use: pulmonary fibrosis, renal impairment, liver impairment
- increased risk of infections
- headache, fatigue
- elevated liver function parameters (GOT, GPT, alkaline phosphatase)
- do not vaccinate with live vaccines during therapy; dead vaccines may become ineffective
- patients taking drugs that are potentially liver damaging (e.g. Leflunomide, Azathioprine, Sulfasalazine, Retinoids) should undergo regular medical check-ups; the same is required for patients concurrently taking Sulfonamides, Trimethoprim/Sulfamethoxazole, Chloramphenicol, Pyrimethamine
- increased toxicity in current folic acid deficiency or concurrent intake of drugs that cause folic acid deficiency (e.g. Sulfonamides, Trimethoprim/Sulfamethoxazole)
- enhanced effect caused by Penicillins, Salicylates, Phenytoin, barbiturates, tranquilizers, oral contraceptives, tetracyclines, Amidopyrine derivatives, sulfonamides, p-aminobenzoic acid, p-aminohippuric acid, probenecid, NSAR

Approval status:

- depends on the specific product (see SPC)

Sources:
- **Germany – SPC:**
  - **antineoplastic**
    - IV, IM
      - **note:** treatment of children only under specialist's supervision
      - no additional information to T or United Kingdom – BNFC
- **USA – T:**
  - consult local treatment protocols for details
- **United Kingdom – BNFC:** does not specify any dosage: consult local treatment protocol for details

Comments:
- for Methotrexate poisoning: administer carboxypeptidase G2 (breaks down Methotrexate by removing the glutamic acid ester)
- Intake of folic acid 24–48 h after each Methotrexate administration reduces the side effects without decreasing efficacy.

Methsuximide

Dosage:
▶ usually: 10–20(–30) mg/kg/d (SPC)
▶ absences 10–40 mg/kg/d as 2 separate doses; target level: 20–35 mg/l

Neuropaediatric indications:
- absences

Mechanism of action:
- exact mechanism of action is unknown
- is broken down to the active metabolite N-desmethylmethsuximide

Relevant contraindications:
- hepatic porphyria
- known haematological disease
- concurrent intake of soporifics or alcohol
- careful use: patients with a history of psychiatric diseases, liver or renal disorders

Relevant side effects and interactions:
- nausea, vomiting, hiccup, fatigue, headache, vertigo, weight loss, appetite disorder
- exanthema up to Stevens-Johnson syndrome
- lupus erythematodes
- depression, movement disorder, psychoses
- rare: blood count changes (aplastic anemia, thrombocytopenia, leukopenia, pancytopenia, eosinophilia)
- enhanced effect of Phenytoin caused by elevated plasma levels
- decreased plasma levels caused by Carbamazepine
- increased plasma levels caused by Valproic acid

Approval status:
- **childhood absence** or petit mal in "mixed" epilepsies, absences

Sources:
- **Germany – SPC:**
  - **childhood absence (or petit mal) epilepsy, absences**
    - oral
    - no published paediatric dosage
    - dosing has to be adjusted according to response; titrate gradually.
  - **adults,** usual dosing: week 1, 150 mg/d; if necessary increase by 150 mg weekly within 7 weeks up to max. 1200 mg/d
    - maintenance: 9.5–11 mg/kg/d, max. 15 mg/kg/d
    - children and adolescents may be compromised in their abilities while using Methsuximide.
- **USA – T:** –
- **United Kingdom – BNFC:** –
- **Drugdex®:**
  - **absences,** median oral children dose: 15–30 mg/kg/d as 3–4 separate doses

Methylphenidate

Dosage:
▶ daily dose: 0.3–1 mg/kg/d, but max. 60 mg/d as 2 separate doses
▶ sustained release products: administer once daily in the morning (duration of effect see below)

Neuropaediatric indications:
- spectrum ADHD

Mechanism of action:
- inhibition of the presynaptic dopamine and noradrenalin reuptake; thus, the concentration of both neurotransmitters is increased in the synaptic cleft

Relevant contraindications:
- heart diseases, arterial hypertension
- agitation, psychoses

Relevant side effects and interactions:
- decreased appetite, stomach pain, vomiting
- increased sweating, dermatitis, pruritus, Quincke's oedema, effluvium

- tachycardia, palpitations, arrhythmias, changes in blood pressure, both up and down
- nervousness, insomnia, drowsiness, vertigo, may exacerbate tic disorders, psychoses
- long-term treatment: growth retardation, reduced weight gain
- do not combine with MAOIs
- can reduce the effect of antihypertensive drugs (primarily guanethidine)
- can enhance the initial sympathomimetic effect of guanethidine and Amantadine
- inhibits breakdown of coumarins, antiepileptics (e.g. Phenobarbital, Phenytoin, Primidone), neuroleptics, tricyclic antidepressants (e.g. Imipramine, Desipramine), Phenylbutazone → dose reduction of these drugs if concurrently administering Methylphenidate
- no concurrent intake with antacids

Approval status:

- depends on the specific product (see SPC)

Sources:

- **Germany – SPC:**
  - **ADHD**
    - oral
      - **children ≥ 6 years:** When starting treatment, carefully titrate the dose, beginning with lowest possible dose.
      - patients who are not currently taking Methylphenidate or any other stimulants: initially 18 mg/d as a SD. Doses may be increased in 18-mg increments at weekly intervals; max. 54 mg/d as a SD.
      - **children < 6 years:** not approved
      - dose conversion

Previous Methylphenidate daily dose	Recommended preparation CONCERTA® dose (extended release)
5 mg Methylphenidate 3 times daily	18 mg once daily
10 mg Methylphenidate 3 times daily	36 mg once daily
15 mg Methylphenidate 3 times daily	54 mg once daily

- **USA – T:**
  - **note:** discontinue medication if no improvement is seen after appropriate dosage adjustments over a one-month period
  - **ADHD (preparation Ritalin®)**
    - oral
      - **children ≥ 6 years:** initially 0.3 mg/kg/dose or 2.5–5 mg/dose before breakfast and lunch; increase by 0.1 mg/kg/dose or 5–10 mg/d at weekly intervals; usual dose, 0.3–1 mg/kg/d, max. 2 mg/kg/d or 60 mg/d; some patients may require 3 doses/d (e.g., 1 additional dose at 4 PM)
  - **ADHD (preparation Ritalin LA®)**
    - **children ≥ 6 years**, Methylphenidate-naive patients: initially 20 mg/d as a SD; may be increased by increments of 10 mg/d at weekly intervals; max. 60 mg/d as a SD

- **note:** If a lower initial dose is desired, patients may begin with Ritalin LA® 10 mg once daily. Alternatively, patients may begin therapy with an immediate release product, and switch to Ritalin LA® once immediate release dosage is titrated to 10 mg/d as 2 separate doses.
- **patients currently receiving Methylphenidate:** see table for initial dose; may be increased by increments of 10 mg/d at weekly intervals; max. 60 mg/d as a SD

Previous Methylphenidate dose	Recommended Ritalin LA® dose
5 mg Methylphenidate twice daily	10 mg once daily
10 mg Methylphenidate twice daily or 20 mg Methylphenidate sustained release	20 mg once daily
15 mg Methylphenidate twice daily	30 mg once daily
20 mg Methylphenidate twice daily or 40 mg Methylphenidate sustained release	40 mg once daily
30 mg Methylphenidate twice daily or 60 mg Methylphenidate sustained release	60 mg once daily

- **United Kingdom – BNFC:**
  - **attention deficit hyperactivity disorder**
    - oral
      - **children 4–6 years:** 5 mg/d as 2 separate doses, increase if necessary at weekly intervals by 2.5 mg/d to max. 1.4 mg/kg/d as 2–3 separate doses; discontinue if no response after 1 month
      - **children 6–18 years:** initially 5 mg/dose 1–2 times daily, increase if necessary at weekly intervals by 5–10 mg/d; licensed max. 60 mg/d as 2–3 divided doses, but may be increased to 2.1 mg/kg (max. 90 mg/d) under direction of a qualified specialist; discontinue if no response after 1 month
      - **note:** If effect wears off in the evening (with rebound hyperactivity) a dose at bedtime may be appropriate (establish need with trial bedtime dose). Treatment may be started using a modified release preparation.

Comments:

- duration of effect: 3–5 h; sustained release products: CONCERTA® 12 h, Medikinet retard® 8 h, Ritalin LA® 8 h, Equazym retard® 8 h
- no isolated drug administration, multimodal therapy concept!
- consider possible withdrawal symptoms: increased hyperactivity, petulance, depressive mood
- for long-term treatment assess blood count and blood pressure (CAUTION: hypertension)

Methylprednisolone

Dosage:

- ▶ progressive GBS or secondary deterioration after 4–6 weeks (especially SIDP or CIDP): pulse therapy with 20 mg/kg/d Methylprednisolone for 3–5 d
- ▶ pseudotumor cerebri: 20–30 mg/kg/d over 3–5 d, no (gradual) titration; max. 500–1000 mg/d
- ▶ idiopathic NNO: 20–30 mg/kg/d, max. 1 g/d for 3 d
- ▶ MS-relapse therapy: 20–30 mg/kg/d, max. 1 g/d for 3 d
- ▶ PACNS, pulse therapy: infusion with 20–30 mg/kg/d for 3 d
- ▶ Henoch Schönlein purpura: infusion with 20–30 mg/kg/d for 3 d
- ▶ radiotherapy-associated cerebral oedema: 1000 mg/d as 2 separate doses for 3 d
- ▶ myositis: initially IV 20–30 mg/kg short-term infusion over 3 d, then oral Prednisone
- ▶ West syndrome: pulse therapy 20 mg/kg/d as separate doses for 3–5 d

Neuropaediatric indications:

- non-infectious inflammation of the CNS, including demyelinating and vasculitis
- SIDP and CIDP
- pseudotumor cerebri
- idiopathic NNO
- radiotherapy-associated cerebral oedema
- severe myositis
- West syndrome

Mechanism of action:

- synthetic glucocorticoid

Relevant contraindications:

- systemic infection

Relevant side effects and interactions:

- nausea, vomiting
- frequent: arterial hypertension and hyperglycemia
- irritability, insomnia
- increased appetite and weight gain
- increased infection risk
- gastrointestinal bleeding
- iatrogenic Cushing's syndrome
- sudden stop of a long-term treatment (> 3 weeks) results in a secondary Addison's disease
- long-term intake: weight gain up to central obesity, osteoporosis, cataract, diabetes mellitus, psychoses

Approval status:

- depends on the specific product (see SPC)

Sources:

- Germany – SPC:
  - acute life-threatening conditions
    - IV
      - children: 4–20 mg/kg. For several indications up to 30 mg/kg; injection intervals differ between 30 min and 24 h, depending on indication.
  - cerebral oedema (caused by cerebral tumor, neurological procedures, cerebral abscess, bacterial meningitis)
    - No published paediatric dose
    - adults: acute or severe cerebral oedema: initially 250–500 mg, followed by 32–64 mg/dose three times daily over several days (same dosage is recommended for treating moderate or chronic cerebral oedema). If necessary, reduce dose gradually and switch to oral application.
- USA – T:
  - anti-inflammatory or immunosuppressive
    - oral, IM, IV
      - children: 0.5–1.7 mg/kg/d or 5–25 mg/m²/d as 2–4 separate doses; "pulse" therapy: 15–30 mg/kg ≥ 30 min as a SD for 3 d
  - acute spinal cord injury:
    - IV
      - children: 30 mg/kg over 15 min followed after 45 min by a continuous infusion of 5.4 mg/kg/h for 23 h;
      - note: Due to insufficient evidence of clinical efficacy (i.e., preserving or improving spinal cord function), the routine use of Methylprednisolone in the treatment of acute spinal cord injury is no longer recommended. If used in this setting, dosing should not be initiated > 8 h after the injury; not effective in penetration trauma (e.g. gunshot).
  - note: also further indications are listed in this source.
- United Kingdom – BNFC:
  - inflammatory and allergic disorders
    - oral, slow IV injection, IV infusion
      - children 1 month–18 years: 0.5–1.7 mg/kg/d as 2–4 separate doses depending on condition and response

Comments:

- steroid pulse therapy has an excellent benefit-/risk-ratio
- Vaccination with dead vaccines is possible. However, highly dosed glucocorticoids may interfere with the immune response and thus success of the vaccination.
- not effective in conventional acute GBS

- in combination with IVIG, marginal efficacy in the high risk group of elderly and ventilated patients
- highly effective (80 %) in previously treated patients and CIDP

Metoprolol

Dosage:
▶ migraine prophylaxis: 0.5–2 mg/kg/dose, max. 160 mg/d
▶ chronic substance abuse (overdosing or severe withdrawal symptoms): 23.75–95 mg/d

Neuropaediatric indications:
- migraine prophylaxis
- chronic substance abuse (overdosing or severe withdrawal symptoms)

Mechanism of action:
- β1-adrenoreceptor blocker

Relevant contraindications:
- concurrent administration of MAO-A inhibitors
- heart failure NYHA III and IV
- AV block II. and III. degree, SA block, sick sinus syndrome
- cardiogenic shock, distinctive hypotension
- bradycardia (< 50/min)
- obstructive bronchial diseases, bronchial asthma
- late stage of peripheral blood flow disorders
- metabolic acidosis
- IV application of verapamil and diltiazem
- careful use: AV block I. degree, impaired liver function, diabetes with greatly fluctuating blood glucose levels, strict fasting, history of severe hypersensitivity reactions, patients on desensitization therapy, pheochromocytoma (only after treatment with alpha receptor blockers), family or patient's history of psoriasis

Relevant side effects and interactions:
- due to decrease of blood pressure: ear noises, vertigo
- activation of psoriasis
- CNS changes (fatigue, hallucination)
- bronchial spasms, erectile dysfunction and urinary voiding dysfunction
- increased effect of drugs that lower blood glucose (insulin, sulfonylurea); Metoprolol can hide the signs of a hypoglycemia (tremor, tachycardia)
- enhancement of the effect of other anti-hypertensive drugs

- when Metoprolol is administered IV, do not combine with Calcium antagonists (certain types of verapamil or diltiazem) or other antiarrhythmics (e. g. disopyramide) (exception: intensive care medicine)

Approval status:
- depends on the specific product (see SPC)

Sources:
- Germany – SPC:
  - **prophylaxis of migraine**
    - no published paediatric dosage
    - **adults, oral:** 100–200 mg/dose, 1–2 times daily as Metoprolol tartrate
- USA – T:
  - **hypertension**
    - oral
      - **children 1–17 years, immediate release tablets:** initially 1–2 mg/kg/d as 2 separate doses; adjust dose based on patient's response; max. 6 mg/kg/d (≤ 200 mg/d)
      - **children ≥ 6 years, extended release tablets:** the manufacturer recommends to use initially 1 mg/kg/d as a SD (max. initial dose: 50 mg/d); adjust dose based on patient's response (max. 2 mg/kg/d or 200 mg/d; higher doses have not been studied).
      - note: the SPC does not specify this indication of interest
- **United Kingdom – BNFC:** this indication of interest is not specified

Mexiletine

Dosage:
▶ infusion IV: 2–5 mg/kg (max. 250 mg) over 15 min, then 5–20 mcg/kg/min (max. 250 mg/h) (off-label)
▶ p.o.: 8 mg/kg (max. 400 mg) as a SD, then 12–24 mg/kg/d (max. 400 mg/dose) as 3 separate doses, start 2 h after initial dose (off-label)

Neuropaediatric indications:
- myotonic dystrophy (functional disability in myotonia)

Mechanism of action:
- antiarrhythmic drug from the group 1b
- inhibition of fast transmembrane sodium channels and slow Calcium influx, which is responsible for the plateau of the action potential
- no sympatholytic or anticholinergic effect
- does not prolong the QT interval

Relevant contraindications:
- no absolute contraindication
- within first 3 months of myocardial infarction
- cardiogenic shock
- AV block II. or III. degree
- sick sinus syndrome
- bradycardia
- hypotension
- heart failure
- Parkinson's disease
- liver or renal disorders
- pregnancy

Relevant side effects and interactions:
- vomiting, nausea, diarrhea, constipation, dry mouth
- vertigo, double vision
- paresthesia, tremor
- tonic-clonic seizures
- bradycardia, hypotension, cardiac arrhythmias
- thrombocytopenia
- supra-additive effects when concurrently taken with local anesthetics, beta blockers and other antiarrhythmics
- decreased effect of Mexiletine when concurrently taken with Phenytoin, Phenobarbital and Rifampicin (CAUTION when stopping any of these drugs due to toxicity)
- can increase the effect of Theophylline
- chinidin inhibits CYP2D6 and thus, slows the breakdown of Mexiletine
- antacids and Atropine decrease the bowel resorption
- Metoclopramide increases the bowl resorption

Approval status:
- approved for antiarrhythmia

Sources:
- **Germany – SPC:** –
- **USA – T:**
- **Management of serious ventricular arrhythmias, suppression of premature ventricular contractions, diabetic neuropathy**
  - Oral
    - **children:** range 1.4–5 mg/kg/dose (mean: 3.3 mg/kg/dose) given every 8 h; start with lower initial dose and increase according to effects and serum levels
- **United Kingdom – BNFC:** –

Comments:
- prior to start of the therapy: cardiac assessment

Midazolam (MDL)

Dosage:
- ▸ fever convulsion: 0.1(–0.3) mg/kg/dose IV
- ▸ sedation in increased cranial pressure: 0.1–0.5 mg/kg/h IV
- ▸ sedation (e.g. lumbar puncture): 0.3–0.5 mg/kg p.o. (≥ 0.5 mg/kg may cause respiratory depression; monitor for 30–60 min)
- ▸ dystonic status: initially 0.1–0.2 mg/kg IV, then 0.05 mg/kg/h, increase according to response
- ▸ status epilepticus:
  - initially 0.2 mg/kg nasal/buccal administration of the IV solution
  - after > 60 min: administration during emergency conditions under EEG-monitoring bolus: 0.2–0.5 mg/kg, then 1–5 mcg/kg/min (0.1–0.5 mg/kg/h); (dosing according to EEG)

Neuropaediatric indications:
- status epilepticus
- fever convulsion
- sedation in increased cranial pressure
- dystonic status
- sedation (e.g. lumbar puncture)

Mechanism of action:
- benzodiazepine
- opens chloride channels and thus enhances GABAergic neuronal inhibition, especially in the limbic system

Relevant contraindications:
- known hypersensitivity to benzodiazepines
- medication-, drug-, alcohol addiction
- acute angle-closure glaucoma
- myasthenia gravis
- careful use: severe liver damage, ataxia, acute poisoning with alcohol, analgesics or soporifics, neuroleptics, antidepressants, Lithium, severe chronic respiratory insufficiency, sleep apnea syndrome, pregnancy

Relevant side effects and interactions:

- hypersensitivity reactions
- muscle weakness, dry mouth, gastrointestinal disorders
- temporary elevation of liver function parameters
- fatigue, drowsiness, weakness, vertigo
- headache, confusion, anterograde amnesia, depressive mood
- paradox reactions (e.g. acute agitation, anger)
- libido reduction
- decrease in blood pressure, respiratory depression
- sedation (increased when combined with other medication, e.g. Phenobarbital)
- high dosing and long-term treatment:
  - unstable walking
  - articulation disorders
  - vertigo
  - addiction, withdrawal syndrome (sudden stop after long-term treatment): sleeping disorder and increased dreaming, tonicity, agitation, anxiety, shivering, sweating, increased tendency of seizures or symptomatic psychosis
  - impaired vision, double vision, nystagmus
- mutually enhanced effect with concurrent intake of centrally depressant drugs and alcohol
- enhanced effect of muscle relaxants, analgesics and laughing gas
- enhanced and prolonged effect of certain benzodiazepines by delayed breakdown when combined with cimetidine
- unpredictable side effects in long-term treatment with centrally depressant anti-hypertensives, beta blockers and anticoagulants when combined with benzodiazepines

Approval status:

- approved for inducing sleep and as a sedative drug in children and adults

Sources:

- **Germany – SPC:**

Indication	children < 12 years	children > 12 years
Analog sedation	IV 6 months–5 years: initially 0.05–0.1 mg/kg, total dose < 6 mg IV 6–12 years: initially 0.025–0.05 mg/kg, total dose < 10 mg rectal > 6 months: 0.3–0.5 mg/kg IM 1–15 years: 0.05–0.15 mg/kg	IV initially 2–2.5 mg IV, titrate in 1 mg-increments IV, total dose 3.5–7.5 mg

Indication	children < 12 years	children > 12 years
sedation in the intensive care unit	IV neonates < 32 weeks, 0.03 mg/kg/h IV neonates > 32 weeks and children ≤ 6 months, 0.06 mg/kg/h IV > 6 months, bolus dose of 0.05–0.2 mg/kg, maintenance with 0.06–0.2 mg/kg/h	IV bolus dose of 0.03–0.3 mg/kg; titrate in steps of 1–2.5 mg to the maintenance dose of 0.03–0.2 mg/kg/h
Premedication prior to anesthesia	**children** > 6 months, 0.3–0.5 mg/kg rectal 1–15 years, 0.08–0.2 mg/kg IM	

- **note:** in children < 6 months, use is not recommended. Rectal application is preferred over IM. Do not give > 1 mg/ml Midazolam to children weighing < 15 kg. Initial dose should be infused over 2–3 min; wait another 2–5 min to assess sedation.
- **USA – T:**
  - **note:** dosage has to be chosen according to the patient's age, underlying diseases, concurrent medications, and desired effect; decrease dose by ~ 30 % if narcotics or other CNS depressants are administered concomitantly.
  - **status epilepticus**
    - IV
      - **neonates:** Dosage regimens vary. Reported doses are higher than those reported for sedation.
      - **note:** consider omitting loading dose in patients receiving benzodiazepine IV; begin continuous IV infusion at lower end of range and titrate to lowest effective dose: loading dose: 0.06–0.15 mg/kg/dose followed by a continuous infusion of 0.06–0.4 mg/kg/h (1–7 mcg/kg/min); max. reported rate: 1.1 mg/kg/h (18 mcg/kg/min).
      - **note:** Patients receiving ECMO may require higher doses due to drug absorption in the ECMO circuit.
      - **children, infants > 2 months:** loading dose, 0.15–0.2 mg/kg/dose followed by continuous infusion with initially 1 mcg/kg/min; increase in increments of 1 mcg/kg/min every 15 min until seizures stop (max. 5 mcg/kg/min); mean infusion rate required in a study with 24 children was 2.3 mcg/kg/min with a range of 1–18 mcg/kg/min
      - **note:** use multiple small doses and titrate to desired sedative effect; allow 3–5 min between doses to decrease risk of oversedation
  - **sedation, anxiolysis, and amnesia prior to procedure or before inducing anesthesia**
    - oral
      - **children, infants ≥ 6 months:** single dose of 0.25–0.5 mg/kg, depending on patient status and desired effect, usually 0.5 mg/kg, max. 20 mg
      - **infants, children ≥ 6 months–< 6 years and less cooperative patients:** higher doses (up to 1 mg/kg) may be required
      - **children 6–< 16 years or cooperative patients:** 0.25 mg/kg may be sufficient
      - **note:** also further indications are listed in this source

- United Kingdom – BNFC:
  - **status epilepticus, febrile convulsions**
    - buccal
      - **neonates:** 0.3 mg/kg, repeat once after 10 minutes if necessary
      - **children 1–6 months:** 0.3 mg/kg (max. 2.5 mg), repeat once after 10 minutes if necessary
      - **children 6 months–1 year:** 2.5 mg, repeat once after 10 minutes if necessary
      - **children 1–5 years:** 5 mg, repeat once after 10 minutes if necessary
      - **children 5–10 years:** 7.5 mg, repeat once after 10 minutes if necessary
      - **children 10–18 years:** 10 mg, repeat once after 10 minutes if necessary
    - IV
      - **neonates:** initially, IV injection of 0.15–0.2 mg/kg, followed by continuous IV infusion of 0.06 mg/kg/h (increased by 0.06 mg/kg/h every 15 min until seizure is controlled); max. 0.3 mg/kg/h
      - **children 1 month–18 years:** initially, IV injection of 0.15–0.2 mg/kg, followed by continuous IV infusion of 0.06 mg/kg/h (increased by 0.06 mg/kg/h every 15 min until seizure is controlled); max. 0.3 mg/kg/h
  - **conscious sedation for procedures**
  - **note:** not licensed for use in children under 6 months for premedication and conscious sedation; not licensed for use by mouth, or by buccal administration)
    - oral
      - **children 1 month–18 years:** 0.5 mg/kg (max. 20 mg), 30–60 min before procedure
    - buccal
      - **children 6 months–10 years:** 0.2–0.3 mg/kg (max. 5 mg)
      - **children 10–18 years:** 6–7 mg (max. 8 mg, if ≥ 70 kg)
    - rectal
      - **children 6 months–12 years:** 0.3–0.5 mg/kg, 15–30 min before procedure
    - IV injection over 2–3 min, 5–10 min before procedure
      - **children 1 month–6 years:** initially 0.025–0.05 mg/kg, increase if necessary in small steps (max. total dose 6 mg)
      - **children 6–12 years:** initially 0.025–0.05 mg/kg, increase if necessary in small steps (max. total dose 10 mg)
      - **children 12–18 years:** initially 0.025–0.05 mg/kg, increase if necessary in small steps (max. total dose 7.5 mg)

Comments:

- buccal administration highly effective
- subtherapeutic blood level: < 0.04 mcg/ml
- half-life: 1.5–3 h
- status epilepticus nasal/buccal:
  - advantage: there are good current studies on efficacy, which is equal to or better than that of Diazepam (rectal)
- status epilepticus, continuous infusion:
- advantage:
  - effect (71–97 %) is comparable to other coma-inducing antiepileptics
  - onset of action after 0.3–1.1 h (Ulvi 2002)

- fewer side effects even when using high dosages. This allows relatively fast titration.
- disadvantage:
  - "break through" seizures frequently reported (approximately 50 %), titration after EEG meaningful
  - seizure relapse (low dosages) 6–19 % reported

Mirtazapine

Dosage:

▶ chronic substance abuse (in overdosing or severe withdrawal symptoms): 15–60 mg/d (off-label), titrate gradually

Neuropaediatric indications:

- chronic substance abuse (in overdosing or severe withdrawal symptoms)

Mechanism of action:

- noradrenergic and specific serotonergic antidepressant drug (tetracyclic antidepressant)
- block of central presynaptic α_2-receptors and consecutive increased release of serotonin, noradrenaline and dopamine
- inhibition of 5-HT$_2$ and 5-HT$_3$-receptors and thus enhanced effect of serotonin at the 5-HT$_1$ receptor
- strong inhibition of H$_1$ receptors (fatigue)

Relevant contraindications:

- acute intoxication with hypnotic drugs, analgesics, psychotropic drugs, alcohol
- organic psychosyndrom (OPS)
- increased tendency of seizures, epilepsy
- liver or renal insufficiency, jaundice
- bradycardia, hypotension, other clinically significant cardiac disorders
- schizophrenia or other psychotic disorders
- acute angle-closure glaucoma
- MAOIs (stop at least 2 weeks prior to onset of therapy)
- diabetes mellitus

Relevant side effects and interactions:

- severe fatigue
- increased appetite, weight gain, oedema
- very young patients: aggressiv behaviour and increased suicidal tendency
- very rare: agranulocytosis
- paresthesia

- extrapyramidal motoric symptoms
- sudden stop of treatment: anxiety, sleeping disorder, sweating
- enhanced sedation with concurrent intake of benzodiazepines, neuroleptics, other sedatives and alcohol
- Carbamazepine and Phenytoin increase the Mirtazapine clearance (45–60 % lower plasma levels of Mirtazapine)
- MAOIs (stop at least 2 weeks prior to start of therapy)
- concurrent intake of SSRI: serotonin syndrome
  - nausea, vomiting and diarrhea
  - restlessness, hallucination, loss of coordination
  - tachycardia, variation in blood pressure, elevated body temperature
- increased reflexes catecholamines and catecholamine-containing local anesthetics enhance the sympathomimetic effect of Mirtazapine
- drugs with anticholinergic effect enhance the anticholinergic effect of Mirtazapine
- increased cardiac conduction disorders when combined with antiarrhythmic drugs (chinidin derivatives and digitalis glycosides)

Approval status:
- not approved for patients under the age of 18 years

Sources:
- **Germany – SPC:**
  - **depressive disorders**
    - **children < 18 years:** not recommended
- **USA – T:** –
- **United Kingdom – BNFC:** –
- **Uptodate.com:** no published paediatric dosage

Mitoxantrone

Dosage:
- ▶ MS: initially 12 mg/m^2/dose every 3 months

Neuropaediatric indications:
- relapsing MS

Mechanism of action:
- intercalates into deoxyribonucleic acid (DNA) through hydrogen bonding, causes cross-links and strand breaks
- potent inhibitor of topoisomerase II, an enzyme responsible for uncoiling and repairing damaged DNA

- cytocidal effect on both proliferating and non-proliferating cultured human cells, suggesting lack of cell cycle phase specificity

Relevant contraindications:
- vaccination with live vaccines
- pregnancy
- previous treatment with cardiocytotoxic cytostatics
- radiotherapy of the thorax or mediastinum
- severe liver insufficiency
- previously administrated total dose > 160 mg Mitoxantrone/m^2 BSA
- acute infections
- severe bone marrow depression
- myocardial damages

Relevant side effects and interactions:
- nausea, vomiting
- loss of appetite, weakness, fever
- hair loss, mucositis
- anemia, thrombocytopenia, leukopenia
- infections due to leukopenia and neutropenia
- elevation of liver enzymes and bilirubin
- blue colouration of the skin, oncholysis, green colouration of the urine
- significant cardiotoxicity: cardiac arrhythmias (reversible), toxic cardiac myopathies (irreversible)
- thrombophlebitis or local necrosis in paravenous application
- especially in combination with etoposide or teniposide, mixantrone can lead to a therapy-associated leukemia (secondary leukemia as secondary malignant neoplasm) (0.05–0.1 % of patients treated with mixantrone)
- no vaccination with live vaccines during therapy; dead vaccines may become ineffective
- enhanced effect of other cytostatics, cardiotoxic drugs (e.g. Cyclophosphamide, anthracyclines) and hepatotoxic drugs (e.g. Methotrexate)
- increased hyperuricemia caused by substances with retarded elimination of uric acid (e.g. sulfonamide, certain diuretics)

Approval status:
- depends on the specific product (see SPC)

Sources:
- **Germany – SPC:**
- **note:** no published paediatric dosage

- USA – T:
  - **multiple sclerosis**
    - oral
      - **adults:** 12 mg/m²/dose every 3 months; maximum cumulative dose is 140 mg/m²/dose (discontinue use with left ventricular ejection fraction < 50 % or clinically significant reduction in LVEF)
  - **solid tumors**
    - **children:** 18–20 mg/m² once every 3–4 weeks or 5–8 mg/m² every week
- **United Kingdom – BNFC:** this indication of interest is not specified

Comments:

- Avoid contact with skin or mucous membranes when you handle anthracyclines. Safety instructions apply for medical staff due to the potential mutagenic and carcinogenic effects. The injection solution has to be prepared in special safety facilities. Be sure to avoid touching excrements or vomitus of patients.
- pregnant staff must be excluded from contact with cytostatics
- cardiotoxicity:
  - continuous echocardiography (at least once a year)
  - consider cumulative total dose
  - especially careful use in patients with known heart diseases

Morphine

Dosage:

- ▶ oral solution 0.5 %, 2 % every 4 h, < 50 kg: 0.15–0.3 mg/kg; > 50 kg: 5–10 mg
- ▶ tablets every 4 h, < 50 kg: 0.15–0.3 mg/kg; > 50 kg: 5–10 mg
- ▶ sustained-release tablets every 8–12 h, < 50 kg: 0.5 mg/kg; > 50 kg: 30–60 mg
- ▶ sustained-release granules every 8–12 h, < 50 kg: 0,5 mg/kg; > 50 kg: 30–60 mg
- ▶ sustained-release capsules every 12–24 h
- ▶ suppository every 4 h
- ▶ injection solution, < 50 kg: 0.05 mg/kg every 2–4 h, continuous infusion: 0.02–0.03 mg/kg/h; > 50 kg: 5–15 mg every 4 hours, continuous infusion: 1 mg/h

Neuropaediatric indications:

- strong and severe pain (i.e. palliative)

Mechanism of action:

- main alkaloid of opium
- pure agonist with a high affinity to μ-receptors and lesser affinity to κ-receptors

Relevant contraindications:

- decompensated respiratory insufficiency
- acute abdomen of unknown origin
- severe hepatic impairment
- uncontrolled seizures, increased tendency of cerebral seizures
- careful use: children < 1 year
- addiction to opioids
- unconsciousness
- disorders of the respiratory center and respiratory function
- raised intracranial pressure
- hypotension in hypovolemia
- biliary tract diseases
- obstructive and inflammatory bowel diseases
- pancreatitis
- myxoedema

Relevant side effects and interactions:

- risk of cumulation in renal insufficiency
- respiratory depression/apnea, bronchial spasms
- sweating, miosis, dry mouth, constipation, spasms of the pancreas or bile ducts, renal colics
- elevated tonicity of the urinary bladder, voiding dysfunction
- nausea, vomiting, headache, vertigo, pruritus, exanthema, peripheral oedema
- hallucination, loss of time feeling/amnesia, depression, euphoria, dysphoria
- apathy, somnolence, coma
- cerebral seizures (primarily with high dosages in children)
- hypotension, orthostatic regulation disorders, bradycardia
- addiction, development of tolerance, withdrawal syndrome
- muscular rigidity
- blurred vision, diplopia, nystagmus, loss of appetite, taste changes

Approval status:

- depends on the specific product (see SPC)

Sources:

- **Germany – SPC:**
  - **moderate and severe pain**
    - oral (as Morphine hydrochloride)

Age, body weight	Single dose	Total daily dose
children < 2 years, < 12.5 kg	2.5 mg	22.5 mg
children 2–6 years, 12.5–20 kg	2.5–5 mg	15–30 mg
children 6–12 years, 20–40 kg	5–10 mg	30–60 mg

Age, body weight	Single dose	Total daily dose
adolescents 12–16 years, 40–50 kg	10–20 mg	60–120 mg
adolescents > 16 years	10–60 mg	Up to 360 mg

- note: Use in children < 1 year requires special care due to possible effect on the respiratory system.
- USA – T:
  - relief of moderate to severe acute and chronic pain
    - note: neonatal doses should be titrated to appropriate effect; when changing routes of administration in chronically treated patients, please note that oral doses are approximately one-half as effective as parenteral dose; use preservative-free formulations
    - IM, IV, SC
      - neonates: initially 0.05 mg/kg/dose every 4–8 h; titrate dose carefully to effect; max. 0.1 mg/kg/dose
      - continuous IV infusion, neonates: initially 0.01 mg/kg/h; do not exceed infusion rates of 0.015–0.02 mg/kg/h due to decreased elimination, increased CNS sensitivity, and adverse effects; note: some centers may use slightly higher doses, especially in neonates who develop tolerance.
      - International Evidence-Based group for neonatal Pain recommendation: intermittent dose, 0.05–0.1 mg/kg; continuous infusion, 0.01–0.03 mg/kg/h
      - infants and children: 0.1–0.2 mg/kg/dose every 2–4 h as needed; may be initiated at 0.05 mg/kg/dose
      - usual max. dose
        - infants: 2 mg/dose
        - children 1–6 years: 4 mg/dose
        - children 7–12 years: 8 mg/dose
        - adolescents: 15 mg/dose
      - note: infants < 3 months are more susceptible to respiratory depression; use with caution and in reduced doses in this age group.
    - oral (prompt release)
      - infants and children: 0.2–0.5 mg/kg/dose every 4–6 h as needed
      - note: The American Pain Society (2008) recommends an initial oral dose of 0.3 mg/kg for children with severe pain.
    - oral (controlled release)
      - children: 0.3–0.6 mg/kg/dose every 12 h
  - sickle cell or cancer pain
    - IV, SC continuous infusion
      - infants: initially 0.02 mg/kg/h
      - children: 0.03 mg/kg/h
      - Conversion from intermittent IV Morphine: administer the total daily IV Morphine dose over 24 h as a continuous infusion; titrate dose to appropriate effect; in one study children with severe pain from terminal cancer required a median dose of 0.04–0.07 mg/kg/h, range: 0.025–2.6 mg/kg/h
  - postoperative pain
    - IV, SC, continuous infusion
      - infants and children: 0.01–0.04 mg/kg/h

- sedation/analgesia for procedures
  - IV
    - infants and children: 0.05–0.1 mg/kg 5 min before the procedure
    - children > 12 years: 3–4 mg; may be repeated after 5 min if necessary
    - note: further indications are listed in this source
- United Kingdom – BNFC:
- pain
  - SC injection
    - neonates: initially 0.1 mg/kg/dose every 6 h, adjusted according to response
    - children 1–6 months: initially 0.1–0.2 mg/kg/dose every 6 h, adjusted according to response
    - children 6 months–2 years: initially 0.1–0.2 mg/kg/dose every 4 h, adjusted according to response
    - children 2–12 years: initially 0.2 mg/kg/dose every 4 h, adjusted according to response
    - children 12–18 years: initially 2.5–10 mg/dose every 4 h, adjusted according to response
  - IV inject over at least 5 min
    - neonates: initially 0.05 mg/kg/dose every 6 h, adjusted according to response
    - children 1–6 months: initially 0.1 mg/kg/dose every 6 h, adjusted according to response
    - children 6 months–12 years: initially 0.1 mg/kg/dose every 4 h, adjusted according to response
    - children 12–18 years: initially 5 mg/dose every 4 h, adjusted according to response
  - IV
    - neonates: initially by IV injection (over at least 5 min) 0.05 mg/kg, then by continuous IV infusion 0.005–0.02 mg/kg/h, adjusted according to response
    - children 1–6 months: initially by IV injection (over at least 5 min) 0.1 mg/kg, then by continuous IV infusion 0.01–0.03 mg/kg/h, adjusted according to response
    - children 6 months–12 years: initially by IV injection (over at least 5 min) 0.1 mg/kg, then by continuous IV infusion 0.02–0.03 mg/kg/h, adjusted according to response
    - children 12–18 years: initially by IV injection (over at least 5 min) 5 mg, then by continuous IV infusion 0.02–0.03 mg/kg/h, adjusted according to response
  - rectal, oral
    - children 1–3 months: initially 0.05–0.1 mg/kg/dose every 4 h, adjusted according to response
    - children 3–6 months: initially 0.1–0.15 mg/kg/dose every 4 h, adjusted according to response
    - children 6–12 months: initially 0.2 mg/kg/dose every 4 h, adjusted according to response
    - children 1–2 years: initially 0.2–0.3 mg/kg/dose every 4 h, adjusted according to response
    - children 2–12 years: initially 0.2–0.3 mg/kg/dose (max. 10 mg) every 4 h, adjusted according to response
    - children 12–18 years: initially 5–10 mg/dose every 4 h, adjusted according to response
  - continuous SC infusion
    - children 1–3 months: 0.01 mg/kg/h, adjusted according to response
    - children 3 months–18 years: 0.02 mg/kg/h, adjusted according to response
- neonatal opioid withdrawal (under specialist's supervision)
- oral
  - neonates: initially 0.04 mg/kg/dose every 4 h until symptoms controlled, increase dose if necessary; reduce frequency gradually over 6–10 d, and stop when 0.04 mg/kg once daily achieved; dose may vary, consult local guidelines

M

Comments:
- opioid with the most experience in paediatrics
- no ceiling effect
- Naloxone is a competitive antagonist

Mycophenolate mofetil

Dosage:
- ▶ up to 2 g/d (positive effects in some cases are reported) (off-label)

Neuropaediatric indications:
- therapy-resistant severe myositis

Mechanism of action
- is converted to mycophenolic acid (MPA)
- MPA is a selective, non-competitive and reversible inhibitor of inosine monophosphate dehydrogenase and thereby inhibits guanosine synthesis and thus formation of DNA.
- Because T- and B-lymphocytes depend for proliferation on de novo synthesis from purines, these cell types are selectively suppressed.

Relevant contraindications:
- hypersensitivity to mycophenolic acid
- fast injection or bolus injection
- use special care when using in patients with phenylketonuria, hereditary fructose intolerance, renal transplant patients < 2 years, heart and liver transplant patients

Relevant side effects and interactions:
- candidiasis at different locations
- diarrhea, sepsis, vomiting, stomach pain, nausea, anorexia
- urinary tract infections
- herpes simplex, herpes zoster
- leukopenia, thrombocytopenia, anemia
- pneumonia, influenza, airway infections
- gastrointestinal infections
- bronchitis, pharyngitis, sinusitis
- fungal dermatitis, rhinitis,
- benign and malignant neoplasia of the skin
- pancytopenia, leukocytosis
- acidosis, hyperkalemia, hypokalemia, hyperglycemia, hypomagnesemia, hypocalcemia, hypercholesterolemia, hyperlipidemia, hypophosphatemia, hyperuricemia, gout
- agitation, confusion, depression, anxiety, abnormal thinking, insomnia, convulsions
- tremor, somnolence, pseudomyasthenic syndrome, drowsiness, headache, paresthesia, dysgeusia
- tachycardia, hypotension, hypertension
- pleural effusion, dyspnea
- peritonitis, ileus, colitis, gastrointestinal ulcer, gastritis, esophagitis, stomatitis, obstipation, dyspepsia, flatulence
- hepatitis, jaundice, hyperbilirubinemia
- hypertrophy of the skin, exanthema, acne, alopecia,
- renal insufficiency, oedema, raised liver function parameters, raised creatinine, elevated LDH, elevated blood urea, elevated alkaline phosphatase
- fever, shivering, pain, malaise, asthenia, weight loss
- elevated plasma levels of Aciclovir and Valaciclovir
- antacids containing Magnesium or aluminium hydroxide decrease the resorption of Mycophenolate mofetil
- the area under the curve of MPA increases when Mycophenolate mofetil is concurrently used with cyclosporine
- decreased MPA exposure when Mycophenolate mofetil is concurrently used with Rifampicin, Norfloxacin and Metronidazole
- intake of Mycophenolate mofetil 1 h prior or 3 h after intake of sevelamer
- drugs that interfere with enterohepatic circulation reduce the efficacy of Mycophenolate mofetil

Approval status:
- approved as add-on medication for the prophylaxis of graft rejection

Sources:
- **Germany – SPC:**
- **prophylaxis of transplant rejection**
  - IV
    - **children < 18 years:** Efficacy and safety have not been established, therefore the use in this age group is not recommended.
- **USA – T:**
- **nephrotic syndrome**
  - oral
  - **note:** preparation CellCept® tablets, capsules and suspension should not be interchanged with the delayed-release tablet formulation (Myfortic®) due to differences in the rate of absorption
    - **children:** nephrotic syndrome frequently relapsing: 25–36 mg/kg/d as 2 separate doses; max. 2 g/d for 1–2 years with a tapering dose of Prednisone

- Steroid-dependent (secondary in the setting of glucocorticoid toxicity); 24–36 mg/kg/d or 1200 mg/m²/d as 2 separate doses; max. 2 g/d
  - **note:** further indications are listed in this source, but indication of this interest is not specified
- **United Kingdom – BNFC:** this indication of interest is not specified

N

Natalizumab

Dosage:

▶ 300 mg/dose every 4 weeks (off-label)

Neuropaediatric indications:

- MS

Mechanism of action:

- humanized, monoclonal IgG_4 antibody
- antibody against α_4-integrin (molecule for cell adhesion on leukocytes)
- inhibits diapedesis of leukocytes from the vessels into the tissue. Therefore, participation of leukocytes in inflammatory reactions is suppressed.

Relevant contraindications:

- patients with increased risk of opportunistic infections
- combination with interferon β or Glatiramer acetate
- known active malignant neoplasm (exception: basalioma)
- be sure to allow a sufficient time interval to any previous immunosuppressive therapies

Relevant side effects and interactions:

- progressive multifocal leukoencephalopathy
- headache, urinary tract infections
- depression, fatigue
- mild respiratory infections, pharyngitis
- limb and joint pain
- very rare: severe liver damage
- there may be an increased risk of opportunistic infections
- development of neutralizing antibody in 6 % of all treated patients

Approval status:

- not approved for treatment of children and adolescents

Sources:

- **Germany – SPC:**
  - **monotherapy for the treatment of relapsing forms of multiple sclerosis**
  - see comments, not approved for children and adolescents < 18 years of age
- **USA – T:** –
- **United Kingdom – BNFC:** –
- **Uptodate.com:**
- no published paediatric dosage
- **Multiple sclerosis**
  - **adults** IV: 300 mg infused over 1 hour every 4 weeks

Comments:

- CAUTION: patients may develop a progressive multifocal leukoencephalopathy
- AFFIRM study (phase III) that led to approval (no paediatric patients):
  - 67 % reduced relapse frequency
  - 42 % delayed onset of chronic clinical disability
  - 92 % reduced number of gadolinium-enhanced lesions in MRT
  - 83 % reduced number of new or expanding T2 lesions
  - 44 % reduced black hole

Neostigmine

Dosage:

▶ test of response in myasthenic syndrome: 0.04 mg/kg IM

Neuropaediatric indications:

- short-term (parenteral) therapy of myasthenia gravis and further disorders of neuromuscular transmission

Mechanism of action:

- acetylcholinesterase inhibitor; increased acetylcholine concentration in the synaptic cleft

Relevant contraindications:

- intestinal obstruction, urinary retention
- bradycardia, hypotension, heart failure
- acute iritis
- bronchial asthma and other pulmonary diseases

- careful use: epilepsy, peptic ulcers, cardiac arrhythmias, hyperthyroidism, vagotonia, megacolon

Relevant side effects and interactions:
- nausea, vomiting, abdominal cramps, diarrhea
- drooling, miosis, elevated lacrimation
- raised bronchial secretion, bronchial spasm, hypotension
- muscle cramps and weakness
- anxiety and anxiety conditions

Approval status:
- approved for myasthenia gravis and for the antagonistic effect on non-depolarizing muscle relaxants

Sources:
- Germany – SPC:
  - reversal of muscle relaxing effect of non depolarizing muscle relaxants
    - slow IV injection (as Neostigmine methylsulfate)
      - **children < 20 kg:** 0,05 mg/kg
      - **children > 20 kg:** 0.5–2 mg, max. 5 mg
      - **note:** give 0.5–1 mg Atropine sulfate (IV) to avoid muscarinic side effects.
- USA – T:
  - myasthenia gravis (diagnosis)
    - IM
      - **note:** All cholinesterase medications should be discontinued at least 8 h before; Atropine should be administered IV immediately prior to, or IM 30 min before Neostigmine.
      - **children:** 0.025–0.04 mg/kg as a SD
  - myasthenia gravis (treatment)
    - oral
      - **children:** 2 mg/kg/d or 60 mg/m²/d as separate doses every 3–4 h, max. 375 mg/d
      - **note:** dosage requirements are variable; adjust dosage such that patient takes larger doses at times of greatest fatigue.
    - IM, IV, SC
      - **children:** 0.01–0.04 mg/kg/dose every 2–4 h
  - reversal of non-depolarizing neuromuscular blockade after surgery in conjunction with Atropine or Glycopyrrolate
    - IV
      - **infants:** 0.025–0.1 mg/kg/dose
      - **children:** 0.025–0.08 mg/kg/dose
- United Kingdom – BNFC:
  - reversal of non-depolarizing muscle block
    - IV injection over 1 min
      - **neonates:** 0.05 mg/kg, after or with Glycopyrronium or Atropine; a further dose of 0.025 mg/kg may be required
      - **children 1 month–12 years:** 0.05 mg/kg (max. 2.5 mg) after or with Glycopyrronium or Atropine; a further dose of 0.025 mg/kg may be required
      - **children 12–18 years:** 0.05 mg/kg (max. 2.5 mg) after or with Glycopyrronium or Atropine; a further dose of 0.025 mg/kg (max. 2.5 mg) may be required
  - treatment of myasthenia gravis
    - oral (as Neostigmine bromide)
      - **neonates:** initially 1–2 mg, then 1–5 mg/dose every 4 h; give 30 min before feeds
      - **children < 6 years:** initially 7.5 mg, repeated at suitable intervals throughout the day, max. 15–90 mg/d
      - **children 6–12 years:** initially 15 mg repeated at suitable intervals throughout the day, max. 15–90 mg/d
      - **children 12–18 years:** initially 15–30 mg repeated at suitable intervals throughout the day, max. 75–300 mg/d (however, the max. most patients can tolerate is 180 mg/d)
    - SC or IM injection (as Neostigmine methylsulfate)
      - **neonates:** 0.15 mg/kg/dose every 6–8 h, 30 min before feeds; increase to max. 0.3 mg/kg/dose every 4 h, if necessary [unlicensed]
      - **children 1 month–12 years:** 0.2–0.5 mg/dose; repeat at suitable intervals throughout the day
      - **children 12–18 years:** 1–2.5 mg/dose, repeat at suitable intervals throughout the day

Comments:
- strong muscarinergic effect, which may necessitate subsequent Atropine administration to treat abdominal cramps, drooling and diarrhea

Nitrazepam (NZP)

Dosage:
▶ 2.5–5 mg/d as a SD (SPC)

Neuropaediatric indications:
- myoclonic epilepsy
- alternative therapy of therapy-resistant infantile spasms (West syndrome)
- short-term treatment of sleeping disorders

Mechanism of action:
- benzodiazepine
- opens chloride channels and thus enhances GABAergic neuron inhibition (especially in the limbic system)

Relevant contraindications:
- known hypersensitivity to benzodiazepines
- addiction to medication, drugs or alcohol
- acute angle-closure glaucoma

- myasthenia gravis
- careful use: severe liver damage, ataxia, acute poisoning with alcohol, soporifics or analgesics, neuroleptics, antidepressants, lithium, severe chronic respiratory insufficiency, sleep apnea syndrome, pregnancy

Relevant side effects and interactions:

- hypersensitivity reactions
- muscle weakness, dry mouth, gastrointestinal disorder
- temporary elevation of liver function parameters
- fatigue, drowsiness, weakness, vertigo, drowsiness
- headache, confusion, anterograde amnesia, depressive mood
- paradox reactions (e.g. acute agitation, anger)
- libido reduction
- blood pressure decrease, respiratory depression
- sedation (increasing in combination with other medication, e.g. Phenobarbital)
- high dosages and long-term treatment:
  - unstable walking
  - articulation disorders
  - vertigo
  - addiction, withdrawal syndrome (when sudden stop after long-term use): sleeping disorder and increased dreaming, anxiety, state of stress, agitation, shivering, sweating, increased tendency of seizures or symptomatic psychoses
  - impaired vision, double vision, nystagmus
- mutually enhanced effect with concurrent intake of centrally depressant drugs and alcohol
- enhanced effect of muscle relaxants, analgesics and laughing gas
- enhanced and prolonged effect of certain benzodiazepines by delayed breakdown when combined with cimetidine
- unpredictable side effects in long-term treatment with centrally depressant antihypertensives, beta blockers and anticoagulants when combined with benzodiazepines

Approval status:

- BNS seizures

Sources:

- **Germany – SPC:**
  - **BNS seizures (West syndrome)**
    - oral
      - **infants and young children:** 2.5–5 mg/d as a SD
- **USA – T: –**

- **United Kingdom – BNFC:**
  - **infantile spasms**
    - oral
      - **children 1 month–2 years:** initially 0.125 mg/kg/dose twice daily; adjust according to response over 2–3 weeks to 0.25 mg/kg/dose twice daily; max. 0.5 mg/kg/dose (not exceeding 5 mg) twice daily; alternatively, total daily dose may be given as 3 separate doses
- **Uptodate.com:**
  - **myoclonic seizures:**
    - oral
      - **children ≤ 30 kg:** usual dosage is 0.3–1 mg/kg/d as 3 separate doses;
      - **note:** Therapy should be initiated below the usual dosage range and titrated carefully based on response. If inadequate response to usual dosage, gradually increase dose further. Manufacturer's labeling does not specify a maximum dosage.

O

Orphenadrine

Dosage:

▶ 3–6 mg/kg/d (max. 100 mg) as 3 separate doses p.o. (off-label)

Neuropaediatric indications:

- dystonia

Mechanism of action:

- diphenylmethane derivative
- interneuron blocker; cellular mechanism of action is unknown
- high affinity to glycinergic and GABAergic interneurons of the CNS
- anxiolytic effect goes together with the decreased release of serotonin in the brain
- mild anticholinergic effects

Relevant contraindications:

- porphyria
- myasthenia gravis
- urinary retention, angle-closure glaucoma, intestinal obstructions, megacolon
- acute pulmonary oedema, tachyarrhythmia

Relevant side effects and interactions:

- urinary retention, constipation, anhidrosis, hyperpyrexia, dry mouth
- tachycardia
- blurred vision, confusion, agitation, hallucination
- increases the anti-parkinson effect of L-dopa

Approval status:

- no explicit approval for children

Sources:

- **Germany – SPC:**
- **muscle relaxant**
  - **children < 16 years:** use is not recommended.
- **USA – T:** –
- **United Kingdom – BNFC:** –
- **Uptodate.com:** no published paediatric dosage muscle spasms
  - **adults:** oral: 200 mg/d as 2 separate doses
  - **adults:** IM, IV: 60 mg every 12 hours

Oxcarbazepine (OXC)

Dosage:

- ▶ mainly: maintenance dose 20–45 mg/kg/d as 2 separate doses p.o.; increase weekly by 5–10 mg/kg/d (SPC/off-label)
- ▶ vestibular paroxysm: 4–8 mg/kg/d as 2 separate doses

Neuropaediatric indications:

- focal epilepsy
- alternative therapy of Rolandic epilepsy
- some paroxysmal movement disorders (e.g. vestibular paroxysm)
- neurogenic pain
- mood stabilizer (incl. bipolar disorder)
- in case of good response to Carbamazepine, but limitations of therapy with Carbamazepine due to its side effects

Mechanism of action:

- reduces the increasing response after repeated stimulus of the afferences, probably by blocking axonal sodium channels

Relevant contraindications:

- pregnancy
- possible deterioration of the signs and symptoms of primary generalized epilepsy (primarily JME), tonic, atonic and absence epilepsy
- careful use in patients who developed skin rashes when previously treated with Carbamazepine (for approximately 25 % additionally rash)
- careful use in hyponatremia, heart failure, conduction disturbances

Relevant side effects and interactions:

- drowsiness, vertigo, weakness, headache
- nausea, vomiting, constipation, diarrhea, stomach pain
- apathy, ataxia, attention disorders, emotional instability
- diplopia
- temporary mild, but clinically not important elevation of liver enzymes
- do not use OXC together with MAOIs
- reduced efficacy of oral contraceptives
- elevated risk of neurotoxicity when combined with Lithium
- decreased AUC of Felodipine when OXC is combined with Felodipine
- increases Phenytoin plasma level
- Carbamazepine, Phenytoin, and Phenobarbital decrease OXC plasma levels

Approval status:

- monotherapy or adjunctive therapy: patients > 6 years with focal and secondary generalized seizures

Sources:

- **Germany – SPC:**
  - **focal seizures with or without secondary generalized tonic-clonic seizures**
    - oral
      - **children ≥ 6 years**, mono- and adjunctive therapy: initially 8–10 mg/kg/d as 2 separate doses
      - maintenance (adjunctive therapy): approximately 30 mg/kg/d; if necessary increase by max. 10 mg/kg/d in weekly intervals, up to max. 46 mg/kg/d
      - **children < 6 years:** not recommended
- **USA – T:**
  - treatment of partial seizures in patients with epilepsy
    - oral
    - adjunctive therapy
      - **neonates and children < 2 years:** not approved for use
      - **children 2–< 4 years:** initially 8–10 mg/kg/d as 2 separate doses, max.: 600 mg/d; < 20 kg: initially: 16–20 mg/kg/d as 2 separate doses, increase dose slowly over 2–4 weeks; do not exceed 60 mg/kg/d as 2 separate doses
      - **children 4–16 years:** initially 8–10 mg/kg/d as 2 separate doses, max. 600 mg/d, increase dose slowly over 2–4 weeks to the following weight-dependent target dose for maintenance: 900 mg/d (20–29 kg), 1200 mg/d (29,1–39 kg), 1800 mg/d (> 39 kg) as 2 separate doses

- conversion to monotherapy
  - **children 4–16 years:** initially 8–10 mg/kg/d given as 2 separate doses, with a simultaneous dose reduction of any concomitant antiepileptic drugs; withdraw concomitant undivided doses completely over 3–6 weeks, while increasing the Oxcarbazepine dose as needed by no more than 10 mg/kg/d at approximately weekly intervals; increase the Oxcarbazepine dose to the monotherapy maintenance dose recommended for the applicable weight of the patient as listed below:
- initiation of monotherapy
  - **children 4–16 years:** initially 8–10 mg/kg/d as 2 separate doses; increase dose every third day by 5 mg/kg/d to achieve the recommended monotherapy maintenance dose appropriate for the patient's weight, as follows: **20 kg:** 600–900 mg/d as 2 separate doses; **25–30 kg:** 900–1200 mg/d as 2 separate doses; **35–40 kg:** 900–1500 mg/d as 2 separate doses; **45 kg:** 1200–1500 mg/d as 2 separate doses; **50–55 kg:** 1200–1800 mg/d as 2 separate doses; **60–65 kg:** 1200–2100 mg/d as 2 separate doses; **70 kg:** 1500–2100 mg/d as 2 separate doses
- **United Kingdom – BNFC:**
  - **monotherapy and adjunctive therapy of focal seizures with or without secondary generalized tonic-clonic seizures**
    - oral
      - **children 6–18 years:** initially 4–5 mg/kg/dose (max. 300 mg) twice daily; increase according to response in steps of up to 5 mg/kg twice daily at weekly intervals (usual maintenance dose for adjunctive therapy is 15 mg/kg/dose twice daily); max. 23 mg/kg/dose twice daily

Comments:

- closely related to Carbamazepine, but with fewer side effects (e. g. no interaction with macrolides)
- no washout period required before switching from Carbamazepine to Oxcarbazepine (usually beginning with a dose that corresponds to about 150 % of the previous Carbamazepine dose)

Oxybutynin

Dosage:

▶ 0.3 mg/kg/d as 2–3 separate doses (max. 15 mg/d) (off-label)

Neuropaediatric indications:

- urinary incontinence in children

Mechanism of action:

- tertiary amine with anticholinergic effect and, additionally, direct relaxation of the smooth muscles
- reduces detrusor muscle contraction
- competitive antagonist at muscarinic acetylcholine receptors (M_1, M_2 and M_3) and Calcium antagonist with direct spasmolytic effect on smooth muscle cells

Relevant contraindications:

- angle-closure glaucoma
- voiding dysfunction with residual urine
- mechanic stenosis in the gastrointestinal tract, megacolon
- tachyarrhythmia
- acute pulmonary oedema
- careful during the third trimester of pregnancy

Relevant side effects and interactions:

- reduction of the sweat-glands-secretion
- flush
- CNS disorders
- accommodation impairment, may provoke glaucoma
- dry mouth
- tachycardia
- micturition disorder
- enhanced anticholinergic effect when combined with Amantadine, Chinidin, tri- and tetracyclic antidepressants, neuroleptics
- mutually reduced effect on gastrointestinal motility with concurrent administration of dopamine antagonists

Approval status:

- depends on the specific product (see SPC)

Sources:

- **Germany – SPC:**
  - **urinary incontinence**
    - oral (as Oxybutynine hydrochloride)
      - **children > 5 years:** initially 5 mg/d as 2 separate doses. Titrate to lowest effective dose.

Age	Body weight	Daily dose
5–9 years	20–30 kg	7.5 mg as 3 separate doses
9–12 years	30–38 kg	10 mg as 2 separate doses
≥ 12 years	> 38 kg	15 mg as 3 separate doses

- Max. 0.3–0.4 mg/kg/d (max. 15 mg). Use is not recommended in children < 5 years
- **USA – T:**
  - **urinary incontinence**
    - oral
      - immediate release formulation:
        - **children 1–5 years:** 0.2 mg/kg/dose 2–3 times daily
        - **children > 5 years:** 10 mg/d as 2 separate doses up to 15 mg/d as 3 separate doses

- extended release formulation:
  - **children ≥ 6 years:** 5 mg/d as a SD, increase as tolerated in 5-mg increments to max. 20 mg/d
- United Kingdom – BNFC:
  - **urinary frequency, urgency and incontinence, neurogenic bladder instability**
    - oral
      - **children 2–5 years:** 1.25–2.5 mg/dose 2–3 times daily
      - **children 5–12 years:** 2.5–3 mg/dose twice daily, increase to 5 mg 2–3 times daily
      - **children 12–18 years:** 5 mg/dose 2–3 times daily, increase if necessary to max. 20 mg/d as 4 separate doses
    - intravesicular instillation
      - **children 5–18 years:** 5 mg/dose 2–3 times daily
  - **nocturnal enuresis associated with overactive bladder**
    - oral
      - **children 5–18 years:** 2.5–3 mg/dose twice daily, increased to 5 mg/dose 2–3 times daily (last dose before bedtime)
  - **neurogenic bladder instability (Lyrinel® XL)**
    - oral
      - **children 6–18 years:** initially 5 mg/d as a SD adjusted according to response in steps of 5 mg at weekly intervals; max. 15 mg/d as a SD

Pamidronate

Dosage:
- ▶ calcinosis: 1 mg/kg/d IV
- ▶ ostealgia: 1 mg/kg every 4 weeks IV infusion

Neuropaediatric indications:
- development of calcinosis as a complication of dermatomyositis
- ostealgia in osteolysis; osteoporosis

Mechanism of action:
- bisphosphonates are stored in the bone matrix and continuously released at sites of bone resorption, which results in inhibition of the osteoclasts and thus reduced bone resorption

Relevant contraindications:
- severe renal insufficiency
- severe hypocalcemia

Relevant side effects and interactions:
- during infusion: fever, flu-like symptoms
- complex formation with Calcium: hypocalcemia, disturbed mineralization up to osteomalacia, renal insufficiency, acute renal failure
- ulceration of the esophagus, esophagitis
- osteonecrosis of the jaw

Approval status:
- treatment of tumor induced hypercalcemia, reduction of the skeletal morbidity rate in patients suffering from osteolytic bone metastases in chemotherapy or hormone therapy of mamma carcinoma
- for the reduction of the skeletal morbidity rate (e.g. Paget's disease), in conjunction with chemotherapy in patients with multiple myeloma (stage III) with osteolytic lesions

Sources:

Germany – SPC:
- **diseases associated with increased activity of osteoclasts**
  - IV
    - **children and adolescents:** there is no clinical experience with this age group

USA – T:
- **hypercalcemia**
  - IV
    - **children (limited experience):** 0.5–1 mg/kg, max. 90 mg/dose
    - note: due to increased risk of nephrotoxicity, single doses should not exceed 90 mg
- United Kingdom – BNFC: –

Comments:

therapy option in febrous dysplasia

Paracetamol (or Acetaminophen)

Dosage:

▶ acute therapy of tension-type headache: 10–15 mg/kg/dose; temporomandibular arthrosis (or temporomandibular joint dysfunction), TMD: children < 2 years of age, max. 60 mg/kg/d; > 2 years, max. 90 mg/kg/d
▶ acute therapy of migraine: 10–15 mg/kg/dose p.o./supp.
▶ fever in febrile convulsion, suppository: < 1 year of age, 125 mg; 1–5 years, 250 mg; > 6 years, 500 mg; p.o.: 10–15 mg/kg/dose, max. every 4 h
▶ intestinal sings and symptoms in Henoch Schonlein purpura: doses of 10–15 mg/kg
▶ headache in radiotherapy: 2000–4000 mg/d as 4 separate doses

Neuropaediatric indications:

– mild to moderate pain (tension-type headache, migraine, headache in radiotherapy)
– fever in febrile convulsion
– intestinal symptomatic in Henoch Schonlein purpura

Mechanism of action:

– has not been completely understood
– very mild anti-inflammatory effect, not anticoagulant
– main effect: inhibition of cyclooxygenase II (COX II) and thus, reduced synthesis of prostaglandins. In contrast to the majority of the COX inhibitors, Paracetamol does not block the active center, but prevents the oxidation of COX, with the result that COX remains in the not-activated form
– additionally modulates the endocannabinoid system, while the metabolite AM404 inhibits the uptake of endogenous cannabinoids into the neurons and sodium channels

Relevant contraindications:

– severe hepatic insufficiency (Child-Pugh score ≥ 9)
– tachyarrhythmia
– hepatic cirrhosis
– hyperthyroidism
– anxiety syndrome
– severe renal insufficiency (creatinine clearance < 10 ml/min, adhere to a dosing interval of at least 8 h)
– Gilbert's syndrome

Relevant side effects and interactions:

– rare undesirable effects
– > 200 mg: muscle tremor, headache, irritability
– insomnia, anxiety
– gastrointestinal disorders
– tachycardia
– increase of liver transaminases (in overdosing: hepatotoxic)
– hemolytic anemia in glucose-6-phosphate dehydrogenase deficiency
– sudden stop after long-term use of high dosages: headache, fatigue, muscle pain, nervousness, vegetative symptoms

Approval status:

– depends on the specific product (see SPC)

Sources:

– **Germany – SPC:**
  – **mild to moderate pain, fever**
    – oral

Bodyweight, age	single dose	max. daily dose (24 h)
3 kg, 0–3 months	40 mg	160 mg
4 kg, 0–3 months	60 mg	240 mg
5 kg, 0–3 months	60 mg	300 mg
6 kg 3–6 months	80 mg	320 mg
7 kg, 6–9 months	100 mg	400 mg
8–9 kg 6–12 months	120 mg	480 mg
10 kg, 1–2 years	140 mg	560 mg
11–12 kg, 1–2 years	160 mg	640 mg
13–15 kg, 2–3 years	200 mg	800 mg
16–18 kg, 3–5 years	240 mg	960 mg
19–21 kg, 5–6 years	300 mg	1200 mg
22–25 kg, 6–8 years	320 mg	1280 mg
26–29 kg, 8–11 years	400 mg	1600 mg
30–32 kg, 8–11 years	440 mg	1760 mg
33–43 kg, 11–12 years	500 mg	2000 mg

- **infants < 3 months, 3–6 kg:** preparation Ben-u-ron® 75 mg suppositories (status: 10/2009)
  - mild to moderate pain and fever
    - rectal

Age	Body weight	Initial dose	Maintenance dose	Daily dose (24 h)
< 3 months	3–4 kg	75 mg	75 mg every 8–12 h	150 mg
	4–5 kg	75 mg	75 mg every 6–8 h	225 mg
> 3 months	4 kg	75 mg	75 mg every 6–8 h	225 mg
	5–6 kg	75 mg	75 mg every 6 h	300 mg

- **USA – T:**
  - mild to moderate pain, fever
    - oral, rectal
      - **neonates:** 10–15 mg/kg every 6–8 h
      - **children ≥ 12 years:** 325–650 mg/dose every 4–6 h or 1000 mg/dose 3–4 times daily, max. 4 g/d
    - oral
    - International Evidence-Based Group for Neonatal Pain Recommendations
      - **gestational age 28–32 weeks:** 10–12 mg/kg/dose every 6–8 h, max. 40 mg/kg/d
      - **gestational age 32–36 weeks or term-neonates < 10 d:** 40–60 mg/kg/d as 4 separate doses, max. 60 mg/kg/d
      - **term-neonates ≥ 10 d:** 10–15 mg/dose every 4–6 h, max. 90 mg/kg/d
      - **infants, children:** 10–15 mg/dose 4–6 h as needed; do not exceed 5 doses in 24 h
      - international Evidence-Based Group for neonatal Pain recommendation
    - rectal
      - **gestational age 28–32 weeks:** 40 mg/kg/d as 2 separate doses, max. 40 mg/kg/d
      - **gestational age 32–36 weeks or term-neonates < 10 d:** loading dose of 30 mg/kg, then 45 mg/kg/d as 3 separate doses, max. 60 mg/kg/d
      - **term-neonates ≥ 10 d:** loading dose of 30 mg/kg, then 20 mg/kg/dose every 6–8 h, max. 90 mg/kg/d
      - **infants, children:** 10–20 mg/dose every 4–6 h as needed; do not exceed 5 doses in 24 h
- **United Kingdom – BNFC:**
  - pain, pyrexia with discomfort
    - oral
      - **neonates 28–32 weeks postmenstrual age:** 20 mg/kg as a SD, then 10–15 mg/kg/dose every 8–12 h as necessary; max. 30 mg/kg/d as separate doses
      - **neonates > 32 weeks postmenstrual age:** 20 mg/kg as a SD, then 10–15 mg/kg every 6–8 h as necessary; max. 60 mg/kg/d as separate doses
      - **children 1–3 months:** 30–60 mg/dose every 8 h as necessary
      - **children 3–12 months:** 60–120 mg/dose every 4–6 h (max. 4 doses in 24 h)
      - **children 1–6 years:** 120–250 mg/dose every 4–6 h (max. 4 doses in 24 h)
      - **children 6–12 years:** 250–500 mg/dose every 4–6 h (max. 4 doses in 24 h)
      - **children 12–18 years:** 500 mg/dose every 4–6 h
    - rectal
      - **neonates 28–32 weeks postmenstrual age:** 20 mg/kg as a SD, then 15 mg/kg/dose every 12 h as necessary; max. 30 mg/kg/d as separate doses
      - **neonates > 32 weeks postmenstrual age:** 30 mg/kg as a SD, then 20 mg/kg/dose every 8 h as necessary; max. 60 mg/kg/d as separate doses
      - **children 1–3 months:** 30–60 mg/dose every 8 h as necessary
      - **children 3–12 months:** 60–125 mg/dose every 4–6 h as necessary (max. 4 doses in 24 h)
      - **children 1–5 years:** 125–250 mg/dose every 4–6 h as necessary (max. 4 doses in 24 h)
      - **children 5–12 years:** 250–500 mg/dose every 4–6 h as necessary (max. 4 doses in 24 h)
      - **children 12–18 years:** 500 mg/dose every 4–6 h
  - IV infusion over 15 min
    - **preterm neonates over 32 weeks postmenstrual age:** 7.5 mg/kg/dose every 8 h; max. 25 mg/kg/d
    - **neonates:** 10 mg/kg/dose every 4–6 h, max. 30 mg/kg/d
    - **children < 50 kg:** 15 mg/kg/dose every 4–6 h; max. 60 mg/kg/d
    - **children > 50 kg:** 1000 mg/dose every 4–6 h; max. 4 g/d
  - **BfArM** (last update: 05/2008): max. 60 mg/kg/d

Comments:

- onset of action: oral, 30–60 min; rectal, 3–4 h
- duration of action: 4(–6) h, note: therapeutic range, consider max. allowable daily dose
- (one of the safest analgesics during pregnancy)

Peppermint oil

(here: topical administration)

Dosage:

▶ apply evenly to forehead and temples (and muscles of the neck)
▶ repeat as necessary several times in 15-minute intervals

Neuropaediatric indications:

- acute therapy of migraine
- acute therapy of tension-type headache
- acute therapy of muscle tensions in primary headache

Mechanism of action:

- stimulates the blood flow: menthol binds to cold-sensitive receptors thus triggering a cooling sensation

Relevant contraindications:

- infants and little children, because asthma-like symptoms may develop during inhaling the aerosols

- skin diseases and exanthematous lesions that typically accompany childhood infections
- open wounds, injured skin
- administration near eyes

Relevant side effects and interactions:

- contact allergy (rare)
- hypersensitivity in sensitive persons (burning and flush)

Approval status:

- not available

Sources:

- **Germany – SPC:**
  - **mild to moderate headache**
    - topical
      - **children ≥ 6 years:** Apply evenly on temples and forehead with the applicator. If necessary repeat several times in intervals of 15 min. If no effect is seen after 2 h, discontinue treatment.
- **USA – T:** –
- **United Kingdom – BNFC:** –
- **Uptodate.com:** –

Petasites extract

(Butterbur)

Dosage:

▶ 6–12 years: 50 mg/d as 2 separate doses; ≥ 12 years: 100 mg as 2 separate doses (SPC)

Neuropaediatric indications:

- migraine prophylaxis

Mechanism of action:

- unknown

Relevant contraindications:

- pregnancy

Relevant side effects and interactions:

- rare: mild stomach trouble
- very rare: dose-independent hepatic failure

Approval status:

- spasmolytic analgesic from 6 years of age

Sources:

- **Germany – SPC:** –
- **USA – T:** –
- **United Kingdom – BNFC:** –

Comments:

in Germany no longer available (see side effects)

Pethidine (or Meperidine)

Dosage:

▶ 0.5–1 mg/kg/dose IV (off-label)

Neuropaediatric indications:

- analgesia (e.g. lumbar puncture, interventions with Botulinum toxin)

Mechanism of action:

- completely synthetic opioid; active metabolite: Norpethidine
- agonist at μ-receptors
- only for acute therapy, it is not recommended for long-term treatment, because Norpethidine can accumulate
- it is not spasmogenic to smooth muscles (therefore, treatment of colics and pancreatitis is possible)

Relevant contraindications:

- addiction to opioids
- unconsciousness
- disorders of respiratory function
- raised intracranial pressure
- hypotension at hypovolemia
- biliary tract diseases
- obstructive or inflammatory bowel disease
- pheochromocytoma
- elevated risk of seizures
- pancreatitis
- myxoedema
- concurrent administration of MAOIs

Relevant side effects and interactions:
- sweating
- pruritus, exanthema
- rigidity
- sedation, vertigo, headache
- respiratory depression, bronchial spasms
- orthostatic circulation disorder, hypotensive reaction of the circulation, bradycardia
- cerebral seizures (particularly with high dosages used in children)
- euphoria, sometimes dysphoria, changes of cognitive and sensoric motivation, changes in allerteness (mostly dulling)
- addiction, development of tolerance, withdrawal syndrome
- miosis, dry mouth
- nausea, vomiting, constipation, increased urinary bladder tone, voiding dysfunction
- enhanced effect and increased side effects (primarily respiratory depression) if combined with centrally depressant drugs and alcohol
- reduced effect caused by opioids with agonistic/antagonistic characteristics
- enhanced effect if combined with Pancuronium and Vecuronium
- increased side effects if combined with MAOIs

Approval status:
- analgesics are contraindicated for children < 1 year of age and there are limitations of administration in children < 16 years of age

Sources:
- **Germany – SPC:**
  - **severe pain**
    - oral (as Pethidine hydrochloride)
      - **children:** SD: 0.6–1.2 mg/kg; do not use in children < 1 year of age
- **USA – T:**
  - **moderate to severe pain**
    - oral, IM, IV, SC
      - **children:** 1–1.5 mg/kg/dose every 3–4 h as needed; 1–2 mg/kg as a SD preoperatively, max. 100 mg/dose
    - continuous IV infusion
      - **children:** loading dose of 0.5–1 mg/kg, followed by 0.3 mg/kg/h; titrate dose to effect, may require 0.5–0.7 mg/kg/h
      - **note:** when changing route of administration, oral doses are about half as effective as parenteral doses
- **United Kingdom – BNFC:**
  - **obstetric analgesia**
    - IM or SC injection
      - **children 12–18 years:** 1 mg/kg (max. 100 mg); repeat 1–3 h later if necessary; max. 400 mg in 24 h

Comments:
- duration of effect: 2–4 h
- IV administration, max. effect after 3–10 min, IM administration after 20–40 min; oral or rectal also possible
- 0.1–0.2 times the potency of Morphine

Phenobarbital (PhB)

Dosage:
- mainly: maintenance dose of 3–4 mg/kg/d as 2 separate doses (SPC)
- loading dose: 10(–20) mg/kg/dose
- rescue-strategy: up to > 100 mg/kg/d (intensive care)
- therapeutic serum level: 10–40 mg/l
- status epilepticus:
  - after 20–60 min: 15–20 mg/kg over 8–10 min (= 2 mg/kg/min); max. 100 mg/min
- juvenile myoclonic epilepsy: 1 mg/kg/d
- seizures in neonates, maintenance dose: 3–5 mg/kg/d as 2 separate doses (2 weeks after last seizure or when clinically significant seizure-free, but continue up to 3 months if there is a conspicuuous EEG and a neurologic medical finding)
- seizures in neonate encephalopathy: 20 mg/kg slow IV injection and diluted at least to 20 mg/ml
- preanesthesia: 20–30 mg/kg IM or IV over 30 min
- hyperekplexia/primary Startle-syndrome/congenital Stiff person syndrome: 5–10 mg/kg/d according to severity
- secondary Startle-syndrome in drug withdrawal: start with 10–20 mg/kg/d; maintenance dose, 5 mg/kg/d

Neuropaediatric indications:
- seizures in neonates
- seizures in neonatal encephalopathy
- epilepsy
  - status epilepticus (injection)
  - (juvenile myoclonic epilepsy)
- hyperekplexia/primary Startle syndrome/congenital Stiff person syndrome
- secondary Startle syndrome in drug withdrawal:

Mechanism of action:
- binding to $GABA_A$ receptor and thus enhanced inhibitory effect of GABA

block of AMPA receptors and thus decreased excitatory effect of the neurotransmitter glutamate

Relevant contraindications:

- absolute:
  - acute alcohol, sleeping drugs or analgesics intoxication
  - Intoxication caused by excitatory or depressant psychotropic drugs
- relative:
- acute hepatic porphyria
  - severe renal or liver function disorders
  - severe heart failure
  - airway diseases
  - medical history of addiction
  - medical history of affective disorders (also in direct relatives)
  - unconsciousness

Relevant side effects and interactions:

- vertigo
- circulatory disorder up to syncope
- respiratory depression
- skin reactions
- long-term use: megaloblastic anemia
- decreased effect caused by folic acid
- mutually enhanced effect when combined with centrally depressant drugs (psychotropic drugs, hypnotic drugs) and alcohol
- decreased effect of: oral contraceptives, oral anticoagulants, digitoxin, Doxycycline, chloramphenicol, cytostatics, griseofulvin, glucocorticoids
- enhancement of the Methotrexate toxicity
- Valproic acid and MAOIs enhance the effect of Primidone

Approval status:

- generalized tonic-clonic (or grand mal), myoclonic epilepsy (impulsive petit mal), grand mal protection in petit mal seizures in children, status epilepticus (injection)
- no limitation in age

Sources:

- **Germany – SPC:**
  - **epilepsy, status epilepticus**
    - slow IV, IM
      - **children:** usually 3–4 mg/kg; children ≥ 15 kg, 150 mg; young children, 60 mg; infants, 20–60 mg
      - 2–3 times daily

- **USA – T:**
- **anticonvulsant**
  - **status epilepticus**
  - IV
    - **neonates**, loading dose: 15–20 mg/kg as a SD; further doses of 5–10 mg/kg may be given every 15–20 min as needed (max. total dose: 40 mg/kg).
    - **infants and children**, loading dose: 15–20 mg/kg (max. 1000 mg/dose); further doses may be given after 15 min as needed (max. total dose: 40 mg/kg)
    - **note:** additional respiratory support may be required, especially when maximizing loading dose.
  - maintenance dose (12 h after loading dose): oral, IV
    - **neonates:** 3–4 mg/kg/d as a SD; assess serum concentration, increase to 5 mg/kg/d if needed (usually by second week of therapy)
    - **infants:** 5–6 mg/kg/d as 1–2 separate doses
    - **children 1–5 years:** 6–8 mg/kg/d as 1–2 separate doses
    - **children 5–12 years:** 4–6 mg/kg/d as 1–2 separate doses
    - **children > 12 years:** 1–3 mg/kg/d as 1–2 separate doses
  - **premedication**
    - oral, IV, IM
    - **children:** 1–3 mg/kg 1–1.5 h before procedure
- **United Kingdom – BNFC:**
  - **all forms of epilepsy except typical absence seizures**
    - oral, IV injection
      - **neonates:** initially 20 mg/kg by slow IV injection, then 2.5–5 mg/kg/d as a SD either by slow IV injection or orally; adjust dose and frequency according to response
    - oral
      - **children 1 month–12 years:** initially 2–3 mg/kg as 2 separate doses; increase by 2 mg/kg/d as required; usual maintenance with 2.5–4 mg/kg/dose once ore twice daily
      - **children 12–18 years:** 60–180 mg/d given as a SD
  - **status epilepticus (Phenobarbital sodium)**
    - slow IV injection (not faster than 1 mg/kg/min)
      - **neonates:** initially 20 mg/kg, then 2.5–5 mg/kg/dose once or twice daily
      - **children 1 month–12 years:** initially 20 mg/kg, then 2.5–5 mg/kg/dose once or twice daily
      - **children 12–18 years:** initially 20 mg/kg (max. 1 g), then 600 mg/d as 2 separate doses

Comments:

- note: West syndrome and absences: not effective
- subtherapeutic blood level: < 10 mcg/ml
- half-life: 60–130 h
- advantage:
  - long-term experience, is not cytotoxic even when used in high doses
  - fast IV-application feasible, onset of action in 5–10 minutes
  - in one study with 36 children: more effective than Phenytoin + Diazepam

- disadvantage:
  - decrease in blood pressure (in status-management)
  - respiratory depression (only for high dosages)
  - high potential of interaction with other drugs

Phenprocoumon

Dosage:
- individual dosing, according to INR
- chronic atrial fibrillation: target INR = 2.0–3.0, if there are no reasons against (risk of falling, compliance etc.), therapy can be started after 3–5 d, if the infarct is small
- mechanical heart valves: INR: 2.5–3.5, biological heart valves: INR: 2.0–3.0
- dissection of arteries supplying the brain without SAH: secondary prophylaxis INR 2.0–3.0 for at least 3 months
- Patients of African ethnicity need higher dosages than patients of Asian ethnicity to achieve the same effect (the concept of racial definition is a tricky one).

Neuropaediatric indications:
- prophylaxis and therapy of thromboembolic disorders
- chronic atrial fibrillation
- mechanical heart valves

Mechanism of action:
- coumarin; Vitamin K antagonist
- inhibits synthesis of functional Vitamin K-dependent clotting factors (factors II, VII, IX, and X) by limiting γ-carboxylation of N-terminal glutamic acid residues in these proteins. As a result, these clotting factors are unable to bind via Calcium ions to phospholipid layers of the vascular endothelium and thus remain functionally inactive.

Relevant contraindications:
- cerebrovascular bleeding in the recent past
- dissection of the aorta
- diseases with increased risk of bleeding (e.g. hemorrhagic diathesis, injured parenchyma of the liver, manifest renal insufficiency, severe thrombocytopenia)
- hypertension (> 200/105 mmHg)
- any diseases, where of blood vessel lesions may be suspected
- large open wounds (also wounds after recent surgery)
- cavernous pulmonary tuberculosis
- intramuscular injection (risk of massive muscle bleeding)
- lumbar puncture, bone marrow biopsy, scheduled anesthesia and any other diagnostic or therapeutic procedures with a chance of uncontrolled bleeding
- angiography

Relevant side effects and interactions:
- higher risk of haematoma, increased gum bleeding, gastrointestinal bleedings, retinal haemorrhage, epistaxis
- nausea, loss of appetite, vomiting, diarrhea
- hepatitis with or without jaundice
- macro-hematuria
- cerebral bleeding
- urticaria, exanthema, pruritus, dermatitis, reversible alopecia capitis totalis, dermal necrosis, purpura
- long-term treatment: osteopenia
- burning pain with concurrent discolouration of the big toes ("purple toes")
- teratogenic if permanently taken
- enhanced effect of other anticoagulants with increased risk of bleeding
- strong binding to plasma proteins: any drug with high-affinity plasma protein binding can displace coumarins from their binding sites, resulting in increased coumarin plasma levels and bioavailability. Conversely, coumarins may displace drugs bound with lower affinity.
- breakdown by the cytochrome P-450 system mutually influences all inhibitors and inductors of the CYP450 enzymes involved

Approval status:
- depends on the specific product (see SPC)

Sources:
- **Germany – SPC:**
  - **prophylaxis of thrombosis and embolism**
  - oral
  - **children < 14 years:** no data is available for the use in this age group
- **USA – T:** –
- **United Kingdom – BNFC:** –
- **Uptodate.com: no published paediatric dosage**

Comments:
- plasma half-life is 160 h and thus, approximately 14 times higher than Warfarin half-life
- closely monitor prothrombin time and INR
- children: coumarins are only indicated for long-term and lifelong treatment, otherwise LMWH are preferred (better management/compliance, less complications)
- normalization of coagulation:

- After discontinuation it takes 10–14 d until the necessary level of fully functional coagulation factors is restored in the patient.
- This lag phase can be reduced to 6–10 h by administering high-dosed Vitamin K.
- In case of emergency, the coagulation factor deficiency can be reversed by temporary administration of a coagulation factor concentrate (PPSB).

Phenytoin (DPH)

Dosage:

▶ epilepsy:
- maintenance dose: 5–7 mg/kg/d as 2–4 separate doses p.o. (SPC)
- children up to 12 years IV: d 1: max. 30 mg/kg/d, d 2: max. 20 mg/kg/d, d 3: max. 10 mg/kg/d (max. injection rate: 1 mg/kg/min) (SPC), then continue with 5–7 mg/kg/d depending on serum level
- target serum level: 10–20(–25) mcg/ml

▶ status epilepticus:
- after 20–60 min: 15–20 mg/kg (max. 1.5 g) over 15–20 min (= 1 mg/kg/min); max. 50 mg/min
- anticonvulsive prophylaxis after traumatic brain injury: 5 mg/kg/d

▶ myotonic dystrophy: 4 mg/kg/d as 2 separate doses

Neuropaediatric indications:

- focal simple or complex epilepsy
- generalized tonic-clonic seizures
- status epilepticus
- neurogenic pain
- prophylaxis of posttraumatic early seizures (head injury)
- myotonic dystrophy

Mechanism of action:

- blocks high frequency repetitive firing of action potentials. This is probably caused by inhibiting axonal sodium channels.

Relevant contraindications:

- hypersensitivity to hydantoin
- AV block II. and III. degree
- sick sinus syndrome
- not before 3 months after myocardial infarction

- heart failure (left ventricular ejection fraction < 35 %), except for the indication of severe cardiac glycoside-conditioned ventricular and supraventricular cardiac arrhythmias
- preexisting impairement of blood cells and bone marrow
- careful use in manifest heart failure, pulmonary insufficiency, severe hypotension (systolic blood pressure < 90 mmHg), bradycardia (< 50/min), sinuatrial block, AV block I. degree, atrial fibrillation, atrial flutter
- pregnancy
- porphyria

Relevant side effects and interactions:

- perceptual disorder, confusion, memory disorder, cognitive performance disorder
- vertigo, headache, fatigue
- ataxia, nystagmus, tremor
- dyskinesia in children with history of neurologic impairment
- gingival hyperplasia (can be minimized by good oral hygiene), hypertrichosis (both are completely reversible)
- rash, osteomalacia
- cardiac arrhythmias if administered IV
- reduced Phenytoin serum levels after oral administration with concurrent administration of antacids
- reduced effect with concurrent administration of folic acid
- reduced Phenytoin serum levels with concurrent administration of Phenobarbital, Primidone, Carbamazepine, Vigabatrin and alcohol
- increased Phenytoin serum levels with concurrent administration of oral anticoagulants, benzodiazepines, Cimetidine, Chloramphenicol, Cycloserine, Disulfiram, Halothane, Isoniazid, Methylphenidate, NSAR, PAS, Sulfonamides, Sulthiame, tricyclic psychotropic drugs, Valproic acid
- increased rifampicin serum levels
- reduction of the active ingredient concentration of oral anticoagulants, Verapamil, Doxycycline, Itraconazole, corticosteroids, oral contraceptives, tricyclic psychotropic drugs, Carbamazepine, Valproic acid
- enhanced Methotrexate toxicity
- dermal necrosis, necrotic extravasation, "Purple glove syndrome"

Approval status:

- mono or adjunctive therapy of focal, secondary generalized and primary generalized seizures and anticonvulsive prophylaxis (craniocerebral trauma; neurosurgery) for children and adults

Sources:
- Germany – SPC:
  - neurogenic pain
    - IV
      - **adolescents ≥ 12 years:** 250–500 mg/d IV; max. injection rate is 25 mg/min
      - **prophylaxis of seizures**
    - IV
      - **children ≤ 11 years:** 5–6 mg/kg; adjust injection rate according to age and body weight
      - **children ≥ 12 years:** 250–500 mg; max. injection rate is 25 mg/min
  - status epilepticus
    - IV
      - **children ≤ 11 years:** day 1, max. 30 mg/kg/d; day 2, 20 mg/kg/d; day 3, 10 mg/kg/d, max. injection rate: 1 mg/kg/min
      - **children ≥ 12 years:** initially 250 mg; max. injection rate is 25 mg/min
      - If seizures do not subside after 20–30 min, dose can be repeated. If cessation of seizures is achieved, a dose of 17 mg/kg (approximately 1500 mg) every 1.5–6 h can be administered.
- USA – T:
  - status epilepticus
    - IV
      - loading dose:
        - **neonates:** 15–20 mg/kg as a SD or separate doses
        - **infants, children:** 15–18 mg/kg as a SD or separate doses
      - maintenance dose (12 h after the loading dose):
        - **neonates:** initially 5 mg/kg/d as 2 separate doses; range, 5–8 mg/kg/d as 2 separate doses; some patients may require dosing every 8 h
        - **infants and children:** initially 5 mg/kg/d as 2–3 separate doses; range:
          - **½–3 years:** 8–10 mg/kg/d
          - **4–6 years:** 7.5–9 mg/kg/d
          - **7–9 years:** 7–8 mg/kg/d
          - **10–16 years:** 6–7 mg/kg/d
        - some patients may require dosing every 8 h
  - anticonvulsant
    - oral
      - **loading dose: infants and children:** 15–20 mg/kg, based on Phenytoin serum levels and recent dosing history; administer oral loading dose as 3 separate doses given every 2–4 h to decrease GI adverse effects and to ensure complete oral absorption.
      - maintenance dose: same as IV maintenance dose listed above. Divide daily dose into 3 doses/d when using suspension, chewable tablets, or non-extended release preparations.
- United Kingdom – BNFC:
  - all forms of epilepsy except absence seizures
    - oral, IV infusion over 20–30 min
      - **neonates:** initial loading dose by slow IV injection is 18 mg/kg, then orally 5–10 mg/kg/d as 2 separate doses, adjusted according to response and plasma Phenythoin concentration (usual max. 15 mg/kg/d as 2 separate doses)
    - oral
      - **children 1 month–12 years:** initially 3–5 mg/kg/d as 2 separate doses, then adjusted according to response and plasma Phenytoin concentration to 5–10 mg/kg/d as 2 separate doses (usual max. 15 mg/kg/d as 2 separate doses or 300 mg/d)
      - **children 12–18 years:** initially 150–300 mg/d as 2 separate doses, then adjusted according to response and plasma Phenytoin concentration to 300–400 mg/d as 2 separate doses (usual max. 600 mg/d as 2 separate doses)
  - status epilepticus, acute symptomatic seizures associated with trauma or neurosurgery
    - slow IV injection or infusion (with blood pressure and ECG monitoring)
      - **neonates:** initially 20 mg/kg as a loading dose, then 5–10 mg/kg/d as 2 separate doses
      - **children 1 month–12 years:** loading dose of 20 mg/kg, then 5–10 mg/kg/d as 2 separate doses
      - **children 12–18 years:** loading dose of 20 mg/kg, then up to 100 mg/dose 3–4 times daily

Comments:
- narrow therapeutic range, therefore, plasma levels have to be monitored regularly (therapeutic: 5–20(–25) mg/l)
- CAUTION: too high dosages may lead to irreversible cerebellar damages (Purkinje cells)
- inconsistent gastrointestinal absorption after oral administration in children up to school age, with the youngest patients showing the greatest variability
- teratogenic
- spectrum of efficacy and mechanism of action are similar to that of Carbamazepine. However, Phenytoin shows higher rates of long-term side effects and is slightly less effective in complex/partial seizures; IV applicable
- IV infusion is strongly alkaline. Therefore, it is important to select a large vein for infusion, administer slowly, and take special care to avoid any paravenous application.
- status epilepticus:
  - advantage:
  - long-term and broadly based experience
  - different mechanism of action than benzodiazepines (theoretically an advantage)
  - less respiratory depression/decrease of blood pressure
- disadvantage:
  - difficult IV-application (separate route, risk of necrosis)
  - onset of action only after 20 minutes (slow administration)
  - cardiac arrhythmias possible (consider contraindications!)
  - deterioration genetically conditioned/generalized status forms are possible (e.g. Dravet syndrome)
  - CAUTION: necrosis (see above)

Pimozide

Dosage:

▶ Tic disorder: 2–12 years, 1–4 mg/d as 2 separate doses (off-label)

Neuropaediatric indications:

– Tic disorder

Mechanism of action:

– neuroleptic drug
– strong inhibitor of D_2-,D_3-, α_1-, 5-HT 2A receptors
– moderate inhibitor of D_1-, D_4-, α_2-receptors and of the presynaptic dopamine reuptake
– in addition, moderate inhibition of Ach-, H_1- and 5-HT_{1A}-receptors

Relevant contraindications:

– acute intoxication with centrally depressant drugs or alcohol
– coma
– congenital QT syndrome or cardiac arrhythmias in anamnesis, bradycardia
– concurrent intake of medication that leads to hypokalemia or other electrolyte disorders
– concurrent intake of CYP3A4 or CYP2D6 inhibitors
– concurrent intake of SSRI
– careful use: severe liver function disorders, endogenous depression, diseases of the brain stem (e.g. Parkinson's disease), cardiovascular disorders, QT extension, medical history of seizures

Relevant side effects and interactions:

– extrapyramidal motoric symptoms (tremor, rigor, drooling, bradykinesia, akathisia, acute dystonia, tardive dyskinesia)
– neuroleptic malignant syndrome
– EEG changes, fatigue, insomnia, anxiety
– headache, drowsiness, vertigo, weakness
– dry mouth, sweating, sialorrhea, regulation disorders of the body temperature
– nausea, constipation, voiding disorder and impaired vision
– hyperprolactinemia (galactorrhea, gynecomastia, oligo- or amenorrhea, erectile dysfunction)
– very rare: hyponatremia (SIADH or psychogenic polydipsia), hypotension, QT extension, ventricular arrhythmias
– withdrawal symptoms for Pimozide: nausea, vomiting, temporal dyskinesia, insomnia

Approval status:

– approved for maintenance therapy of chronic schizophrenic psychosis in children and adults

Sources:

– **Germany – SPC:**
  – **chronic schizophrenic psychoses**
    – oral
      – **children:** initially 1–2 mg/d; increase by 1–2 mg in weekly intervals to the usual maintenance dose of 3 mg/d (range: 1–6 mg/d); max. 8 mg/d
– **USA – T:**
  – **suppression of severe motor and phonic tics in patients with Tourette syndrome**
    – oral
      – **children ≤ 12 years:** initially 0.05 mg/kg/d as a SD (max. 1 mg/dose) preferably at bedtime; gradually titrate dose every 1–2 weeks as tolerated; if necessary, increase dose every third day; maintenance dose of 2–4 mg/d as a SD, max. 10 mg/d or 0.2 mg/kg/d (whichever is less)
      – **children ≥ 12 years:** initially 1–2 mg/d as separate doses; gradually titrate dose every 1–2 weeks as tolerated; may increase dose every other day if needed; maintenance: 7–10 mg/d as separate doses; max. 10 mg/d or 0.2 mg/kg/d (whichever is less)
      – **note:** use lowest effective dose
– **United Kingdom – BNFC:**
  – **Tourette syndrome**
    – oral
      – **children 2–12 years:** 1–4 mg/d
      – **children 12–18 years:** 2–10 mg/d

Piracetam

Dosage:

▶ 30–40 mg/kg/d as 3 separate doses p.o. (off-label)

Neuropaediatric indications:

– severe distal myoclonic twitches in Angelman syndrome
– Lance-Adams syndrome (posthypoxic myoclonia)
– myoclonic seizures

Mechanism of action:

– cyclic derivative of GABA
– antidementive drug
– possibly increases blood flow in the brain
– precise mechanism of action is unknown

Relevant contraindications:
- hypersensitivity to other pyrrolidone derivatives
- cerebral bleeding
- terminal renal insufficiency
- Huntington's chorea
- careful use: psychomotor anxiety, renal insufficiency, hemostasis disorder, major clinical procedures, severe bleeding, pregnancy

Relevant side effects and interactions:
- allergic reactions
- nausea, abdominal pain, diarrhea, weight gain
- increased libido and sexuality
- hypertension, hypotension
- increased psychomotor activity, sleeping disorder, insomnia, nervousness, aggressive behaviour, somnolence, hallucination
- depressive mood, anxiety
- vertigo, asthenia
- headache, ataxia, disturbances of equilibrium
- increased risk of seizures
- additional side effects and interactions associated with IV administration: reduced blood pressure, pain at the injection site, thrombophlebitis, fever
- enhanced effect of CNS-stimulating drugs, neuroleptics, thyroid hormones given for hypothyroidism, and coumarin derivatives

Approval status:
- depends on the specific product (see SPC)

Sources:
- **Germany – SPC:**
  - **adjunctive therapy of myoclonic syndrome (cortical origin)**
  - oral
    - no published paediatric dosage
    - **adults:** initially 8–12 g/d as 2–3 separate doses, followed 7–14 days after the initial period by a longer period of gradual dose reduction. Treat until myoclonic seizures disappear. Primary treatment with other drugs can be continued as usual and gradually reduced after response.
- **USA – T:** –
- **United Kingdom – BNFC:** –
- **Uptodate.com:**
  - no published paediatric dosage
  - **Enhance cognition in the elderly, cortical myoclonus, sickle cell anemia**
    - oral
      - **adults:** 2400 mg/d as 3 separate doses; doses up to 24 g/d reported

Comments:
- variable published dosage recommendations for adults (no paediatric dosing mentioned)

Pleconaril

Dosage:
▶ 15 mg/kg/d as 3 separate doses (only in phase II studies; reports about infants)

Neuropaediatric indications:
- encephalitis caused by enteroviruses (reports about infants)

Mechanism of action:
- oral anti-capsid-binding drugs of the third generation
- competes with pocket factor (a fatty acid) for binding to the hydrophobic pocket of the VP1 protein within the capsid of rhino- and enteroviruses (picornaviruses)
- the binding of Pleconaril to the hydrophobic pocket results in conformational changes, which inhibits viral attachment to the host cell and/or uncoating of the viral genome, thus preventing viral replication

Relevant contraindications:
- insufficient experiences with Pleconaril

Relevant side effects and interactions:
- abdominal pain, nausea, diarrhea
- headache
- long-term administration: combination with antiasthmatic drugs, virostatic agents and oral contraceptives can lead to menstruation disorders and tachycardia
- reduced effect of oral contraceptives
- increased occurrence of side effects when combined with Theophylline
- probably: CYP3A4 induction
- decreased effect in smokers
- overall insufficient experiences with Pleconaril

Approval status:
- no approval

Sources:
- **Germany – SPC:** –
- **USA – T:** –
- **United Kingdom – BNFC:** –
- **Uptodate.com:** –

Comments:

– The replication of almost all entero- and rhinoviruses and 90 % of all clinically examined isolates could be inhibited by Pleconaril (0,01–1 μM) in vitro.

Prednisolone

Dosage:

▶ progressive GBS or secondary deterioration after 4–6 weeks (primarily SIDP or CIDP): 1 mg/kg/d
▶ West syndrome: 2–5 mg/kg/d as a SD; decision between conventional (gradual reduction) or pulsatile (no gradual reduction) therapy
▶ PACNS: 0.1–0.2 mg/kg/d (max. 5 mg/d)
▶ Henoch Schonlein purpura: 0.1–0.2 mg/kg/d (max. 5 mg/d); intestinal symptoms, 1–2 mg/kg/d as separate doses (only for a few days)
▶ Takayasu's arteritis: 0.1–0.2 mg/kg/d (max. 5 mg/d)

Neuropaediatric indications:

– GBS
– West syndrome
– epileptic encephalopathies
– non-infectious CNS infections (demyelinating, vasculitis)
– immunomodulating therapy in Chorea minor
– chemotherapy of CNS tumors

Mechanism of action:

– synthetic glucocorticoid and active metabolite of Prednisone

Relevant contraindications:

– acute infection
– for oral intake: hereditary intolerance of galactose, deficiency of lactase, glucose-galactose malabsorption

Relevant side effects and interactions:

– frequent: arterial hypertension and hyperglycemia
– irritability
– increased appetite and weight gain
– increased risk of infection
– gastrointestinal bleedings
– iatrogenic Cushing's syndrome

– sudden stop of a long-term therapy (> 3 weeks) leads to secondary Addison's disease
– for long-term intake: weight gain up to central obesity, osteoporosis, cataract, diabetes mellitus, psychoses

Approval status:

– depends on the specific product (see SPC)

Sources:

– **Germany – SPC:**
– **severe acute asthma attack**
  – IV
    – **children:** initially 2 mg/kg, then 1–2 mg/kg/dose every 6 h until improvement; a concomitant administration of bronchodilators is recommended
– **USA – T:**
– **anti-inflammatory or immunosuppressive**
  – oral
    – **children:** 0.1–2 mg/kg/d as 1–4 separate doses
– **United Kingdom – BNFC:**
  – **infantile spasms**
    – oral
      – **children 1 month–2 years:** initially 40 mg/d as 4 separate doses for 14 d (if seizures not controlled after 7 d, increase to 60 mg/d as 3 separate doses for 7d); reduce dose gradually over 15 d until stopped (patients taking 40 mg/d, reduce dose in steps of 10 mg every 5 d, then stop; patients taking 60 mg/d, reduce dose to 40 mg/d for 5 d, then 20 mg/d for 5 d, then 10 mg/d for 5 d, then stop)
– **Uptodate.com:**
– **bronchopulmonary dysplasia**
  – **infants:** treat with 2 mg/kg/d as 2 separate doses for 5 d, followed by 1 mg/kg/d once daily for 3 d, followed by 1 mg/kg/dose every other day for 3 doses. This was used in 131 former premature neonates, postmenstrual age: ≥ 36 weeks) with BPD; results showed weaning off supplemental oxygen was facilitated in patients with capillary pCO2 < 48.5 mm Hg and pulmonary acuity score < 0.5
  – note: Dose depends on condition being treated and response of patient; dosage for infants and children should be based on disease severity and patient response, rather than rigidly adhering to dosage guidelines by age, weight, or body surface area. Consider alternate day therapy for long-term therapy. Discontinuation of long-term therapy requires gradual withdrawal by tapering the dose.
– **anti-inflammatory or immunosuppressive**
  – **children:** 0.1–2 mg/kg/d as 1–4 separate doses

Comments:

– The bone density has to be monitored when long-term use is necessary. Calcium and Vitamin D supplements are recommended for the prophylaxis of osteoporosis
– Vaccination with dead vaccines is possible. High dosages of glucocorticoids can interfere with the immune response and thus the success of vaccination. Not effective in conventional acute GBS.

- in combination with IVIG, only marginally effectiv in the high risk group of elder and ventilated patients
- highly effective (80 %) for protracted cases and CIDP

Prednisone

Dosage:
- ▶ progressive GBS or secondary deterioration after 4–6 weeks (suspected SIDP or CIDP): 1 mg/kg/d Prednisone
- ▶ Duchenne muscular dystrophy: 0.75 mg/kg/d
- ▶ facioscapulohumeral muscular dystrophy: 0.75 mg/kg/d (in one study without any effect, in some cases with "Duchenne-like" course partially effective)
- ▶ myositis:
  - start with 2 mg/kg/d as 2–3 separate doses
  - after clinical improvement within 6–12 weeks, slow dose reduction, e.g. every 2 months by 0.5 mg/kg; once reaching 0.5 mg/kg/d, reduce in steps of 0.1 mg or alternating

Neuropaediatric indications:
- GBS, SIDP and CIDP (progressive GBS)
- Duchenne's muscular dystrophy
- facioscapulohumeral muscular dystrophy
- mild to moderate myositis

Mechanism of action:
- synthetic glucocorticoid
- is metabolized to the active form (Prednisolone) in the liver

Relevant contraindications:
- acute infections
- diabetes
- severe heart failure
- children (growth in length has to be closely monitored)
- immunocompromised children and persons without a history of a infection with measles or varicella
- hypothyroidism, hepatic cirrhosis (consider reduced dose)
- gastrointestinal ulcers
- severe osteoporosis
- badly manageable hypertension
- psychiatric disorders
- angle-closure and open-angle glaucoma
- severe ulcerative colitis, diverticulitis

Relevant side effects and interactions:
- frequent: arterial hypertension and hyperglycemia
- irritability
- increased appetite and weight gain
- increased risk of infection
- gastrointestinal bleedings
- Iatrogenic Cushing's syndrome
- sudden discontinuation of long-term therapy (> 3 weeks) leads to secondary Addison's disease
- for long-term intake: weight gain up to central obesity, osteoporosis, cataract, diabetes mellitus, psychoses
- increased risk of gastrointestinal bleeding with concomitant intake of NSAR
- Atropine and other anticholinergic agents lead to further increase of intraocular pressure
- enhanced effect of cardiac glycosides possibly caused by potassium deficiency
- increased risk of blood count changes with concomitant administration of ACE inhibitors
- increased risk of cardiac myopathies with concomitant intake of Chloroquine, Hydroxychloroquine, Mefloquine
- elevated risk of epileptic seizures with concurrent intake of Cyclosporine
- estrogen-containing contraceptives enhance the effect of Prednisone
- less effective blood glucose reduction by oral antidiabetics and insulin

Approval status:
- depends on the specific product (see SPC)

Sources:
- Germany – SPC:
  - **chronic Guillain-Barré syndrome**
    - oral
      - **children:**

Dosing	Dose in mg/kg/d
High dose	2–3
Medium dose	1–2
Maintenance dose	0.25

- Administer according to response, type and severity of disease. Treatment should be alternated or intermittent for children. Start dose reduction after onset of clinical effect. High doses administered over a few days may be interrupted without gradual dose reduction (depending on disease type).
- **USA – T:**
- **anti-inflammatory or immunosuppressive**
  - oral
    - **children:** 0.05–2 mg/kg/d as 1–4 separate doses
- **United Kingdom – BNFC: –**

Comments:

- long-term therapy (over months): bone density has to be monitored and Calcium and Vitamin D supplements are recommended for the prophylaxis of osteoporosis
- inactivated vaccines are possible. High dosages of glucocorticoids can interfere with the immune response and thus the success of vaccination.

Pregabalin (PGB)

Dosage:

- ▶ limited experience in children (off-label)
- ▶ adults:
  - initially 150 mg/d as 2–3 separate doses p.o.
  - if needed, titrate after 3–7 d up to 300 mg/d; max. 600 mg/d

Neuropaediatric indications:

- neuropathic pain and paraesthesia
- adjunctive therapy of focal epilepsy

Mechanism of action:

- GABA analog, but does not act either as GABA agonist or as antagonist
- mechanism of action: binds to and inhibits voltage-dependent Calcium channels

Relevant contraindications:

- severe heart failure
- pregnancy
- no studies on use in children and adolescents under the age of 18 years
- careful use: hereditary intolerance to galactose, lactase deficiency, glucose-galactose malabsorption
- dose adjustment in renal failure

Relevant side effects and interactions:

- drowsiness (particularly at the beginning), euphoria, confusion, irritability

- ataxia, coordination disorders, tremor, dysarthria, disturbances of memory, attention disorders
- vertigo, blurred vision, vomiting
- paresthesia
- appetite and weight gain
- oedema, digestion disorder, sweating
- rare: muscle twitching and muscle cramps, dyskinesia
- there are only a few interactions, no influence on oral contraceptives
- effect of benzodiazepines and alcohol is enhanced
- respiratory insufficiency is possible if combined with centrally depressant drugs
- enhanced impairment of the cognitive and gross sensory motor function induced by oxycodone

Approval status:

- adjunctive therapy: > 18 years of age, focal and secondary generalized seizures
- no approval for children and adolescents

Sources:

- **Germany – SPC:**
  - **children < 18 years:** is not recommended, because efficacy and safety have not been established
- **USA – T: –**
- **United Kingdom – BNFC: –**
- **Uptodate.com:**
  - no published paediatric dosage
    - **neuropathic pain, diabetes associated**
      - oral
        - **adults:** initially 150 mg daily as separate doses (50 mg 3 times daily); may be increased within 1 week based on tolerability and effect; maximum dose is 300 mg daily (dosages up to 600 mg daily were evaluated with no significant additional benefit but increased adverse effects)
    - **partial-onset seizures (adjunctive therapy)**
      - oral
        - **adults:** initially 150 mg daily as separate doses (75 mg twice daily or 50 mg 3 times daily); may be increased based on tolerability and effect (optimal titration schedule has not been defined). Maximum dose is 600 mg daily.
        - **note:** discontinuation of therapy: Pregabalin should not be abruptly discontinued; taper off dosage over at least 1 week

Comments:

- well tolerated, quick dose titration is possible
- no serum level evaluation
- accumulation of epileptic seizures after sudden discontinuation
- efficacy is controversially discussed

Primidone (PRM)

Dosage:
- essential tremor: 1–20 mg/kg; individualized, slowly titrated dosage (off-label)
- epilepsy:
  - maintenance with 15–20 mg/kg/d as 2 separate doses (SPC)
  - therapeutic plasma levels: 4–15 mcg/ml

Neuropaediatric indications:
- epilepsy
  - grand mal (generalized clonic-tonic seizures)
  - impulsive petit mal epilepsy (myoclonic epilepsy)
  - juvenile myoclonic epilepsy
- essential tremor

Mechanism of action:
- Primidone is quickly metabolized, mainly to Phenobarbital and to a much lesser extent to Phenylethylmalonamide
- effect of Phenobarbital:
  - binds to $GABA_A$-receptor and thus enhances the inhibitory effect of GABA
  - blocks AMPA receptors and thus reduces the effect of the excitatory neurotransmitter glutamate

Relevant contraindications:
- poor general health condition
- deficient liver, renal- or breathing function (consider reduced dose)
- acute intoxications with centrally depressant drugs and alcohol
- medical history of known or latent and acute porphyria
- severe liver function disorders
- severe myocardial damages
- severe renal damages (half-life for most of the barbiturates remains the same; impairs renal function)
- hypovolemic, cardiac, septic, anaphylactic shock
- status asthmaticus
- careful use: hyperkinetic children (paradoxical reactions), bronchopulmonary diseases with dyspnea, bronchial asthma, cor pulmonale, cardiac arrhythmias, severe septic diseases, severe metabolic diseases, intense anemia, pregnancy
- chronic renal diseases: elimination of barbiturates can be substantially delayed (dose reduction is necessary)

Relevant side effects and interactions:
- fatigue, slowdown, vertigo, blurred vision, disturbances of equilibrium
- depression
- allergic rash in 5–10 % of patients
- chronic intake: cognitive impairment, behavioural disorder, depressive mood, concentration disorders, disorders of Calcium metabolism with osteoporosis
- long-term use: megaloblastic anemia
- folic acid lowers the effect
- mutually enhanced effect if combination with centrally depressant drugs (psychotropic and hypnotic drugs) and alcohol
- decreased effect of oral contraceptives, oral anticoagulants, Digitoxin, Doxycycline, Chloramphenicol, cytostatics, Griseofulvin, glucocorticoids
- enhanced Methotrexate toxicity
- Valproic acid and MAOIs enhance the effect of Primidone
- enhanced metabolism of Phenobarbital, Carbamazepine, Phenytoin, Clonazepam, Diazepam

Approval status:
- focal and generalized epilepsy, incl. absence epilepsy and myoclonic seizures in adolescents, without age limit

Sources:
- Germany – SPC:
  - epilepsy (grand mal, focal seizures, impulsive petit mal)
    - oral
      - children ≥ 2 years:

Daily dose						
	2–5 years		6–9 years		≥ 9 years	
Schedule	Morning	Evening	Morning	Evening	Morning	Evening
Day 1–3	–	62.5 mg	62.5 mg	62.5 mg	62.5 mg	62.5 mg
Day 4–7	–	125 mg	62.5 mg	125 mg	125 mg	125 mg
Week 2	62,5 mg	125 mg	125 mg	250 mg	250 mg	250 mg
Week 3	125 mg	250 mg	250 mg	250 mg	375 mg	375 mg
After week 3	250 mg	250 mg	250 mg	500 mg	375 mg	375 mg
Maintenance dose	500–750 mg		750–1000 mg		750–1500 mg	

– **epileptic and myoclonic seizures, absences (impulsive petit mal)**
  – oral
    – **children < 2 years:**

Schedule	Infants		Children < 2 years	
	Morning	Evening	Morning	Evening
Day 1–3	–	62.5 mg	–	62.5 mg
Day 4–7	62.5 mg	62.5 mg	–	125 mg
Week 2	62.5 mg	62.5 mg	125 mg	125 mg
Week 3	62.5 mg	125 mg	125 mg	187.5 mg
After week 3	125 mg	125 mg	125 mg	187.5 mg
Maintenance dose	250–500 mg		500–750 mg	

– **USA – T:**
  – **seizure disorder**
    – oral
      – **neonates:** 12–20 mg/kg/d as 2–4 separate doses; start with lower dosage and titrate upward
      – **children < 8 years:** initially 50–125 mg/d at bedtime; increase by 50–125 mg/d every 3–7 d; usual dose 10–25 mg/kg/d as 3–4 separate doses
      – **children ≥ 8 years:** initially 125–250 mg/d at bedtime; increase by 125–250 mg/d every 3–7 d; usual dose 750–1500 mg/d as 3–4 separate doses with max. 2 g/d
– **United Kingdom – BNFC:**
  – **all types of epilepsy except absence seizures**
    – oral
      – **children < 2 years:** initially 125 mg/d at bedtime; increase by 125 mg every 3 d according to response; usual maintenance with 250–500 mg/d as 2 separate doses
      – **children 2–5 years:** initially 125 mg/d at bedtime; increase by 125 mg every 3 d according to response; usual maintenance with 300–750 mg/d as 2 separate doses
      – **children 5–9 years:** initially 125 mg/d at bedtime; increase by 125 mg every 3 d according to response; usual maintenance with 750–1000 mg/d as 2 separate doses
      – **children 9–18 years:** initially 125 mg/d at bedtime; increase by 125 mg every 3 d to 500 mg/d as 2 separate doses, then increase according to response by 250 mg every 2 d to max. 1500 mg/d as 2 separate doses

Comments:

– subtherapeutic blood level: < 10 mcg/ml
– half-life: 60–130 h
– slow titration is recommended due to frequent incidence of vertigo

Procyclidine

Dosage:
▶ 0.15–0.8 mg/kg/d as 3–4 separate doses p.o.; max. 10 mg/dose (off-label)

Neuropaediatric indications:

– emergency treatment of acute dystonia or oculogyric crisis

Mechanism of action:

– anticholinergic agent

Relevant contraindications:

– myasthenia gravis
– tardive dyskinesia
– psychiatric diseases
– careful use: angle-closure glaucoma, obstructive gastrointestinal diseases, voiding disorders, renal or liver function disorders

Relevant side effects and interactions:

– common: dry mouth, blurred vision, mydriasis, constipation, urinary retention
– occasional: nausea, vomiting, gingivitis, fatigue, nervousness, rash
– rare: confusion, impairment of cognitive functions and loss of memory, disorientation and hallucinations
– in combination with neuroleptics, potentiated symptoms of tardive dyskinesia
– MAOIs or anticholinergic drugs (e.g. Amantadine, antihistamines, phenothiazines, tricyclic antidepressants, chinidin, disopyramide) can enhance the anticholinergic effect of Procyclidine
– can reduce effect of L-dopa
– antacids can reduce the resorption
– when combined with neuroleptics: reduced plasma concentration of neuroleptics

Approval status:

– not approved in the paediatric patient group

Sources:

– **Germany – SPC:**
  – **early dyskinesia, extrapyramidal signs and symptoms**
    – oral (as Procyclidine hydrochlorid)
      – **children:** not recommended, only if benefits outweigh the risks
      – **adults:** initially 7.5 mg/d as 3 separate doses. Increase dose every 2–3 d by 2.5–5 mg/d to maintenance dose:

- symptoms of Parkinson's disease: 10–20 mg/d
- tremor in Parkinson's disease: 30 mg/d, in exceptional cases up to 60 mg/d
- Interrupt treatment of medication-induced Parkinson's disease after 3–4 months and re-start treatment only if symptoms reappear. Interval treatment is also indicated in patients receiving Procyclidine longer than 3–4 months.
- **United Kingdom – BNFC:**
  - **acute dystonia**
    - IM or IV injection
      - **children < 2 years:** 0.5–2 mg as a SD
      - **children 2–10 years:** 2–5 mg as a SD
      - **children 10–18 years:** 5–10 mg (occasionally > 10 mg)
      - **note:** usually effective in 5–10 min but may need 30 min for relief
  - **dystonia**
    - oral
      - **children 7–12 years:** 3.75 mg/d as 3 separate doses
      - **children 2–10 years:** 7.5 mg/d as 3 separate doses

Comments:
- no sudden complete discontinuation
- effect after 5–10 min, max. effect after about 30 min
- variable published dosage recommendations in common paediatric sources

Promethazine

Dosage:
▶ acute dystonic reaction: IV 0.5–1 mg/kg/dose (max. every 4–6 h) (off-label)
▶ sedation: 0.5–1.5 mg/kg/dose (max. 100 mg) (off-label)

Neuropaediatric indications:
- acute dystonic reaction

Mechanism of action:
- antihistaminic agent
- competitive antagonist at peripheral and central H_1 receptors
- anticholinergic effect

Relevant contraindications:
- absolute: acute intoxication with centrally depressant drugs and alcohol, preexisting severe impairement of blood cells or bone marrow, circulatory shock, anamnestic known malignant neuroleptic syndrome
- severe liver function disorders
- preexisting cardiac impairement
- renal impairment
- hypotension, orthostatic circulation disorder
- diseases of the brain stem
- chronic breathing disorder, asthma
- voiding dysfunction with residual urine, gastrointestinal stenosis

Relevant side effects and interactions:
- fatigue, weakness, sleeping disorder and drowsiness, lethargy, anxiety, vertigo
- movement disorders: oculomotor cramps, suddenly protruding tongue, dyskinesias, akathisia
- symptoms of Parkinson's disease such as tremor, slowed and restricted movement, loss of automatic movement, stiff muscles
- hypotension, orthostatic circulation disorder, tachycardia, cardiac arrhythmias, cardiac conduction disorders
- elevation of prolactin level, chest tightness, galactorrhea, menstruation disorder up to amenorrhea, erectile dysfunction
- asthma
- dry mouth, accommodation impairment, constipation, voiding disorders, weight gain
- headache, depression, agitation conditions, seizures, speech disorder, disturbances of memory
- pruritus, elevated liver function parameters, leukopenia, hyperglycemia

Approval status:
- depends on the specific product (see SPC)

Sources:
- **Germany – SPC:**
- **USA – T:**
  - **sedation**
    - oral, IM, IV, rectal
      - **children:** 0.5–1 mg/kg/dose (max. 25 mg) every 6 h as needed
- **United Kingdom – BNFC:** this indication of interest is not specified
- **Uptodate.com:**
  - **children ≥ 2 years** (use with extreme caution, utilizing the lowest effective dose):
  - **antihistamine**
    - oral: 0.1 mg/kg/dose (do not exceed 12.5 mg) every 6 hours during the day and 0.5 mg/kg/dose (do not exceed 25 mg) at bedtime as needed
  - **antiemetic**
    - oral, IM, IV, rectal: 0.25–1 mg/kg (do not exceed 25 mg) 4–6 times/d as needed
  - **motion sickness**
    - oral, rectal: 0.5 mg/kg (do not exceed 25 mg) 30 minutes to 1 hour before departure, then every 12 hours as needed

- **preoperative analgesia/hypnotic adjunct**
  - IM, IV: 1.1 mg/kg once in combination with an analgesic or hypnotic (at reduced dosage) and with an Atropine-like agent (at appropriate dosage). **note:** Promethazine dosage in children should not exceed half of the suggested adult dosage.
  - sedation: oral, IM, IV, rectal: 0.5–1 mg/kg/dose (do not exceed 25 mg) every 6 hours as needed

Comments:

- variable published dosage recommendations, overall "old-fashioned"

Propiverine

> **Dosage:**
> ▶ children: 0.4–0.8 mg/kg/d as 2 separate doses (SPC)
> ▶ adults: 30–45 mg/d

Neuropaediatric indications:

- urinary incontinence in children

Mechanism of action:

- anticholinergic agent: competitive antagonist at muscarinic acetylcholine receptors
- spasmolytic agent: inhibition of Calcium influx through the Calcium channels (L-type) in smooth muscle cells

Relevant contraindications:

- angle-closure glaucoma
- voiding dysfunction with residual urine
- mechanic stenosis in the gastrointestinal tract, megacolon
- tachyarrhythmia
- acute pulmonary oedema
- note: careful indication in the third trimester of pregnancy

Relevant side effects and interactions:

- reduced sweating
- flush
- disorders of the central nervous system
- accommodation impairment, release of glaucoma
- dry mouth
- tachycardia
- micturition disorder
- enhanced anticholinergic effect when combined with Amantadine, chinidin, tri- and tetracyclic antidepressants, neuroleptics

- mutually decreased effect on gastrointestinal tract motility when used together with dopamine antagonists

Approval status:

- neurogenic bladder dysfunction in children and adults

Sources:

- **Germany – SPC:**
  - **urinary incontinence**
    - oral

children > 5 years:	mean: 0.8 mg/kg/d in 2–3 divided doses
12–16 kg	4.55 mg–0 mg–4.55 mg
17–22 kg	4.55 mg–4.55 mg–4.55 mg
23–28 kg	9.1 mg–0 mg–9.1 mg
29–34 kg	9.1 mg–4.55 mg–9.1 mg
> 35 kg	9.1 mg–9.1 mg–9.1 mg
or	13.65 mg–0 mg–13.65 mg

- The treatment of neurogenic detrusor overactivity caused by spinal cord injury is also indicated for patients < 5 years of age. But use in children < 1 year is not recommended.
- **USA – T:** –
- **United Kingdom – BNFC:** –
- **Uptodate.com:**
  - no published paediatric dosage
  - **management of urinary frequency, urgency, and incontinence in neurogenic bladder disorders in idiopathic detrusor instability**
    - oral
      - **adults:** usually 15 mg 2–3 times/d; may be increased to 4 times/d, some patients may respond to 15 mg/d
- **Drugdex®:**
  - **urinary incontinence**
    - oral
      - **children 4.5–11 years:** 0.2–0.4 mg/kg/d (Propiverine hydrochloride) as 2 separate doses was clinically effective and well tolerated; daily doses of 0.8 mg/kg Propiverine produced further clinical improvement in one study, but a higher incidence of adverse effects was reported.

Comments:

- is better tolerated than Oxybutynin

Propofol

Dosage:
- ▸ administration under emergency conditions (including EEG monitoring)
- ▸ bolus: 1–2 mg/kg, then 1–4 mg/kg/h (dosing after EEG)

Neuropaediatric indications:
- therapy-resistant status epilepticus (after > 60 min)
- anesthesia

Mechanism of action:
- hypnotic, not analgesic
- short plasma half-life
- low risk of cumulation

Relevant contraindications:
- hypersensitivity to peanuts or soy beans
- children < 3 years of age (anesthesia) and adolescents > 16 years of age (sedation)
- concurrent administration of Lidocaine for hereditary acute porphyria
- careful use: lipid metabolism disorders, diseases where fatty emulsions are not clearly recommended, heart failure, circulation, respiratory insufficiency, hypovolemia, high vagotonia (or sympathetic imbalance), combination with drugs that lead to bradycardia, epilepsy

Relevant side effects and interactions:
- respiratory depression, apnea
- decrease in blood pressure
- agitation
- anaphylaxis
- local pain during injection
- seizures (up to 6 h after application)
- Propofol infusion syndrome is possible after long-term treatment (severe metabolic disorders like rhabdomyolysis and lactic acidosis possible)
- after extended infusions, brown and green discolouration of urine is possible
- additive effects with drugs, which could lead to hypotension or respiratory depression

Approval status:
- depends on the specific product (see SPC)

Sources:
- Germany – SPC:
  - Sedation, anesthesia
    - IV
    - no published paediatric dosage
- USA – T:
  - general anesthesia
  - IV induction
    - **children (healthy) 3–16 years, ASA I or II:** 2.5–3.5 mg/kg over 20–30 sec; use a lower dose for children ASA III or IV
    - **maintenance, infants (healthy) ≥ 2 months and children < 16 years, ASA I or II:** initially (immediately following induction): 200–300 mcg/kg/min; decrease dose after 30 min if clinical signs of light anesthesia are absent; usual infusion rate is 125–150 mcg/kg/min; younger paediatric patients may require higher infusion rates compared to older children.
- **United Kingdom – BNFC:** this indication of interest is not specified
- Uptodate.com:
  - General anesthesia
    - IV induction
      - **children (healthy) 3–16 years, ASA I or II**: 2.5–3.5 mg/kg over 20–30 seconds; use a lower dose for children ASA III or IV
    - maintenance: IV infusion
      - **infants (healthy) ≥ 2 months to children 16 years, ASA I or II:** initially (immediately following induction) 200–300 mcg/kg/minute; decrease dose after 30 minutes if clinical signs of light anesthesia are absent; usual infusion rate is 125–150 mcg/kg/minute; younger paediatric patients may require higher infusion rates compared to older children
- Drugdex®:
- General anesthesia
- Safety and efficacy of Propofol injection has not been established for use in the intensive care unit, sedation, or for monitored anesthesia care (MAC) sedation in paediatric patients. In a study of 327 patients, an increase in the number of deaths in patients receiving Propofol compared to standard sedative agents (i.e., Lorazepam, Fentanyl, Ketamine) was reported.
- Induction
- 1) Dosage should be individualized and titrated: Healthy paediatric patients (older than 3 years of age) – The majority of patients require 2.5 to 3.5 mg/kg, administered over 20 to 30 seconds. Although induction with Propofol is appropriate in the paediatric population, the high frequency of pain upon injection may limit its usefulness for anesthetic induction in paediatrics.
- 2) The mean Propofol anesthetic induction dose has been determined to be 2.28 mg/kg (range 2 to 2.78) for children aged 1 to 5 years, and the mean dose to be 2.1 mg/kg (range, 2 to 2.4) in children aged 5 to 10 years.
- 3) A mean Propofol induction dose of 2.8 mg/kg intravenously was required for the loss of the eyelash reflex in 90 % of medicated children. The study was conducted in 144 children between the ages of 1 to 12 years of age. Children who had been premedicated with oral Trimeprazine 3 mg/kg required a mean Propofol dose of 2 mg/kg.
- Maintenance
- 1) A variable rate infusion should be titrated to the desired clinical effect:

2) Healthy paediatric patients (older than 2 months) – the recommended maintenance dose of Propofol for general anesthesia ranges from 125 to 300 mcg/kg/min (7.5 to 18 mg/kg/hour). Requirements for total intravenous anesthesia using Propofol and Alfentanil in 59 children (aged 3 to 12 years) have been the following: patients receiving a loading dose of Alfentanil 85 mcg/kg and Alfentanil infusion of 65 mcg/kg, of Propofol 6 mg/kg/hour; patients receiving a loading dose of Alfentanil 65 mcg/kg and Alfentanil infusion of 50 mcg/kg of 7.5 mg/kg/hour.

Comments:

- be careful concerning bacterial contamination, if the bottle is already open and stays open until injection/infusion
- subtherapeutic blood levels: < 2 mcg/ml
- half-life: 3–8 h
- status epilepticus:
  - advantage:
    - fast effect (burst suppression in the EEG within 35 min)
    - easy titration, easy to control (short half-life)
    - 33 children: retrospectively better than Thiopental (64 % vs. 55 % effectiveness), fewer pulmonary problems than with Thiopental
  - disadvantage:
    - Propofol infusion syndrome (cardiac failure, rhabdomyolysis, acidosis, renal failure, partially fatal; however, this concerns primarily doses > 5 mg/kg/d and administration over multiple days)
    - therefore, clear indication for the treatment of malignant status epilepticus
    - decrease in blood pressure ranges between 50 and 70 %

Propranolol

Dosage:
- ▶ migraine prophylaxis: 0.5–1.5(–2) mg/kg/d
- ▶ essential tremor: individual target dosing 30–300 mg/d as 3 separate doses (off-label)

Neuropaediatric indications:
- migraine prophylaxis
- essential tremor

Mechanism of action:
- beta-blocker
- no intrinsic activity
- non-cardioselective beta-blocker, which binds to β_1- and β_2-receptors

Relevant contraindications:
- severe asthma
- clinically manifest heart failure, AV block II. or III. degree
- bradykardia
- acidosis
- severe circulation disorder in extremities
- careful use: AV block I. degree, diabetes mellitus, liver or renal impairment

Relevant side effects and interactions:
- initial increase in blood pressure; high dosages may lead to hypotension, syncopes, bradycardia
- provocation of heart failure or aggravation of present heart failure symptoms
- diarrhea
- lethargy, depression
- bronchial spasms
- no combination with MAOIs
- can enhance or extend the effect of insulin and can mask signs of hypoglycemia
- strong decrease in blood pressure when combined with the following drugs:
  - other beta-blockers
  - tri- and tetracyclic antidepressants
  - barbiturates
  - diuretics
  - vasodilators
  - narcotics
  - Nitroglycerin
- bradycardia and conduction disturbances when combined with:
  - cardiac glycosides
  - with cerebral acting blood pressure-decreasing drugs: Reserpine, Methyldopa, Guanfacine, Clonidine
- enhanced effect of antiarrhythmic drugs
- cimetidine (H2 receptor blocker) enhances the effect of Propranolol
- indometacin (Novalgin) can decrease the effect of Propranolol

Approval status:
- depends on the specific product (see SPC)

Sources:
- **Germany – SPC:**
  - **prophylaxis of migraine**
    - no published paediatric dosage – off label

- USA – T:
  - migraine headache prophylaxis
    - oral
      - **children:** 0.6–1.5 mg/kg/d as 3 separate doses, max. 4 mg/kg/d or ≤ 35 kg: 30–60 mg/d as 3 separate doses, > 35 kg: 60–120 mg/d as 3 separate doses
- United Kingdom – BNFC:
  - migraine prophylaxis
    - oral
      - **children 2–12 years:** initially 0,4–1 mg/kg/d as 2 separate doses; usually 20–40 mg/d as 2 separate doses; max. 4 mg/kg/d as 2 separate doses
      - **children 12–18 years:** initially 40–80 mg/d as 2 separate doses; usually 80–160 mg/d as 2 separate doses; max. 2 mg/kg/dose (max. 120 mg) twice daily

Comments:
- used as racemate

Pyridostigmine

> **Dosage:**
> - ▸ has to be individually adjusted to clinical response
> - ▸ 2–18 mg/kg/d as 2–6 separate doses; max. 200 mg/d as separate doses (off-label)

Neuropaediatric indications:
- myasthenia gravis

Mechanism of action:
- acetylcholinesterase inhibitor; increased acetylcholine concentration at the synaptic cleft

Relevant contraindications:
- intestinal obstruction, urinary retention
- bradycardia, hypotension, heart failure
- acute iritis
- asthma and other pulmonary diseases
- careful use: epilepsy, peptic ulcers, cardiac arrhythmias, hyperthyroidism, vagotonia, megacolon

Relevant side effects and interactions:
- nausea, vomiting, abdominal cramps, diarrhea
- drooling, miosis, lacrimation
- elevated bronchial secretion, bronchial spasms, hypotension
- muscle pain and weakness
- anxiety attacks and anxiety disorders
- enhanced effect of opiates, barbiturates, benzodiazepines, beta blockers
- prolonged effect (suxamethonium) or inhibition (curare-like muscle relaxants) of muscle relaxants

Approval status:
- depends on the specific product (see SPC)

Sources:
- Germany – SPC:
  - myasthenia gravis
  - oral
    - **children:** initially 4 mg/kg/d as Pyridostigmine bromide as 4 separate doses; increase to response, max. 360 mg/d
- USA – T:
  - myasthenia gravis
  - oral
    - **neonates:** 5 mg/dose every 4–6 h
    - **children:** 7 mg/kg/d as 5–6 separate doses
  - IM, IV
    - **neonates and children:** 0.05–0.15 mg/kg/dose, max. 10 mg/dose
- United Kingdom – BNFC:
  - treatment of myasthenia gravis
  - oral
    - **neonates:** initially 1–1.5 mg/kg; increase gradually to max. 10 mg, repeat throughout the day, giving 30–60 min before feeds
    - **children 1 month–12 years:** initially 1–1.5 mg/kg/d, increase gradually to 7 mg/kg/d as 6 separate doses, usually 30–360 mg/d
    - **children 12–18 years:** 30–120 mg, repeat throughout the day; usually 300–600 mg/d (but consider immunosuppressant therapy if total daily dose exceeds 360 mg; if total daily dose exceeds 450 mg, down-regulation of acetylcholine receptors is possible)

Comments:
- less muscarinergic effect compared to Neostigmine, but longer time of effect and fewer side effects
- various dosages published in common paediatric sources

Pyridoxal phosphate (PALP, PLP, P5P)

Dosage:
- ▶ therapy attempt for cryptogenic, therapy-resistant seizures in neonates: 30–50 mg/kg/d as 3–5 separate doses p.o. over 3 d (off-label)
- ▶ West syndrome: 15–30(–40) mg/kg/d as 3–4 separate doses (off-label)

Neuropaediatric indications:
- cryptogenic, therapy-resistant seizures in neonates
- epilepsy, particularly West syndrome

Mechanism of action:
- = active form of Pyridoxine (Vitamin B_6)
- Phosphorylated Vitamin B_6 derivatives are coenzymes in about 100 different enzymatic reactions (primarily in amino acid metabolism)
- cofactor for the synthesis of δ-aminolevulinic acid (intermediate product of heme synthesis)
- cofactor in glycogen break down
- cofactor in the elimination of cysteine, threonine, and serine
- the Vitamin B_6 group (Pyridoxines) consists of Pyridoxamine, Pyridoxal, and Pyridoxine, together with their 5'-phosphate-esters, and the catabolite 4-pyridoxate (eliminated via urine)
- except for pyridoxate, all of these water-soluble vitamin forms are interconvertible; biologically active is pyridoxal-5'-phosphate (PLP)

Relevant contraindications:
- isolated folic acid deficiency

Relevant side effects and interactions:
- vomiting, loss of appetite, constipation or diarrhea, gastritis, colics that could lead to disturbances
- polyneuropathy. This is dose-related and may develop only after several weeks or months of administration (peripheral, sensory neuropathy with atactic gait disorder, impaired reflexes and disorders concerning tactile, vibration and temperature sensation).
- all described adverse events are reversible
- only when overdosing: photosensitivity, dermatitis; infants given ≥ 1 g Pyridoxine per day may develop tachycardia, peripheral circulation disorder, areflexia
- isoniazid and D-penicillinamine is able to displace Pyridoxal phosphate from its binding sites on various enzymes.

Approval status:
- not applicable

Sources:
- Germany – SPC: –
- USA – T: -
- United Kingdom – BNFC: –
- Uptodate.com: –

Comments:
- Vitamin B_6 naturally occurs in most kinds of food, whether of plant or animal origin
- Manifestation of Pyridoxine-dependent epilepsy is possible until the age of 18 months, under special circumstances also as status epilepticus. Thus, administration is recommended until the age of 2 to confirm diagnosis if no other aetiology of the status has been established.
- Elevated risk of hypotension and apnea with bolus administration of Pyridoxine (under EEG control) to children who are Pyridoxine dependent. Therefore, children with West syndrome should be given multiple oral dosages during the day or a continuous infusion.
- even using diluted drug solutions does not prevent side effects (40–70 %), especially gastrointestinal problems, stressful for both the children and their parents
- In a prospective study concerning Sulthiame and Pyridoxine as a basic medication, Pyridoxine did not show any significant effect (initially given for 3 d as monotherapy); therefore, a longer lasting therapy does not seem to have any benefits and is no longer recommended due to the possible side effects.
- in the treatment of West syndrome, the response rates to the two Vitamin B_6 derivatives Pyridoxine and Pyridoxal phosphate do not significantly differ
- signs of Vitamin B_6 deficiency are rare and often unspecific:
  - seborrheic dermatitis
  - glossitis
  - seizures, neuritis, depression, irritability
  - growth disturbance
  - anemia

Pyridoxine

Dosage:
- West syndrome: 100–300 mg/kg/d as 3–4 separate doses
- oral administration for the prophylaxis of Vitamin B_6 deficiency signs: 1.5–25 mg/d
- cryptogenic, therapy-resistant seizures in neonates: 100–500 mg/dose IV, then 30 mg/kg/d as 2–3 separate doses p.o. over 3 d
- oral administration for the treatment of Vitamin B_6-deficiency-conditioned seizures in neonates and infants: 0.5–4 mg/kg/d
- status epilepticus: convulsive status epilepticus, children < 2 years: 100 mg IV

Neuropaediatric indications:
- cryptogenic, therapy-resistant seizures in neonates
- epilepsy, particularly West syndrome
- signs of Vitamin B_6 deficiency
- status epilepticus

Mechanism of action:
- = Vitamin B_6
- phosphorylated Vitamin B_6 derivatives are coenzymes in about 100 different enzymatic reactions (primarily in amino acid metabolism)
- the Vitamin B_6 group (Pyridoxines) consists of Pyridoxamine, Pyridoxal and Pyridoxine, together with their 5'-phosphate-estersandin, and the catabolite 4-Pyridoxate (eliminated via urine)
- except for pyridoxate, all of these water-soluble vitamins are interconvertible, biologically active is pyridoxal-5'-phosphate (PLP)

Relevant contraindications:
- isolated folic acid deficiency

Relevant side effects and interactions:
- vomiting, loss of appetite, constipation or diarrhea, gastritis, colics that could lead to disturbances
- polyneuropathy. This is dose-related and may develop only after several weeks or months of administration (peripheral, sensory neuropathy with atactic gait disorder, impaired reflexes and disorders concerning tactile, vibration and temperature sensation).
- all described adverse events are reversible
- only when overdosing: photosensitivity, dermatitis; infants given ≥ 1 g Pyridoxine per day: tachycardia, peripheral circulation disorder, areflexia
- Pyridoxine administration can reduce the effect of L-Dopa
- intake of oral contraceptives can promote the development of Pyridoxine deficiency

Approval status:
- depends on the specific product (see SPC)

Sources:
- Germany – SPC:
  - initial therapy for Vitamin-B_6 deficiency caused seizures
    - IV
      - **neonates and infants:** usually 100–200 mg Pyridoxine hydrochloride IV; maintenance dose is usually given via oral route
      - **note:** sedation, hypotension and respiratory disorders (apnea, dyspnea) can occur. Therefore, provide for prompt reanimation when needed.
- USA – T:
  - Pyridoxine-dependent seizures
    - oral, IM, IV
      - **infants:** initially 50–100 mg, preferably IV; maintenance preferably oral, usually with 50–100 mg/d; range 10–200 mg
  - dietary deficiency
    - oral, IM, IV
      - **children:** 5–25 mg/d for 3 weeks, then 1.5–2.5 mg/d in a multivitamin product
- United Kingdom – BNFC: Pyridoxine hydrochloride
  - Pyridoxine-dependent seizures
    - oral, IV injection
      - **neonates:** initial test dose of 50–100 mg by IV injection, may be repeated; if patient responds, follow with an oral maintenance dose of 50–100 mg/d given as a SD, adjusted to response as necessary
      - **children 1 month–12 years:** initial test dose 50–100 mg; if patient responds, follow with an oral dose of 20–50 mg/dose 1–2 times daily, adjusted to response as necessary; doses up to 30 mg/kg or 1 g/d have been used

Comments:
- Vitamin B_6 naturally occurs in most kinds of food, whether of plant or animal origin.
- Manifestation of Pyridoxine-dependent epilepsy is possible until the age of 18 months, under special circumstances also as SE. Thus, administration is recommended until the age of 2 to confirm diagnosis if no other aetiology of the status has been established.
- Elevated risk of hypotension and apnea with bolus administration of Pyridoxine (under EEG control) to children who are Pyridoxine dependent. Therefore, children with West syndrome should be given multiple oral dosages during the day or a continuous infusion.
- Even using dilutions does not prevent side effects (40–70 %), especially gastrointestinal problems, stressful for both the children and their parents.

- In a prospective study concerning Sulthiame and Pyridoxine as a basic medication, Pyridoxine did not show a significant effect (initially given for 3 days as a monotherapy); therefore, a longer lasting therapy does not seem to have any benefits and is no longer recommended due to the possible side effects.
- In the treatment of West syndrome, the response rates to the two Vitamin B_6 derivatives Pyridoxine and Pyridoxal phosphate do not significantly differ.
- various published dosages recommended in common paediatric sources
- signs of Vitamin B_6 deficiency:
  - rare and often unspecific
  - seborrhoeic dermatitis
  - glossitis
  - seizures, neuritis, depression, irritability
  - growth disturbance
  - anemia

R

Risperidone

Dosage:
▶ 0.5–4(–9) mg/d as 2 separate doses (off-label)

Neuropaediatric indications:
- tic disorder
- behavioural disorder
- chorea

Mechanism of action:
- atypical neuroleptic drug
- antagonist at the dopamine D_2 receptors (about ⅓ as effective as Haloperidol)
- high-affinity 5-hydrotryptamine ($5\text{-}HT_2$) antagonist (much higher affinity than for the dopamine receptors)
- additionally, antagonist to adrenoreceptors and histamine H_1 receptors (primary cause for side effects)

Relevant contraindications:
- hyperprolactinemia
- acute intoxication with centrally depressant drugs
- known neuroleptic malignant syndrome
- cerebral disorders, predisposition for seizures
- careful use:
  - bradycardia, congenital long QT syndrome, other cardiac disorders
  - pathologic changes in blood count
  - diabetes mellitus

Relevant side effects and interactions:
- extrapyramidal disorders
- early dyskinesia (reversible)
- tardive dyskinesia (sometimes only incompletely reversible): swallowing and pharyngeal cramps, "problematic" speech, dystonic movement
- fatigue, akathisia
- hypotension (especially if volume deficiency is present), orthostatic dysregulation, cardiac conduction disorders (AV block, bundle branch block)
- speech disorder
- neuroleptic malignant syndrome (very rare)
- ischaemic events and TIA
- weight gain
- elevation of prolactin serum levels
- combination with other psychotropic drugs increases side effects
- do not combine with Furosemide

Approval status:
- depends on the specific product (see SPC)

Sources:
- **Germany – SPC:**
- **Behavioral disorder**
  - oral
    - **children 5–18 years, ≥ 50 kg:** initially 0.5 mg/d as a SD. If necessary, increase every other day by 0.5 mg/d as a SD. Usual dose is 1 mg/d as a SD; range from 0.5–1.5 mg/d as a SD.
    - **children 5–18 years, < 50 kg:** initially 0.25 mg/d as a SD. If necessary, increase every other day by 0.25 mg/d as a SD. Usual dose is 0.5 mg/d as a SD; range from 0.25–0.75 mg/d as a SD.
- **note:** Evaluate treatment continuously. Use in children < 5 years is not recommended.
- **USA – T:**
- **Tourette syndrome**
  - oral: limited information is available
    - Study from 2001: (n = 26, age 11–50 years, median age 20 years, 10 patients < 18 years) A fixed dose titration from 0.5 mg/d to 2 mg/d was used for the first week. This was followed by a flexible dosing

period of 7 weeks. Doses were increased by ≤ 1 mg/week to max. 6 mg/d in a SD (final dose range: 0.5–6 mg/d). **note:** a slower dosing schedule and lower long-term doses (e.g., 1–2 mg/d) may be needed.
- Study from 1995: (n = 7, age 11–16 years, mean age 12.9 ± 1.9 years. Patients with chronic tic disorders, 5 of them with Tourette syndrome) initially 0.5 mg at bedtime; doses were increased in 5 of the 7 patients by 0.5 mg/d every 5–7 d.
- **United Kingdom – BNFC:** This indication of interest is not specified.

Comments:
- various recommended dosages published in common paediatric sources

Rituximab

Dosage:
- ▶ myositis: 2 schemes are possible:
  - 100 mg/m² body surface area on the 1st, 8th, 15th and 22nd day
  - 375 mg/m² body surface area/week (off-label)
- ▶ Opsoclonus Myoclonus Ataxia Syndrome (OMAS): no dose scheme

Neuropaediatric indications:
- therapy-resistant severe myositis
- Opsoclonus Myoclonus Ataxia Syndrome, OMAS (individual attempt of therapy)

Mechanism of action:
- chimeric monoclonal antibody that binds to CD20
- CD20 is widely expressed on B cells and B cell tumors and is responsible for B cells activation
- binding of Rituximab results in killing of pathogenic and normal B cells by the immune system
- hematopoetic stem cells do not express CD20 and therefore are not affected by Rituximab

Relevant contraindications:
- active severe infection
- immunocompromised patients
- hypersensitivity to murine proteins
- severe heart failure (NYHA IV), uncontrollable severe heart diseases
- careful use: pregnancy, hypotension, bronchial spasm, heart diseases, neutrophils < 1,5 × 10 9/l, thrombocytes < 75 × 10 9/l, past HBV infection, moderate heart failure (NYHA III), relapsing/chronic infections

Relevant side effects and interactions:
- pain, oedema, infections
- fever, shivering, asthenia, cold, sore throat
- multiple organ failure, abdominal extension
- nervousness, depression, fatigue, hot flushes
- vertigo, paresthesia, anxiety, insomnia, hypoesthesia, agitation, cranial neuropathy, peripheral neuropathy, facial nerve paralysis, loss of other sensory perceptions, migraine
- impaired sense of taste
- (orthostatic) hypotension, hypertension, arrhythmia (atrial fibrillation, ventricular/supraventricular tachycardia), bradycardia, tachycardia, heart failure, angina pectoris (also aggravation of pre-existing similar disorders), myocardial infarction
- coagulation disorders
- thromboembolic cerebrovascular events, vasculitis (mainly cutaneous)
- nausea, vomiting, diarrhea, dyspepsia, anorexia, dysphagia, stomatitis, constipation, gastrointestinal perforation
- leukopenia, neutropenia, thrombocytopenia, (hemolytic/aplastic/transient aplastic) anemia, hypoxia, lymphadenopathy, pancytopenia, temporary increase of IgM plasma levels
- hypercholesterolemia, hyperglycemia, LDH increase, hypocalcemia
- myalgia, arthralgia, rigor, muscle cramps, osteoarthritis
- bronchial spasms, rhinitis, increased coughing, dyspnea, interstitial pneumonia, asthma, pulmonary diseases, bronchiolitis fibrosa obliterans, pulmonary infiltration, respiratory insufficiency, nasopharyngitis
- pruritus, exanthema, urticaria, night sweats, sweating, flush, alopecia, severe bullous skin reactions, toxic epidermal necrolysis (TEN)
- tinnitus, loss of hearing, severe loss of vision
- hypersensitivity reactions
- tumor lysis syndrome
- reactivation of hepatitis B (including fulminant hepatitis)
- renal failure
- temporary hyperuricemia, elevated phosphate levels, hyperkalemia, hypocalcemia

Approval status:
- approved for chemotherapy, particularly for the treatment of lymphoma

Sources:
- **Germany – SPC:**
  - **children:** efficacy and safety have not been established
- **USA – T:**
  - **note:** Refer to individual protocols. Pretreatment with Acetaminophen and an antihistamine is recommended for all indications.

- **refractory SLE**
  - IV infusion
    - **children:** 375 mg/m² once weekly for 2–4 weeks; or 750 mg/m² on days 1 and 15 (maximum dose: 1000 mg)
    - **note:** further indications are listed in this source
- **United Kingdom – BNFC:** no dosage recommendation specified: consult local treatment protocol for details
- **Uptodate:** –
- **Drugdex®: Post-transplant lymphoproliferative disorder children:** 375 mg/m² once weekly has been used in paediatric patients in retrospective studies
  - **children:** the safety and effectiveness has not been established in paediatric patients

Comments:

- originally developed for the treatment of lymphatic malignant diseases

Rizatriptan

Dosage:

- ▶ acute therapy of migraine after insufficient success with NSAID: 5–10 mg as a SD (off-label)
- ▶ headache during radiation therapy: 10 mg as a SD (off-label)

Neuropaediatric indications:

- reducing symptoms of migraine attacks after insufficient success with NSAID
- headache during radiation therapy

Mechanism of action:

- selective agonist of the serotonin receptors 5-HT$_{1B}$ and 5-HT$_{1D}$
- at the activation of these receptors leads to constriction of the dilated cerebral vessels and to a decreased release of inflammatory mediators

Relevant contraindications:

- vasospasm, prior cerebrovascular problems or TIA
- peripheral vascular disease, arterial hypertonia, angina pectoris, severe heart diseases
- concurrent administration of MAOIs (contraindicated for up to 2 weeks after discontinuation of Rizatriptan)
- severe liver and renal impairment
- Prinzmetal angina
- careful use: hemiplegic, basilar or ophthalmoplegic migraine, other severe neurologic diseases, obesity, hypercholesterolemia, diabetes mellitus

Relevant side effects and interactions:

- angina-pectoris-like disorders, change in blood pressure
- vertigo, fatigue, sedation
- awareness of heart beat, feeling of tightness in the throat and neck region
- erythema
- using high dosages: green-black colour change of the blood (sulfhemoglobinemia)
- serotonin syndrome with concurrent administration of a triptan together with SSRI or SNRI antidepressants:
  - nausea, vomiting and diarrhea
  - restlessness, hallucinations, loss of coordination
  - tachycardia, variation in blood pressure, elevated body temperature
  - increased reflexes
- no concomitant administration of MAOIs
- Propranolol increases the serum level of Rizatriptan (waiting period after Propranolol administration: at least 2 h)

Approval status:

- ≥ 6 yrs., USA, see below

Sources:

- **Germany – SPC:** –
- **USA – T: labeling ≥ 6 yrs.**
- **United Kingdom – BNFC:** –
- **Uptodate.com:**
  - **Migraine, acute treatment**
    - oral
      - **children and adolescents ≥ 6 years, CAUTION:** safety and efficacy of multiple Rizatriptan doses in a 24-hour period has not been established for paediatric patients.
      - **< 40 kg:** 5 mg as a SD
      - **≥ 40 kg:** 10 mg as a SD

Comment:

Established combination of Rizatriptan and Naproxen

Rufinamide

Dosage:

Single dosages
< 30 kg: 200 mg every 2nd–3rd d
> 30–50 kg: 400 mg every 2nd–3rd d
Max. maintenance dose
< 30 kg: 1000 mg; with additional administration of Valproic acid, 600 mg
30–50 kg: 1800 mg
50–70 kg: 2400 mg
> 70 kg: 3200 mg
Each dose as 2 separate doses/d

Neuropaediatric indications:

- adjunctive treatment of seizures associated with Lennox-Gastaut syndrome in children 4 years and older and in adults

Mechanism of action:

- involves stabilization of sodium channels in their inactive state, effectively keeping these ion channels closed

Relevant contraindications:

- known hypersensitivity to Rufinamide, derivatives of Triazole or other ingredient

Relevant side effects:

- drowsiness, headache, vertigo
- nausea, vomiting
- fatigue
- pneumonia, influenza, nasopharyngitis, ear infections, sinusitis, rhinitis
- anorexia, eating disorder, loss of appetite
- anxiety, insomnia
- status epilepticus, convulsion, abnormal coordination, nystagmus, psychomotor agitation, hyperactivity, tremor
- diplopia, blurred vision
- vertigo
- epistaxis
- abdominal pain, constipation, dyspepsia, diarrhea
- rash, acne
- back pain
- oligomenorrhea
- motion disorder
- weight loss
- allergic reactions
- Increase of hepatic enzymes

Interactions:

- potential for other drugs to affect Rufinamide
  - Other antiepileptic drugs: Rufinamide concentrations are not subject to clinically relevant changes on co-administration of antiepileptic drugs with known enzyme-inducing activity. In patients on Rufinamide (e.g. Inovelon®) treatment who receive Valproic acid for the first time, significant increases in Rufinamide plasma concentrations may occur. The most pronounced increases were observed in patients of low body weight (< 30 kg). Therefore, consideration should be given to a dose reduction of Rufinamide in patients < 30 kg who are initiated on Valproic acid therapy. The addition or withdrawal of either of these drugs or any dose adjustments during Rufinamide therapy may require dose adjustments of the respective comedication. No significant changes in Rufinamide concentration are observed following co-administration with Lamotrigine, Topiramate or benzodiazepines.
- potential for Rufinamide to affect other drugs
  - Other antiepileptic drugs: The pharmacokinetic interactions between Rufinamide and other antiepileptic drugs have been evaluated in patients with epilepsy using population pharmacokinetic modeling. Rufinamide appears not to have clinically relevant effects on Carbamazepine, Lamotrigine, Phenobarbital, Topiramate, Phenytoin or Valproic acid steady state concentrations.
  - Oral contraceptives: Co-administration of Rufinamide 800 mg b.i.d. and a combined oral contraceptive (ethinyl estradiol 35µg and Norethindrone 1 mg) for 14 d resulted in a mean decrease in the ethinyl estradiol AUC 0–24 of 22 % and in Norethindrone AUC 0–24 of 14 %. Studies with other oral or implant contraceptives have not been conducted. Women of child-bearing potential using hormonal contraceptives are advised to use an additional safe and effective contraceptive method.
  - Cytochrome P450 enzymes: Rufinamide is metabolized by hydrolysis, and is not metabolized to any notable degree by cytochrome P450 enzymes. Furthermore, Rufinamide does not inhibit the activity of cytochrome P450 enzymes. Thus, clinically significant interactions mediated through inhibition of the cytochrome P450 system by Rufinamide are unlikely to occur. Rufinamide has been shown to induce the cytochrome P450 enzyme CYP3A4 and may therefore reduce the plasma concentrations of substances which are metabolized by this enzyme. The effect was modest to moderate. The mean CYP3A4 activity, assessed as clearance of Triazolam, was increased by 55 % after 11 days of treatment with Rufinamide 400 mg b.i.d. The exposure of Triazolam was reduced by 36 %. Higher Rufinamide

doses may result in a more pronounced induction. It may not be excluded that Rufinamide may also decrease the exposure of substances metabolized by other enzymes, or transported by transport proteins such as P-glycoprotein. It is recommended that patients treated with substances that are metabolized by the CYP3A4 enzyme system are to be carefully monitored for two weeks at the start of, or after the end of treatment with Rufinamide, or after any marked change in the dose. A dose adjustment of the concomitantly administered drugs may need to be considered. These recommendations should also be considered when Rufinamide is used concomitantly with substances with a narrow therapeutic range such as Warfarin and Digoxin. A specific interaction study in healthy subjects revealed no influence of Rufinamide at a dose of 400 mg b.i.d on the pharmacokinetics of olanzapine, a CYP1A2 substrate.

- No data on the interaction of Rufinamide with alcohol are available.

Approval status:

adjunctive treatment of seizures associated with Lennox-Gastaut syndrome in children 4 years and older and in adults

Sources:

Germany – SPC:
- **adjunctive therapy of Lennox-Gastaut syndrome**
  - oral
  - no additional information to USA – T or United Kingdom – BNFC
- **USA – T:**
- **Lennox-Gastaut syndrome**
  - oral
    - **children ≥ 4 years:** initially 10 mg/kg/d as 2 separate doses; increase dose by ~ 10 mg/kg increments every other day to a target dose of 45 mg/kg/d as 2 separate doses (max. 3200 mg/d); effectiveness of doses lower than the target dose is unknown
- **United Kingdom – BNFC:**
- **adjunctive treatment of seizures in Lennox-Gastaut syndrome**
  - oral
    - **children 4–18 years (< 30 kg):** initially 100 mg/dose twice daily, increase according to response in steps of 100 mg twice daily up to every 2 d; max. 1000 mg/d as 2 separate doses (max. 600 mg/d as 2 separate doses if adjunctive therapy with Valproic acid)
    - **children 4–18 years (> 30 kg):** initially 200 mg/dose twice daily, increase according to response in steps of 200 mg/dose twice daily up to every 2 d
    - **30–50 kg:** max. 900 mg/dose twice daily;
    - **50–70 kg:** max. 1200 mg/dose twice daily;
    - **> 70 kg:** max. 1600 mg/dose twice daily

S

Scopolamine

Dosage:
- ▶ 1.5 mg/72 h

Neuropaediatric indications:
- sialorrhea

Mechanism of action:
- vagolytic drug; belongs to the natural alkaloids of various plants in the Solanaceae family
- exerts its effects by acting as a competitive antagonist at muscarinic acetylcholine receptors
- using high dosages inhibits nicotinic acetylcholine receptors and consequently the transfer to autonomic ganglia and the neuromuscular junction
- therapeutic dosages have a centrally depressant effect on the CNS (in contrast to Atropine)

Relevant contraindications:
- angle-closure glaucoma

Relevant side effects and interactions:
- accommodation impairment, elevated intraocular pressure
- dry mouth, nausea
- voiding disorders
- anxiety, apathy, hallucinations, paramnesias
- coordination disorders
- tachycardia
- local skin reactions
- mutually reduced effect of Scopolamine and dopamine antagonists (e.g. Metoclopramide)
- enhanced effect with antihistamines
- H_2 receptor block (e.g. Ranitidine) results in an additional reduction of gastric acid production

Approval status:
- contraindicated in children under the age of 10 due to the increased risk of intoxication

Sources:
- Germany – SPC:
  - indication of interest is not mentioned
- USA – T:
  - **preoperatively and antiemetic**
    - IM, IV, SC
      - **children:** 0,006 mg/kg/dose (max. 0.3 mg/dose); may be repeated every 6–8 h
- United Kingdom – BNFC:
  - **excessive respiratory secretions**
    - transdermal
      - **children 1–3 months:** 0.25 mg/72 h
      - **children 3 months–10 years:** 0.5 mg/72 h
      - **children 10–18 years:** 1 mg/72 h
    - oral, sublingual
      - **children 2–12 years:** 0.01 mg/kg, max. 0.3 mg/dose 4 times daily
      - **children 12–18 years:** 1.2 mg/d as 4 separate doses
  - **drooling associated with Clozapine therapy**
    - oral
      - **children 12–18 years:** 0.3 mg up to 3 times daily; max. 0.9 mg/d

Comments:
- rarely sufficiently effective
- various dosages published in common paediatric sources

Stiripentol

Dosage:
- ▶ max. maintenance dose
- ▶ children: 50 mg/kg/d as 2 separate doses
- ▶ adults: 2000–3000 mg/d as 2 separate doses

Neuropaediatric indications:
- Stiripentol is indicated for use in conjunction with Clobazam and Valproic acid as adjunctive therapy of refractory generalized tonic-clonic seizures in infants with severe myoclonic epilepsy (SMEI, Dravet's syndrome) whose seizures are not adequately controlled with Clobazam and Valproic acid

Mechanism of action:
- antiepileptic drug
- precise mechanism of action is not clear

Relevant contraindications:
- Carbamazepine, Phenytoin and Phenobarbital
- These substances should not be used in conjunction with Stiripentol in the management of Dravet's syndrome. The daily dosage of Clobazam and/or Valproic acid should be reduced according to the onset of side effects whilst on Stiripentol therapy.
- growth rate of children
- given the frequency of gastrointestinal adverse reactions to treatment with Stiripentol and Valproic acid (anorexia, loss of appetite, nausea, vomiting), the growth rate of children under this combination of treatment should be carefully monitored.
- neutropenia
- may be associated with the administration of Stiripentol, Clobazam and Valproic acid
- Blood counts: Should be assessed prior to starting treatment with Stiripentol. Unless otherwise clinically indicated, blood counts should be checked every 6 months.
- liver function: Should be assessed prior to starting treatment with Stiripentol. Unless otherwise clinically indicated, liver function should be checked every 6 months.
- hepatic or renal impairment: In the absence of specific clinical data in patients with impaired hepatic or renal function, Stiripentol is not recommended for use in patients with impaired hepatic and/or renal function.
- substances interfering with CYP enzymes: Stiripentol is an inhibitor of the enzymes CYP2C19, CYP3A4 and CYP2D6 and may markedly increase the plasma concentrations of substances metabolized by these enzymes and increase the risk of adverse reactions. In vitro studies suggested that Stiripentol phase 1 metabolism is catalyzed by CYP1A2, CYP2C19 and CYP3A4 and possibly other enzymes. Caution is advised when combining Stiripentol with other substances that inhibit or induce one or more of these enzymes.
- The pivotal clinical studies did not include children younger than 3 years. As a consequence, it is recommended that children between 6 months and 3 years of age are carefully monitored whilst on Stiripentol therapy.

Relevant side effects:
- anorexia, loss of appetite, weight loss (especially when combined with sodium Valproic acid)
- insomnia
- drowsiness, ataxia, hypotension, dystonia
- neutropenia (severe neutropenia usually resolves spontaneously when Stiripentol is stopped)
- thrombocytopenia
- aggressiveness, irritability, behavioural disorders, opposing behaviour, hyperexcitability, sleep disorders
- hyperkinesias
- nausea, vomiting

- raised γ-GT (notably when combined with Carbamazepine and Valproic acid)
- diplopia (when used in combination with Carbamazepine)
- photosensitivity, rash, cutaneous allergy, urticaria
- fatigue
- liver function parameters
- pathologic

Interactions:

- potential drug interactions affecting Stiripentol
  - the influence of other antiepileptic drugs on Stiripentol pharmacokinetics is not well established. The impact of macrolides and azole antifungal agents on Stiripentol metabolism that are known to be inhibitors of CYP3A4 and substrates of the same enzyme, is not known. Likewise, the effect of Stiripentol on their metabolism is not known.
  - in vitro studies suggested that Stiripentol phase 1 metabolism is catalyzed by CYP1A2, CYP2C19 and CYP3A4 and possibly other enzymes. Caution is advised when combining Stiripentol with other substances that inhibit or induce one or more of these enzymes.
  - effect of Stiripentol on cytochrome P450 enzymes: Many of these interactions have been partially confirmed by in vitro studies and in clinical trials. The increase in steady state levels with the combined use of Stiripentol, Valproic acid, and Clobazam is similar in adults and children, though inter-individual variability is marked. At therapeutic concentrations, Stiripentol significantly inhibits several CYP450 isoenzymes: for example, CYP2C19, CYP2D6 and CYP3A4. As a result, pharmacokinetic interactions of metabolic origin with other medicines may be expected. These interactions may result in increased systemic levels of these active substances that may lead to enhanced pharmacological effects and to an increase in adverse reactions.
  - caution must be exercised if clinical circumstances require combining Stiripentol with substances metabolized by CYP2C19 (e.g. Citalopram, Omeprazole) or CYP3A4 (e.g. HIV protease inhibitors, antihistamines such as Astemizole, Chlorpheniramine, Calcium channel blockers, statins, oral contraceptives, Codeine) due to the increased risk of adverse reactions (see further in this section for antiepileptic medicines). Monitoring of plasma concentrations or adverse reactions is recommended. A dose adjustment may be necessary. Co-administration with CYP3A4 substrates with a narrow therapeutic index should be avoided due to the markedly increased risk of severe adverse reactions. Data on the potential for inhibition of CYP1A2 are limited, and therefore, interactions with Theophylline and Caffeine cannot be excluded because of the increased plasma levels of Theophylline and Caffeine which may occur via inhibition of their hepatic metabolism, potentially leading to toxicity. Use in combination with Stiripentol is not recommended. This warning is not only restricted to drugs but also to a considerable number of foods and nutritional products aimed at children, such as cola drinks, which contain significant quantities of Caffeine or chocolate, which contains trace amounts of Theophylline.
  - as Stiripentol inhibited CYP2D6 in vitro at concentrations that are achieved clinically in plasma, substances that are metabolized by this isoenzyme like beta blockers (Propranolol, Carvedilol, Timolol), antidepressants (Fluoxetine, Paroxetine, Sertraline, Imipramine, Clomipramine), antipsychotics (Haloperidol), analgesics (Codeine, Dextromethorphan, Tramadol) may be subject to metabolic interactions with Stiripentol. A dose adjustment may be necessary for substances metabolized by CYP2D6 and that are individually dose titrated.
  - potential for Stiripentol to interact with other drugs: In the absence of available clinical data, caution should be taken with the following clinically relevant interactions with Stiripentol:
- undesirable combinations (to be avoided unless strictly necessary)
  - Rye ergot alkaloids (Ergotamine, Dihydroergotamine): Ergotism with possibility of necrosis of the extremities (inhibition of hepatic elimination of rye ergot)
  - Cisapride, Halofantrine, Pimozide, Quinidine, Bepridil: Increased risk of cardiac arrhythmias and torsades de pointes/wave burst arrhythmia in particular.
  - immunosuppressants (Tacrolimus, Cyclosporine, Sirolimus): Raised blood levels of immunosuppressants (decreased hepatic metabolism).
  - Statins (Atorvastatin, Simvastatin, etc.): Increased risk of dose-dependent adverse reactions such as rhabdomyolysis (decreased hepatic metabolism of cholesterol-lowering agent). Combinations requiring precautions.
  - Midazolam, Triazolam, Alprazolam: Increased plasma benzodiazepine levels may occur via decreased hepatic metabolism leading to excessive sedation.
  - Chlorpromazine: Stiripentol enhances the central depressant effect of Chlorpromazine.
  - effects on other AEDs: Inhibition of CYP450 isoenzyme CYP2C19 and CYP3A4 may provoke pharmacokinetic interactions (inhibition of their hepatic metabolism) with Phenobarbital, Primidone, Phenytoin, Carbamazepine, Clobazam, Valproic acid, Diazepam (enhanced myorelaxation), Ethosuximide, and Tiagabine. The consequences are increased plasma levels of these anticonvulsants with potential risk of overdose. Clinical monitoring of plasma levels of other anticonvulsants when combined with Stiripentol with possible dose adjustments is recommended.
  - Topiramate: In a French compassionate use program for Stiripentol, Topiramate was added to Stiripentol, Clobazam and Valproic acid in 41 % of 230 cases. Based on the clinical observations in this group of patients, there is no evidence to suggest that a change in Topiramate dose and dosage schedules is needed if co-administered with Stiripentol. With regard to Topiramate, it is considered that potential competition of inhibition on CYP2C19 should not occur because it probably

requires plasma concentrations 5–15 times higher than plasma concentrations obtained with the standard recommended Topiramate dose and dosage schedules.
- Levetiracetam: Levetiracetam does not undergo hepatic metabolism to a major extent. As a result, no pharmacokinetic metabolic drug interaction between Stiripentol and Levetiracetam is anticipated.

Approval status:

- use in conjunction with Clobazam and Valproic acid as adjunctive therapy of refractory generalized tonic-clonic seizures in patients with severe myoclonic epilepsy in infancy (SMEI, Dravet's syndrome), whose seizures are not adequately controlled with Clobazam and Valproic acid
- children > 3 years of age

Sources:

- **Germany – SPC:**
- **Preparation Diacomit® is indicated for use in conjunction with Clobazam and Valproic acid as adjunctive therapy of refractory generalized tonic clonic seizures in patients with severe myoclonic epilepsy in infancy (SMEI, Dravet's syndrome) whose seizures are not adequately controlled with Clobazam and Valproic acid.**
  - oral
  - **note:** only under an appropriately qualified specialist's supervision
  - initial therapy is recommended for 3 d followed by a gradual increase of doses to the recommended 50 mg/kg/d as 2–3 separate doses (during meal), administered with Clobazam and Valproic acid. There is no data available for use of doses > 50 mg/kg/d.
  - dose adjustments of other antiepileptics used in combination with Stiripentol
  - despite the absence of comprehensive pharmacological data on potential drug interactions, the following advice regarding modification of the dose and dosage schedules of other antiepileptic drugs administered in conjunction with Stiripentol is provided based on clinical experience.
  - Clobazam: In the pivotal studies, when the use of Stiripentol was initiated, the daily dose of Clobazam was 0.5 mg/kg/d usually administered as separate doses, twice daily. In the event of clinical signs of adverse reactions or overdose of Clobazam (i.e., drowsiness, hypotonia, and irritability in young children), this daily dose was reduced by 25 % every week. Approximately two to three-fold increases in Clobazam and five-fold increases in norClobazam plasma levels respectively have been reported with co-administration of Stiripentol in children with Dravet's syndrome.
  - Valproic acid: The potential for metabolic interaction between Stiripentol and Valproic acid is considered modest and thus no modification of Valproic acid dosage should be needed when Stiripentol is added, except for clinical safety reasons. In the pivotal studies in the event of gastrointestinal adverse reactions such as loss of appetite, loss of weight, the daily dose of Valproic acid was reduced by around 30 % every week.
    - **children < 3 years:** the pivotal clinical evaluation of Stiripentol was done in children of 3 years of age and older with SMEI. The clinical decision for use of Stiripentol in children with SMEI less than 3 years of age needs to be made on an individual patient basis taking into consideration the potential clinical benefits and risks. In this younger group of patients, adjunctive therapy with Stiripentol should only be started when the diagnosis of SMEI has been clinically confirmed. Data are limited about the use of Stiripentol under 12 months of age. For these children the use of Stiripentol will be done under the close supervision of the specialist.
- **USA – T:** –
- **United Kingdom – BNFC:**
  - **severe myoclonic epilepsy in infancy**
    - oral
      - **children 3–18 years:** initially 10 mg/kg as 2–3 separate doses; titrate dose over a minimum of 3 d to max. 50 mg/kg/d as 2–3 separate doses

Sulthiame (STM)

Dosage:
- Rolandic epilepsy: (3–)5–10 mg/kg/d (SPC)
- [West syndrome: 5–15 mg/kg/d as 2(–4) separate doses (off-label)]

Neuropaediatric indications:

- Rolandic epilepsy
- West syndrome
- focal epilepsy

Mechanism of action:

- Sulfonamide, but without antimicrobial effect
- no structural similarity with other anticonvulsants
- potential inhibitor of carbonic anhydrase primarily in the CNS
- mechanism of action is not completely understood
- leads to increased carbon dioxide levels and thus mild acidification of extracellular fluid, which may partly explain the anticonvulsive effectiveness of Sulthiame
- inhibitory effect on voltage-gated sodium channels resulting in depressed neuronal excitation
- interaction with neurotransmitters has not been clearly established so far

Relevant contraindications:

- porphyria
- hyperthyroidism
- arterial hypertension
- careful use: renal impairment, medical history or present psychiatric diseases, women in child-bearing age and girls > 11 years, hereditary intolerance of galactose, deficiency of lactase, glucose-galactose malabsorption, pregnancy

Relevant side effects and interactions:

- in over 40 years of clinical treatment, no life-threatening side effects that have been related to Sulthiame alone
- but reversible adverse events are relatively frequent
- most frequent: hyperventilation (caused by metabolic acidosis), paresthesia, gastro-intestinal disorders (stomach trouble, weight loss, loss of appetite) and vigilance disorders
- dyspnea, vertigo, headache, double vision, arthralgias, muscle weakness, hiccup
- hallucinations, anxiety, avolition, status epilepticus, higher frequency of seizures
- allergic reaction: fever, swelling of lymph nodes, sore throat, flu-like symptoms
- side effects of the carbonic anhydrase inhibition: kidney stones, acidosis
- Primidone can enhance the side effects of Sulthiame
- plasma level of Phenytoin can be elevated

Approval status:

- alternative treatment of Rolandic epilepsy

Sources:

- **Germany – SPC:**
  - **alternative treatment of Rolandic epilepsy, if treatment failed with other antiepileptic drugs**
    - oral
    - Dosing is individual and the physician has to decide the amount of intake. Maintenance dose: about 5–10 mg/kg/d as 3 separate doses (attained over a titration period of one week). Constant plasma levels after 5–6 d.
- **USA – T:** –
- **United Kingdom – BNFC:** –
- **Drugdex®:** –
- **Uptodate.com:** –

Comments:

- in Germany (practice) first choice to treat Rolandic epilepsy
- one of the oldest approved antiepileptics (approval in 1960 by Bayer)
- in two studies, Sulthiame was 30–35 % efficacious for short-term treatment of West syndrome. The advantage of this medication is the short time required for assessment of the effectiveness (1–2 weeks) and only few and less serious side effects (indication West remains controvers).

Sumatriptan

Dosage:

- ▶ acute migraine therapy after unsatisfactory success with NSAID: nasal 10–20 mg/dose
- ▶ emergency situation of migraine: SC max. 6 mg/dose
- ▶ (velum tremor: experimental, no established dose for children)

Neuropaediatric indications:

- acute symptom treatment during migraine attacks after unsatisfactory success with NSAID
- velum tremor

Mechanism of action:

- a selective agonist of serotonin receptors 5-HT_{1B}, 5-HT_{1D} and 5-HT_{1F} (cerebral vessels and presynaptic neuronal cleft)
- activation of these receptors leads to vasoconstriction of dilated cerebral arteries and to a decreased release of inflammatory mediators

Relevant contraindications:

- vasospasm, prior cerebrovascular disorders or TIA
- peripheral vascular diseases, arterial hypertonia, angina pectoris, severe heart diseases
- concomitant intake of MAOIs (contraindicated for up to two weeks after discontinuation of Sumatriptan therapy)
- severe liver and renal impairment

Relevant side effects and interactions:

- unpleasant taste
- angina-pectoris-like disorders, change in blood pressure
- vertigo, fatigue, sedation
- awareness of heart beat, feeling of tightness in throat and neck
- erythema
- high dosages can lead to green-black colour of blood (sulfhemoglobinemia)
- serotonin syndrome when combining triptan with antidepressants (either SSRI or SNRI):
  - nausea, vomiting and diarrhea
  - restlessness, hallucinations, loss of coordination
  - tachycardia, variation in blood pressure, elevated body temperature
  - Increased reflexes

- no concomitant intake of MAOIs
- ergotamine increases the risk of coronary spasms

Approval status:
- depends on the specific product (see SPC)

Sources:
- **Germany – SPC:**
  - **acute treatment of migraine with or without aura**
    - **children ≥ 12 years:** 10–20 mg intranasal/dose
    - **children 12–18 years:** 10–20 mg as a SD; repeat once after > 2 h if migraine reoccurs, max. 40 g in 24 h
    - **note:** child not responding to initial dose should not receive a second dose for same attack
- **USA – T:**
  - **acute treatment of migraine with or without aura**
    - **note:** for children < 18 years of age not recommended by manufacturer
    - Study: (n = 17, age: 6–16 years, patients with juvenile migraine): SC, 6 mg in 15 children (30–70 kg), 3 mg/dose in 2 patients (22 and 30 kg)
- **United Kingdom – BNFC:**
  - **treatment of acute migraine**
    - oral
      - **children 6–10 years:** 25 mg as a SD; repeat once after > 2 h if migraine reoccurs
      - **children 10–12 years:** 50 mg as a SD; repeat once after > 2 h if migraine reoccurs
      - **children 12–18 years:** 50–100 mg as a SD; repeat once after > 2 h if migraine reoccurs
    - SC injection:
      - **children 12–18 years:** 6 mg as a SD; repeat once after > 1 h if migraine recurs, max. 12 mg in 24 h
    - intranasal:
      - **children 12–18 years:** 10–20 mg as a SD; repeat once after > 2 h if migraine recurs, max. 40 mg in 24 h
    - **note:** child not responding to initial dose should not receive a second dose for same attack
  - **treatment of acute cluster headache (under specialist supervision)**
    - SC injection
      - **children 10–18 years:** 6 mg as a SD; repeat once after > 1 h if headache recurs; max. 12 mg in 24 h
    - intranasal
      - **children 12–18 years:** 10–20 mg as a SD; repeat once after > 2 h if headache recurs; max. 40 mg in 24 h

T

Tacrolimus

(also called FK-506, or Fujimycin)

Dosage:
▶ local administration: apply twice daily over 4–6 weeks (positive effects are reported in some cases with continuing skin symptoms in good muscle condition)

Neuropaediatric indications:
- severe therapy-resistant myositis

Mechanism of action:
- macrolide from Streptomyces tsukubaensis
- binds to immunophilin FKBP12 (FK506 binding protein) and creates a new complex
- this FKBP12-FK506 complex interacts with and inhibits calcineurin thus inhibiting both T-lymphocyte signal transduction and IL-2 transcription
- similar mechanism of action as Ciclosporin

Relevant contraindications (only as ointment formulation):
- hypersensitivity against macrolides
- prior to start of the treatment, local infection should be healed
- careful use: herpes simplex infection, genetically determined impairement of the epidermis-barrier (e.g. Netherton's syndrome), concomitant administration of other topical drugs, concomitant consumption of systemic steroids, immunosuppressive drugs or CYP3A4 inhibitors, skin diseases

Relevant side effects and interactions:
- up to 50 % of the patients: skin burning, pruritus, flush
- skin prickling, folliculitis, acne, herpes simplex, hyperesthesia, intolerance of alcohol

Approval status:
- in children younger than 2 years

Sources:
- **Germany – SPC:**
- SPC does not specify this indication of interest
- **USA – T:**
- **Prevention of organ rejection**
  - oral

- liver transplant
  - **children:** initially 0.15–0.2 mg/kg/d as 2 separate doses
  - **note:** further indications are listed in this source
- **United Kingdom – BNFC:** indication of interest is not mentioned
- **Uptodate.com:** indication of interest is not mentioned
  - **moderate to severe atopic dermatitis**
  - **dermal (preparation Protopic®)**
  - **note:** Discontinue use when symptoms have cleared. If no improvement occurs within 6 weeks, patients should be re-examined to confirm diagnosis.
  - **children and adolescents ≥ 2–15 years:** apply a thin layer of 0.03 % ointment to affected area twice daily; rub in gently and completely
  - **adolescents ≥ 16 years:** apply a thin layer of 0.03 % or 0.1 % ointment to affected area twice daily; rub in gently and completely

Comments:

- various dosages published in common paediatric sources

Tetrabenazine

> **Dosage:**
> ▶ initially 25 mg, increase by 25 mg/week up to max. 100–200 mg/d as 3 separate doses (off-label)

Neuropaediatric indications:

- dystonia
- heredodegenerative or secondary dystonia
- hyperkinetic movement disorders in Huntington's disease and Sydenham's chorea
- therapy-resistant moderate to severe tardive dyskinesia

Mechanism of action:

- inhibits reversibly the vesicular monoamine transporter 2 (VMAT2)
- promotes the early metabolic degradation of dopamine (less dopamine in the presynaptic vesicles), which leads to a decreased signaling

Relevant contraindications:

- prolactin-dependent tumors
- pheochromocytoma
- depressive mood
- concomitant intake of MAOIs (contraindicated for up to 2 weeks after discontinuation of Tetrabenazine)
- careful use: medical history of tumor, hereditary intolerance of galactose, lactase deficiency, glucose-galactose malabsorption

Relevant side effects and interactions:

- frequent: drowsiness, depression, agitation, confusion, anxiety, insomnia, symptoms of Parkinson's diseases (e. g. vestibular disorder, drooling, tremor)
- rare: leukopenia, neuroleptic malignant syndrome, oculogyric crisis, photophobia, disorientation, ataxia, akathisia, dystonia, disturbance of memory, vertigo, bradycardia, hypotension, dysphagia, dry mouth, sweating, weakness
- hyperprolactinemia (galactorrhea, gynecomastia, oligo- or amenorrhea, erectile dysfunction)
- inhibits effect of L-dopa
- enhanced effect of alcohol and centrally acting drugs
- combination with MAOIs can result in severe side effects

Approval status:

- no explicit paediatric approval

Sources:

- **Germany – SPC:**
  - **hyperkinetic disorders due to Huntington's chorea, moderate to severe tardive dyskinesia**
    - oral
      - **children:** There have not been any controlled clinical trials. Limited clinical experience is available and suggests a 50 % reduced adult dose to start with, then titrate gradually to response.
  - **Huntington's chorea**
    - **adults:** initially: 75 mg/d as 3 separate doses. May be increased every 3–4 d by 25 mg/d to response or side effects; max. 200 mg/d.
    - If no response with max. dose after 7 d, this medication is unlikely to be useful for the patient.
  - **tardive dyskinesia**
    - **adults:** Initially 12.5 mg/d; increase according to response. Interrupt treatment if no response is seen or side effects occur.
- **USA – T:** –
- **United Kingdom – BNFC:** –
- **Uptodate.com:**
- no published paediatric dosage
  - **chorea associated with Huntington's disease**
    - oral
      - **adults:** initially 12.5 mg once daily; may be increased to 12.5 mg twice daily after 1 week
      - maintenance: may be increased by 12.5 mg/d at weekly intervals; doses > 37.5 mg/d separated to 3 doses (maximum single dose: 25 mg)
      - patients requiring doses > 50 mg/d: genotype for CYP2D6:
      - extensive/intermediate metabolizers: maximum of 100 mg/d; 37.5 mg/dose
      - poor metabolizers: maximum of 50 mg/d; 25 mg/dose
      - Concomitant use with strong CYP2D6 inhibitors (e. g., Fluoxetine, Paroxetine, Quinidine): Dose of Tetrabenazine should be reduced by 50 % in patients receiving strong CYP2D6 inhibitors; follow dosing for poor CYP2D6 metabolizers. Use caution when adding a CYP2D6 inhibitor to patients already taking Tetrabenazine.

- **note:** If treatment is interrupted for > 5 d, retitration is recommended. If treatment is interrupted for < 5 d resume at previous maintenance dose.
- **Drugdex®:**
  - **spontaneous dyskinesia**
    - oral
      - in two children (8 and 13 years of age), some improvement was seen with doses of 50 mg and 150 mg daily
      - safety and efficacy have not been established in children

Comments:
- release of dopamine from synaptic vesicles; reversible effect after 24 h

Tetrazepam

Dosage:
- ▶ loading dose: 2 mg/kg/d
- ▶ prolonged treatment: 4 mg/kg/d

Neuropaediatric indications:
- generalized spasticity/dystonia with cerebral palsy

Mechanism of action:
- benzodiazepine
- opens chloride channels and therefore conditional enhancement of the inhibitory function of GABA neurons
- chiefly a muscle relaxant; compared to other benzodiazepines less anxiolytic, sedative, hypnotic and anticonvulsive

Relevant contraindications:
- drug-, alcohol-addiction
- acute angle-closure glaucoma
- < 1 year of age
- careful use:
  - myasthenia gravis
  - cerebellar and spinal ataxia (disorders of balance and movement coordination)
  - acute poisoning with alcohol, analgesics, sleep-inducing drugs, neuroleptics, antidepressants, Lithium
  - severe impairement of liver function
  - severe respiratory insufficiency
  - sleep apnea
  - severe chronic hypercapnia
- risk of addiction
- pregnancy

Relevant side effects and interactions:
- respiratory depression especially by IV administration in status epilepticus, risk of respiratory depression is higher when given several low doses than one high bolus dose
- fatigue, drowsiness, lack of concentration, anterograde amnesia
- headache, confusion, articulation disorders, vertigo
- muscle weakness, unstable walking
- impaired vision, double vision, nystagmus
- dry mouth, gastrointestinal disorders
- depressive mood
- increase of libido
- addiction with chronic administration
- temporary increase of liver function parameters
- decrease in blood pressure
- mutually enhanced effect when combined with other centrally acting drugs or alcohol
- enhanced effect of muscle relaxants, analgesics and laughing gas
- Cimetidine results in enhancement and prolonging of the effect of Tetrazepam
- prolonged treatment: type and severity of interaction with centrally acting anti-hypertensives, beta blockers and anticoagulants not predictable

Approval status:
- depends on the specific product (see SPC)

Sources:
- **Germany – SPC:**
  - **severe spastic syndromes**
    - oral
      - **children ≥ 1 year:** usual max. 4 mg/kg/d as 3 separate doses
      - **CAUTION:** do not use in children < 1 year
- **USA – T:** –
- **United Kingdom – BNFC:** –
- **Uptodate.com:**
  - no published paediatric dosage
  - **treatment of painful muscular contractions**
    - oral
      - adults: 50 mg at bedtime; may be increased by 25 mg/d until the maximum dose of 150 mg/d is reached; may be taken as 2–3 separate doses with the larger dose given in the evening

Theophylline

(Aminophylline)

Dosage:

▸ 3–4 mg/kg/d

Neuropaediatric indications:

– breathing disorders with hypoxemia

Mechanism of action:

– competitive, non-selective cAMP-specific inhibition of two phosphodiesterase isozymes (PDE3 and PDE4)

Relevant contraindications:

– current myocardial infarction
– acute cardiac arrhythmias
– careful use: unstable angina pectoris, cardiac arrhythmia related to substance abuse, severe hypertension, hypertrophic obstructive cardiomyopathy, hyperthyroidism, epilepsy, gastrointestinal ulcera, porphyria, hepatic or renal disorders

Relevant side effects and interactions:

– headache, agitation, tremors or shaking, irritability, insomnia
– seizures (Theophylline plasma levels > 25 mcg/ml)
– nausea, vomiting, diarrhea
– increase of gastroesophageal reflux disease
– gastrointestinal bleeding (Theophylline plasma levels > 25 mcg/ml)
– tachycardia, palpitations, hypotension
– changing serum electrolytes (primarily hypokalemia, increased Calcium serum levels), increase of serum creatinine, hyperglycemia, hyperuricemia
– increased diuresis
– ventricular arrhythmia, sudden decrease of blood pressure (Theophylline plasma levels > 25 mcg/ml)
– allergic reactions
– synergistic effect with other xanthines, beta sympathomimetics, Caffeine, diuretics
– elevated Theophylline plasma levels with concurrent use of macrolides, oral contraceptives, gyrase inhibitors, Imipenem, Isoniazid, Tiabendazole, Calcium antagonists, Propranolol, Mexiletine, Propafenone, Ticlopidine, Cimetidine, Allopurinol, alpha-interferon, influenza-vaccines, Ranitidine, Ciprofloxacin, Enoxacin

– reduced Theophylline plasma levels with concurrent use of barbiturates, Carbamazepine, Phenytoin, Rifampicin, Primidone, Sulfinpyrazone
– reduced plasma levels of concurrently used Lithium carbonate and beta blockers
– severe cardiac arrhythmia in combination with Halothane

Approval status:

– depends on the specific product (see SPC)

Sources:

– Germany – SPC:
  – **treatment of symptoms and reversible airway obstruction due to chronic asthma, chronic bronchitis, or COPD**
    – **note:** only in special cases should **children < 1 year** be treated with Theophylline. **children ≥ 6 months** need higher body weight related doses than adults who are non-smokers. By contrast, in **infants < 6 months**, Theophylline elimination is reduced.
    – IV
    – **depending on age and comorbidities, the initial dose for patients without prior Theophylline treatment is** 4–5 mg/kg over 20–30 min, **for patients with prior Theophylline treatment** 2–2.5 mg/kg over 20–30 min
    – maintenance dose
    – **children 6 months–9 years:** 1 mg/kg/h for 1–12 h; then 0.8 mg/kg/h (19 mg/kg/d)
    – **children 9 years–16 years:** 0.8 mg/kg/h for 1–12 h; then 0.65 mg/kg/h (15 mg/kg/d)
– USA – T:
  – **apnea of prematurity**
    – oral (fast release product should be used)
      – **neonates:** loading with 5–6 mg/kg/dose; maintenance with 2–6 mg/kg/d as 2–3 separate doses
      – **manufacturer's recommendation:**
      – **neonates:** Loading with 4.6 mg/kg/dose
      – premature neonates, postnatal age < 24 d: 1 mg/kg/dose every 12 h
      – premature neonates, postnatal age ≥ 24 d: 1.5 mg/kg/dose every 12 h
      – full-term infants: total daily dose (mg)= [(0.2 × age in weeks) + 5] × (weight in kg); separate dose into 3 equal amounts and administer at 8-h intervals
– **United Kingdom – BNFC:** as Aminophylline
  – **neonatal apnea**
    – IV injection over 20 min
      – **neonates:** initially 6 mg/kg, then 2.5 mg/kg/dose every 12 h (increased if necessary to 3.5 mg/kg/dose every 12 h)
      – **note:** optimum response with plasma Theophylline levels of 8–12 mcg/ml

Thiopental

Dosage:
- ▶ decrease of intracranial pressure: 1–5 mg/kg as bolus or 1–5 mg/kg/h by infusion
- ▶ CAUTION: decrease of blood pressure (careful monitoring)
- ▶ status epilepticus:
  - administration in emergency condition including EEG monitoring
  - bolus 5 mg/kg, then 3–5 mg/kg/h (dosing along EEG)

Neuropaediatric indications:
- reducing intracranial pressure
- therapy-resistant status epilepticus (over > 60 min)
- anesthesia

Mechanism of action:
- short-term acting barbiturate without analgesic effect
- binding to the $GABA_A$ receptor and thus enhanced inhibitory effect of GABA
- block of AMPA receptors and thus reduced effect of the excitatory neurotransmitter glutamate

Relevant contraindications:
- intoxication with alcohol, hypnotic drugs, analgesics, psychotropic drugs
- acute hepatic porphyria
- shock
- status asthmaticus
- malignant hypertension
- careful use: obstructive respiratory diseases, hypovolemia, severe myocardial impairement, severe liver and renal function disorders, infants < 1 year

Relevant side effects and interactions:
- allergic dermal reactions, nausea, vomiting
- phlebitis, thrombosis, venous pain
- coughing, sneezing, bronchial spasms, laryngospasms, respiratory depression
- euphoria, nightmares
- mutually enhanced effect when administered with central nervous system depressants and alcohol
- decreased effect of cumarines, griseofulvin, glucocorticoids and oral contraceptives
- enhanced effect of Methotrexate and anticonvulsants

Approval status:
- depends on the specific product (see SPC)

Sources:
- **Germany – SPC:** -
- **USA – T:**
  - increased intracranial pressure
    - IV
      - **children:** 1.5–5 mg/kg/dose; repeat as needed to control intracranial pressure; larger doses (30 mg/kg) to induce coma after hypoxic-ischaemic injury do not appear to improve neurologic outcome
  - seizures
    - IV
      - **children:** 2–3 mg/kg/dose, repeat as needed
- **United Kingdom – BNFC:**
  - **prolonged status epilepticus**
    - slow IV injection and infusion
      - **neonates:** initially up to 2 mg/kg by IV injection, then up to 8 mg/kg/h by continuous IV infusion, adjusted according to response
      - **children 1 month–18 years:** initially up to 4 mg/kg by IV injection, then up to 8 mg/kg/h by continuous IV infusion, adjusted according to response

Comments:
- CAUTION: avoid paravenous or intraarterial injections (risk of severe tissue necrosis and local necrosis)
- subtherapeutic blood levels: < 1 mcg/ml
- half-life: 3–8 hrs
- status epilepticus:
- advantage:
  - about 74–100 % effective
  - for adults: better than Midazolam + Propofol
  - compared to high dosages of Phenobarbital, faster acting on the CNS, better manageable due to shorter half-life
- disadvantage:
  - liposoluble, therefore accumulation in fatty tissues possible
  - considerable adverse events: respiratory depression, decreased blood pressure, reduced cardiac output
- various dosages published in common paediatric sources

Tiagabine

Dosage:
- ▶ 0.25–1.5 mg/kg/d as 2–3 separate doses p.o. (off-label)
- ▶ increase daily dose, e.g. weekly, by 0.25 mg/kg (off-label)

Neuropaediatric indications:
- adjunctive therapy of focal epilepsy

Mechanism of action:
- blocks GABA uptake

Relevant contraindications:
- severe liver function disorders
- pregnancy
- careful use: behavioural disorder, anxiety, depression, galactosemia, lapp lactase deficiency, glucose-galactose malabsorption, generalized epilepsy (especially idiopathic forms with absences, LGS or similar disorders)

Relevant side effects and interactions:
- nausea, diarrhea
- drowsiness, vertigo, somnolence, concentration disorders, depressive mood
- tremor, ataxia, nystagmus
- rare event: non-convulsive status epilepticus
- CYP450-inducing drugs (Phenytoin, Phenobarbital, Primidone, Carbamazepine, Rifampicin) accelerate metabolism of Tiagabine

Approval status:
- anticonvulsive adjunctive therapy: patients > 12 years with focal and secondary generalized seizures

Sources:
- **Germany – SPC:**
  - **adjunctive therapy in the treatment of partial seizures with or without secondary generalization, when other antiepileptic drugs are not sufficiently effective**
    - oral
    - **together with enzyme-inducing comedication:**
      - **children > 12 years:** initially 5–10 mg/d as a SD. Titrate dose in weekly intervals by 5–10 mg/d up to maintenance with 30–50 mg/d as 2–3 separate doses; doses up to 70 mg/d were well tolerated.
    - **together with non-enzyme-inducing comedication:**
      - **children > 12 years:** initially 5–10 mg/d as a SD. Titrate dose in weekly intervals by 5–10 mg/d up to maintenance with 15–30 mg/d as 2–3 separate doses.

- **USA – T:**
  - **adjunctive therapy in the treatment of partial seizures**
    - oral
    - **note:** doses were determined in patients receiving enzyme-inducing comedication; use of these doses in patients not receiving any enzyme-inducing comedication may result in serum concentrations more than twice those of patients receiving enzyme-inducing comedication; lower doses are required in patients not receiving any enzyme-inducing comedication; a slower titration may also be necessary in these patients. Consider Tiagabine dosage adjustment if enzyme-inducing comedication is introduced, discontinued, or its dose is changed. Do not use loading doses of Tiagabine in any patient; do not use a rapid dosage escalation or increase the dose in large increments.
      - **children < 12 years:** only limited data available
      - **children 12–18 years:** initially 4 mg/d as a SD for 1 week, then 8 mg/d as 2 separate doses for 1 week, then increase weekly by 4–8 mg/d; administer as 2–4 separate doses per day; titrate dose to response; max. 32 mg/d (doses > 32 mg/d have been used in selected adolescent patients for short periods of time)
- **United Kingdom – BNFC:**
  - **adjunctive treatment for focal seizures with or without secondary generalization not satisfactorily controlled by other antiepileptics**
    - oral
    - **with enzyme-inducing comedication**
      - **children > 12 years:** initially 5–10 mg as 1–2 separate doses, increase in steps of 5–10 mg/d at weekly intervals; usual maintenance with 30–45 mg/d as 2–3 separate doses
    - **without enzyme-inducing comedication**
      - **children > 12 years:** initial: 5–10 mg as 1–2 separate doses, increase in steps of 5–10 mg/d at weekly intervals; initial maintenance with 15–30 mg/d as 2–3 separate doses

Comments:
- possible aggravation of generalized tonic-clonic, atonic and myoclonic seizures
- no influence on the effect of oral contraceptives
- various dosages published in common paediatric sources

Tiapride

Dosage:
- ▶ 7–12 years: 50–100 mg/dose 2–3 times daily

Neuropaediatric indications:
- tic disorder

Mechanism of action:
- neuroleptic
- selectively blocks D_2 dopamine receptors in the caudate nucleus and the putamen

Relevant contraindications:
- prolactinoma
- breast cancer
- pheochromocytoma
- simultaneous treatment with L-dopa
- neuroleptic malignant syndrome

Relevant side effects and interactions:
- weakness, fatigue, drowsiness, agitation, indifference, insomnia
- vertigo, headache
- increased plasma levels of prolactin (chest pain, chest tightness, gynecomastia, galactorrhea, menstruation disorders, erectile dysfunction)
- extrapyramidal movement disorders (e.g. drug-induced parkinsonian syndrome, dyskinesia after treatment of antidopaminergic drugs = early dyskinesia; tardive dyskinesia after long-term treatment)
- neuroleptic malignant syndrome
- sometimes weight gain

Approval status:
- approved for the treatment of neuroleptic-induced tardive dyskinesia

Sources:
- **Germany – SPC:**
  - **Huntington's Chorea**
    - oral
      - **children:** 150–300 mg/d as 3 separate doses
- **USA – T:** –
- **United Kingdom – BNFC:** –
- **Drugdex®:**
  - **Tic disorder**
    - oral
      - **children 7–12 years:** usually 50–100 mg/dose 3 times daily (product information preparation Tiapridex® 1992)

Tizanidine

Dosage:
- ▶ initially: 1 mg/d (off-label)
- ▶ maintenance dose: 0.3–0.5 mg/kg/d; maximum: 36 mg/d (off-label)

Neuropaediatric indications:
- generalized spasticity (cerebral palsy)

Mechanism of action:
- α_2 adrenergic agonist
- centrally acting muscle relaxant (main target: spinal cord)
- presumably reduces spasticity by increasing presynaptic inhibition of motor neurons (α_2 adrenergic receptors) and therefore inhibits the release of glutamate
- thus, the polysynaptic signaling to the interneuron in the spinal cord is blocked and the elevated myotonus is reduced

Relevant contraindications:
- reduced liver function
- concomitant fluvoxamine or ciprofloxacin
- pregnancy
- careful use: hereditary intolerance of galactose, lactase deficiency, glucose-galactose malabsorption, children, epilepsy, myasthenia gravis, disorders of the cardiovascular system, coronary insufficiency, combination with other CYP1A2 inhibitors, liver or renal disorders

Relevant side effects and interactions:
- dry mouth, gastrointestinal disorders, nausea
- fatigue, weakness, muscle weakness, insomnia, sleeping disorder
- vertigo, bradycardia
- hallucinations
- temporary elevation of transaminase
- decreasing blood pressure and bradycardia with concomitant administration of diuretics and antihypertensive drugs
- mutually enhanced effect when co-administered with other centrally active drugs, muscle relaxants and alcohol
- increased plasma level of Tizanidine when administered together with CYP1A2 inhibitors

Approval status:
- in infants and children contraindicated

Sources:
- **Germany – SPC:**
  - **neurogenic spastic conditions**
    - **infants and children:** the efficacy and safety have not been established
- **USA – T:** –
- **United Kingdom – BNFC:** –

Comments:
- off-label use in spastic crises, e.g. NCLF

Tolperisone

Dosage:

- ▶ 2–4 years: 60–180 mg/d as 2–3 separate doses (off-label)
- ▶ 5–8 years: 60–270 mg/d as 2–3 separate doses (off-label)
- ▶ 9–14 years: 200–600 mg/d as 2–3 separate doses (off-label)

Neuropaediatric indications:

- – generalized spasticity (cerebral palsy)

Mechanism of action:

- – central and peripheral inhibition of voltage-dependent sodium and Calcium channels

Relevant contraindications:

- – myasthenia gravis
- – pregnancy

Relevant side effects and interactions:

- – allergic reactions
- – sleeping disorders, confusion, depression, concentration disorders
- – vertigo, headache
- – tachycardia
- – dry mouth, epigastric pain, nausea, diarrhea
- – myasthenia
- – enhanced effect of NSAID
- – metabolized via CYP2D6: no interactions reported so far, but these cannot be excluded

Approval status:

- – not approved in children younger than 15 years of age

Sources:

- – **Germany – SPC:**
  - – **spasticity due to neurological diseases**
    - – oral
      - – **children < 15 years:** not recommended due to lack of data
      - – **children > 15 years:** 150–450 mg Tolperisone hydrochloride/d as 3–9 separate doses
- – **USA – T:** –
- – **United Kingdom – BNFC:** –
- – **Uptodate.com:** –

Comments:

- – various dosages published in common paediatric sources

Topiramate (TPM)

Dosage:

- ▶ epilepsy: monotherapy maintenance dose 3(–6) mg/kg/d p.o. as 2 separate doses (leaflet instruction)
- ▶ prophylaxis of migraine: 1(–3) mg/kg/d as 2 separate doses
- ▶ prophylaxis of tension-type headache (chronic daily headache): 1(–3) mg/kg/d as 2 separate doses
- ▶ essential tremor: 1(–3) mg/kg/d as 2 separate doses
- ▶ cerebellar (intention) tremor: 1–3 mg/kg/d as 2 separate doses

Neuropaediatric indications:

- – focal and generalized epilepsy
- – seizures in neonates (only limited number of cases)
- – prophylaxis of tension-type headache, prophylaxis of migraine
- – essential tremor
- – cerebellar (intention) tremor

Mechanism of action:

- – inhibition of AMPA receptors
- – blockage of voltage-dependent sodium channels
- – increased gamma-aminobutyric acid activity at some subtypes of the $GABA_A$ receptors

Relevant contraindications:

- – angle-closure glaucoma
- – children < 2 years
- – prior kidney stones, or diseases that are related to a higher risk of kidney stones

Relevant side effects and interactions:

- – nausea, weight loss
- – paresthesia (numbness & tingling) (elevation of symptoms due to increased intake of potassium), ataxia, tremor, problems with speech
- – insomnia, cognitive disorders, depression, tiredness, nightmares, enhanced excitability
- – glaucoma
- – kidney stones
- – agitation, constipation, hyperventilation (probably due to a Topiramate-caused metabolic acidosis), excitability
- – hypohidrosis with elevated body temperature
- – decreased effect of oral contraception

- Phenytoin and Carbamazepine lower the plasma level of Topiramate
- increase in plasma levels of Phenytoin possible
- possible decrease in dioxin plasma levels
- Propranolol, Diltiazem, Hydrochlorothiazide and Metformin increase plasma levels of Topiramate
- possibly elevated plasma levels of Metformin
- decreased plasma levels of Pioglitazone
- increased risk of kidney stones when using concomitant medication that increase the risk of kidney stones (Acetazolamide, Triamterene, Zonisamide, > 2 g Vitamin C/D)
- some observations suggest that Topiramate may interact with: Flunarizine, Diltiazem, Amitryptiline, Haloperidol, Propranolol, Risperidone, Glibenclamide
- hyperammonemia possible with concomitant use of Valproic acid
- monitor Lithium levels
- CAUTION: metabolic acidosis

Approval status:
- monotherapy: > 3 years in newly diagnosed epilepsy
- adjunctive therapy: > 3 years in focal seizures with and without generalization, primary generalized tonic clonic seizures and Lennox-Gastaut syndrome

Sources:
- Germany – SPC:
  - **focal seizures with or without secondary generalization and primary generalized tonic-clonic seizures**
    - oral
    - **monotherapy**
      - **children > 6 years:** week 1, 0.5–1 mg/kg in the evening, then increase according to response in steps of 0.5–1 mg/kg/d as 1–2 separate doses in 1 or 2 week intervals, usual maintenance with 100 mg/d (e.g., 2 mg/kg/d for the age of 6–16-years)
    - **adjunctive therapy**
      - **children ≥ 3 years:** 5–9 mg/kg/d as 2 separate doses; week 1, titrate by 25 mg (or less, range: 1–3 mg/kg/d) and start in the evening. In intervals of 1 or 2 weeks increase dose by 1–3 mg/kg/d as 2 separate doses. Doses up to 30 mg/kg/d were well tolerated.
      - **note:** not recommended for treatment or prophylaxis of migraine in children
- USA – T:
  - **anticonvulsant, adjunctive therapy**
    - oral
    - **partial onset seizures or Lennox-Gastaut syndrome**
      - **children 2–16 years:** initially 1–3 mg/kg/d (max. 25 mg) given nightly for 1 week; increase at 1- to 2-week intervals by 1–3 mg/kg/d as 2 separate doses; titrate dose to response; usual maintenance with 5–9 mg/kg/d as 2 separate doses
      - **children ≥ 17 years:** initially 25–50 mg/d for 1 week; increase at weekly intervals by 25–50 mg/d as 2 separate doses; titrate dose to response; usual maintenance with 200–400 mg/d as 2 separate doses; max. 1600 mg/d
  - **primary generalized tonic-clonic seizures**
    - **children 2–16 years:** use initial dose as listed above, but use slower initial titration rate; titrate to 6 mg/kg/d by the end of 8 weeks
    - **children ≥ 17 years:** use initial dose as listed above, but use slower initial titration rate; titrate upwards to recommended dose by the end of 8 weeks; usual maintenance with 400 mg/d as 2 separate doses; max. 1600 mg/d
  - **anticonvulsant monotherapy**
    - **children ≥ 10 years:** initially 50 mg/d as 2 separate doses; increase at weekly intervals by 50 mg/d up to a dose of 200 mg/d as 2 separate doses (week 4 dose); thereafter, if required, increase at weekly intervals by 100 mg/d up to the recommended max. 400 mg/d as 2 separate doses
- United Kingdom – BNFC:
  - **monotherapy of generalized tonic-clonic seizures of focal seizures with or without secondary generalization**
    - oral
      - **children 6–18 years:** initially 0.5–1 mg/kg (max. 25 mg) at night for 1 week, then increase in steps of 0.25–0.5 mg/kg (max. 25 mg) twice daily at intervals of 1–2 weeks; initial target dose 50 mg/dose twice daily; max. 7.5 mg/kg/dose (max. 250 mg) twice daily
  - **adjunctive treatment on generalized tonic-clonic seizures of focal seizures with or without secondary generalization, adjunctive treatment of seizures in Lennox-Gastaut syndrome**
    - oral
      - **children 2–18 years:** initially 1–3 mg/kg (max. 25 mg) at night for 1 week, then increase in steps of 0.5–1.5 mg/kg (max. 25 mg) twice daily at intervals of 1–2 weeks; usual dose is 2.5–4.5 mg/kg/dose twice daily; max. 7.5 mg/kg/dose (max. 200 mg) twice daily
  - **migraine prophylaxis**
    - oral
      - **children 16–18 years:** initially 25 mg/d at night for 1 week, then increase in steps of 25 mg/d at intervals of 1 week; usual dose is 50–100 mg/d as 2 separate doses; max. 200 mg/d

Comments:
- lower initial doses decrease the risk of side effects
- West syndrome: so far only investigated in open or retrospective studies with few patients
- reason for higher dose tolerance in infants is related to the higher clearance rate of this medication in this age group
- CAUTION: aggravation of psychiatric disorders, negative cognition

Trazodone

Dosage:

▶ 1.5–2 mg/kg/d as 3 separate doses, maximum: 6 mg/kg/d (off-label)

Neuropaediatric indications:

– "rage attacks" in Opsoclonus-Myoclonus-Ataxia-Syndrome (OMAS)

Mechanism of action:

– antidepressant activity, probably by inhibiting serotonin reuptake
– acts predominantly as a 5-HT$_{2A}$ receptor antagonist
– no extrapyramidal effects, has no affinity for the mACh receptors and therefore does not produce any anticholinergic side effects

Relevant contraindications:

– hypnotics, analgesics, psychotropics, alcohol
– carcinoid syndrome
– MAO inhibitors (up to 2 weeks after discontinuation of treatment)
– careful use: arrhythmia, cardiac insufficiency, decompensated heart failure, renal impairment, < 18 years, severe liver disorders, increased risk of seizures

Relevant side effects and interactions:

– headache, tiredness, sleeping disorders, vertigo, dry mouth, akathisia
– stomach pain
– arrhythmias, hypotension
– priapism
– rare events: hypertension, constipation, agitation, trembling, weight gain, weight loss, confusion, visual impairment, serotonin syndrome (sweating, diarrhea, changing blood pressure, tachycardia, agitation, fever, tremor, confusion), epileptic seizures, hepatitis, changes in blood count, increased transaminase, hyperbilirubinemia

Approval status:

– depends on the specific product (SPC)

Sources:

– **Germany – SPC:** –
– **USA – T:** –
– **United Kingdom – BNFC:** –
– **uptodate.com: depression (off-label use)**
  – oral
    – **children 6–12 years:** initially 1.5–2 mg/kg/d as separate doses; increase gradually every 3–4 d as needed; max. 6 mg/kg/d as 3 separate doses
    – **adolescents:** initially 25–50 mg/d; increase to 100–150 mg/d as separate doses

Trihexyphenidyl

(Benzhexol)

Dosage:

▶ primary generalized dystonia (after relapse during treatment with L-dopa), progressively degenerative or secondary dystonias: p.o.: 0.5 mg/d as 3 separate doses, increase in steps of 0.5 mg weekly up to a maximum of 30–60 mg (off-label)
▶ focal dystonia after Botulinum toxin failure: p.o.: 0.5 mg/d as 3 separate doses, increase in steps of 0.5 mg weekly up to a maximum of 30–60 mg (off-label)
▶ sialorrhea: 5–15 mg/d as 3 separate doses (off-label)

Neuropaediatric indications:

– extrapyramidal movement disorders (e.g. primary generalized dystonia, progressively degenerative or secondary dystonia, focal dystonia after Botulinum toxin failure)
– sialorrhea

Mechanism of action:

– anticholinergic
– muscarinic receptor antagonist, decreases the acetylcholine release

Relevant contraindications:

– intestinal obstruction, urinary retention
– diseases that could lead to tachycardia, heart diseases
– brain diseases
– myasthenia gravis
– glaucoma
– liver or kidney disorders

Relevant side effects and interactions:

– urinary retention, constipation
– bradycardia, anhidrosis and hyperpyrexia
– blurred vision, mydriasis, dry mouth, photophobia
– anxiety, hallucinations, confusion, agitation, insomnia, speech disorders
– dyskinesias
– increased occurrence of side effects when used in combination with other anticholinergic, antihistaminic, spasmolytic drugs or alcohol
– L-dopa enhances dyskinesias

Approval status:

- contraindicated in children and adolescents (for medicolegal, not medicobiologic reasons), Off-label use!

Sources:

- **Germany – SPC: –**
- **USA – T:**
  - **dystonia in cerebral palsy**
    - oral
      - **children 2 -17 years:** initially 0.1–0.2 mg/kg/d as 3 separate doses for 1 week; increase by 0.05–0.3 mg/kg/d as 3 separate doses for the second week; thereafter, titrate up weekly by 0.05–0.5 mg/kg/d as 3 separate doses as clinically tolerated; dosage is based on a prospective trial of 23 patients.
- **United Kingdom – BNFC:**
  - **dystonia**
    - oral
      - **children 3 months–18 years:** initially 1–2 mg/d as 1–2 separate doses; increase every 3–7 d by 1 mg/d; adjuste according to response and side effects; max. 2 mg/kg/d

Comments:

- gradual titration leads to tolerance of very high dosages in children

Valproic acid

Dosage:

- ▶ regularly for epilepsy: maintenance with 20–30 mg/kg/d p.o. as 2–3 separate doses (SPC)
- ▶ therapeutic target level: 50–120 mg/l
- ▶ juvenile myoclonic epilepsy: 10–30 mg/kg/d as 2 separate doses or as a SD at night
- ▶ West syndrome: 20–60 mg/kg/d as 2 separate doses
- ▶ absences: monotherapy as a first choice therapy/adjunctive therapy (with Lamotrigine/Ethosuximide): 15–30 mg/kg/d as 2 separate doses
- ▶ epilepsy in Angelman syndrome: 20–30(–60) mg/kg/d
- ▶ status epilepticus:
  - after 20–60 min, 20–40 mg/kg over 3–5 min (max. 6 mg/kg/min)
- ▶ hyperekplexia (also known as primary startle syndrome or congenital stiff person syndrome): 20–60 mg/kg/d

Neuropaediatric indications:

- focal and generalized epilepsy
- anticonvulsive therapy in Angelman syndrome
- prophylaxis of migraine
- chronic substance abuse (overdosage or severe withdrawal symptoms)
- (non-convulsive) status epilepticus
- hyperekplexia (primary startle syndrome, congenital stiff person syndrome)

Mechanism of action:

- blocks the voltage-gated sodium channels and T-type Calcium channels
- believed to affect the function of the neurotransmitter GABA
- inhibitor of the enzyme histone deacetylase 1

Relevant contraindications:

- pre-existing severe hepatic impairement or known severe liver dysfunction in the family history
- known or suspected Alpers' syndrome
- porphyria
- bleeding disorders
- diseases that can be exacerbated by Valproic acid, have to be excluded first:
  - urea cycle disorders
  - mitochondrial and peroxisomal disorders
  - β-oxidation disorders
- careful use: small children receiving more than one antiepileptic drug, disabled children and adolescents with severe seizures, spinal cord injuries, metabolic disorders, renal insufficiency and hypoproteinemia, SLE, concomitant Acetylsalicylic acid (especially in infants and small children)
- monitor coagulation; when using Vitamin K antagonists, carefully monitor pro-thrombin time
- before starting therapy in children aged < 15 years: clinical assessment, and close monitoring especially in the first 6 weeks of therapy
- adolescents and adults: monitoring in the first 6 month of therapy
- CAUTION: pregnancy – see updated national guidelines

Relevant side effects and interactions:

- in the beginning: stomach ache, nausea, vomiting, weariness
- dose related thrombocytopenia, increased bleeding
- hepatotoxicity and pancreatic toxicity
- somnolence, tremor, stupor, ataxia, hyperactivity, dementia
- decreased or increased appetite, diarrhea, sialorrhea, oedema
- hair loss

- coagulation disorders, e.g. von-Willebrand disease
- hearing loss, headache, muscle hardening/hypotonia
- encephalopathy (especially in long-term treatment, with increasing number of seizures and severe changes in the EEG)
- polycystic ovary disease
- fanconi's syndrome
- reduced effect in comedication with enzyme inducing antiepileptic drugs (Phenobarbital, Primidone, Phenytoin, Carbamazepine), Mefloquine, Meropenem
- mutually increased plasma levels by concurrent with Felbamat
- enhanced effect in comedication with MAO inhibitors, Cimetidine, Erythromycin
- Fluoxetine can increase or lower Valproic acid serum levels
- increased bleeding risk with concurrent use of anticoagulants or Acetylsalicylic acid
- increased Phenobarbital plasma levels
- increased plasma levels of free Phenytoin (increased risk of side effects, particularly brain damage)
- increased toxic effect of Carbamazepine
- increased plasma levels of free Diazepam, decreased plasma clearance and distribution volume, half-life remains the same
- reduced plasma clearance of Lorazepam
- increased Phenytoin plasma levels in children taking Phenytoin and Clonazepam
- inhibits metabolism of Lamotrigine
- influences metabolism and protein binding of codeine
- enhances the effect of barbiturates, neuroleptics and antidepressive drugs
- interaction with other anticonvulsants regarding the plasma levels is possible
- increased plasma levels of Zidovudine
- possibly increased liver toxicity in combination with hepatotoxic medications
- in patients with a history of absences, concomitant Clonazepam may induce absence status
- Chloroquine and Carbapenem antibiotics reduce the plasma levels of Valproic acid
- changes in thyroid hormones (abnormal thyroid function tests)

Approval status:
- generalized seizures, focal and secondary generalized seizures, as well as mixed epilepsy
- no limitation in age

Sources:
- **Germany – SPC:**
  - **seizures (absences, myoclonic, tonic-clonic), focal and secondary generalized seizures, adjunctive therapy for all other types of seizures**
    - oral
      - **preparation Convulex® 150:**

age	Body weight (in kg)	Mean Valproic acid dose in mg/d
3–6 years	about 15–25	300–600
7–14 years	about 25–40	450–1500

      - **preparation Convulex solution®:**

age	Body weight (in kg)	Mean Valproic acid dose in mg/d
3–6 months	about 5.5–7.5 kg	173 mg sodium Valproic acid (i.e. 150 mg Valproic acid)
6–12 months	about 7.5–10 kg	173–346 mg sodium Valproic acid (i.e. 150–300 mg Valproic acid)
1–3 years	About 10–15 kg	346–518 mg sodium Valproic acid (i.e. 300–450 mg Valproic acid)
3–6 years	about 15–25 kg	346–692 mg sodium Valproic acid (i.e. 300–600 mg Valproic acid)

  - **note:** the use of Valproic acid in small children is only indicated for special cases
- **USA – T:**
  - **refractory seizures**
    - oral
      - **neonates:** loading dose of 20 mg/kg, followed by a maintenance dose of 5–10 mg/kg/dose every 12 h; adjust dose according to serum concentrations;
      - **note:** limited data available; due to increased risk of Valproic acid-associated hepatotoxicity, Valproic acid is not a preferred agent for use in neonates
  - **refractory status epilepticus**
    - IV
      - **neonates:** loading dose of 20–40 mg/kg, followed by a continuous infusion of 5 mg/kg/h was used in five neonates; once patients were seizure-free for 12 h and no longer showed any seizure activity on EEG, the infusion rate was decreased every 2 h by 1 mg/kg/h
      - **infants and children:** optimal dosage is not established; paediatric studies have used initial loading doses of 20–40 mg/kg
      - **maintenance dose:** optimal dosage is not established; paediatric studies used continuous infusions of 5 mg/kg/h after the loading dose; once patients were seizure-free for 6 h, the infusion rate was decreased by 1 mg/kg/h every 2 h.

- seizure disorders
  - oral
    - **children:** initially 10–15 mg/kg/d as 1–3 separate doses; increase by 5–10 mg/kg/d at weekly intervals until therapeutic levels are achieved; maintenance with 30–60 mg/kg/d as 2–3 separate doses.
    - **note:** children receiving more then 1 anticonvulsant may require doses up to 100 mg/kg/d as 3–4 separate doses.
  - rectal
    - **children:** dilute syrup 1:1 with water for use as a retention enema; loading dose, 17–20 mg/kg once; maintenance with 10–15 mg/kg/dose every 8 h
  - IV
    - total daily IV dose is equivalent to the total daily oral dose; however, the daily IV dose should be administered as 4 separate doses spaced 6 h apart; if the IV form is administered 2–3 times/d, close monitoring of trough levels is recommended; switch patients to oral product as soon as clinically possible (IV use has not been studied for > 14 d)
    - **note:** Valproic acid is not a preferred agent in patients < 2 years of age
- **United Kingdom – BNFC:**
- **all forms epilepsy**
  - oral, rectal
    - **neonates:** initially 20 mg/kg/d as a SD; usual maintenance with 20 mg/kg/d as 2 separate doses
    - **children 1 month–12 years:** initially 10–15 mg/kg/d as 1–2 separate doses; usual maintenance with 25–30 mg/kg/d as 2 separate doses (up to 60 mg/kg/d as 2 separate doses in infantile spasms; monitor clinical chemistry and haematological parameters if dose exceeds 40 mg/kg/d)
    - **children 12–18 years:** initially 600 mg/d as 1–2 separate doses increased gradually (in steps of 150–300 mg) every 3 d; usual maintenance with 1–2 g/d as 2 separate doses; max. 2.5 g/d as 2 separate doses
  - IV
    - **neonates:** IV injection of 20 mg/kg/d as 2 separate doses
    - **children 1 month–12 years:** initially by IV injection of 10 mg/kg; then 20–40 mg/kg/d by continuous IV infusion, or by intermittent IV infusion or IV injection as 2–4 separate doses
    - **children 12–18 years:** initially 10 mg/kg by IV injection, then up to max. 2.5 g/d by continuous IV infusion, or by intermittent IV infusion or IV injection as 2–4 separate doses.
    - **note:** if switching from oral therapy to IV therapy give current oral daily dose by IV injection or intermittent IV infusion as 2–4 separate doses, or by continuous IV infusion

Comments:

- monitoring of liver values is not necessary in asymptomatic children
- parents should immediately contact the physician if nausea, vomiting, dark urine, icterus or impaired consciousness are observed life-threatening liver failure has occurred in patients taking Valproic acid (risk: 1 : 20 000–50 000). Children younger than 2 years are at increased risk of developing life-threatening liver damage, especially those on more than 1 drug (risk: 1 : 600).
- the development of a liver failure can not be predicted by continuous control of Valproic acid blood levels

- Valproic acid interferes with the metabolism of carnitine. Carnitine can be life saving in acute liver failure, if it is recognized early and administered IV. Some authors recommend substitution with carnitine in children suffering from West syndrome and proceedingly treated with Valproic acid.

Vigabatrin

Dosage:

▶ 40–100(–150) mg/kg/d as 2 separate doses (SPC)

▶ patients should be continuously monitored. Dosing and duration of Vigabatrin treatment as well as possible alternatives should be carefully considered because the risk of adverse events may increase with the amount and duration of medication.

Neuropaediatric indications:

- monotherapy for West syndrome, particularly for symptomatic epilepsy in case of a tuberous sclerosis complex (TSC)
- adjunctive therapy for refractory complex partial seizures with or without secondary generalization

Mechanism of action:

- GABA analogue
- irreversible inhibition of γ-aminobutyric acid transaminase (GABA-T) resulting in increased levels of GABA in the central nervous system

Relevant contraindications:

- loss of vision, patients unable to undergo periodic vision assessment (children < 7 years)
- reduced renal function
- psychosis, depression, behavioural disturbance
- myoclonic seizures
- pregnancy

Relevant side effects and interactions:

- mostly mild hypotension, somnolence or nervousness
- headache, memory impairment and disorders of attention and concentration
- blurred vision, vertigo, nystagmus, abnormal coordination, paresthesia
- agitation (more likely in children), depression or psychosis (more likely in adults)
- for long-term treatment: weight gain, exacerbation of the effect of generalized epilepsy like absences or myoclonic absences

- irreversible loss of vision in 30–50 % of all adults who received treatment for over 1 year (independent of dose, age, duration of epilepsy and comedication with other antiepileptic drugs); no clear data available on children
- reduced hemoglobin levels
- do not combine with retinotoxic drugs
- reduced Phenytoin plasma levels
- reduced GPT plasma activity, and sometimes also reduced GOT levels
- increased level of amino acids in urine

Approval status:
- adjunctive therapy: resistant focal and secondary generalized seizures
- monotherapy: West syndrome

Sources:
- Germany – SPC:
  - **adjunctive therapy for refractory complex partial seizures with or without secondary generalization**
    - oral
      - **children:**
        - initially 40 mg/kg/d.

body weight (kg)	doses up to maximum (g/d)
10–15 kg	0.5–1 g/d
15–30 kg	1–1.5 g/d
30–50 kg	1.5–3 g/d
> 50 kg	2–3 g/d

  - **monotherapy for treatment of infantile spasms (West syndrome)**
    - **children:** initially 50 mg/kg/d; treatment effect may be achieved within one week. Doses up to 150 mg/kg/d were well tolerated.
- USA – T:
  - **infantile spasms**
    - oral
      - **infants and children 1 month–2 years:** initially 50 mg/kg/d as 2 separate doses; may be titrated upwards by 25–50-mg/kg/d increments every 3 d, depending on response and tolerability; max. 150 mg/kg/d as 2 separate doses
      - **note:** to taper off, decrease dose by 25–50 mg/kg/d every 3–4 d
  - **adjunctive treatment of refractory complex partial seizures**
    - oral
      - **children ≥ 10 kg:** initially 40 mg/kg/d as 2 separate doses; maintenance dosages based on patient weight:
        - **10–15 kg:** 0.5–1 g/d as 2 separate doses
        - **16–30 kg:** 1–1.5 g/d as 2 separate doses
        - **31–50 kg:** 1.5–3 g/d as 2 separate doses
      - **> 50 kg:** 2–3 g/d as 2 separate doses
      - **adolescents ≥ 16 years:** initially 1000 mg/d as 2 separate doses; increase daily dose by 500 mg increments at weekly intervals based on response and tolerability; recommended dose: 3 g/d as 2 separate doses.
      - **note:** to taper off, decrease dose by 1 g/d on a weekly basis
- United Kingdom – BNFC:
  - **adjunctive treatment of focal seizures with or without secondary generalization not satisfactorily controlled with other antiepileptics**
    - oral
      - **neonates:** initially 30–40 mg/kg/d as 2 separate doses increased over 2–3 weeks to usual maintenance dose 60–80 mg/kg/d as 2 separate doses; max. 150 mg/kg/d as 2 separate doses
      - **children 1 month–2 years:** initially 30–40 mg/kg/d as 2 separate doses, increase over 2–3 weeks to usual maintenance with 60–80 mg/kg/d as 2 separate doses; max. 150 mg/kg/d as 2 separate doses
      - **children 2–12 years:** initially 30–40 mg/kg/d (max. 500 mg) as 2 separate doses, increase over 2–3 weeks to usual maintenance with 60–80 mg/kg/d (max. 3 g) as 2 separate doses
      - **children 12–18 years:** initially 500 mg/d as 2 separate doses, increase over 2–3 weeks to usual maintenance with 2–3 g/d as 2 separate doses
    - rectal
      - **children 1 month–18 years:** dose as for oral therapy
  - **infantile spasm as monotherapy**
    - oral
      - **neonates:** initially 30–50 mg/kg/d as 2 separate doses, adjust according to response over 7 d to usual maintenance with 80–100 mg/kg/d as 2 separate doses; max. 150 mg/kg/d as 2 separate doses
      - **children 1 month–2 years:** initially 30–50 mg/kg/d as 2 separate doses, adjust according to response over 7 d to usual maintenance with 80–100 mg/kg/d as 2 separate doses; max. 150 mg/kg/d as 2 separate doses

Comments:
- closely monitor any CNS side effects
- control field of vision continuously, a VGT-associated limitation of the field of vision is irreversible
- may increase the amount of amino acids in the urine, possibly leading to a false positive test for certain rare genetic metabolic diseases (e.g. alpha aminoadipic aciduria)
- may exacerbate generalized tonic clonic seizures, absences and myoclonic epilepsy
- West syndrome: In most of the studies, response rates of 50 % (26–81 %) have been achieved, but it took at least two weeks of treatment before response was observed. Symptomatic West syndrome patients showed better response towards medication than the others did. Relapse rates varied up to a maximum of 50 %.
- Tuberous sclerosis complex (TSC) has been very effectively treated. Response rates of 95 % were reported in a review of Hancock and Osborne (studies included until 1999). In the only randomized trial, the efficacy was 100 % in the treatment of children with TSC. This is more effective than treatment with hydrocortisone (45 %). A similar efficacy has been achieved in children with trisomy 21.

Voriconazole

Dosage:
▶ maintenance dose (2–12 years): 14 mg/kg/d as 2 separate doses (SPC)

Neuropaediatric indications:
- aspergillus meningoencephalitis

Mechanism of action:
- synthetic triazole with a broad spectrum, which has a similar structure as Fluconazole
- inhibition of fungal cytochrome P-450-mediated 14 alpha-lanosterol demethylation, an essential step in fungal ergosterol biosynthesis
- the accumulation of 14 alpha-methyl sterols correlates with the subsequent loss of ergosterol in the fungal cell membrane and may be responsible for the antifungal activity of Voriconazole
- Voriconazole inhibits the 14-alpha-demethylation up to 160 times stronger than Fluconazole does
- susceptible:
  - candida spp. (C. albicans, C. dubliniensis, C. glabrata, C. guilliermondii, C. krusei, C. lusitaniae, C. parapsilosis, C. tropicalis, etc.) including the majority of the Fluconazole-resistant Candida spp.
  - cryptococcus neoformans
  - aspergillus spp. (A. flavus, A. fumigatus, A. nidulans, A. niger, A. terreus, etc.) including many Amphotericin-B-resistant species
  - fusarium spp., Trichosporon spp., Scedosporium apiospermum (Pseudallescheria boydii), Acremonium spp.
  - dimorphic fungi like Blastomyces dermatitidis, Coccidioides immitis, Paracoccidioides brasiliensis, Penicillium marneffei or Histoplasma capsulatum
  - cladophialophora bantiana or Exophilala dermatitidis
  - several dermatophytes
- resistant: Zygomycetes such as Mucor spp. or Rhizopus spp., Sporothrix schenckii, Paecilomyces variotii, Scedosporium prolificans

Relevant contraindications:
- concurrent administration of CYP3A4 substrates
- concurrent administration of rifampicin, Carbamazepine, Phenobarbital, ritonavir, hypericum, sirolimus, efavirenz
- note: cardiac arrhythmia, cardiomyopathy, bradycardia, concurrent administration of medication that prolongs the QT interval

Relevant side effects and interactions:
- exanthema, alopecia, angiooedema, face oedema, rash
- headache, vertigo, peripheral neurological disorders
- nausea, vomiting, stomach pain, diarrhea, meteorism
- seizures
- disorders of taste sensation
- increased alkaline phosphatase, increased SGO, increased SGPT, elevated total bilirubin; severe liver dysfunctions, hepatitis, jaundice
- hypercholesterolemia, hyperglyceridemia, hypokalemia
- leukopenia, neutropenia, agranulocytosis, thrombocytopenia
- impairement of renal function parameters
- enhanced effect and side effects of anticoagulants, benzodiazepines, oral antidiabetic drugs (Glibenclamide, Glipizide, Tolbutamide), Rifabutin, Tacrolimus, Sirolimus, Phenythoin, Cyclosporine, Theophylline, Terfenadine, Zidovudine
- reduced effect of Rifampicin
- elevated Fluconazole serum levels conditioned by hydrochlorothiazide
- probably no negative impact on the efficacy of oral contraceptives
- inhibition of glucocorticoid metabolism
- elevated risk of myopathy or rhabdomyolysis when used in combination with HMG-CoA reductase inhibitors (i.e. statins)

Approval status:
- antifungal agent for children and adults

Sources:
- **Germany – SPC:**
  - **invasive aspergillosis**
    - **children < 2 years:** is not recommended
    - **children 2–12 years:**

	IV	Oral
Initial dose	A special oral initial dosage is not recommended; IV: 9 mg/kg/dose every 12 h	
Maintenance dose	9 mg/kg twice daily	350 mg twice daily

  - **children > 12 years:**

	IV	Oral	Oral
		Patient > 40 kg	**Patient < 40 kg**
Initial dose within the first 24 h	6 mg/kg every 12 h (within the first 24 h)	400 mg every 12 h (within the first 24 h)	200 mg every 12 h (within the first 24 h)
Maintenance dose after the first 24 h	4 mg/kg twice daily	200 mg twice daily	100 mg twice daily

- **USA – T:** indication of interest is not specified
- **United Kingdom – BNFC:**
  - **invasive aspergillosis; serious infections caused by Scedosporium spp., Fusarium spp., or invasive Fluconazole -resistant Candida spp. (including C. krusei)**
    - oral
      - **children 2–12 years (oral suspension recommended):** 200 mg/dose every 12 h
      - **children 12–18 years, < 40 kg:** 200 mg/dose every 12 h for 2 doses then 100 mg/dose every 12 h, increased if necessary to 150 mg/dose every 12 h
      - **children 12–18, ≥ 40 kg:** 400 mg/dose every 12 h for 2 doses then 200 mg/dose every 12 h, increased if necessary to 300 mg/dose every 12 h
    - IV infusion
      - **children 2–12 years:** 7 mg/kg/dose every 12 h (reduced to 4 mg/kg/dose every 12 h if not tolerated) for max. 6 months
      - **children 12–18 years:** 6 mg/kg/dose every 12 h for 2 doses, then 4 mg/kg/dose every 12 h (reduced to 3 mg/kg/dose every 12 h if not tolerated) for max. 6 months
- **Uptodate.com:** no published paediatric dosage
  - **children 2 to < 12 years:**
  - **note:** Limited information regarding paediatric dosing exists. The dosing specified below represents small studies and expert opinion; children ≤ 12 years appear to require higher dosing than adults.
  - **aspergillosis, invasive, including disseminated and extrapulmonary infection: Duration of therapy should be a minimum of 6–12 weeks or throughout period of immunosuppression:**
    - IV
    - IDSA Guidelines: 5–7 mg/kg/dose every 12 hours (Walsh, 2008)
    - CDC Opportunistic Infections Guidelines (CDC, 2009): loading dose: 6–8 mg/kg/dose (maximum: 400 mg/dose) every 12 hours (2 doses on day 1). Maintenance dose: 7 mg/kg/dose (maximum: 200 mg/dose) every 12 hours; change to oral administration when clinically possible; duration of therapy (IV and oral combined): ≥ 12 weeks, but should be individualized.
    - Oral (CDC, 2009): Loading dose: 8 mg/kg/dose (maximum: 400 mg/dose) every 12 hours (2 doses on day 1). Maintenance dose: 7 mg/kg/dose (maximum: 200 mg/dose) every 12 hours
  - **children ≥ 12 year Aspergillosis, invasive, including disseminated and extrapulmonary infection: Duration of therapy should be a minimum of 6–12 weeks or throughout period of immunosuppression (Walsh, 2008):**
    - IV
    - initial: Loading dose: 6 mg/kg every 12 hours for 2 doses; followed by maintenance dose of 4 mg/kg every 12 hours
    - oral: Maintenance dose:
      - Manufacturer's labeling:
      - Patients < 40 kg: 100 mg every 12 hours; maximum: 300 mg/d
      - Patients ≥ 40 kg: 200 mg every 12 hours; maximum: 600 mg/d
      - IDSA recommendations: consider oral therapy in place of IV with dosing of 4 mg/kg (rounded up to convenient tablet dosage form) every 12 hours; however, IV administration is preferred in serious infections since comparative efficacy with the oral formulation has not been established
  - **Drugdex®:** no additional information

Warfarin

Dosage:

- individual dosing, adjust according to INR
- cardioembolic stroke: INR 2.5–3.5
- chronic atrial fibrillation: target INR = 2.0–3.0, if there are no reasons against it (risk of falling, compliance etc.). Therapy can be started after 3–5 d, if the infarct is small
- mechanical heart valves: INR 2.5–3.5; biological heart valves: INR 2.0–3.0
- dissection of arteries supplying the brain without SAH: secondary prophylaxis INR 2.0–3.0 for at least 3 months
- patients of African ethnicity need higher dosages than patients of Asian ethnicity to achieve the same effect

Neuropaediatric indications:

- prophylaxis and therapy of thromboembolic disorders
- chronic atrial fibrillation
- mechanical heart valves

Mechanism of action:

- coumarin; Vitamin K antagonist
- inhibits the synthesis of functional Vitamin K-dependent clotting factors (factors II, VII, IX, and X)
- inhibits Vitamin K reductase, thereby limiting formation of the reduced form of Vitamin K, which in turn limits γ-carboxylation of N-terminal glutamic acid residues. Without sufficient carboxylation, the Vitamin K-dependent clotting factors are unable to bind via Calcium ions to the phospholipid layers on the vascular endothelium and thus remain functionally inactive.

Relevant contraindications:

- cerebrovascular bleeding in recent history
- dissection of the aorta
- diseases with a high risk of bleeding (e.g. hemorrhagic diathesis, parenchymal liver disease, renal insufficiency, severe thrombocytopenia)
- hypertension (> 200/105 mmHg)
- diseases that are associated to lesions of the vascular system
- large open wounds (surgical wounds)
- cavernous tuberculosis of the lung
- intramuscular injections (risk of bleeding into the muscles)

- lumbar puncture, epidural anesthesia and other diagnostic or therapeutic procedures could result in uncontrolled bleeding
- angiography
- hereditary intolerance of galactose, deficiency of lactase, glucose-galactose-malabsorption

Relevant side effects and interactions:

- occult and overt bleeding or haemorrhage, gastrointestinal haemorrhage, increased gum bleeding, retina bleeding, nose bleed
- trauma, and other serious bleeding events have been reported
- nausea, loss of appetite, vomiting, diarrhea
- hepatitis with or without jaundice
- hematuria
- cerebral bleeding
- urticaria, exanthema, pruritus, dermatitis, reversible alopecia diffusa, dermal necrosis, purpura
- long-term treatment: osteopenia
- pain and change of colour of the big toe ("purple toes")
- teratogenic when used frequently
- enhanced effect with concurrent use of other anticoagulation drugs
- strong binding to plasma proteins: any drug with high-affinity plasma protein binding can displace coumarins from its binding sites, resulting in increased coumarin plasma levels. Conversely, coumarins may displace drugs bound with lower affinity.
- metabolized by CYP3A4 and CYP2C9; influences all inhibitors and inductors of these enzymes

Approval status:

- contraindicated in children younger than 14 years of age

Sources:

- **Germany – SPC:**
  - **heart valves (prophylaxis/treatment of thromboembolic complications)**
    - oral
      - **children ≥ 14 years:** For patients with a bileaflet mechanical valve or a Medtronic Hall tilting disc valve in the aortic position who are in sinus rhythm and without left atrial enlargement, therapy with Warfarin to a target INR of 2.5 (range, 2.0–3.0) is recommended.
      - For patients with tilting disc valves and bileaflet mechanical valves in the mitral position, therapy with Warfarin to a target INR of 3.0 (range, 2.5–3.5) is recommended.
      - For patients with caged ball or caged disc valves, concomitant aspirin dosage of 75–100 mg/d is recommended.
      - For patients with a bioprosthetic valve in the mitral position, therapy with Warfarin to a target INR of 2.5 (range, 2.0–3.0) for the first 3 months after valve insertion is recommended. If additional risk factors are present, additional 3 months treatment could be justified.

- **atrial fibrillation (Prophylaxis/treatment of thromboembolic complications)**
  - **children ≥ 14 years:** target INR of 2.5 (range, 2.0–3.0)
  - **long-term treatment of myocardial infarction**
  - **children ≥ 14 years:** with aspirin, target INR of 2.5 (range, 2.0–3.0)
  - without aspirin, target INR of 3.0–4.0
  - **usual: children ≥ 14 years**, initially 2.5–5 mg/d, adjust according to INR, maintenance with 2.5–10 mg/d; monitor INR closely
- **USA – T:**
  - oral
    - **note:** dosing must be individualized. New product labeling identifies genetic factors, that may increase a patient's sensitivity to Warfarin. Specifically, genetic variations in the proteins CYP2CP and VKORC1, responsible for Warfarin's primary metabolism and pharmacodynamic activity, respectively, have been identified as predisposing factors associated with decreased dose requirements and increased bleeding risk. A genotyping test is available and may provide important guidance on initiation of anticoagulant therapy.
    - **infants and children:** to maintain an INR between 2–3:
      - initial loading dose, d 1 (if baseline INR 1–1.3): 0.2 mg/kg (max. 10 mg/dose); 0.1 mg/kg if patient has liver dysfunction or has undergone a fontan procedure
      - loading dose, d 2–4: doses are dependent on patient's INR
        - INR (1.1–1.3): repeat the initial loading dose
        - INR (1.4–1.9): 50 % of initial loading dose
        - INR (2–3): 50 % of initial loading dose
        - INR (3.1–3.5): 25 % of initial loading dose
        - INR (> 3,5): withhold the drug until INR < 3.5, then restart at 50 % of previous dose
      - maintenance dose guidelines for d 5 of therapy and beyond: doses depend on patient's INR:
        - INR (1.1–1.4): increase dose by 20 % of previous dose
        - INR (1.5–1.9): increase dose by 10 % of previous dose
        - INR (2–3): do not change the dose
        - INR (3.1–3.5): decrease dose by 10 % of previous dose
        - INR (> 3.5): withhold the drug and check INR daily until INR < 3.5, then restart at 20 % less than the previous dose
  - usual maintenance dose ~ 0.1 mg/kg/d, range 0.05–0.34 mg/kg/d (age related)
- **United Kingdom – BNFC:** as Warfarin sodium
  - **treatment and prophylaxis of thrombotic episodes**
    - oral
      - **neonates (under specialist supervision)**, d 1: 0.2 mg/kg as a SD, reduced to 0.1 mg/kg/d for following 3 d (but if INR still below 1.4, use 0.2 mg/kg once daily, or if INR above 3, use 0.05 mg/kg once daily, if INR above 3.5, omit dose); then adjust according to INR; usual maintenance with 0.1–0.3 mg/kg/d as a SD (max. required, up to 0.4 mg/kg/d as a SD, especially if bottle fed)
      - **children 1 month–18 years**, d 1: 0.2 mg/kg (max. 10 mg) as a SD, reduced to 0.1 mg/kg/d (max. 5 mg) for following 3 d (but if INR still below 1.4, use 0.2 mg/kg (max. 10 mg) once daily, or if INR above 3, use 0.05 mg/kg (max. 2.5 mg) once daily; omit dose if INR above 3.5); then adjust according to INR; usual maintenance with 0.1–0.3 mg/kg/d as a SD (max. required, up to 0.4 mg/kg/d as a SD, especially if bottle fed)

- **note:** induction dose may have to be adjusted according to condition, concomitant interacting drugs, and if baseline INR above 1.3

Comments:
- Mainly used in the USA. In Europe, Phenprocoumon is the more commonly used drug.
- regularly monitor prothrombin time; to ensure standardized comparison, INR (international normalized ratio) is the preferred parameter
- effect is different in each patient due to polymorphism of the VKORC1-gen or cytochrome P450 (CYP2P9)
- monitoring of the anticoagulation: INR
- Oral anticoagulation with coumarins is only indicated for long-term treatment over 3 years up to lifelong. Otherwise LMWH is preferred (superior compliance, co-ordination and less complications).

Z

Zolmitriptan

Dosage:
- ▶ migraine therapy after poor effect of NSAID: 2.5 mg or 5 mg in 1 dose as (orodispersible) tablet or nasal spray (off-label)

Neuropaediatric indications:
- alleviation of migraine attack symptoms after treatment failure with NSAID

Mechanism of action:
- selective agonist for the vascular serotonin receptor subtypes $5\text{-}HT_{1B}$ and $5\text{-}HT_{1D}$
- vasoconstriction of cranial arteries and inhibition of pro-inflammatory neuropeptide release

Relevant contraindications:
- vasospasm, prior cerebrovascular disorders or TIA
- angina pectoris, history of myocardial infarction, peripheral vascular diseases, arterial hypertension, severe heart diseases, Prinzmetal angina, myocardial infarction
- concurrent administration of MAOI within 2 weeks, ergotamine-containing or ergot-type medication
- creatinine clearance < 15 ml/min
- prophylaxis of migraine
- orodispersible tablet: phenylketonuria
- tablets: hereditary galactose intolerance, lactase deficit, glucose-galactose-malabsorption
- careful use: symptomatic Wolff-Parkinson-White syndrome, hemiplegic, ophthalmologic or basilar migraines, other serious neurological disorders, children and adolescents < 18 years (limited experience), ergotamine-containing or ergot-like medication (administration at the earliest 6 h after Zolmitriptan, and administration of Zolmitriptan 24 h after ergotamines)

Relevant side effects and interactions:
- dizziness
- angina-pectoris-like disorders, changes in blood pressure
- vertigo, drowsiness, sedation
- heart palpitation, feeling of constriction in pharynx and throat
- erythema
- using high dosages: colour changes of the blood to green/black (sulfhemoglobinemia)
- serotonin syndrome when using triptans with an antidepressant (SSRI or SNRI):
  - nausea, emesis, diarrhea
  - agitation, hallucinations, loss of coordination
  - tachycardia, elevated body temperature
  - elevated reflexes
- elevated risk of coronary spasms with concurrent administration of ergotamines or ergotamine derivates (administration at the earliest 6 h after Zolmitriptan, and administration of Zolmitriptan 24 h after ergotamines)

Approval status:
- nasal spray ≥ 12 years of age

Sources:
- **Germany – SPC:**
  - **acute treatment of migraine with or without aura**
  - **children ≥ 12 years:** intranasal 2.5–5 mg (1 puff) into 1 nostril, repeated after not less than 2 h if migraine recurs; max. 10 mg in 24 h
  - **note:** child not responding to initial dose should not receive a second dose for same attack
- **USA – T:** –
- **United Kingdom – BNFC:**
  - **treatment of acute migraine**
    - oral
      - **children 12–18 years:** 2.5 mg, repeated after not less than 2 h if migraine recurs (if response unsatisfactory after 3 attacks, consider increasing dose to 5 mg or switching to alternative treatment); max. 10 mg in 24 h

- intranasal
  - **children 12–18 years:** 5 mg (1 puff) into 1 nostril, repeated after not less than 2 h if migraine recurs; max. 10 mg in 24 h
  - **note:** child not responding to initial dose should not receive a second dose for same attack
- **treatment of acute cluster headache**
  - intranasal
    - **children 12–18 years:** 5 mg (1 puff) into 1 nostril, repeated after not less than 2 h if headache recurs; max. 10 mg in 24 h

Zonisamide

Dosage:

▶ 4–12 mg/kg/d p.o. as 2 separate doses (off-label)

Neuropaediatric indications:

- a therapy of partial-onset seizures with or without generalization
- West syndrome

Mechanism of action:

- the precise mechanism is unknown
- inhibits sodium and Calcium channels
- carbonic anhydrase inhibitor

Relevant contraindications:

- patients weighing < 40 kg
- hepatic and renal disorders

Relevant side effects and interactions:

- generally, frequent psychiatric and neurologic side effects
- agitation, irritability, confusion, depression
- ataxia, vertigo, difficulty with memory, drowsiness
- diplopia
- anorexia, diarrhea, nausea
- allergic reactions, neuroleptic malignant syndrome, rhabdomyolysis
- no influence on oral contraceptives
- teratogenic
- see table: interactions of anticonvulsive drugs
- renal calculus, in particular when given in addition to Topiramate
- rifampicin reduces effect of Zonisamide

Approval status:

- adjunctive therapy: patients > 18 years with focal and secondary generalized seizures

Sources:

- **Germany – SPC:**
  - **adjunctive therapy for the treatment of seizures with or without secondary generalization**
    - **children < 18 years:** not recommended
- **USA – T:**
  - **adjunctive therapy of partial seizures**
    - oral
      - **infants and children:** a review article considering 20 Japanese paediatric studies suggests: initially 1–2 mg/kg/d as 2 separate doses, titrate dose upwards if needed every 2 weeks; usual dose is 5–8 mg/kg/d (higher initial and maximum doses have been recommended by others); to treat infantile spasm, several studies used a faster titration
      - **children > 16 years:** initially 100 mg/d as a SD; dose may be increased to 200 mg/d after 2 weeks; further increases in dose should be made in increments of 100 mg/d and only after a minimum of 2 weeks between adjustments; usual effective dose is 100–600 mg/d
      - **note:** There is no evidence of increased benefits with doses > 400 mg/d
- **United Kingdom – BNFC:** –

Comments:

- efficacy in children was seen in children with partial and generalized seizures in some studies in particular in the Middle East. There, Zonisamide has been used since the end of the 1980's. The response rates in patients with West syndrome in open studies have been reported to range between 20 and 38 %. Serious side effects have not been observed. Relapse rate under therapy was reported to be 36 %.

Notes

Notes

Notes

Notes

Notes